QUALITATIVE INQUIRY
IN CLINICAL AND EDUCATIONAL SETTINGS

QUALITATIVE INQUIRY
in Clinical
and Educational Settings

DANICA G. HAYS
ANNELIESE A. SINGH

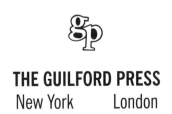

THE GUILFORD PRESS
New York   London

© 2012 The Guilford Press
A Division of Guilford Publications, Inc.
72 Spring Street, New York, NY 10012
www.guilford.com

Printed in the United States of America

This book is printed on acid-free paper.

Last digit is print number: 9   8   7   6   5   4   3   2   1

Library of Congress Cataloging-in-Publication Data
Hays, Danica G.
  Qualitative inquiry in clinical and educational settings / Danica G. Hays,
Anneliese A. Singh.
    p. cm.
  ISBN 978-1-60918-245-8 (pbk.)–ISBN 978-1-60918-485-8 (hardcover)
    1. Qualitative research.   2. Qualitative research—Data
processing.   3. Qualitative research—Moral and ethical aspects.   I. Singh,
Anneliese A.   II. Title.
  H61.H34 2012
  001.4′2—dc22

                                                    2011002823

For my mother—
a model of balance, strength, and unconditional love.
—D. G. H.

For my mom—who taught me rules can be transformed
and that we should all live like we are in heaven.
I love you!
—A. A. S.

For Dr. Joel Meyers, our first qualitative teacher.
Your mentorship, passion, empowerment,
and attention to practice and justice are inspiring.
Thank you for throwing wild cards our way.
—D. G. H. and A. A. S.

Preface

Relationships are at the heart of qualitative inquiry. As you engage in qualitative research, you will build relationships with participants and your research team. You will also build a relationship with your research topic itself. As with any relationship, this relationship can vary in time, focus, energy, and outcomes. Regardless, we wrote this book because we want you to have a healthy relationship with qualitative designs.

As we ourselves learned about qualitative inquiry, we experienced every emotion that exists. At times we were confused, surprised, frustrated, hopeful, hopeless, saddened, and ultimately inspired as we investigated phenomena from a qualitative approach. Fortunately, as we built our relationship with qualitative research, we already had a wonderful friendship that we could draw on, wherein we shared all of the thoughts and feelings we had with one another. We could challenge and support one another, and through this process we ultimately discovered that our relationship with qualitative design was one of adventure, where we discovered ways to engage in qualitative research that had integrity, were ethical, and were exciting. We wanted to write this book to share this adventure with you—and to challenge and support you in the twists and turns that become the "road" of a qualitative study.

Relationships are also central to how we interact as professionals with those with whom we work in clinical and educational settings. Research has shown time and time again that relationships provide the foundation upon which human potential is actualized. Because qualitative research involves relationship building, this type of inquiry provides immense potential for positive growth and liberation of the people with whom we work along the way—and also for ourselves. This potential can feel overwhelming for researchers who are new to qualitative inquiry. However, we encourage you to remember that qualitative research is less overwhelming and more of an adventure when you build your relationship with your topic one step at a time.

So, we invite you to become immersed in this text and experience the significant ideas of traditional scholars, "radical" thinkers from a variety of educational backgrounds, and those of our beloved colleagues and students. First, we think it is important for you to understand our training background and a few of our assumptions about research in general and qualitative research more specifically.

We received training in ethnographic methods in our doctoral programs (Counselor Education and Counseling Psychology) at Georgia State University. We identify as counselor educators, with training in mental health counseling (Hays) and mental health counseling and counseling psychology (Singh). As educators, we teach qualitative research and advise on research projects of master's and doctoral students of a variety of disciplines. We hold licenses in our respective specialty areas and adamantly support the integration of knowledge within and across disciplines.

During our training our mentor, Dr. Joel Meyers—an ethnographer and school psychologist—emphasized the importance of context, advocacy, and application in qualitative inquiry. In both his formal and informal instruction, he was always there to throw his students wild cards—thought-provoking questions or challenges—as they navigated qualitative research. We hope to provide some of these throughout the text. One of our more vivid memories of learning from him is his message that research *is* practice: That is, it is important to conduct research that benefits clients and/or students across disciplines. This work can relate to training practitioners, developing or improving interventions, and building theory and giving voice to under-researched populations, to name just a few applications. In our publications since our graduate training, involving a broad range of research traditions and topics, we still attend to the importance of application and context when reporting or presenting findings.

Relatedly, we believe that our clinical orientation is integral to our research orientation. A common theoretical framework from our clinical practice is feminism. Although we value other theoretical orientations in understanding and intervening with clients, a feminist lens shapes these perspectives. Thus, a focus on shared power, collaboration, and personal and political activism is infused in our research approach and recommended often throughout the text.

We assume that clinical and educational disciplines use a variety of research paradigms and traditions; the decision when developing a research design is not a discipline issue but a concern of the research purpose and process. So, you will not find a prescriptive view in this text of *who* should do *what* kind of qualitative research to address *what* problem or issue.

And we don't view quantitative research as a polar-opposite "enemy" of qualitative research. In fact, many of our quantitative studies have qualitative beginnings, and we affirm an equal partnership of qualitative and quantitative approaches in discipline research: There is no "better" approach, and the two should not be evaluated or applied in the same manner.

This text is most suitable for graduate-level students, practitioners, and educators in a variety of social science and education disciplines. For graduate students, this book is structured to include proposal development exercises, in-class and field activities, journal exercises, and other tools to complete a quality proposal or report. We include a glossary of key terms and sample qualitative proposals for your reference as you embark in probably unfamiliar research territory. For practitioners and educators, this text also offers several case examples, perspectives, and activities aimed toward enhancing the research agenda. For all, development as a culturally relevant scientist-practitioner conducting qualitative inquiry is the overarching goal.

Some of the features of the text include:

- *Activities:* Class and field activities to apply qualitative concepts;
- *Reflexive Activities:* Journaling exercises for reflecting on qualitative practices;
- *Case Examples:* Exemplar qualitative studies and proposals in clinical and educational settings;

- *Perspectives:* Practitioner and student perspectives on various qualitative concepts;
- *Proposal Development Activities:* Concrete activities to assist students in developing qualitative proposals;
- *Wild Cards:* Cautionary notes about potential pitfalls in conducting qualitative research;
- *Graphs and illustrations* that help to organize chapters and present concepts; and
- *Tables* to summarize concepts and present helpful tips.

Although we believe that qualitative inquiry is by no means a linear process, an aim of this text is to present ideas that build upon one another, beginning with foundational concepts as you consider what your initial research design and process will look like. Then we discuss things you might actually do in qualitative inquiry, the hands-on work with data. As we hope you will find in this text, we intentionally focus on the foundations of research *first* and doing research *second*. We wanted to create a text that addresses issues, reflections, and actions throughout the research process; however, this text is by no means a comprehensive model for qualitative inquiry. To this end, we refer you to various readings to supplement your understanding of each chapter. We hope that you will find helpful the way in which we organized and presented the materials, to try to capture complex constructs and simplify them.

We use diverse examples of works, as we believe that the research process, shared perspectives, and lessons learned from any one discipline can be readily applied to your project. Part of our choice in including several disciplines, rather than just our own home disciplines, is to highlight the notion that researchers from various backgrounds can learn from one another when addressing a research problem.

We assume that our readers have some basic background knowledge in quantitative research and the scientific method. Although we mention quantitative research throughout the text, we do not fully describe the characteristics of this approach.

Now let's talk about how the text is organized.

PART I: FOUNDATIONS OF QUALITATIVE INQUIRY

Part I of this text offers some of the foundations of qualitative research: Key definitions and uses of qualitative research, research paradigms and traditions, and research ethics are introduced. This section introduces the use of clusters for later design considerations, as well as data collection, management, and analysis.

Chapter 1, *Introduction to Qualitative Inquiry*, describes the characteristics and history of qualitative research and explores the role of qualitative inquiry in clinical and educational settings. We also provide a description of how you can establish a research agenda and use qualitative research as a powerful tool in school and community settings to create change in various systems.

Chapter 2, *Qualitative Research Paradigms and Traditions*, outlines various research paradigms and traditions that help to shape design decisions. These can be conceptualized as the "theoretical orientation" of a study: which assumptions and blueprints you use to conceptualize and carry out a study.

Chapter 3, *Ethical Issues in Qualitative Research*, introduces the reader to some of the major ethical concepts that influence the entire qualitative research process. In addition to meta-ethical principles that frame ethical decision making, the concepts of informed consent, confidentiality, multiple relationships, and competence are presented. Finally, special considerations in qualitative inquiry are outlined.

PART II: QUALITATIVE RESEARCH DESIGN

With a sense of the value of conducting qualitative inquiry and a primer on research paradigms and traditions, Part II moves forward with some "behind-the-scenes" components of qualitative inquiry. These activities include selecting a topic, understanding the researcher's role, entering the field, and maximizing trustworthiness. These undertakings are considered "behind the scenes" for two reasons: (1) They are heavily considered and strategized upon before any data collection occurs; and (2) they are at the forefront of the researcher's mind throughout data collection and analysis.

To help you understand them more clearly, Part II treats each of these components as separate goals in qualitative inquiry, and thus each is discussed in a separate chapter. However, these components interact and are interdependent in actual practice. A "good" qualitative researcher is constantly reflecting on the relationship among the four components described in this section: How is my research topic affected by the literature as well as the research questions I am using as a lens to study that topic? How does my topic yield various sampling and fieldwork decisions? What role do I and others play in the study as a whole and in relation to topic selection and sampling methods? What strategies can I use now as well as later to maintain a rigorous research design with valid findings?

Based on the complexity of these ongoing reflections, you can see that qualitative inquiry is an active decision-making process, even before the first data collection.

Chapter 4, *Selecting a Topic*, addresses using the literature and other sources of information to arrive at a general research topic and more specific research questions. In this chapter we explore three key facets of topic selection: research goals, conceptual framework, and research questions. In addition, considerations for selecting a mixed methods approach are offered.

Chapter 5, *Understanding the Researcher's Role*, outlines several efforts of reflection a qualitative researcher needs to undertake to conduct rigorous qualitative research. These efforts include reflexivity, subjectivity, participant "voice," peer debriefing, and use of research teams.

Chapter 6, *Entering the Field*, describes the initial actions involved in launching the study. In this chapter we discuss purposeful sampling methods, sample size considerations, as well as steps for selecting, entering, and exiting a site. The role of gatekeepers, stakeholders, and key informants is discussed throughout the process of entering the field.

Chapter 7, *Maximizing Trustworthiness*, presents a general discussion of what constitutes quality research. We discuss the quantitative research bias evident in evaluating qualitative research and outline several criteria and strategies for establishing trustworthiness in qualitative research.

PART III: DATA COLLECTION AND ANALYSIS

The first two sections of the text serve as a backdrop for what we actively do as qualitative researchers: collecting and analyzing data derived from a sound research design. Although data collection and analysis are presented as separate topics, we emphasize that they should occur simultaneously. Further, neither can occur without proper data management along the way.

There are so many decisions involving qualitative data: How and from whom do we collect it? How do we know when we have "enough"? How do we manage and store the massive amounts of data that are produced? Is there a generic process to data analysis, or are there variations based on research design components? What are the most important data collection and analysis methods for your study?

Qualitative data collection, data management, and data analysis are addressed across four chapters:

Chapter 8, *Data Collection via Fieldwork, Interviewing, and Focus Groups*, presents a description of interviewing and observational strategies. Specifically, fieldwork activities (e.g., participant observation, individual interviews, focus group interviews) and related records (e.g., field notes, memos, contact summary sheets) are outlined.

Chapter 9, *Data Collection Using the Internet, Documents, or Arts-Based Methods*, reviews the use of various media for data collection. Attention is given to innovative media data collection methods, such as e-mail and chat room interviewing. The use of arts-based media is also discussed, highlighting photography and participant artwork as a data collection method. Data collection involving written materials and personal and public documents is also presented.

Chapter 10, *The Basics of Qualitative Data Management and Analysis*, outlines some universal steps of qualitative data analysis, several coding considerations, and outlines qualitative data management strategies. Special attention is given to a key data management strategy used in data collection and analysis: the case display. Furthermore, the use of qualitative software is discussed.

Chapter 11, *Qualitative Data Analysis by Research Tradition*, reviews the differences and similarities of data analysis among the research traditions. Five categories of analytic approaches are highlighted: case study, experience and theory formulation (grounded theory, consensual qualitative research, phenomenology, heuristic inquiry), meaning of symbol and text (narratology, biography, and hermeneutics), cultural expressions of process and experience (ethnography, ethnomethodology, autoethnography), and participatory action research.

PART IV: PRESENTING YOUR QUALITATIVE RESEARCH

Chapter 12, *Writing and Presenting Qualitative Research*, is the final chapter of the text. We dedicate this chapter to the nuances of reporting data and reflecting on the research process. Guidelines for developing a research proposal are provided, with special attention to proposal components such as the conceptual framework, purpose statement, selected research paradigm and tradition, research questions, researcher bias, and "thick" descriptions of methods and analysis. Finally, we discuss considerations for presenting and publishing your qualitative report.

Now, let's begin the adventure of qualitative research. We hope you have a sense of the organization of the text, beginning with discussions of foundational elements of qualitative research, traveling through components of qualitative research design and data collection and analysis, and continuing on to data reporting. We are encouraged that your journey into qualitative inquiry will allow for deeper relationships with your research interests, participants, research teams and peers, and, most important, yourself. Enjoy the ride!

Acknowledgments

We thank C. Deborah Laughton for her tireless effort and investment in making this book a reality, providing great flexibility and trust in crafting it. What a wonderful experience and privilege it has been writing this book with you by our side! We are grateful as well to Senior Production Editor Laura Specht Patchkofsky.

We thank the reviewers who provided significant feedback and recommendations on earlier drafts of all or part of this text, including Cray Mulder, School of Social Work, Grand Valley State University; Kathleen Burns-Jager, Family and Child Clinic, Michigan State University; Ruth Chao, Department of Counseling Psychology, University of Denver; Thomas Schram, Department of Education, University of New Hampshire; Wendy Troxel, Department of Educational Administration and Foundations, Illinois State University; Lisa Harrison, Department of Psychology, California State University, Sacramento; Rajeswari Natrajan-Tyagi, Marriage and Family Therapy Program, California School of Professional Psychology, Alliant International University; William Kline, Department of Counseling Education, University of Mississippi; Lee Duemer, Department of Educational Psychology, Texas Tech University; Hema Genapathy-Coleman, Department of Educational and School Psychology, Indiana State University; Phil Cusick, Department of Educational Administration, Michigan State University; and Tanner Wallace, Department of Developmental Psychology, University of Pittsburgh.

Finally, we thank our colleagues and students who constantly inspire and remind us of the value of qualitative research in our practice, pedagogy, and scholarship.

Brief Contents

Extended Contents

PART II. QUALITATIVE RESEARCH DESIGN

PART III. DATA COLLECTION AND ANALYSIS

PART IV. PRESENTING YOUR QUALITATIVE RESEARCH

PART I

FOUNDATIONS OF QUALITATIVE INQUIRY

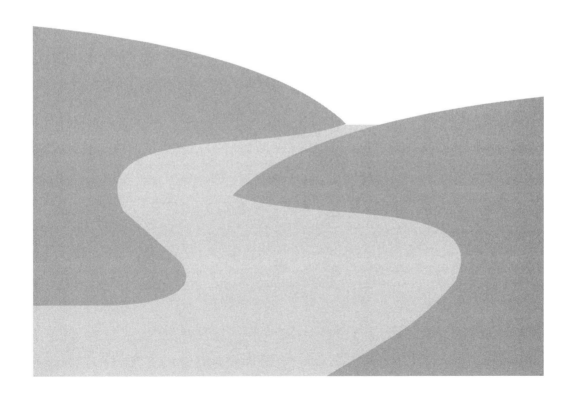

CHAPTER 1

Introduction to Qualitative Inquiry

CHAPTER PREVIEW

Qualitative inquiry, the process of conducting qualitative research, is being increasingly applied today by educators and practitioners in a variety of social science disciplines. This chapter provides a general introductory overview of qualitative research and discusses ways in which qualitative inquiry can become a part of your research agenda. First, we define qualitative inquiry and outline a rationale for its use in clinical and educational settings. Then we describe several characteristics of qualitative research. Following this foundational information we briefly discuss uses of qualitative research throughout history as well as in the present day. Finally, we outline strategies for establishing a successful research agenda.

A RATIONALE FOR QUALITATIVE RESEARCH

Several years ago we took a road trip to Louisiana, a state we proudly call home. We were driving from Atlanta to New Orleans to celebrate Mardi Gras (Fat Tuesday) with a few friends. It was February 2006, 6 months following the levee failures of Hurricanes Katrina and Rita, and we wanted to be a part of the resurgence of New Orleans life. National news anchors, including Anderson Cooper of CNN (one of our personal favorites!), were there covering the important revival of the city and showing the world that a city could thrive after adversity. If you have ever visited New Orleans or experienced Mardi Gras really anywhere in the Gulf Coast region, you probably can relate to how important a cultural marker the celebration is to natives. If you haven't, it's something to experience directly. Our friend Michele (who has lived in New Orleans 40+ years) reminded us to always "be a tourist in your own city." To understand the city and its people, you have to talk to them and get their perspective and "expertise."

New Orleans could be Anytown, U.S.A., or any context or setting in the disciplines to which we belong. The example underscores the importance of context, process, and direct quality experience; the limited importance at times of numbers, isolated events, and quantity; and the constant motivation we have to explore our surroundings. To understand a phenomenon, whether it is Mardi Gras or some other cultural event, or something in disciplines such as a therapy or classroom process, you have to talk to or observe those individuals affected by the phenomenon and directly experience it in the most comprehensive and engaged way possible. This is the task of qualitative research.

Qualitative research is the study of a phenomenon or research topic in context. Phenomena tend to be exploratory in nature, as researchers examine topics that have not been investigated or need to be investigated from a new angle. Because topics are exploratory, qualitative design tends to include research questions that address the *how* or *what* (i.e., a process) versus *why* (i.e., etiology of outcome) aspects of a phenomenon. There is a tendency to focus on narratives and words over numbers, quality over quantity: "The word *qualitative* implies an emphasis on the qualities of entities, on processes and meaning that are not experimentally examined or measured (if measured at all) in terms of quantity, amount, intensity, or frequency" (Lincoln & Guba, 1985, p. 8).

Qualitative research often occurs in a natural setting with researchers spending extensive and intensive time collecting and analyzing data. Language is an important conduit for obtaining information about phenomena that aren't always directly observable, easily defined, or previously explored (Morrow, 2007). Qualitative researchers approach the setting with an intention to become immersed and to rid themselves of an expert status. They are accepting of and empathic toward individuals, groups, and communities within that context. They listen to individuals' accounts of a phenomenon, engaging actively, and integrating new perspectives into their own ways of understanding participants, the context, phenomenon, or all three. Miles and Huberman (1994) referred to this as *local groundedness*: studying phenomena in context rather than at a distance. In some cases of qualitative inquiry, direct, sustained experience with participants in context becomes a source of knowledge and takes into account the ones who produce the knowledge; both researchers and participants (Haverkamp & Young, 2007). The guiding purposes of qualitative research in generating knowledge, then, are description, attention to process, and collaboration within a social structure and with its people.

In clinical and educational disciplines, practitioners and educators interact daily with students, clients, peers, colleagues, or administrators and encounter phenomena that need to be understood in context to guide our work as well as influence policy. Disciplines thus parallel the purposes of qualitative research quite well: Qualitative inquiry involves remaining flexible within the environment, attending to cultural considerations, understanding another's perspective, building trust and rapport, and relying on techniques that elicit participant meanings and understandings (Manning, 1992; Morrow, 2007).

From this brief introduction to qualitative research, we hope you are beginning to see why the approach is so important for clinical and educational settings. Practitioners and educators draw conclusions and make decisions that are hopefully framed in relation to those individuals and contexts that a phenomenon impacts. Research findings need to be comprehensive and relevant for a particular population if practitioners and educators are to apply them to disciplines. This form of research aims to inform practice by providing thick description (discussed shortly) of processes within a particular context—understandings from those who have not previously contributed to knowledge (Haverkamp & Young, 2007). Thus, qualitative inquiry is well suited to help bridge the gap between research and practice within a particular discipline.

CHARACTERISTICS OF QUALITATIVE RESEARCH

In this section we highlight several key characteristics of qualitative research. They include:

- Inductive and abductive analysis
- Naturalistic and experimental settings
- The importance of context
- The humanness of research
- Purposive sampling
- Thick description
- Interactive, flexible research design

Inductive and Abductive Analysis

Since qualitative research is exploratory in nature, often researchers use inductive reasoning or a "bottom-up" approach. **Inductive analysis** refers to the notion that data drive theory or a deeper understanding of an issue or phenomenon. The research process involves collecting data to refine research questions and build theory, not to test hypotheses. As the research study progresses, patterns and themes are identified and a phenomenon is understood more fully.

The research process, however, is not entirely inductive. Patton (2002) noted that qualitative research is both inductive and recursive, involving "discovery and verification"—moving back and forth between the research process and reflection on the process and findings.

An example might help illustrate inductive analysis. A community agency administrator notes that several substance abuse counselors have left the agency within a year and decides she wants to investigate what factors promote retention of substance abuse counselors. Since there is minimal literature on the topic and qualitative inquiry is warranted, the administrator collects pilot data, makes adjustments in her design, and generates an initial list of factors. With more data collection and analysis, a theory of what factors promote retention is identified. Additional adjustments are made in the research process to verify that the theory holds for future data.

In Agar's (2006) exploration of the epistemology—or ways of knowing—that qualitative research proposes to explore, he discussed the role of **abductive analysis**, noting that "deductive logic was the way to get new conclusions from old premises. Inductive logic was the way to see how well new material fit the available concepts. But both those kinds of logic were closed with reference to the concepts in play" (p. 10). Abductive logic, from the Latin word meaning to "lead away," would provide an additional perspective on qualitative research. Agar encouraged qualitative researchers to acknowledge the ways in which their analyses might also generate what he termed "new concepts."

Naturalistic and Experimental Settings

Qualitative researchers often investigate phenomena in social settings, where participants—also known as *informants*—interact with their environments to derive personal meaning. Qualitative inquiry in a **naturalistic setting** is important because researchers are interested in the role of context. The naturalistic setting affords practitioners and researchers with opportunities to examine how individuals interact with their environment through symbols, social roles, and social structures, to name a few. Not all qualitative research is conducted in a naturalistic setting. Qualitative approaches can be integrated into experimental research designs, in some forms of mixed method designs (Creswell & Plano Clark, 2011). An **experimental setting** that integrates qualitative research, for instance, might be a classic experimental–control quantitative research design in which an experimental group receives some type of treatment, whereas the control group does not in order to measure the effect of that treatment.

Qualitative researchers immerse themselves in the culture being studied, investing time in participants and the community (Manning, 1992). Data collection tends to occur within sustained contacts with participants, in places where they spend their time normally—a classroom, neighborhood, counseling office, university, hospital, and so forth. Qualitative research as a naturalistic inquiry means, then, that practitioners and educators study the real world "as it unfolds" for participants in their everyday environments (Patton, 2002). Naturalistic inquiry is a discovery-oriented approach in which researchers are open to ongoing change as it happens within a setting. Terms used to describe this work include *fieldwork, prolonged engagement, qualitative interviewing,* and *participant observation.* These terms are discussed in more detail in Chapter 8.

The Importance of Context

Take a moment and think about your experiences in graduate school. Perhaps even more specifically recall sitting in a qualitative research course and spending week after week learning about the topic. If you are currently enrolled in such a course, you probably expect that your experience in that course will be affected by many things, including time and location of the course, setting, content, activities, and interactions among peers as well as with the instructor, to name a few. If we were investigating your experience in a graduate-level qualitative research course, we could make the assumption that your experience is affected by environment, that to understand your perspective, we should also understand what the course and perhaps the graduate program are like.

The **importance of context** as a characteristic of qualitative research refers to how participants create and give meaning to social experience. Phenomena are created and maintained by those in an environment, and individuals self-organize activities within social settings. "By observing the sequential actions that occur when students interact, the investigator is able to witness how they understand each others' prior actions and what they do with that understanding in their subsequent actions" (Patton, 1991, p. 393). To this end, individuals interact with one another in context, and patterns emerge that illustrate phenomena.

The importance of context also includes the research context itself: Our ability to collect and interpret data fully relies on the researcher–participant relationship and on situational constraints and opportunities of the design. Practitioners and educators are sensitive to the natural and research environment when collecting and analyzing data, as well when determining the degree to which findings are transferable (Patton, 2002). Participants and researchers cannot be understood in isolation from the research relationship and design. It is also essential to recognize that participants may be not only individuals, but also may be conceptualized as groups, families, partnerships, and communities. Understanding a phenomenon fully may entail that the qualitative researcher thinks broadly about "who" the participants are within a context.

A key assumption underlying the notion of the importance of context is that participants are best understood holistically versus as a sum of their parts. Although in qualitative research you often lose "control" of variables by not isolating them or manipulating conditions, adding contextual data provides a more comprehensive picture with which to address a research problem (Borland, 2001). Some answers in counseling and education cannot be directly observed and measured; these unquantifiable data can be accessed only by exploring participants' perspectives through interacting with them or examining "traces" (e.g., letters, photographs) in their environments. Just as when you read an article in your local newspaper, or hear a client's story, or evaluate a student's behavior in a classroom, you understand that the "truth" of that perspective or action is bounded by the time and context in which it was observed, as well as by how others may perceive it. "Taking things out of context" only leads to limited and often inaccurate interpretations. The wide variety of ways in which researchers can explore phenomena allow better understanding of how participants make meaning of themselves, their environment, and some social phenomena.

The Humanness of Research

The fact that we as researchers are human, that we allow our subjectivity to be integrated with our skill set in qualitative inquiry, is a great strength *and* challenge. We refer to this characteristic as the **humanness of research**, or *Verstehen*. It relates to the researcher's competence and to his or her impact on the design and participants—that is, to the nature of being studied and of studying humans (Patton, 2002).

A researcher often has direct contact with people and settings, and is therefore an instrument of the study. Patton (2002) noted, "The credibility of qualitative methods ... hinges to a great extent on the skill, competence, and rigor of the person doing fieldwork" (p. 14). The qualitative researcher is an important part of the design itself and thus must have a wide range of interpersonal, organizational, and technical skills. Some of the key skills qualitative researchers need to possess include the following (Morrow, 2007; Patton, 1991, 2002):

- Attending to a rigorous research design, including a focus on research paradigms and traditions throughout the study;
- Using a multitude of strategies, techniques, and approaches in a creative and innovative manner to explore a phenomenon;
- Displaying **empathic neutrality**, which means communicating understanding and care, remaining neutral to the extent needed to maintain study integrity, and being nonjudgmental toward participants and their experiences;
- Reflecting on the research process and being mindful of voice and representation;

- Valuing a research relationship that promotes egalitarianism, cultural sensitivity, collaboration and respect; and

- Understanding that knowledge presented to researchers in the research process is ultimately re-presented by us (Patton, 1991), and that self-reflection is necessary to recognize the benefits and challenges of subjectivity.

Purposive Sampling

Because participants are experts in relation to the phenomenon under study, and thus are partners in qualitative research, practitioners and educators seek information-rich cases that will best address a research question. The intention in **purposive sampling** is to select participants for the amount of detail they can provide about a phenomenon, and not simply selecting participants to meet a certain sample size.

Sample size in purposive sampling is relative to the research goals and tradition, and thus it is very difficult to establish the "right" number of participants. Typically, you need more participants if you are interested in theory development and/or heterogeneity in perspectives (Sandelowski, 1995). Purposive sampling is discussed in more depth in Chapter 6.

Thick Description

The term **thick description** is used when there is ample detail about the research process, the context, and the participants. Qualitative researchers aim for insight and deeper understanding to illustrate a phenomenon fully, rather than for generalizability to a larger sample (i.e., depth versus breadth). A common misconception of thick description is that it is simply providing more detail or description. Thick description, however, refers to providing a comprehensive and focused picture of a behavior or occurrence that includes relevant psychosocial, affective, and cultural undertones (see Geertz, 1973). The end goal of thick description is to provide enough interpretive depth and detail that the reader can generalize findings to a narrowed context or can replicate the study in another setting. The truth is that qualitative research can be so descriptive and systematic that collection methods and findings may be easily replicated and generalized to a specific setting (Berg, 2004).

Qualitative research is named for its reference to "quality"—to the detailed accounts and description of data. Qualitative researchers are interested in the *who, what, when, where, why,* and *how* of a phenomenon. Thus, the detailed report typically involves words and pictures more so than numbers. The report often describes and tells a story, and typically includes participant quotes. Thick description is discussed in more depth in Chapter 7.

An Interactive, Flexible Research Design

Designing qualitative research is not a linear, sequential process. Patton (2002) described the process as one of being open to discovering new paths. Maxwell (2005) also argued that it should be reflexive, and that different components of the design are reactive to the ongoing research process. A design should interact with the environment, allowing a mutual influence. Maxwell developed an interactive model of qualitative research design that we believe best captures the evolving nature of qualitative inquiry. There are five major, interrelated components (see Figure 1.1):

- *Goals.* The intention and focus of the research study, and how the expected outcomes might affect various stakeholders. Three types of goals are identified and discussed for the researcher in more detail in Chapter 4: personal, practical, and scholarly goals. Additionally, participant concerns and funder goals influence research design goals.

- *Conceptual framework.* A network of significant constructs from guiding theories based on personal and professional experience as well as previous literature. Essentially, the conceptual framework constitutes an evolving literature review and theoretical model of personal and professional assumptions that collectively build a study rationale. Personal experience, existing theory and prior research, exploratory and pilot research/preliminary conclusions, and thought experiments are primary contextual factors that influence (and are influenced by) the conceptual framework, and are further discussed in Chapter 4.

- *Research questions.* Referred to as the "hub" of the interactive model, research questions are the "what do you want to know" component of qualitative research design. They are influenced by the other four components and related contextual factors. Research questions are discussed primarily in Chapters 2 and 4.

- *Methods.* Actions taken in the design. Methods involve four components: the researcher–participant relationship (see Chapter 5); site and participant selection (sampling; see Chapter 6); data collection methods (see Chapters 8 and 9); and data analysis (see Chapters 10 and 11).

- *Validity.* The limitations or "how you might be wrong" aspects of research design. Commonly referred to as *trustworthiness*, validity impacts primarily data collection, management, and analysis. Validity is discussed further in Chapter 7.

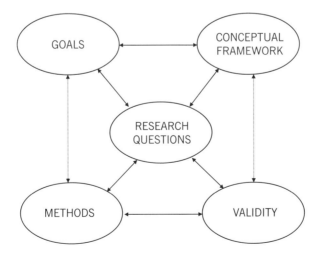

FIGURE 1.1. The interactive model of qualitative research design. *Source*: Maxwell (2005). Reprinted with permission from Sage Publications.

We address each of these components, as well as the contextual factors associated with the model, in more detail throughout this text. Finally, Maxwell (2005) noted that ethics is a component of the model infused in all other components. Ethics in qualitative research design is discussed further in Chapter 3.

THE QUALITATIVE–QUANTITATIVE "DEBATE"

"Qualitative research is easier than quantitative research."

"Qualitative research is nonscientific, 'fluff,' and invalid."

"Qualitative research is subjective, and quantitative research is objective."

These are just a few of the comments you might overhear as you engage in qualitative inquiry and discuss your design with others. We do! One reason for these misconceptions is lack of understanding of how qualitative inquiry can be conducted in clinical and educational settings. This lacuna could be due to a minimal emphasis historically on qualitative research in counseling specifically (see Brief History section below). There are also stereotypes about qualitative approaches—for example, that they are suited only to the study of human processes and are not useful in basic research as well. Relatedly, there have not been many training materials (e.g., texts, empirical articles) available to serve as models for conducting qualitative inquiry, particularly for counseling-related professions.

Regardless, it is important to understand the differences between qualitative and quantitative approaches. The overall purpose of social science is to explore basic human processes, develop and verify theory, and enact social change. Qualitative and quantitative methods are both "tools" of science that allow us to answer research questions. Before discussing the debate between qualitative and quantitative camps, we would like to highlight some characteristics of each (see Table 1.1). The characteristics of qualitative research are outlined in greater depth throughout the text.

In this section we highlight aspects of a **qualitative–quantitative debate** that have been occurring since qualitative research was introduced in a variety of disciplines. Traditionally, the two sides of the debate (qualitative and quantitative) are thought of as types of researchers rather than as methodologies. So, it's almost like you have a qualitative or quantitative personality that is destined to guide your research process! We think that this is a false dichotomy that has created much of the current debate. After presenting the two sides, we discuss ways in which qualitative and quantitative methods are *methods*, not *people*, and are similar or mutually beneficial and may be used together to address a phenomenon.

The quantitative side has quoted some of the above in their arguments against qualitative research. Qualitative research has been labeled "soft" because, although it involves rich, contextual descriptions, it is not easily translated into statistical procedures (Bogdan & Biklen, 2003). That is, the absence of numbers often has led to a traditional view of qualitative research as anecdotal or nonscientific (Maxwell, 2010). Because the "gold standard" in scientific research—that is, achieving validity, reliability, and generalizability (Kvale & Brinkmann, 2009; see Chapter 7)—is not produced by qualitative research, it is labeled as nonscientific or invalid.

TABLE 1.1. Characteristics of Qualitative and Quantitative Research

	Qualitative	Quantitative
Descriptors	Naturalistic Depth and detail Exploratory Context Participant perspective Words Images	Confirmatory Outer perspective Numbers
Goals	Process Understanding	Outcome Causes
Research paradigms	Constructivism Critical theory Feminism Queer theory	Positivist/postpositivist
Research design	Interactive Evolving Research traditions (e.g., grounded theory, phenomenology, case study)	Experimental Quasi-experimental Nonexperimental Predetermined
Data collection methods	Interviews Observations Documents Archival data	Survey research Structured interviews Structured observations
Research setting and relationships	Trust Empathy Egalitarian Participant as expert Intense Idiographic/emic based on a specific case	Short-term Detachment Subject Studies relationships among variables, not humans Nomothetic/etic perspective from large samples
Data collection tools	Digital recorder Videorecorder Transcriber Computer	Standardized data collection Questionnaires Scales Test scores Inventories Computer
Data analysis	Ongoing Inductive Concurrent with data collection Constant comparison Models, themes Thick description to present individual holistically	Postdata collection Deductive Statistical Create knowledge by testing theory Thin description to maximize generalizability

(cont.)

TABLE 1.1. *(cont.)*

	Qualitative	Quantitative
Report writing	Tentative conclusions and ongoing Use of first person	Generalizations made at the end of study Use of third person
Limitations of approach	Time-consuming Reliability Unstandardized procedures Small samples	Difficulty controlling variables Validity

Sources: Bogdan and Biklen (2003); Borland (2001); and Patton (2002).

The qualitative side has defended its methodology and discussed how quantitative research is flawed. Qualitative research is often cited as more intensive and time-consuming at all stages of design (Berg, 2004) and seeks to represent the voices of those typically not represented in research (Morrow, 2007). Maxwell (2010) indicated that a focus on variables in quantitative research assumes regularity or linearity, which challenges the notion that constructs are process-oriented, dynamic, and socially constructed. That is, generalizable results from a quantitative study are valid only to the extent that they represent a comprehensive picture of a phenomenon and include a truly representative sample. Qualitative researchers have argued that some experimental research creates artificial experiences and environments that render participant reactions and findings not useful (Borland, 2001; Gnisci, Bakeman, & Quera, 2008). Furthermore, experimental designs have been traditionally critiqued for their lack of practical significance, their inattention to individual variation, and their use of inappropriate measures (Sandelowski, 1996). In researchers' efforts, then, to control conditions to make more "accurate" statements about a phenomenon to generalize to a population, they may limit participant authenticity and construct description. Finally, as long as quantitative research does not randomize a sample or contains results with little variability (e.g., most participants score at one end of a survey), generalizability is threatened.

Even with the polarization between quantitative and qualitative approaches, qualitative researchers across disciplines are using numbers to supplement their studies. As Becker (1970) noted, researchers using terms such as *most, often,* or *many* are assuming some quantitative value to a theme or construct; quasi-statistics, then, influence qualitative data presentation in many cases. Maxwell (2010) cited several advantages to using quantitative approaches to qualitative data: numbers can help identify patterns not apparent from singular constructs or codes, may indicate evidence to refute criticisms that qualitative research is too "soft," and can facilitate internal generalizability (i.e., achieved when information is comprehensive and characteristic of a specific case; see Maxwell, 1992) and check for diversity of variability in this process. Maxwell cautioned, however, that numbers during data presentation and interpretation carry meanings: "more" or "less" often signify—sometimes unconsciously—to the reader "better" or "worse."

Ercikan and Roth (2006) added several points about how several aspects of quantitative research can use description beyond numbers. First, in designs using statistics, many of the reported statistics are descriptive. For example, I (Hays) conducted a survey of dating violence prevalence on a college campus in 2009 and 2010. Although the survey contained quantitative items and I computed descriptive statistics, such as measures of central tendency and variability, the results were discussed both in terms of prevalence rates *and* how participants responded to particular survey items. Yes, it was important to discover that approximately one-third of the sample experienced dating violence, and it was important to outline specific dating violence experiences. Researchers consistently provide qualitative information about a data set in the Discussion or Conclusion section of any manuscript they develop.

Another example of how quantitative research has qualitative findings is in the use of rubrics or scaling methods. When scorers use rubrics, no matter how objective the rubrics are, they are still subjective in their judgments (Ercikan & Roth, 2006). Take, for example, a study that involves clinical supervisors assessing supervisees' skills through observing particular behaviors in a video recording. As each supervisor uses the scale, he or she reflects on the following "qualitative" questions: What does each point mean? How might various supervisors have different thresholds for when a skill has been demonstrated? Am I assessing skill level based on how competent the supervisee should be at this level of training, or am I assessing skill level based on the skills of a counselor who is able to see clients independently?

The reverse is also true. Sometimes in qualitative studies, researchers rely on frequency counts to interpret and present findings (see Part III of this volume). For example, in a program evaluation, a research team may count the number of times a particular need was mentioned in several focus groups. Although these needs could be presented in narrative form, it may be more meaningful in some cases to present them in some order, with the most cited need first.

From this brief discussion of the debate and a couple of examples of how each type of research can contain aspects of the other, we argue against polarizing the two research methodologies. Ercikan and Roth (2006) noted that *qualitative* and *quantitative* are not appropriate divisions because (1) all research has quantitative and qualitative elements or dimensions, whether explicit or not; (2) we interpret data using similar processes, and the distinction between objectivity and subjectivity is artificial and thus not useful; and (3) most constructs in which educational researchers are interested are based on subjective judgments. So, both methodologies can contain characteristics of the other, can be subjective and objective, and can be interpreted collectively to address research problems in clinical and educational settings. Borland (2001) echoed this perspective, stating that these approaches should be considered a continuum of complementary methods that, when used together, produce a comprehensive and useful picture.

One way qualitative research is receiving increasing recognition in traditionally quantitative designs is by contributing to mixed methods studies. Miles and Huberman (1994) highlighted four mixed methods strategies:

1. Qualitative and quantitative data continuously collected and integrated;
2. Continuous qualitative data collection, with intermittent "waves" of quantitative data collection;

3. Qualitative data collected first to explore, followed by quantitative data, then qualitative data again to deepen and verify findings; and

4. Quantitative data collected first, then qualitative data, and then quantitative data.

We encourage you to review their text for additional information on these strategies. Although the mixed methods approach is discussed in Chapter 4, here we would like to highlight some of the contributions of qualitative research (see Table 1.2).

We believe it is better to appreciate the merits of both qualitative and quantitative research, and we hope we have argued that the characteristics of both types of research can be shared. We also encourage you to reflect on your stance toward the qualitative–quantitative debate (see Activity 1.1). Choices about research methodology should not be based on what kind of researcher you are, but on the questions you want to explore: "The purpose of research is to generate knowledge rather than concretely realize one method or another" (Ercikan & Roth, 2006, p. 21). Research questions, not methods, drive research. Thus, collaborations among researchers with varying levels of expertise are necessary to best address a research problem.

TABLE 1.2. Contributions of Qualitative Research to Mixed Methods Studies

- Planning of research for quantitative data collection, data analysis, and data reporting and communication of results
- Giving voice to underrepresented or underresearched individuals
- Providing context for a sample
- Taking account how people feel and construct their experiences
- Developing observation protocols that may be used for more quantifiable observations
- Using qualitative findings to develop surveys to distribute to a larger sample
- Providing information in experimental designs as a first phase of research, as a component of a trial, or to help explain the findings (e.g., "piloting" the trial, understanding the clinical trial postintervention)
- Formulating interventions
- Contributing to community engagement and social change
- Determining what scale points mean (i.e., judgments about categories)
- Exploring surprising findings or unexpected results
- Stimulating theory development for various phenomena to be later tested or refined using quantitative methods
- Explaining quantitative findings
- Helping to explain mechanisms behind relationships
- Exploring constructs or variables that are unknown
- Exploring or confirming research areas

Sources: Borland (2001); Creswell, Shope, Plano Clark, and Green (2006); Ercikan and Roth (2006); Gnisci et al. (2008); Morrow (2007); and Sandelowski (1996).

ACTIVITY 1.1. The Qualitative–Quantitative Debate

As a class or in small groups reflect on the following questions:

- What type of research have you considered more rigorous? Where do these beliefs originate?
- How, if at all, do you think quantitative research contributes to qualitative research?
- How, if at all, do you think qualitative research contributes to quantitative research?
- Are there examples of research topics that might be better suited for one approach or another?

- What are some potential criticisms you see of each approach? How would you address these criticisms?
- Qualitative approaches are often used to study human processes and phenomena. What are some examples of how qualitative approaches are used in basic research as well?

A BRIEF HISTORY OF QUALITATIVE INQUIRY

The earliest roots of qualitative research are found in the work of anthropologists and sociologists beginning as early as the 15th century, as they attempted to understand the "other" (the outsider) and culture (Morrow, 2007; Vidich & Lyman, 2001). We only begin to see this methodology reflected in education and other social sciences beginning in the 1960s and 1970s (Bogdan & Biklen, 2003). In this section we highlight briefly some of the key moments in the history of qualitative research. You should note that these moments in qualitative research are in response to, or coincide with, historical events, and definitions and conceptualizations of qualitative research vary depending on the historical moment. For instance, with colonization comes the idea that qualitative inquiry involves evaluating those "outside" by Western standards and values, and that rigor in research depends on the degree to which the researcher is deemed expert.

It is important to think of these moments not as a linear progression of history, but as lessons that we, as researchers, come back to as we move toward the future. That is, we revisit and celebrate the contributions of these moments:

> We can discover work in the past which challenges us to rethink our assumptions, or to treat them with a little more caution than we are currently inclined to do; so that the past can set us new problems, or cast old problems in a new light. What are not helpful, from this point of view, are histories which treat the past as simply a prelude to the present; or histories where all the loose ends are sewn up … in order to justify present practice and some future line of development. (Hammersley, 2004, p. 25)

Using primarily the works of Lincoln and Guba (1985) and Vidich and Lyman (2001), we discuss the following historical moments: early ethnography, colonial ethnography, traditional period, and modernist phase. You will also note that the first few moments of qualitative research are labeled *ethnography*, as this was the primary tradition used. We highlight key points of these moments in Table 1.3. We direct you to texts in the Recommended Readings section at the end of this chapter for additional information on the history of qualitative research.

TABLE 1.3. Key Historical Moments in Qualitative Research

	Time frame[a]	Key events	Contributions
Early ethnography	15th to 17th centuries	Detached and "objective" study of diversity in "uncivilized" societies using a Eurocentric view of diversity; development of theories of human diversity.	Beginnings of fieldwork.
Colonial ethnography	17th to 19th centuries	Two camps of ethnographers with a focus on colonization or liberation; introduction of constructivism and hermeneutics.	Some attention within one camp to local context in studying groups.
Traditional period	Early 1900s to mid-1940s	Classic ethnography shifting to modern ethnography; focus on decolonization abroad and colonization and conversion within the United States; Chicago School and British School formed to study local and global ethnography; expansion of hermeneutics and introduction of critical theory and phenomenology.	Greater emphasis on conducting fieldwork, taking field notes, and writing theory.
Modernist phase	1940s to 1970s	Emergence of grounded theory, semiotics, ethnomethodology, positivism, postpositivism, and feminism; increased value on rigor (i.e., "golden age of qualitative analysis").	Introduction of additional qualitative methods and strategies.
Blurred genres	1970 to 1986	Blurring of humanities with other disciplines; introduction of narratology.	Attention to interpretivism and the qualitative report; emergence of qualitative research in education and social sciences.
Crisis of representation	Mid-1980s	Increased attention to feminism, constructivism, and critical theory paradigms; view of writing and fieldwork as integrated.	Development of evaluation standards; increased view of phenomena as dynamic social systems influenced by cultural and political factors; discussion of researcher positionality (e.g., researcher bias).
A triple crisis	Mid-1980s to mid-1990s	Questions develop over the best way to represent, evaluate, and report findings.	Attention to the power of disseminating findings and representation.
Postexperimental inquiry and beyond	Mid-1990s to present	Sophistication of methods and focus on alternative and non-Western approaches to qualitative research design.	Introduction of novel forms of data reporting.

[a]Time frame per phase is approximated, and there is some overlap of phases.

Early Ethnography

The **early ethnography** period (15th–17th centuries) is a historical moment that involved a comparison of diversity throughout the globe against an established theory of human diversity, beginning as early as Columbus and the Eurocentric colonialism efforts. Vidich and Lyman (2001) defined **ethnography** as a description of individuals and their social contexts, and in this moment, descriptions were made of how non-Western societies diverged from the "civilized" European nations (Morrow, 2007). Thus, the first ethnographic methods were reported in texts that reflected Western interest in understanding others and their communities (Suzuki, Ahluwalia, Mattis, & Quizon, 2005). This interest was motivated by a need to classify human diversity across the world. During this period inquiry was conceptualized as atheoretical, primarily concerned with description of non-Western countries by Western (European) countries. Terms such as *savage* and *primitive* were used to describe individuals from non-Western societies.

Colonial Ethnography

The **colonial ethnography** period (17th, 18th, and 19th centuries) reflects a time of complexity in qualitative research, with one camp of researchers interested in studying and colonizing the "primitives," and another camp interested in liberating colonized peoples. Thus, ethnographies from this period tell readers much about values and perspectives of those studied as well as of the Western researchers (Vidich & Lyman, 2001).

During the first part of this period, explorers, guided by what has later was described as positivism and postpositivism paradigms (see Chapter 2), searched for scientific "truth" through observation and comparison. These researchers asserted that knowledge was acquired through direct experience and observation of facts. Uncovering truth was influenced by an agenda of colonizing non-Western peoples and interpreting data often through a Christian lens.

During the later part of this period, a division of camps led to value conflicts and moral dilemmas among ethnographers. Those in the second camp, of liberation, began to attend to the importance of the local context of those studied in understanding findings, and *not* the context and standards of Western societies. Researchers were beginning to consider the idea of multiple truths and the notion that context influenced individuals' reality. Kant's *Critique of Pure Reason* (1787) laid the foundation for constructivism and thus influenced the division among ethnographers during this period (Vidich & Lyman, 2001). Constructivism is an important groundwork for most qualitative research to come in later moments and is described more fully in Chapter 2.

Influenced by Kant's work, hermeneutics emerged initially in the 1800s and early 1900s as a philosophy for conducting qualitative research and later as its own research tradition (see Chapter 2). Hermeneutics as a philosophy assumed that texts needed to be interpreted in relation to historical and literature contexts to understand the author's intentions. Hermeneutics eventually extended its purview beyond texts to include understanding of all human behavior and cultural products (Sandage, Cook, Hill, Strawn, & Reimer, 2008). Scholars such as Schleiermacher (1768–1834), Dilthey (1833–1911), and Heidegger (1884–1976) helped shape this research tradition.

Although there is some division among researchers in notions of what constitutes truth and from whose perspective and standard, most of the ethnographers in this period continued to see the mission of their research as efforts to judge the outsider or "other" against some European standard. We continue to see this stance in the traditional period as qualitative research extends to the United States.

Traditional Period

The **traditional period** extends from the early 1900s to the mid-1940s (Lincoln & Guba, 1985). We consider it one of the most foundational periods of qualitative research because the greatest amount of growth in ideas and traditions occurs across a variety of disciplines. Classic ethnography is prevalent at the beginning of this period, slowly shifting to what is known as modern ethnography. A major contribution of this period included a greater emphasis on conducting fieldwork, taking field notes, and writing theory. Classic ethnography continued using the "objective" reports from often what has been termed the *lone ethnographer*, the expert fieldworker returning home with stories of *the other* (Lincoln & Guba). Vidich and Lyman (2001) noted a focus on the American Indian during this period and the idea of "saving Indians" by converting them to Christianity—in other words, colonization. At the same time decolonization movements were forming in Africa and Asia. During the early part of this period, there is an increased value on decolonization efforts abroad and thus a focus more on local context in research and more attention to support of colonization efforts in the United States. Worldwide, the term *primitive* was slowly replaced by *underdeveloped*, and access to tribal societies became more and more difficult.

The qualitative research of modern ethnographers emphasized participant observation and fieldwork as an important way to gain information about people within their communities (Suzuki et al., 2005). In the 1920s through the 1950s Margaret Mead wrote of applied educational phenomena in other parts of the world to those in the United States (Bogdan & Biklen, 2003), and George Herbert Mead, in *Mind, Self, and Society* (Morris, 1934), discussed how the social nature of self, thought, and community was a product of human meaning and interaction.

Researchers see the emergence of the critical theory paradigm (see Chapter 2) from theorists Horkheimer, Adorno, and Marcuse at the Institute of Social Research in Frankfurt, and there is a growing assumption that researchers' values are important to the task, purpose, and methods of research. In 1925 Husserl introduces phenomenology in the psychology discipline, asserting that it is important to understand individuals' subjective experiences of particular life experiences (Jennings, 1986). Scholars such as Piaget, Freud, Horney, Maslow, and Rogers give increased attention to qualitative methods in the form of detailed observations, use of diaries, and case study interviews as these become prevalent in European psychology (Morrow, 2007).

Researchers also see the expansion of hermeneutics to include dialectical hermeneutics by scholars such as Gadamer (1900–2002), Habermas (1929–), and Ricouer (1913–2005). **Dialectical hermeneutics** refers to the examination of meanings created through dialogue and conversation. It is assumed that individuals have a strong interest in praxis and that speech promotes a mutual understanding through social discourse.

The British School

In England an anthropological school of qualitative research, known as the **British School**, emerged in the 1920s and 1930s. The British School is credited with development of the fieldwork method. Bronislaw Malinowski (1884–1942), the first major fieldworker, spoke of the importance of viewing culture from the natives' point of view through sustained contact. Malinowski spent 2 years in the Trobriand Islands and produced the seminal work *Argonauts of the Western Pacific: An Account of Native Enterprise and Adventure in the Archipelagoes of Melanesian New Guinea* (1922).

The British School scholars conceptualized ethnography as requiring being in the presence of the people one is studying, not just their texts or artifacts. They asserted that it was important to evaluate individuals based on behavior versus only verbal statements; to experience prolonged, active engagement with the group being studied; and to consider behaviors in a larger social context. The British School also conducted work within England, examining the processes involved in conflict, urbanization, and imperialism (MacDonald, 2001).

The Chicago School

During this period there is movement within the social sciences of anthropology and sociology in the United States to apply the notions of modern ethnography to "slices of life" in the Chicago area. The movement was known as the **Chicago School** and presented several core ethnographies between 1917 and 1942. The movement began with what William Foote White coined as *participant observation* (discussed in Chapter 8). For instance, White's *Street Corner Society* observed the different individuals and groups in a neighborhood, including the details of where these individuals and groups gathered (e.g., street corners, local shops). Several University of Chicago scholars, originating with Robert Park and Ernest Burgess and others and then later including their students, studied normal, everyday face-to-face interactions within a city. Salient Chicago School methods include conducting local studies of the natural areas or urban structures of the city, and creating a natural history of collective behavior; in addition, the school introduced the concept of radical social change as a natural pattern (Deegan, 2001). The American city, then, became an ideal outlet for examining social behavior via conducting fieldwork in specific locations. Fieldworkers explored aspects of ordinary life for various urban cultural groups that were typically marginalized by society. Social interaction was the source of various realities for urban subgroups, and lived experiences were best understood from the perspectives of the different subgroups. With the Chicago School, ethnography was becoming more localized.

Park and Burgess had a major influence on several core ethnographies and often wrote introductions to the studies. Some of the core ethnographies of this school included a focus on (1) Polish peasants and immigrants to America (*The Polish Peasant in Europe and America, 1918–1920* [Thomas & Znaniecki, 1927]); (2) juvenile delinquency (*The Jack-Roller*, 1930; *The Natural History of a Delinquent Career*, 1931; *Brothers in Crime*, 1938 [Clifford Shaw]); (3) women and the changing division of labor (*The Woman Who Waits*, 1920; *The Saleslady*, 1929 [Frances Donovan]); (4) race relations and the melting pot idea (*The City* [Park, Burgess, & McKenzie, 1925]; *Negro Politicians* [Gosnell, 1935];

The Etiquette of Race Relations in the South [Doyle, 1937]; *Race and Culture* [Park, 1950]; *Society* [Park, 1955]).

Modernist Phase

The **modernist phase** (1940s–1970s) primarily involved the emergence of several new approaches (e.g., ethnomethodology, feminism, positivism, postpositivism, semiotics, grounded theory) applied specifically to qualitative research, as well as the increased attention to rigor and quality (referred to as the "golden age of qualitative analysis" by Lincoln and Guba, 1985). With these changes in methodology, researchers were viewed as cultural romantics, beautifully crafting narratives of those they encountered. The Chicago School continued its study of the "slice of life," with works such as *Boys in White* (Becker, Geer, Hughes, & Strauss, 1961), *Middletown* (Lynd & Lynd, 1929), and *Middletown in Transition: A Study in Cultural Conflicts* (Lynd & Lynd, 1937).

Vidich and Lyman (2001) described this phase in terms of two time periods: ethnography of the "civic other" or community studies/ethnography of the early American immigrants (early 20th century to the 1960s) and studies of ethnicity and assimilation (1950s–1980s). For the former period, they noted that, similar to the American Indian ethnographies, researchers sought to assimilate blacks and Asian and European immigrants into Christianity. In fact, there is a surge of survey methods by churches to understand immigration trends as they increased. During the latter phase, scholars begin to challenge Park's melting pot idea.

Blurred Genres

The **blurred genres** moment occurred from 1970 to 1986 (Lincoln & Guba, 1985). The golden age of researchers as cultural romantics was over, and greater attention was given to the act of writing itself. That is, reports were no longer being viewed as free of the researcher's values; reports were now considered interpretations of interpretations. Clifford Geertz, in two works that seem to sandwich this historical moment (*The Interpretation of Cultures*, 1973; *Local Knowledge*, 1983) best articulates this point when he argues for more interpretive approaches to qualitative research that include thick descriptions of events and rituals to maximize the likelihood that participants' stories are well represented.

Genres such as social sciences and humanities were being blurred, giving rise to new scholars and approaches from education and social science disciplines. Contemporary scholars such as Harry Wolcott, Egon Guba, Robert Stake, and Yvonna Lincoln emerge in education. Research efforts sprout in education and social science disciplines, including social work, psychology, and counseling. Before this period the term *qualitative research* was virtually nonexistent in education and social sciences (Rennie, 2000).

With this blurring of disciplines, we see the tradition of *narratology* develop, shaped by Foucalt's work on narratives as a product of cultural and political practice. Scholars such as Ricouer (1984, 1985), Bakhtin (1984), and MacIntyre (1984) articulate the roles narratives and voice play in identity.

Crisis of Representation

In the mid-1980s qualitative research enters the historical moment termed "**crisis of representation.**" In this period there is a rise in feminism, constructivism, and critical theory paradigms. The crisis comes as a result of an increased realization that qualitative researchers may not be representing themselves and their participants in an accurate way. They realize that they are not experts, that there is an erosion of the notions of objectivism, structured social life, and ethnographies as museum pieces (Lincoln & Guba, 1985). "No longer would ethnography have to serve the interests of a theory of progress that pointed toward the breakup of every ethnos" (Vidich & Lyman, 2001, p. 87).

During this historical moment, researchers begin to examine more closely the role of gender, class, and race in participants as well as in their own lives and work. They question their writings, and see that fieldwork and report writing are blurred activities influencing one another and thus difficult to separate. During this phase, researchers are exposed to new evaluation standards of credibility, dependability, transferability, and confirmability (see Lincoln & Guba, 1985).

A Triple Crisis

A **triple crisis** (mid-1980s to mid-1990s) as a historical moment refers to the postmodern period of ethnography and other forms of qualitative research, a time of struggle with how to best represent the other (Denzin & Lincoln, 2005). Representations of phenomena in the forms of grand narratives about social structures are replaced by context-specific cases. The three crises that make up this moment are the following: (1) the realization that lived experience cannot be directly represented because it is *re*created as it is written (i.e., *representational crisis*); (2) the legitimacy of traditional evaluation criteria in qualitative research is questioned (i.e., *legitimation crisis*); and a combination of both, (3) the question, Is it possible to affect change in society if we only write about it? With this moment qualitative researchers struggle to best represent their participants and phenomena, be flexible in how they evaluate the rigor of qualitative design, and consider alternative methods beyond writing to disseminate their findings.

Postexperimental Inquiry and Beyond

In this last subsection we discuss changes in qualitative research over the past 15 years. Although our understanding of recent history is still evolving, Denzin and Lincoln (2005) identify some major events and tasks yet to come. First, qualitative research continues to help break down discipline boundaries and introduce new traditions. Second, novel forms of writing, such as poetry, autobiography, art, and visual media, are becoming increasingly common. Third, efforts are being made to come to consensus on the several research paradigms and traditions available for conducting research. (Put simply, there are so many choices yet little agreement on the definitions and practices of these choices.) Finally, greater attention is being placed on indigenous studies and non-Western approaches, studies with social purpose, and overall methodological sophistication.

QUALITATIVE INQUIRY TODAY: APPLIED RESEARCH IN CLINICAL AND EDUCATIONAL SETTINGS

Whether you are in clinical or educational settings, potential phenomena to study abound. Qualitative inquiry in these settings opens a window to greater understanding of these phenomena with an in-depth richness that otherwise may not be possible. With the U.S. population becoming increasingly diverse, there are shifting needs, priorities, and demands for individuals and groups who interact with counseling and educational settings (Choudhuri, 2003). Qualitative approaches may help researchers and practitioners illuminate complex phenomena in their settings, specifically as they relate to the daily lived experiences of individuals and groups. Whereas the roots of qualitative inquiry, as discussed in earlier sections of this chapter, were anthropological and sociological in nature, qualitative inquiry has become a powerful method of investigation.

For instance, it is one thing to say that we are living in a more diverse, multicultural society today and that our counseling and educational methods must respond to this societal shift. We can collect survey data, develop assessment instruments, and distribute questionnaires in an attempt to gain knowledge of what the needs of our multicultural nation are. These are important sources of knowledge. It is also important, however, to understand how people *actually experience* and *live* in a multicultural society.

A good example of this need is the qualitative study conducted by Sue, Lin, Tornio, Capodilupo, and Rivera (2009) that sought an in-depth understanding of racial microaggressions during "difficult dialogues" involving multiculturalism within the classroom. From the quantitative literature on multiculturalism and training, we have learned counselor preparation in multicultural competence has been lacking and contributes to ethical issues (e.g., premature termination of clients, harming clients). However, Sue and colleagues' qualitative study provided an in-depth understanding of how students of color experienced microaggressions during difficult dialogues in classroom discussions of multicultural issues. The researchers identified three overarching domains influencing this phenomenon. First, from the perspectives of their participants, racial microaggressions precipitated the difficult dialogues themselves. Second, the participants experienced a broad range of reactions to the difficult dialogues—from overt denial of the experiences of racism by students of color and nonverbal cues by white students indicating their disinterest in the topic (e.g., rolling one's eyes, refraining from eye contact). Third, the authors found that there were certain instructor strategies that either hindered or facilitated the difficult dialogues as they unfolded in the classroom. The thick, rich descriptions of the 14 participants in the study (in two separate focus groups) provided information that even the best multicultural survey never could: the daily *lived experiences* of students of color.

In another example, Johnson (2006) investigated how teacher education methods used with reading specialists prepared them for interactions within an urban setting. She used interviews, written evaluations, participant observation, and her own experiences as the researcher to gain a deeper understanding of this phenomenon. Johnson's qualitative analysis identified several roles performed by the reading specialist (e.g., advocate, collaborator, consultant, and resource for teachers, administrators, and parents). She concluded: "Effective reading educators not only assess and instruct children who struggle with particular literacy problems, but they serve in a powerful capacity-building role, mentoring other school community members" (pp. 421–422). As a result of using an in-depth qualitative inquiry method, Johnson is able to highlight this particular advocacy role reading specialists may likely face in urban settings, in addition to being able to alert training programs to prepare reading specialists to engage in such an advocacy role.

The Role of Action in Qualitative Inquiry

Because advocacy has become such a critical role for counselors and educators in the new millennium of our multicultural society, the use of qualitative approaches has major implications for social change within counseling and educational settings. In this manner, qualitative researchers must recognize that their approaches of inquiry fall along a continuum of the degree to which the role of action is valued in research—whether or not researchers recognize it as such (which we certainly hope you do recognize). For instance, there are qualitative approaches that specifically have *action* as an integral component of their approach, such that the researcher collaborates with community partners to answer a question salient to the community (participatory action research [PAR] is described further in Chapter 2).

Because there is the action involved in the research of connecting with participants, qualitative data collections tend to be intimate and relational in nature. Rather than completing a Likert scale, participants reveal their innermost truths to us as they share their daily lived experiences of a phenomenon. In doing so, we must challenge ourselves not only to uphold the utmost integrity as researchers, but also to recognize (and not minimize) that we as researchers hold significant power in the lives of our participants as they share their experiences with us.

One of our favorite stories about data collection comes from our colleague and friend Dr. Sheneka Williams (see Chapter 6 for her author perspective). She tells the story of her first qualitative data collection, when she was collecting data on African American experiences of education in the South. The participants in this particular study did not have access to significant educational or financial resources and equity. At the time Sheneka was a doctoral student at Vanderbilt. More often than not her participants wanted to talk about how she, as an African American, had "made it" to Vanderbilt. She became a symbol—whether she wanted that status or not—of positive change to her participants, and she was a source of information and hope for them.

As Dr. Williams's story illustrates, even when we are not looking to "make change" or "take action" as qualitative researchers, we do so. Greenwood and Levin (2005) noted both the challenges and opportunities that social science researchers encounter when they decide to value a researcher role that acknowledges the central importance of action. Although the authors are specifically discussing participatory action research, they also discuss the fact that one of the central barriers to action research that is collaborative with communities is the "ivory tower" value system of university academia itself. The authors encourage the use of various ways in which researchers can intentionally transcend these barriers—in addition to discussing the ethical mandates of social science researchers to ensure their research's relevance to the daily lives of people and communities.

It is important to honor this ethical mandate in how we engage with the qualitative research process. We think it is important for current qualitative researchers in counseling and education to be aware of and identify how their qualitative designs constitute action research in themselves. What is the influence of the research process on participants? How will we interact with participants before, during, and after the research process? What will we "leave" with participants, and what do we inevitably "take away" from participants from our mere presence as researchers? Although there are no simple answers to these questions, we do believe that it is important to hold these questions in mind throughout every single step of the qualitative investigation.

A Researcher–Practitioner Model

Often when we engage in qualitative research, we face challenges in the form of what might seem like the competing roles of researcher and practitioner. Indeed, in her exploration of the advantages and challenges inherent in these two roles, Fryer titled her 2004 article "Researcher–Practitioner: An Unholy Marriage?" It is true that as individuals, we may feel more aligned, competent, comfortable, and/or prepared to take on one role more than the other. At the same time, however, how can one truly "backseat" one role over the other when we receive training in both roles in counseling as well as educational settings? So, although you may be naturally drawn to one role more than the other, we encourage you to engage both roles as you conduct qualitative research.

Finding a balance between the two roles of researcher and practitioner definitely is important. Elliott (2003) explored the "space" between researcher and practitioner and found ways to strike this balance. She discussed drawing from her "wisdom" gained as a practitioner and the "authority" she gained as a new academic to find this balance. Elliott resolved to not "remove" herself within her researcher role, instead seeking to understand the emotions of her participants while also using her wisdom as a practitioner to build trusting, ethical relationships with them. She described the value of being present with both herself and her participants as a helpful tool with which to maintain that balance between the "voice" of the practitioner, who is immersed in the settings, and the "voice" of the researcher, whose role may include seeking to understand, interrogate, challenge, support, and so on.

There are ethical issues, as well, with respect to managing this balance between the two roles (discussed further in Chapter 3). From a nursing perspective Arber (2006) discussed how she leveraged her role as a practitioner to underscore for her participants (the audience for her study) her familiarity with the medical care context in which her participants (nurses and patients) were situated. On one hand, her credibility as a researcher was enhanced because of her practitioner background. At the same time, she negotiated a significant ethical challenge of maintaining boundaries in terms of where the role of researcher and practitioner began and ended. In both counseling and educational settings, we are working with people. We hold some knowledge about what may be helpful or not helpful in terms of their needs, in addition to standards and competencies in the field. Much of our own qualitative research has been with survivors of trauma. As we seek to further understand the experiences of participants, we are naturally also tapping into both our innate and acquired skills as practitioners that could (and do) pull us out of that researcher role.

In addition to balancing the roles of practitioner and researcher during the research process, there is a further challenge as the fields of counseling and education move toward a focus on the researcher–practitioner (Hays, 2010). This scientist–practitioner model recognizes that research should inform practice, and vice versa, rather than both being disembodied from one another. Hays (2010) cites Stricker's (2002) four components of the scientist–practitioner role. First, as one engages as a researcher–practitioner, one does so with curiosity and explores evidence for "what works." Second, one is aware of salient research in the field and folds this research into practice. Third, one regularly evaluates individual clinical practice within the framework of research findings. Finally, the generation of research based on practice is a focus (often in collaboration with the individuals, groups, and communities we serve). Greenwood and Levin (2005) also noted that qualitative knowledge that is praxis-oriented and arises from collaborations between communities, individuals, and researchers holds immense potential for societal change because this knowledge is more easily transferable, accessible, and accountable to the needs of everyday people and communities.

Research as a Political Tool

The well-known feminist saying of the 1960s and 1970s—"the personal is political"—is an important one to keep in mind as a qualitative researcher. As we discussed in the previous section on action research, researchers have an impact and influence on the phenomena they investigate. So, knowing that, how do you leverage power as researchers to facilitate social change? In addition, we should be mindful, as the Advocacy Competencies of the American Counseling Association recommend, whether we as qualitative researchers are acting *with* or *on behalf of* participants (Lewis, Arnold, House, & Toporek, 2003). A first step is to seek understanding, from a community's point of view, of the role that qualitative research can serve as a political tool. In Table 1.4 we include an excerpt describing the basic principles of participatory action research from

---

TABLE 1.4. Some Basic Principles of Participatory Action Research

1. We are experts in our own experiences and have many different ways of knowing and getting information about our conditions.

2. We control the gathering and use of information about our communities. We decide what information we need to make the changes we want and how to get it. We decide what questions we need to answer and how. We lead and are integrally involved in all aspects of the design and implementation of the research, and of the analysis and distribution of the information gathered.

3. We gather information to inform our actions for change.

4. We reflect on the information we've gathered and the way in which we are gathering it throughout the process. We also reflect on the action we've taken and decide if we need more information before taking further action.

5. The people we gather information with and from are active and not passive participants in the process. We use information gathering to build community and movement, to develop leadership, and to empower ourselves to make change.

6. We are not trying to "prove" an assumption or hypothesis; we want to learn more about ourselves and our communities as a way to make change.

7. We agree on principles and values that will guide our information gathering, and we will stay accountable to them throughout the process.

Source: INCITE! Women of Color Against Violence. (2008). *Participatory action research*. Retrieved April 10, 2010, from *www.incite-national.org/index.php?s=129.*

the community perspective of INCITE! Women of Color Against Violence, a national activist organization.

We discuss participatory action research (PAR) in more depth in Chapter 2; however, we include Table 1.4 here to encourage you to begin considering the larger community context within which your qualitative research will take place. We find the particular language and manner in which INCITE wrote the basic principles of PAR to be extremely useful for beginning qualitative researchers. We believe that no matter which research tradition you select to use in your study, INCITE's list of principles articulates a level of accountability whereby qualitative researchers value the context within which participants live, in addition to recognizing that research is indeed a political tool for social change. As you read through each chapter in this book, we encourage you to explore ways to invite participants into collaborative roles within your study's design, as well as to specifically seek input from communities where you will conduct your research about what their needs truly are. Formulating your thoughts on qualitative research as a political tool is also an important way to begin to develop your research agenda.

 ACTIVITY 1.2. Exploring Your Role as a Qualitative Researcher

In a small group of two to three individuals, discuss the following:

- What are the opportunities to engage in action research within your field?
- Identify a few topics involving action research in which you might be interested.

- Do you feel more comfortable with the role of *researcher*, *practitioner*, or both?
- Select a topic. What would be the advantages and disadvantages of both roles in a qualitative inquiry of this topic?

BUILDING A RESEARCH AGENDA

The generation of research is both an inductive and deductive process. In the inductive mode, one may gather and explore data and generate theory based on this data. In the deductive mode, one may begin with an established theory and then seek to understand data through this lens. Qualitative research tends to be an inductive process. Building a research agenda, however, can be a deductive or inductive process (or both). Regardless, we encourage you to consider the larger context within which your qualitative study will be conducted. Qualitative work, at its heart, is quite an intimate act. Participants share the salience of their lived experiences with us as researchers. Therefore, we believe it is important to generate knowledge (i.e., publish) to honor the time and energy of participants as well as to align with the ethics standards of research within education and counseling settings.

Establishing a Research Agenda

A good place to begin building a research agenda is to think about why you have engaged in the research process in the first place. What phenomenon are you seeking to understand? How possible is it to study this phenomenon? What relevance does this phenomenon hold for you personally? What has the literature in your field established (or not established) about this phenomenon? Your research agenda can involve deductive, or inductive, or both approaches to generating knowledge. For example, you may begin with a theory of resilience and seek to apply that theory to students or clients in educational and counseling settings (deductive). Or you may begin to collect some data with these same students or clients and from this data generate hypotheses and theories (inductive). Furthermore, you can begin with an established theory of resilience to investigate how individuals of a particular subgroup fit with that theory, discover an alternative theory is to be developed, and test the emerging theory with those individuals (a combination of inductive and deductive processes).

A large component of establishing a research agenda is thinking ahead of where you are now as a researcher. For instance, where do you "see" your research going in 1 year, 5 years, more? And we are not just saying this for those of you who want to secure a faculty position or work in a different research institution. For those of you who are interested in careers in practice (and keeping the values of the researcher–practitioner in mind), it is also important to think ahead in terms of how you will build a research agenda that informs your practice. Within both research and practice settings, a research agenda should be flexible; it should make room for "surprise" turns in focus. If you stringently stay on one path of a research agenda, then your practice *and* your research may become stale. A strong research agenda allows for and welcomes creativity and new lines of inquiry. This creativity should not translate into a scattered focus, however. A simple test to determine if you have a solid focus in your research agenda is whether you can describe it in a few sentences.

Developing a Publication Record

Your research agenda should be evident in a publication record, a document that includes presentations and manuscripts on your topic. We discuss publishing your research in more detail in Chapter 12. For now, as you begin to engage in qualitative inquiry, consider the various public settings in which you might present the different stages of your research—from classroom presentations to professional conferences. Presenting your qualitative work early and often throughout the research process will provide opportunities for you to receive feedback and to strengthen your work. Throughout this book, we ask you to participate in journal activities, small-group discussions, and writing exercises. Use these opportunities to find qualitative authors whom you enjoy and respect. Then take a look at the publication records of these writers and examine their other work. Look at the themes, the phenomena of inquiry, the journals in which they publish, and how they generally have approached an inductive and/or deductive research agenda.

Reflecting on the Research Process

Once you start down the road of research, stop along the way to reflect on your research agenda. What has gone well in your research agenda? What might have gone better—or what might you want to shift? Who or what groups have most influenced your research agenda? Are there researchers in the field with whom you would like to clarify a component of your research agenda—or even with whom you might collaborate? What are the best next steps to take, considering what your findings have been so far? Taking time to consider the answers to these questions ultimately will strengthen your research agenda, and you will become a more effective researcher–practitioner.

In Perspectives 1.1, we each discuss how we have established a research agenda, developed a publication record, and reflected on the next steps of our research process.

• •

Perspectives 1.1. On Building a Research Agenda

"It's funny looking back at my earlier qualitative work now. I was so excited about qualitative inquiry and its potential for social change that I did not really stop to think about establishing a research agenda. I had been a community organizer for so long, and the practitioner role in my approach to investigating phenomena was more salient than the researcher role. I also was thinking I would be a practitioner, and had no idea I would eventually work as a faculty member. As a student, I found myself getting more and more involved in qualitative research due to my interest in historically marginalized groups. I also had training as a traumatologist. I knew from the moment I engaged with participants that I would commit to publish the findings they shared with me because I felt an ethical responsibility to do so. Once I understood the in's and out's of publishing, things like cover letters, revisions of manuscripts, and understanding how to find a good outlet for my work became like second nature to me. Reflecting on my research agenda, it is strange how there is a strong theme throughout all of my work. The "elevator speech" about my research agenda goes something like this: I investigate the resilience and coping patterns of historically marginalized communities, with a specific interest in people of color and LGBTQQ [lesbian, gay, bisexual, transgender, queer, questioning] people. I didn't much plan for this line of inquiry, although looking back, I wish I had thought more about the specific steps of building a research agenda. There are certainly areas of inquiry I might have pursued further or avoided altogether."

—AAS

"I second Anneliese's reflection that a research agenda was developed over time, and through a process of doing research, it became clearer. As a graduate student my interest in social justice issues in counselor preparation was most salient. Specifically, I conducted studies on how trainees and new professionals thought about their cultural privilege in relation to oppression. Back then, it didn't feel like "enough" to just ask about their conceptualization of social justice issues. However, I couldn't figure out how to make the research I was doing feel more comprehensive. Then my clinical experience in a psychiatric hospital and addictions agency really tuned me in to the processes involved in assessing and labeling clients with mental and substance abuse disorders, and how much the assessment and diagnostic process influenced client treatment and outcome. In my clinical work and training I was also exposed to trauma and its prevention and treatment, and I developed an interest in domestic violence. Over the years, with each new clinical, academic, and research experience, I reflected on my evolving research agenda that included these three interest areas: privilege and oppression, assessment and diagnosis, and domestic violence. Over time, my research agenda both expanded and integrated these areas and became more directly applicable to the clients and students with whom I work. Although it is still evolving, I see the work I do having some direct impact, confirming for me, even more, the value of qualitative research."

—DGH

• •

<hr />

REFLEXIVE ACTIVITY 1.1. Research Expectations

Reflect on the following and write one to two paragraphs in response to the following questions:

1. What are your expectations of research in general?

2. What are your expectations of qualitative research?

3. What is your stance on the quantitative–qualitative debate?

4. What are your personal and professional fears and challenges regarding conducting qualitative inquiry?

5. How do you see qualitative inquiry as a fit for your profession?

<hr />

THE TOP 10 POINTS ABOUT QUALITATIVE RESEARCH TO CONSIDER

We hope that this chapter has provided some important foundational information as you begin to think about your qualitative projects. In closing, we present our top 10 points of qualitative research that we hope you will keep in mind throughout your qualitative proposal or report.

1. **It's a journey, not a destination.** Qualitative inquiry is a process and not simply a product in the form of a report or presentation. It is interactive and reflexive based on the context. So, you cannot plan every detail of your study. Issues, problems, and revised research questions will occur as you conduct your study. Ambiguity comes with the territory.

2. **Begin with a strong foundation.** Although a qualitative study is reflexive and evolving, its rationale is often founded in theoretical and philosophical assumptions. You should articulate your perspective on the nature of reality ("truth") and knowledge acquisition. Think of the base of your research endeavor as the historical/philosophical assumptions, research paradigms, and personal and professional experiences that have led to your research design. (We discuss these in the next chapter.) In a cyclical fashion, research questions drive your research design, which influences your choice of methods. If you have a strong foundation of knowledge about why you are asking the questions you are asking, you will be more open to changes in your research.

3. **Keep it as simple as possible.** Select a single idea and a single research paradigm to begin. Go from the particular to the general. Data will pile up and become more difficult to manage the more people and things you include.

4. **Of course, the more people and things involved, the better.** The strength and rigor of qualitative research lies in the number of data sources and researchers. The only way we can achieve rigor as researchers is to immerse ourselves in our fieldwork. However, there is no magic number regarding how many people or things should be involved in the study. Be open to combining approaches and techniques.

5. Let go of your defenses! We are all biased researchers; we may just admit it more often in qualitative inquiry because, as researchers, we serve as instruments of data collection and analysis. You cannot change what you know and/or how you know phenomena. You cannot change who you are or your unique experiences. Strike a balance between knowing that you have biases and being open to the fact that others do too. Accept that most of a qualitative inquiry deals with multiple realities and perspectives. Because researchers offer unique perspectives to studies and engage in collective data analysis, our theories and/or findings are tentative and qualifiable. We as researchers have to be open to change and to criticism. Finally, you cannot claim to know everything about a phenomenon, nor can you necessarily apply your results to other populations. Generalizability is not the goal.

6. It's not just about words. Qualitative research is not "easier" than quantitative research. It's not about identifying keywords and themes. It's a complex effort of attempting to search for patterns in light of the frequency of data occurring. Comprehensive understanding of a particular group or context is the goal. Qualitative research should go beyond description to build theory or to apply findings directly to a discipline. Unfortunately, qualitative research never ends—you have to decide when to stop.

7. Quantity is not always important, and quantitative research is not the enemy. As discussed previously, one major critique of quantitative research is that statistical control (isolation and measurement of variables) and large samples may distort the meaning of process and outcome data and limit "voices" of participants. Thus, counting is not always helpful or necessary. Qualitative and quantitative research can be thought of as legs in a race. It's a team effort; team members and their role may look different, depending on the research question(s). Each adds something essential and unique and can build upon the other. They are complementary in that research designs may combine or use both areas of inquiry at various points of a study.

8. We are all studying and being studied. Researchers and participants influence each other. We are instruments of data collection. Our participants know more than us about a phenomenon, and we affect how much they tell us. "Analysis is the interplay between researchers and data" (Strauss & Corbin, 1998, p. 13). Furthermore, this mutual influence should not stop until data have been analyzed and changes have been implemented for those involved in the research. The research findings should lead to a change in awareness and/or to action on the part of the researcher(s) and/or participant(s).

9. Data collection and analysis occur somewhat simultaneously. Qualitative research is typically an inductive process. Recursiveness is an integral component of asking better questions. You should constantly compare and revise themes and codes as you gather data.

10. Acknowledge your role as a researcher–practitioner and consider the role of your research in social change as you build a research agenda. Balance the roles of practitioner and researcher in qualitative work. Because all research is political, remember the power that you hold in both roles and consistently seek to share that power with participants and to understand their needs. Consider how your qualitative study fits within a larger research agenda.

CHAPTER SUMMARY

This chapter has provided a rationale for qualitative research. As part of this rationale we presented several characteristics of qualitative research, including (1) inductive analysis; (2) naturalistic setting; (3) the importance of context; (4) the humanness of research; (5) purposive sampling; (6) thick description; and (7) an interactive, flexible research design. In essence, qualitative research attends to social interactions and context and honors collaboration and participant voices and perspectives.

Next, we attempted to demystify the so-called qualitative–quantitative debate by presenting arguments that the two approaches can and do work together to address a phenomenon in comprehensive and innovative ways.

Following the discussion of the "debate," we briefly discussed several key moments in the history of qualitative research. These span ethnographies from early colonizing efforts to case studies of urban regions, to attention to cultural diversity and voice, to greater attention to context and method sophistication, and to the interrelated nature of researcher, writing, and fieldwork. Specifically, these moments are early ethnography, colonial ethnography, traditional period, modernist phase, blurred genres, crisis of interpretation, a triple crisis, and postexperimental inquiry and beyond.

The last section of the chapter addressed the issue of bridging the gap between research and practice and the use of research as a tool. Research is a political act. Our recommendation is to consider how to honor your participants and the contexts in which they live in order to identify the political aims of your research and to engage in social change. Always remember that in the highest quality of any research, it seeks to inform practice, and vice versa. Strive to become a strong researcher–practitioner and build a research agenda that reflects on the knowledge you generate, build upon, and seek to illuminate in the future.

RECOMMENDED READINGS

Agar, M. (2006). An ethnography by any other name ... *Forum: Qualitative Social Research, 7*(4), Art. 36. Retrieved February 2, 2011, from *www.qualitative-research.net/index/php/fas/article/view/177/396.*

Arber, A. (2006). Reflexivitiy: A challenge for the researcher as practitioner? *Journal of Research in Nursing, 11*(2), 147–157.

Choudhuri, D. D. (2003). Qualitative research and multicultural counseling competency: An argument for inclusion. In D. B. Pope-Davis, H. L. K. Coleman, W. M. Liu, & R. L. Toporek (Eds.), *Handbook of multicultural competencies in counseling and psychology* (pp. 267–281). Thousand Oaks, CA: Sage.

Elliott, E. (2003). Moving in the space between researcher and practitioner. *Child and Youth Care Forum, 32*(5), 299–303.

Fryer, E. M. (2004). Researcher–practitioner: An unholy marriage? *Educational Studies, 30*(2), 175–185.

Vidich, A. J., & Lyman, S. M. (2001). Qualitative methods: Their history in sociology and anthropology. In N. K. Denzin & Y. S. Lincoln (Eds.), *The landscape of qualitative research* (2nd ed., pp. 55–129). Thousand Oaks, CA: Sage.

CHAPTER 2

Qualitative Research Paradigms and Traditions

CHAPTER PREVIEW

One of the essential features of qualitative inquiry is its focus on the connection between researcher and theoretical framework, or research orientation. This theoretical framework is formed by the researcher's careful and continual exploration of research paradigms and traditions. As you consider a research problem to be investigated, it is important to reflect upon how you define scientific pursuit and which research paradigm(s) and tradition(s) are best suited for your study. A solid research orientation involves understanding and utilizing various research paradigms and traditions to construct your research design. This chapter examines qualitative research paradigms and traditions and describes the roles they play in decisions about research design. Figure 2.1 depicts these "foundational" aspects of qualitative research design.

A CAUTIONARY NOTE

Qualitative inquiry is an evolving practice in counseling and education; thus, there are several ideas in the literature of what constitutes a *research paradigm* and a *research tradition*. Before presenting our construction of what these look like in qualitative inquiry, we would like to highlight some potential challenges that may influence you as you integrate qualitative research into your practice. First, the terms *research paradigm* and *research tradition* are often used interchangeably in the literature. To complicate matters, these terms are also labeled as *theoretical frameworks* or *research methods*. Inattention to the concepts of research paradigm and research tradition independently may be problematic because discussion of a researcher's orientation may be minimized, leaving the reader with little to no information about his or her assumptions, values, and orientations. Thus, research paradigms and traditions may not be adequately described in published studies.

Another challenge with classifying research paradigms and traditions relates to the process of labeling, which is counter to many of the characteristics of qualitative

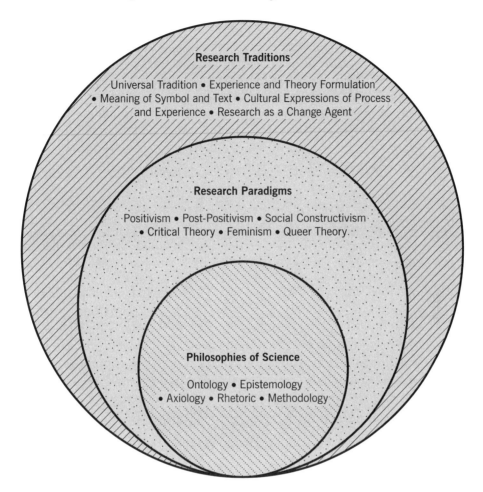

FIGURE 2.1. The foundations of qualitative inquiry.

research. As described in Chapter 1, qualitative inquiry is a holistic approach that often values subjective meaning of a research problem and context as well as collaboration between researcher and participant in constructing and understanding knowledge. Placing an "objective" label on this process is difficult because qualitative researchers have varying ways of conceptualizing their values, assumptions, and orientations for qualitative inquiry, in general, and for a research problem, more specifically.

Because of the complexities with labeling in qualitative inquiry, a related challenge is that several research paradigms and traditions overlap one another. Thus, many share perspectives related to how a research problem should be investigated. Furthermore, research traditions borrow terms from each other in data analysis or, in many cases, label very similar data collection and analytic procedures with different terminology. Because of this overlap, research traditions are not necessarily fixed entities and can change depending on the nature of a study. This adaptation may be helpful because it allows the qualitative researcher some flexibility in situating a research problem or question.

The process of conducting qualitative research within each of the traditions is a final challenge because there is not a unified method among qualitative researchers within a particular research tradition. For instance, there are several divergent ideas about what phenomenological research is as well as competing views of how and when "theory" enters grounded theory research. In sum, we are cognizant of these challenges as we present our construction of the categories of research paradigms and traditions. Before discussing these categories, it is important to reflect on what constitutes science and the pursuit of knowledge and truth in counseling and education (see Activity 2.2 on page 42).

PHILOSOPHIES OF SCIENCE

As noted in Chapter 1, qualitative inquiry has some flexibility in the way data are collected and analyzed, particularly how the researcher and participant view a research question. This flexibility allows for variations in how science is unfolded by the researcher in conducting qualitative research. Science is defined as the systematic search, observation, analysis, and presentation of knowledge (Galuzzo, Hilldrup, Hays, & Erford, 2008). In qualitative research, the pursuit of science involves integrating the assumptions and practices of research paradigms and traditions as the researcher constructs a research design. Scientific pursuit should have some flexibility, as is needed, in qualitative research design. There are several core **philosophies of science** that are embedded within research paradigms and traditions that help construct scientific inquiry in qualitative research. These include ontology, epistemology, axiology, rhetoric, and methodology. Essentially, these core philosophies overlap and build upon each other to describe the relationship between the knower and the known in qualitative inquiry (Creswell, 2006). Before reading these descriptions, complete Reflexive Activity 2.1.

Ontology refers to the nature of reality; in qualitative research the term points to the degree to which a "universal truth" is sought about a particular construct or process in qualitative research. Is reality objective or subjective? Is it universal (*etic*) or contextual (*emic*)? Are there factors that influence the reality of a phenomenon? Reality can be thought of along a continuum, with objective truth (*Truth*) at one end and subjective or multiple truths at the other end (*truth*). Qualitative inquiry in counseling and education generally involves examination of how "real" a phenomenon is through the subjective lenses of both researchers and participants (Guba & Lincoln, 2005; Ponterotto, 2005). Your ontological perspective is characterized by the degree to which you believe that reality is limited or predetermined.

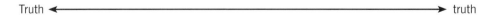

Truth ⟵——————————————————————————⟶ truth

For example, let's consider the construct of family discord. Researchers who fall toward the left side of the continuum (*Truth*) would argue that there is a universal definition or reality of what family discord looks like for families. With enough investigation, information about family discord may be known and thus applied universally to work with families. Alternatively, researchers who fall toward the right side of the continuum (*truth*) would assert that a complete, universal understanding of family discord is im-

---

REFLEXIVE ACTIVITY 2.1. Philosophies of Science

Review the following statements and mark an "**X**" next to those you endorse.

____ There is only one reality or truth for any phenomenon.

____ Multiple truths exist for a phenomenon; however, some truths are more salient than others.

____ Truth does not exist as there are multiple, equally valid, truths.

____ There is a limit to what we can know about a construct.

____ Knowledge acquisition is limitless.

____ Knowledge changes as social interactions change.

____ A researcher should not integrate personal and professional values in a research design.

____ Participant values should be considered in research design.

____ Researcher subjectivity can be an important asset to qualitative research.

____ It is inappropriate to use the first-person voice in a research report.

____ It is inappropriate to use the second-person voice in a research report.

____ Presenting data as numbers is more valuable than presenting participant stories or narratives.

____ Research designs should be selected based on research paradigms and traditions.

____ Methodology drives research questions.

____ Research questions drive methodology.

---

possible, since the construct must be understood in relation to a particular context. That is, multiple notions or beliefs about what constitutes family discord are equally valid and valued.

Epistemology refers to the study of the process of knowing; in qualitative research it refers to the degree to which knowledge is believed to be constructed by the research process, in general, and in the context of the researcher–participant relationship, more specifically. That is, epistemology is the knowledge acquisition process for the phenomenon of interest; it is "how we know what we know" (Guba & Lincoln, 2008; Hansen, 2004; Ponterotto, 2005). Is knowledge limited? A majority of qualitative researchers view knowledge as being essentially unlimited and actively constructed within the context of the research relationship. An epistemological perspective in qualitative inquiry typically involves the notion that knowledge about a research topic is limited only by the quality of the interactions of those involved in the research process.

Limited knowledge 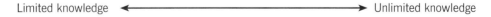 Unlimited knowledge

Let's examine this philosophy of science for the construct of family discord. Researchers with the epistemological stance that knowledge is limited would argue that the research relationship content is likely irrelevant to knowledge acquisition. That is, how we know what we know about family discord comes from a more generic, finite research process. For those who believe that knowledge is unlimited, knowledge about family discord can be continually expanded with changes in research design as well as in research relationships and dynamics.

Axiology encompasses the researcher's values and assumptions in qualitative inquiry and how they influence research questions and research design. Additionally, it includes considering the values of participants and the research setting (Ponterotto, 2005). What is the role of values in qualitative inquiry? Do you think values should be considered in research design? How are our scientific pursuits guided by what we as researchers value as knowledge and reality? Qualitative researchers are encouraged to reflect on what role, if any, their values play in the research process (see Reflexive Activity 2.2.).

Objectivity ◄─────────────────────────────────► Reflexivity

For the family discord example, "objective" researchers would attempt to minimize the influences of values in research and thus try to maintain the research relationship as neutral, uninfluenced by the researchers' assumptions or experiences. Researchers

---

REFLEXIVE ACTIVITY 2.2. Values in Research

Identify values you hold about your profession. List these in the left column. Next, review each of these values and brainstorm ways in which they may influence how you conduct qualitative research. List these in the right column.

Professional values	Influences in qualitative inquiry

would likely not disclose their perspectives related to family discord so as not to "bias" participants. An axiological stance that valued researchers as an instrument in the design would emphasize the importance of relating their experience and assumptions about family discord to the research–participant relationship. The research relationship would likely be a collaborative process of investigating family discord.

Rhetoric encompasses the various formats in which qualitative data are presented. As described in later chapters, data can be presented in various formats depending on the selected research paradigm, tradition, and general study design. How you present data involves decisions about the use of voice (i.e., first, second, third) of the researcher(s) and participants, terminology with which to present data collection and analytic methods, and the degree to which narratives, thematic categories, and/or numbers are presented as findings (Creswell, 2006; Ponterotto, 2005). Should data be presented in narratives or numbers, or both? Generally, the more narratives allowed in qualitative inquiry, the more "voice" participants have in a report. However, the greater degree a researcher takes the "expert stance" in report writing, the less participant voice may be present, no matter the use of voice.

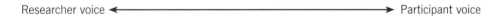

Researcher voice ←———————————————————→ Participant voice

This philosophy of science relates heavily to the role of voice and is discussed in more detail in later chapters. Researchers who value a prominent researcher voice in data presentation would likely present more aggregated data related to family discord; this might involve statistics and/or minimal narratives and discussion of the findings using the third person (e.g., "The researcher found … ") with greater attention to researcher interpretation of the findings. Those who value participant voice in data presentation would likely provide participant quotes and narratives and attempt to represent data from participants' perspectives. When they provide interpretations, researchers use first and second voice (e.g., "We interviewed 21 participants … ").

Methodology as a philosophy of science involves the actual practice of qualitative inquiry. It is heavily influenced by other core philosophies of science. Our ideas about what constitutes truth and knowledge in the context of the values of those involved in the research process shape how we design a qualitative study. Thus, methodology encompasses decisions about aspects such as selection of research paradigms and traditions, research questions, and data collection methods (Creswell, 2006). Should data designs be qualitative, quantitative, or a combination of these (i.e., mixed methods; see Chapter 4)? Thus, a study of family discord could involve qualitative or quantitative data, or both.

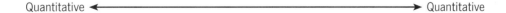

Quantitative ←———————————————————→ Quantitative

In sum, scientific pursuit involves an active and continual reflection on how the researcher envisions the intersection of perspective (ontology), knowledge construction (epistemology), values (axiology), and dissemination of findings (rhetoric). These overlap and influence research design decisions (methodology). Figure 2.2 illustrates these considerations using a research problem as a guide. In addition, complete Activity 2.1 on the next page to practice describing and distinguishing these components of science.

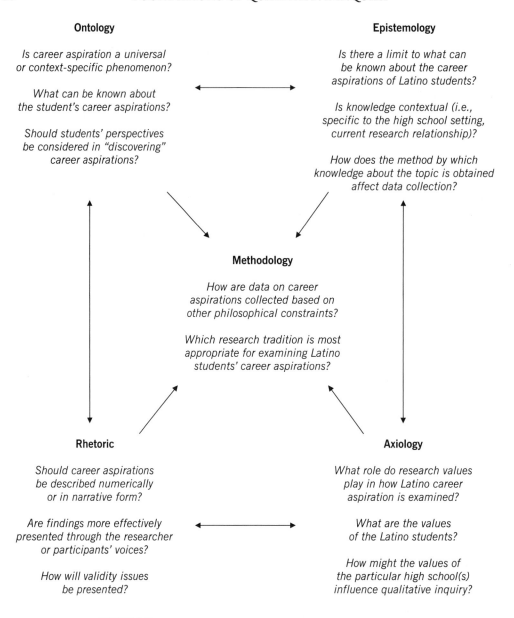

Ontology

*Is career aspiration a universal
or context-specific phenomenon?*

*What can be known about
the student's career aspirations?*

*Should students' perspectives
be considered in "discovering"
career aspirations?*

Epistemology

*Is there a limit to what can
be known about the career
aspirations of Latino students?*

*Is knowledge contextual (i.e.,
specific to the high school setting,
current research relationship)?*

*How does the method by which
knowledge about the topic is obtained
affect data collection?*

Methodology

*How are data on career
aspirations collected based on
other philosophical constraints?*

*Which research tradition is most
appropriate for examining Latino
students' career aspirations?*

Rhetoric

*Should career aspirations
be described numerically
or in narrative form?*

*Are findings more effectively
presented through the researcher
or participants' voices?*

*How will validity issues
be presented?*

Axiology

*What role do research values
play in how Latino career
aspiration is examined?*

*What are the values
of the Latino students?*

*How might the values of
the particular high school(s)
influence qualitative inquiry?*

FIGURE 2.2. Career aspirations of Latino high school students.

 ACTIVITY 2.1. Describing Philosophies of Science

Select a salient research problem in counseling or education. Using the five core
philosophies of science, brainstorm various questions you could explore.

RESEARCH PARADIGMS

Research paradigms can be thought of as belief systems based on the core philosophies of science (Guba & Lincoln, 2005; Ponterotto, 2005). The ways by which you come to conceptualize the five core philosophies of science for various research questions influence and are influenced by various paradigms that include positivism, post-positivism, social constructivism, critical theory, feminism, and queer theory. You may adhere differentially to these belief systems, given their various ideas about what the research process and scientific pursuit look like. Table 2.1 illustrates the relationships among various research paradigms and ideas about scientific pursuit.

Positivism refers to the assumption that researchers can arrive at an objective, universal truth through direct observation and experience of phenomena. Thus, only verifiable claims should be considered genuine knowledge. Positivists are primarily concerned with empirically verifying existing theory through hypothesis testing, with goals of operationally measuring constructs, replicating methods across disciplines, and generalizing knowledge to a population (Patton, 2002). In order to achieve these goals, positivist researchers seek to maintain objectivity in research design by establishing a clear boundary with research participants, avoiding a discussion of values of those involved in the research, and using well-known statistical procedures to control contextual variables that impact a study (Galuzzo et al., 2008). Positivism has dominated and characterized scientific pursuit for several centuries, particularly in quantitative studies.

To illustrate positivism, consider the following research question: Is behavioral therapy effective in the treatment of phobias? To address this question, a researcher would develop hypotheses and establish a research design using treatment and control groups, with randomized sampling procedures, and operationally define and objectively measure phobic responses using a standardized treatment manual for behavioral therapy. Through a controlled design, the researcher might demonstrate that a group of participants that received behavioral interventions (i.e., treatment) had less phobic responses than participants in a control group, who may not have received any counseling intervention.

The belief that theory should be tested to be verified *and* falsified led to the development of **post-positivism**. In this approach theories should be falsified in order to strengthen them (Patton, 2002). Although post-positivists hold similar beliefs about science as positivists, they assert that universal reality can never fully be realized because you cannot say with complete certainty that a theory fully describes a phenomenon or construct. Although post-positivists argue that reality or universal truths exist, they state that you cannot fully measure or understand them. With this paradigm, issues of validity, reliability, and alternative hypotheses are heavily emphasized. Consider again the example of the treatment of phobias. Theories surround both behavioral therapy and phobias, yet the post-positivist would seek to find other therapies that could be effective in the treatment of phobias while exploring potential sources of error in measuring effectiveness across all therapies. If a researcher is able to show that behavioral therapy is most effective for the treatment of phobias, the theory is strengthened.

As scientific inquiry increased in counseling and education, many viewed the approaches of earlier paradigms incongruent with characteristics of qualitative research. They argued that, although these paradigms are effective in understanding general

TABLE 2.1. Research Paradigms and Philosophies of Science

Paradigms and accompanying philosophies of science	Foci in qualitative inquiry
Positivism, post-positivism	
Ontology: There is a universal truth that can be known (positivism) or approximated (post-positivism), and the researchers' findings correspond to that truth in varying degrees. *Epistemology*: Knowledge is obtained through measurable experience with participants and may be applied across a population. These experiences can be directly observed (positivism) or both directly and indirectly measured (post-positivism). *Axiology*: Research relationships have minimal influence on the results, and researchers should remain emotionally neutral. Research may be value-free. *Rhetoric*: "Neutral" report writing and third-person voice are used. *Methodology*: Structured methods and designs help control and manipulate conditions. Research is considered scientific if internal validity, external validity, reliability, and objectivity are addressed.	• What's *really* going on in the real world? • How do the researcher's findings correspond to a truth shared within the scientific community? • What can be known about a particular theory? • To what degree can we measure accurately a phenomenon? • What other hypotheses might explain the research problem?
Social constructivism	
Ontology: Multiple realities of a phenomenon exist. *Epistemology*: Knowledge is co-constructed between researcher and participants. *Axiology*: There is an emphasis on the values of the researcher, participants, and research setting. *Rhetoric*: Data largely reflect the participants' voices and thoroughly describe the roles of the researcher and research setting in understanding the research problem. *Methodology*: Decisions about what and how research problems are studied are largely determined collaboratively between researcher and participants. Research is considered scientific if it is contextually relevant and trustworthiness has been established.	• How do participants conceptualize the research problem? • What contextual factors influence how participants and researchers construct, study, and report research findings?
Critical theory, feminism, and queer theory	
Ontology: Reality is subjective and may be influenced by oppressive experiences. *Epistemology*: Knowledge is co-constructed between the researcher and participants. *Axiology*: The researcher's values are instrumental in acknowledging social injustice and promoting change. *Rhetoric*: Participants' voices are central to reporting findings. *Methodology*: The research design seeks to minimize exploitive processes in qualitative inquiry by using appropriate data collection methods and considering how results may affect the social experiences of participants.	• In what ways has the role of gender been ignored in qualitative inquiry? • What influences do forms of oppression (e.g., racism, classism, sexism, heterosexism) have on understanding the research problem? • How might qualitative inquiry create social and political change within and outside the research process?

Sources: Patton (2002) and Ponterotto (2005).

counseling and educational processes, there were several unanswered questions about these processes. For instance, there was growing concern that findings were not applicable to all and that they minimized and marginalized various groups. As such, several paradigms were introduced to attend to the context in which participants live and experience phenomena and to incorporate participants' and researchers' subjective voices (Guba & Lincoln, 2005). After you review the following paradigms, complete Activity 2.3.

Social constructivism is a belief system that assumes that "universal truth" cannot exist because there are multiple contextual perspectives and subjective voices that can label truth in scientific pursuit. This paradigm also has been referred to as **postmodernism**. Social constructivists argue that reality about counseling and education phenomena should never be labeled as objective since the voices of researchers and participants are biased and seated in different cultural experiences and identities. These researchers seek to construct knowledge through social interactions as well as to understand how individuals construct knowledge. Cultural, historical, and political events and processes influence these interactions. A collaborative dialogue among researcher and participants about defining and understanding the research problem as well as collecting and interpreting findings is highly valued (Patton, 2002; Ponterotto, 2005). Thus, those who identify primarily as social constructivists enter a research setting with **foreshadowed problems** rather than main and alternative hypotheses (McMillan & Schumacher, 2006). With social constructivism, the notion of *trustworthiness* (discussed in Chapter 7) replaces the concepts of *reliability* and *validity* for establishing scientific rigor.

With the phobia example, social constructivists would conceptualize phobia as a relative construct that can be understood only within the social context of the participants who may be experiencing it. Essentially, there is no universal definition of phobia. Furthermore, social constructivists would assert that various therapies to treat phobias are contextual and thus their "effectiveness" largely depends on the environment and situation in which they are implemented, the attitudes of the counselor–researcher and participants related to a particular therapy and to phobias in general, and the interaction between the two.

Critical theory, **feminism**, and **queer theory** are extensions of social constructivism. With these paradigms, researchers not only seek to understand a phenomenon through various subjective lenses, but they also strive to create social and political changes to improve the lives of participants. Thus, they closely examine how social norms are manifested in both positive and negative ways in participants' lives. Followers of these paradigms view researcher objectivity as impossible and subjectivity as something that should be readily acknowledged and valued. The researcher is seen as often changed by the research process (Patton, 2002).

Critical theory can be considered the most influential of the three paradigms, with the largest focus. Specifically, critical theorists assume that participants' experiences, and thus constructions of various phenomena, may be influenced by social injustices. In addition, the research process in general may exploit participants because their voices are often minimized and objectified. Critical theorists strive to make qualitative inquiry a political endeavor that facilitates social action to benefit those without power. Thus, advocacy against various oppressive experiences is a key concept.

In addition to valuing political action, **feminism** as a paradigm places emphasis on the roles of affect and researcher–participant relationship in the research process. Gender is an organizing principle in understanding and reporting research findings. For example, feminists argue that women have largely been excluded from scientific pursuit. When women are included in research, they are often pathologized in some manner. Feminists seek to address and dismantle methods by which "patriarchy" may play into qualitative inquiry. Feminism as a paradigm is expanding to address other forms of oppression beyond sexism. **Queer theory**, a recent paradigm, attends to how sexual orientation as a participant characteristic influences experiences of various phenomena. Furthermore, attention is given to how oppression (i.e., heterosexism), experienced by virtue of being a member of a sexual minority, impacts participants' experiences (Patton, 2002).

Let us consider the phobia research example in relation to these three paradigms. Building upon the ideas that social constructivists might have about the social construction of phobia and clinical treatment, qualitative inquiry within one of these paradigms may seek to (1) understand the degree to which cultural variables (e.g., race/ethnicity, gender, sexual orientation) and related oppression from being a member of a minority status impact the understanding and presentation of phobias; (2) explore how various treatment approaches may be biased for certain groups; and (3) gather information about changes that need to be made in counseling practice to better serve participants.

 ACTIVITY 2.2. Challenges with Research Traditions

Several research traditions are presented throughout this chapter in five major clusters. Review these traditions and discuss them in dyads in relation to the challenges presented earlier in this chapter.

 ACTIVITY 2.3. Researcher Paradigms Debate

Some opponents of social constructivism, feminism, critical theory, and queer theory may argue that since findings are not generalizable to a larger population, they are not significant contributions to the larger scientific community. Divide into two groups and debate both sides of this argument.

PROPOSAL DEVELOPMENT 2.1. Examining Research Paradigms

As you think about developing your research proposal, it is important to consider possible benefits and challenges for each of the research traditions. To what degree do each of the following research traditions "fit" for you as you think of possible professional and research interests? Write down some of your thoughts below.

Tradition	Benefits	Challenges
Positivism		

Tradition	Benefits	Challenges
Post-positivism		
Social constructivism		
Critical theory		
Feminism		
Queer theory		

ACTIVITY 2.4. Interviewing Exercise

Interview a qualitative researcher in your profession about his or her research orientation. How did he or she arrive at this research orientation? What benefits and challenges does he or she perceive as related to the selected research orientation?

RESEARCH TRADITIONS

Building upon decisions of how you conceptualize science and select a research paradigm, choosing a research tradition creates a solid foundation for your research design. In this section, we outline several research traditions that are present in counseling and education qualitative research. These traditions are presented in five primary clusters that share underlying themes in qualitative inquiry:

- The universal tradition
- Experience and theory formulation
- The meaning of symbol and text
- Cultural expressions of process and experience
- Research as a change agent

As noted earlier, these clusters may overlap and be combined depending on the purpose of the qualitative inquiry. Below we provide a brief description of various research traditions. Data collection and analysis procedures are elaborated upon in later chapters. Table 2.2 provides an overview of the clusters' characteristics, and Table 2.3 outlines how a research topic pertaining to dual-career families can be examined based on the selected research tradition.

THE UNIVERSAL TRADITION: CASE STUDY

A **case** is a specific, unique, bounded system, and the **case study** allows the researcher to study individual(s), events, activities, or processes/elements of a bounded system (Creswell, 2003, 2006). For a case to be studied using a case study tradition, it must be *bounded* (i.e., have distinct boundaries), be functioning or have working parts, and indicate patterned behaviors such as sequence or coherence (Stake, 2005). That is, case studies are distinguished from other qualitative traditions because cases are researched in depth and the data are delineated by time period, activity, and place (Plummer, 2001). The organizing principle of a case study is the case itself, and the tradition is both a process and product of inquiry (Stake, 2005).

The emphasis in the case study is on examining a phenomenon as it exists in its natural context in order to identify the boundaries between the two (i.e., between the context and the phenomenon; Yin, 2003). Case studies may be the optimal research tradition to utilize when (1) counselors and educators are seeking to answer "how" and "why" questions, (2) control over events is limited, and (3) a phenomenon can be

TABLE 2.2. Research Tradition Clusters

	General characteristics	Unique characteristics
Cluster 1: The universal tradition		
Case study	• Boundary • Individual(s) • Event(s) • Processes(s) • Can be applied to most of the research traditions below	
Cluster 2: Experience and theory formulation		
Grounded theory	• Discovery • Direct experience • Phenomenon • Subjectivity	• Theory behind experience • Theory generation, primarily inductive, theoretical sampling, constant comparison • Divergent views on how external factors (e.g., researcher bias, previous literature or theory) affect inductive nature
Phenomenology		• Emphasis on universal and divergent aspects of an experience itself • Participants' direct, immediate experience within their worlds • Researcher takes "fresh" perspective and refrains from subjective interpretation (i.e., epoche)
Heuristic inquiry		• Interaction between experience and person • Topic has personal significance for researcher; results primarily increase researcher's self-knowledge with some implications for general field
Consensual qualitative research		• Experience and participants' perspectives useful in generating theory • Emphasis on research rigor and shared power among researchers, participants • Researchers' reflections may be present in initial data collection stages
Cluster 3: The meaning of symbol and text		
Symbolic interaction	• Language • Symbols • Story • Identity • Context	• Active response to symbols (language, cultural artifacts) to facilitate personal and shared meanings
Semiotics		• Search and interpretation of existing codes, signs, and symbols
Life history		• Personal meanings and context • Researcher's story becomes part of the interpretation • Researcher extracts meaning from historical review and applies to current context • May involve "rewriting history"
Hermeneutics		• "Sacred" text (scripture, mythology, history, politics, art) • Interpretation of both current and historical context
Narratology		• Structure of and communication methods in narrative emphasized

(cont.)

TABLE 2.2. *(cont.)*

	General characteristics	Unique characteristics
Cluster 4: Cultural expressions of process and experience		
Ethnography	• Culture • Prolonged engagement • Participant observation • Fieldwork	• Global description of culture or cultural group
Ethnomethodology		• Description of social patterns and rules, "everydayness"
Autoethnography		• First-person account of cultural event or process
Cluster 5: Research as a change agent		
Participatory action research	• Change of conditions, context, researcher, participants • Power analysis • Action research	

studied in its natural context (Denzin, 1989). Plummer (2001) described case studies as establishing "collective memories and imagined communities; and they tell of the concerns of their time and place" (p. 395).

Case studies have long been used in the social sciences as a way to carefully document life stories and events. Case studies have emerged from the tradition of biographical writing within the fields of psychology, sociology, anthropology, political science, and history (Gilgun, 1994). This tradition is particularly useful in counseling and education because practitioners are interested both in unique dimensions of a case (often a client or student) as well as their more generalized applicability to other individuals.

Case selection is an important a priori activity for this tradition. Researchers select cases that offer the greatest opportunity to learn and thus most often the case or cases to which they have greatest accessibility (Stake, 2005). Furthermore, researchers decide whether they will study one or multiple case studies. **Single case studies** involve the examination of one phenomenon that is a single experiment and should meet the criteria for testing a theory with one case: "The single case can be used to determine whether a theory's propositions are correct or whether some alternative set of explanations might be more relevant" (p. 40). For instance, a single case study might be warranted when a case represents a unique case, such as using feminist counseling techniques with an immigrant woman; whereas in **multiple case studies** (i.e., collective case studies), the researcher investigates several phenomena that are similar in nature, such as examining curricula in several counseling graduate programs in response to accreditation changes.

Alternatively, Stake (2005) categorized case studies in three ways: (1) **intrinsic case study**, wherein the researcher has an internally guided, or intrinsic, interest in a particular case; (2) **instrumental case study**, wherein the researcher seeks out cases to assist in an understanding of a particular issue exterior to a specific case; and (3) **collective case study**, wherein multiple cases are used to investigate a more general or broad phenomenon or population. Consider a case study of childrearing practices in stepfamilies where the case is the stepfamily. Depending on the researcher's purpose, the focus of the case study could be on a particularly successful parenting practice of a particular family (intrinsic case study), how conflict in childrearing is addressed in stepfamilies (instrumental case study), or common conflicts occurring in childrearing for several stepfamilies (collective case study). Thus, the degree of applicability often shapes the type of case study.

Stake (2005) noted that the following components are often included in a case study report: the nature of the case; the case's historical background; the physical setting of the case; economic, political, legal, aesthetic, and other contexts; other cases to which this case is attached; and those informants through whom the case be known. Furthermore, researchers have several stylistic options for presenting a case or cases:

- How much to make the report a story;
- How much to compare with other cases;
- How much to formalize generalizations or leave that to readers; and
- Whether or not and how much to disguise case elements (Stake, 2005).

The case study tradition can be considered a universal tradition because it can be applied to several of the traditions described in the remainder of this chapter. The fact that most traditions discussed in this chapter deal with cases is evidence of the natural blending of research traditions. In the beginning of this chapter, we cautioned that traditions overlap one another at times in both purpose and activity. Case study as a tradition offers a distinctive benefit of case description, and thus many qualitative studies are case studies. If the purpose and intention of your research entail more than case description and comparison, however, we suggest that you use other traditions to guide your design.

One such tradition to which the case study tradition can be applied is the life history approach. The similarity between these two approaches is that the case study is often intended to document and interpret a life history. The **autobiographical case study** is one written by researchers about themselves (Reed-Danahay, 2001) and is rarely conducted at the graduate level (Creswell, 2003). The autobiography may involve personal writings and interviews as data sources. In the **biographical case study**, the researcher documents the history of an individual by using primarily archival data and other information sources about the person (Plummer, 2001). In conducting a **life history** the researcher follows the life of an individual, including the cultural norms that shape the person, and uses interviews with him or her as data collection (Denzin, 1989). An **oral history** is a way for the researcher to document events, including cultural themes emerging from individual interviews.

Although case studies may seem simple to conduct, they are in reality one of the most challenging research traditions to undertake (Stake, 1995). Much of the challenge emerges because there is an absence of structured guidelines for the case study inquiry. Yin (2003) identifies several considerations involved in data collection with the case study: (1) researcher skills with the case study format (e.g., attention to bias, listening, flexibility); (2) current training with the case study at hand; (3) protocol that guides the research process; (4) screening of potential case study ideas; and (5) pilot study of the phenomenon. In this preparation for data collection, researchers selecting the case study design should also consider how to identify the researcher perspective and resulting influence on the case study research design and process (Creswell, 2003). This identification allows readers to make decisions about the trustworthiness or quality of the case study results. Complete Activity 2.5 to consider how you might apply the case study tradition.

An example of a single case study involved an African American parent's perceptions of the process and influence of filial therapy, an extension of play therapy in which parents conduct child-centered play sessions (Solis, Meyers, & Varjas, 2004). For this case study, Solis conducted ten 90-minute filial therapy training sessions that included 30-minute play sessions for 7 of the 10 training sessions. Through analysis of interviews, parent questionnaires, and parent journal entries, several themes relating to the structure, content, and congruence of the approach with cultural values and influences on the parent, child, and parent–child relationship were noted. This exploratory research deepened current knowledge of the role of culture in play therapy efficacy.

Koliba, Campbell, and Shapiro (2006) conducted a multiple case study in New England schools in order to gain a comprehensive idea of how service learning was perceived in school and community contexts for three schools. During this case study inquiry, a skilled researcher spent 14 days conducting semistructured interviews with 280 people (e.g., teachers, parents, students, school board members) about the culture of the schools, the relationship between the school and community, and their perceptions of the implementation of service learning at the schools.

 ACTIVITY 2.5. Applying the Universal Tradition

Select a topic of interest in your profession. Consider how the case study tradition might influence how you would study the research topic. How might the topic be addressed by each of the case study types described by Denzin (1989) and Stake (2005)?

EXPERIENCE AND THEORY FORMULATION: GROUNDED THEORY, PHENOMENOLOGY, HEURISTIC INQUIRY, AND CONSENSUAL QUALITATIVE RESEARCH

The second cluster is one of the more popular collections of research traditions. This cluster includes grounded theory, phenomenology, heuristic inquiry, and consensual qualitative research. After reading about these four traditions, complete Activity 2.6.

Grounded Theory

Grounded theory has been described as the most influential research tradition in social science disciplines today (Patton, 2002). The purpose of a grounded theory approach is to generate theory that is *grounded* in data regarding participants' perspectives for a particular phenomenon (Fassinger, 2005). It involves discovering new ways of examining the world, remaining close to the data, and allowing data to guide theory development (McLeod, 2001). The theories that are generated often explain a process or action surrounding an experience or a sequence of events pertaining to a particular topic.

One of the hallmark early characteristics of grounded theory (Glaser, 1978; Glaser & Strauss, 1967) is its **inductive approach**. That is, qualitative researchers approach a phenomenon by setting aside preconceived notions to formulate (but not test) a theory about that phenomenon, moving from simpler to more complex constructions or descriptions. In general, qualitative researchers select methods that allow for rich data collection useful for generating local or grand theories. Throughout data collection, researchers move back and forth to uncover a core category, or **constant comparison**, that will serve as the basis for theory development. Participants are selected based on their congruence with theoretical constructs, a process known as **theoretical sampling**. To allow data to drive new theory, data are often collected without reviewing prior literature extensively. However, qualitative researchers return to the literature as theory is generated. Charmaz and Mitchell (2001) identified six general characteristics of grounded theory: (1) simultaneous data collection and analysis; (2) pursuit of emergent themes through early data analysis; (3) discovery of basic social processes within the data; (4) inductive construction of abstract categories that explain and synthesize these processes; and (5) integration of categories into a theoretical framework that specifies causes, conditions, and consequences of the process(es).

Grounded theory has roots in sociology. In 1967 Barney Glaser and Anselm Strauss introduced the discovery-oriented approach, described above, after conducting research on terminal illness. Although Glaser and Strauss agree with many of the general characteristics of this approach, in the 1990s their ideas diverged regarding how purely inductive grounded theory should be (see Glaser, 1992; Strauss & Corbin, 1998). Glaser maintained that grounded theory as a research tradition serves to generate and validate theory based on present data, and that the approach should rely only on constant comparison (Henwood & Pidgeon, 2006; Rennie, 1998). Strauss and Juliet Corbin believed that the approach could be used to verify existing theory (i.e., select data that might be congruent with preexisting theory or researcher assumptions) and to generate theory based on conditions related to a phenomenon that might not necessarily be grounded in present data. In essence, Strauss and Corbin's approach allows more voice for research subjectivity, existing theory, and potentially related conditions in explaining a phenomenon; Glaser argues that this allowance creates movement away from the "groundedness" of the approach (Rennie, 1998).

More recent work in grounded theory has shifted it from post-positivism to constructivism (see Charmaz, 2005; Clarke, 2005). Clarke (2005) expanded traditional grounded theory by assuming that multiple, contextualized truths and several social processes could explain a particular phenomenon. Essentially, the social world—wherein humans make meaning from interactions with others as well as from the material world—is the starting point for understanding a phenomenon. She acknowledged that the research process and reports are mediated by researchers' perspectives and, to this end, researchers should accentuate the "messiness" of models—that data do not fit perfectly into models, there is "no one right reading" of data (p. 8), and models cannot be oversimplified.

Grounded theory has several benefits, including its high degree of structure, emphasis on collecting large amounts of data to generate and eventually test a developing theory, its ability to fragment and analyze text, and its focus on the researcher's role and acknowledgment of biases. These same strengths also create challenges for grounded theory studies because data collection and analyses often rely on researchers' skills and awareness of the role values play. Also, the large amount of data needed to generate theory is labor- and time-intensive. Finally, an additional challenge relates to determining the degree to which theories will transfer or apply to other settings.

To illustrate grounded theory in studying the therapeutic process, Rennie (1994) conducted interviews with 14 clients on an immediate counseling session to understand the processes and attitudes within the session. Using grounded theory procedures, Rennie discovered eight key categories that indicated client deference to therapists (e.g., meeting the perceived expectations of the therapist, fear of criticizing the therapist). Results helped inform theory about the construct of politeness in the therapeutic relationship. Related to educational reform and training principals, McKenzie and Scheurich (2004) interviewed eight white teachers about the relationship between their perceptions of students of color and their own racial identities. Results indicated four equity traps, or barriers to successful academic outcomes, for students of color (i.e., deficit view, racial erasure, avoidance and employment of the gaze, and paralogical beliefs and behaviors).

Phenomenology

Whereas a grounded theory approach seeks to develop theory, the purpose of **phenomenology** is to discover and describe the meaning or essence of participants' lived experiences, or knowledge as it appears to consciousness. It is the understanding of individual and collective human experiences and how we actively think about experience (Hesse-Biber & Leavy, 2006; Patton, 2002; Wertz, 2005). Qualitative researchers strive to assess participants' *intentionality*, or internal experience of being conscious of something. Phenomenology as a practice involves researchers approaching a phenomenon with a fresh perspective, as if viewing it for the first time, through the eyes of participants who have direct, immediate experience with it. This process begins with understanding the *Lebenswelt* or life-world of a participant and then searching for commonalities across participants to see how lived experiences relate to a phenomenon of interest. There is a unique dialogue between the person and the ordinary world, as self and world cannot be separated according to this approach. Consider the experience of grief. Phenomenologists would interview participants who have experienced grief on their awareness of their grief, how their grief intersects with their life-world, and what universal characteristics can be described about grief.

According to phenomenologists, human experience can be understood only by ignoring or setting aside prior explanations of phenomena found in literature and acknowledging and bracketing off researchers' values and assumptions regarding phenomena. This process is known as **epoche**, a Greek word for refraining from judgment (Moustakas, 1994). Participants are viewed as co-researchers because of their extensive firsthand knowledge of an experience. As researchers encounter experiences of a phenomenon, they move back and forth to assess the **essence** of the experience as well as variations of that experience. The final product is a written representation of the structure of an experience through several participants.

Although phenomenology as a concept was introduced by Kant in the mid-1700s, Edward Husserl (1859–1935) is credited as the father of phenomenology. Husserl's desire to understand better the social crisis in Europe post–World War I led him to phenomenology, with its roots in philosophy. Husserl applied the tradition to mental health because he believed that human experience could not adequately be addressed through the more positivist, laboratory-like approaches being used in mental health disciplines (Hesse-Biber & Leavy, 2006; Wertz, 2005). As Husserl viewed phenomena, anything that was a product of direct, immediate experience could not be understood with complete certainty (Groenewald, 2004).

Since Husserl, many philosophers and schools of thought have extended or slightly diverged from his thoughts on phenomenology, including the Duquesne empirical phenomenological approach (McLeod, 2001), de Rivera's conceptual encounter method (de Rivera, 2006), and the works of Sartre, Heidegger, Merlean-Ponty, Scheler, and Giorgi (Groenewald, 2004; Maso, 2001; McLeod, 2001). A common thread among the divergent thoughts on phenomenology is the value of subjective experience and the connection between self and world.

Applied to counseling research, a phenomenological approach would primarily value clients' perspectives of their problems and the counseling process. Consider two studies that explored participants' resiliency around surviving childhood sexual abuse (Bogar & Hulse-Killacky, 2006; Singh, Hays, Chung, & Watson, 2010). Through interviewing methods, both studies illuminated various resilience strategies that helped adult survivors thrive and make meaning of their abuse. In Bogar and Hulse-Killacky's (2006) study, a sample of primarily white women ($n = 8$ of 10) yielded five determinant clusters (i.e., interpersonally skilled, competent, high self-regard, spiritual, helpful life circumstances) and four process clusters (i.e., coping strategies, refocusing and moving on, active healing, achieving closure) for trauma recovery. From a sample of 13 South Asian women Singh and her colleagues (2010) described a connection between South Asian cultural context (i.e., gender, family, ethnic identity, acculturation) and resilience strategies (i.e., sense of hope, use of silence, social support, social advocacy, self-care). Findings from these studies could be useful for improving counseling practice with trauma survivors.

Phenomenology has also been applied to educational settings, as indicated by two studies (Alerby, 2003; Cornett-DeVito & Worley, 2005). Alerby conducted interviews with 25 11-year-old students on their experiences in school and found that students valued additional time for schoolwork, relationships with peers and teachers, more voice in school policy and rules, and general increased knowledge in school. Cornett-DeVito and Worley (2005) interviewed 21 college students with learning disabilities to understand what types of teacher communication were considered effective. Themes described as most desired for positive academic and social outcomes were teachers' interest, motivation, and competence with respect to instructing students with learning disabilities. With these studies, data based in the life-world of participants indicate ways by which teachers and other stakeholders can create a more effective learning environment for students.

Heuristic Inquiry

Heuristic inquiry has roots in humanistic psychology and was founded by Clark Moustakas. The term *heuristic* originates from the Greek word *heuriskein*, which means to discover or to find. Heuristic inquiry is considered a variation of phenomenology that emphasizes the essence of experience *and* the person in relation to that experience (Moustakas, 1990, 1994). Qualitative researchers using a heuristic approach seek to understand moderately intense experiences of the human condition, such as grief, loss, love, anger, happiness, achievement, and mental health. These phenomena have some personal significance to researchers involved in qualitative inquiry. Heuristic inquiry as a tradition focuses on intense phenomena from the perspective of researchers with attention to how participants' experiences relate to researchers' increased self-awareness and knowledge. Thus, heuristic inquiry is somewhat autobiographical with implications for understanding social phenomena in general (Moustakas, 1990, 1994; Patton, 2002).

Sortino (1999), an educator, used a heuristic approach to understand better the experience of students with behavior disorders. In this dissertation, Sortino presented five vignettes of teaching experiences based on active participation in school activities with 20 students. Through these vignettes, he described a continuous process of reflecting on personal childhood experiences, his increasing insight into the experiences of the students, and methods by which special educators could more effectively work with this population.

Thus, the interaction between person and experience is personally relevant to heuristic researchers, as examined phenomena are experiences that they seek to reflect upon in collaboration with co-researchers and participants. Researchers' voices play an important role in describing and reflecting upon phenomena, with participants' voices as instrumental in facilitating ongoing reflection of the phenomena. Collaboration and sense of connectedness among researchers and participants in discovering and describing the essence of shared experiences are significant. For instance, McNeil (2005) used heuristic inquiry to describe the shared experiences of growing up with a diagnosis of attention-deficit/hyperactivity disorder (ADHD) for the researcher (diagnosed at age 40) and three adolescent females (diagnosed in second grade). The researcher compared themes derived from examining social, academic, and behavioral experiences of the three participants to her experiences with ADHD. Results indicated a need for support groups for students struggling with ADHD as well as professional development opportunities for educators to understand the influence of ADHD on students' sense of social and academic functioning.

Consensual Qualitative Research

Introduced to the social sciences in 1997, **consensual qualitative research** (CQR) integrates phenomenological, grounded theory, and other approaches. Hill and her colleagues (Hill et al., 2005; Hill, Thompson, & Williams, 1997) developed this approach to conduct qualitative inquiry that involves researchers selecting participants who are very knowledgeable about a topic and remaining close to data without major interpretation, with some hopes of generalizing to a larger population. CQR varies slightly from other grounded theory and phenomenological approaches because researchers often reflect on their own experiences with a phenomenon when developing interview questions. *Consensus* is key to this approach, as qualitative researchers use rigorous methods to facilitate agreement in interpretations among themselves and participants, as well as a general audience. Key components of CQR include open-ended questions in semi-structured interviews (see Chapter 8); use of judges for consensus building; use of at least one auditor to evaluate the research (see Chapter 7); and use of domains, core ideas, and cross-analyses in data analysis (see Chapter 11).

● ●

Perspectives 2.1. Dr. Clara Hill on CQR

Dr. Clara Hill and her colleagues have been instrumental in introducing the CQR approach to researchers in the helping professions. In her own words, she describes why CQR was developed and the strengths and challenges to the approach (C. Hill, personal communication, December 4, 2006):

"We wanted to do qualitative research and found that the existing methods were hard to understand and implement. So after receiving extensive consultation from a qualitative expert and then trying out a number of different qualitative methods, we developed CQR and tried to write about it in a clear way so that others could easily use it. As we came to learn, however, qualitative methods are hard to learn and implement. It is probably always wise to work with a mentor on one's first study. In addition, I would add that the CQR method is still evolving and we continue to use it.

"The strengths of this approach are the use of consensus among judges, the use of auditors, and clear guidelines for communicating results. Another clear strength is that CQR is fun to do and it gets you close to the phenomenology of the topic. CQR is a very sociable way to do research because researchers meet together and do everything as a team.

"The challenges are the length of time it takes to complete a CQR project, some difficulty in switching between doing the domains/core ideas and the cross-analysis because these require very different skills, and then making sense of the results. An additional challenge is that the method is best suited for interview data and less suited for other forms of data.

"CQR is very flexible and can easily be used in counseling and education research. Any topic that can be explored in an interview is appropriate for CQR. Interviewees do need to be aware of their experiences of the topic, of course, to provide good interviews."

● ●

Hayes and his colleagues (1998) conducted a study examining therapists' views on countertransference that illustrates the characteristics of CQR. After observing sessions for eight therapy dyads, research assistants conducted 127 interviews with therapists on their perspectives of what constitutes countertransference. The six authors (Hayes et al., 1998) served as auditors and discussed how their values and expected findings influenced interview and data analysis methods. Findings indicated three major themes or domains that helped establish a working theory for better understanding countertransference.

One feature of CQR is its focus on data consistency to inform theory to allow for greater applicability within a setting. Another unique aspect of CQR is its emphasis on power in all aspects of the research process: Researchers share power among each other and via the use of research teams, as well as with participants. Part of the rationale for sharing power in the research process deals with the notion that researcher bias, or assumptions and values about what data are collected and how they are interpreted, is inevitable in qualitative inquiry. Sharing power allows various research team members to discuss how their personal and cultural identities and assumptions about the research topic influence data collection and analysis as well as appreciate the perspectives of participants for better practice. For instance, Kasturirangan and Williams (2003) interviewed nine Latino survivors of domestic violence with the goal of informing counseling practice. As a result of sharing power with participants, counseling researchers discovered from the participants how ethnicity, gender, and family interact with domestic violence interventions.

**ACTIVITY 2.6. Applying the Experience
and Theory Formulation Tradition**

Suppose you are interested in studying the role of technology in your profession. Consider how each
of the traditions discussed in the Experience and Theory Formulation cluster would influence how
you might study the role of technology. Compare the traditions and discuss benefits and challenges
of each for your topic.

THE MEANING OF SYMBOL AND TEXT: SYMBOLIC INTERACTION, SEMIOTICS, LIFE HISTORY, HERMENEUTICS, AND NARRATOLOGY

The third cluster predominantly involves a meaningful "symbol" to us all: language. Researchers adhering to traditions in this cluster typically examine textual documents for the role of language in shaping attitudes and behaviors. However, some traditions, such as symbolic interaction and biography, also rely on verbal and nonverbal communication as a process for learning about social symbols. After reading about these traditions, complete Activity 2.7 to apply them.

Symbolic Interaction

Reflect on a label with which you identify; it can be a self-imposed label or something placed upon you. Labels might include "Asian American," "female," "alcoholic," "schizophrenic," or "gifted." What meanings do you understand as ascribed to the label? How has the label description changed over time? Has your understanding of that label been influenced predominantly by interactions with others? This brief example gives you some indication of what the tradition of symbolic interaction explores.

Symbolic interaction has been credited with influencing many qualitative research traditions, such as phenomenology and ethnography. It is closely aligned with social constructivism in that the interactions between individual and context are seen to create knowledge and truth. Symbolic interactionists believe that only through social experience can individuals become self-identified. That is, individuals interpret their experiences and identities based on social interactions. They actively interact with their environments, making sense of and responding to symbols, including things like language, signs, and cultural artifacts. Common symbols provide meaning to their interactions (Hays & Newsome, 2008). Language is a particularly important symbol for this approach because how individuals label things or processes greatly influences the way they interact with and interpret them. "We can never get beyond our language ... all the questions we ask and words we use to articulate our understandings are embedded in culture" (McLeod, 2001, p. 56). As an illustration, consider the language clinicians and educators have used to describe significantly lower intelligence over the past century. Language describing these individuals has evolved from earlier terms such as *moron* and *imbecile* to *mental retardation* to an emerging term, *intellectual disability*. With changes in language, changes in meaning and general attitudes toward these individuals have created more sensitive assessment and educational practices.

Symbolic interaction has its roots in social psychology, with George Herbert Mead as one of the most recognized contributors to the approach. Mead believed that the "self" was defined primarily through social and behavioral methods with a need for external examination and validation. Thus, Mead viewed individuals as comprising a unique self that considers social interactions in defining the self. Through the consideration of social context, a shared meaning among individuals arises. This shared meaning leads to social organization and an understanding of various social rules and symbols. In social interactions, we respond to ourselves as others do or expect us to do (Farberman, 1985).

Thus, personal and shared meanings are created within and derived from social interactions. This meaning becomes individuals' phenomenological reality and creates a cycle wherein they act upon things based on their meanings of them, which in turn are based on earlier interactions. Context symbols (i.e., language) influence identity, which influences an understanding of identity in context. Consider Pedro's (2005) study on preservice teachers' reflective practices. Pedro examined five preservice teachers' attitudes regarding reflective practice within the context of a teacher preparation program and discovered nine themes that were categorized as one of three components of symbolic interactionism: acquiring perspective on reflective practice (context symbols), achieving individuality (identity), and situating reflective acts within context (identity in context).

Semiotics

A research tradition closely tied to symbolic interaction is **semiotics**. Codes and symbols regarding a culture or context surround the qualitative researcher. Semiotics is the search, description, and interpretation of these codes (Chandler, 2002). Specifically, qualitative researchers using this tradition attempt to understand how rules guide codes and symbols, such as language.

Similar to a symbolic interaction approach, the relationship between language and other symbols and behavior—and how language influences behavior within a particular context—is salient. Symbolic interaction focuses on how language derives personal and collective meanings. Semiotics focuses more on the rules for code or symbol acquisition itself rather than reflecting on its meaning after it is used. For example, Radford (2003) examined the processes by which mathematics students master algebraic syntax. In the study, Radford discovered that language and gestures were important to move students from presymbolic to symbolic algebraic generalizations. The study described the context for learning, how students engaged with symbols, and how learning was transmitted.

Life History

The **life history** tradition presents an account of a person's life couched in a broader social context, a research tradition that seeks to identify personal meanings individuals give to their social experiences. Often, life histories allow qualitative researchers to "rewrite history" and give voice to marginalized groups. The researcher gathers stories and explores meanings for an individual as well as how the stories fit into a broader social or historical context. Although the term *life history* is used interchangeably with those of *biography, autobiography,* and *oral history,* Creswell (2006) defined each of these terms in these ways: biography as a life story of an individual from archival documents written by someone other than the individual; autobiography as a life story written directly by an individual; life history as a presentation of an individual's life derived from interviews and personal conversations in which a researcher accounts the individual's life and how it relates to cultural, social, and/or personal themes; and oral history as personal recollections of events and their impact on the individual taken from taped or written works of living or deceased individuals. Many life history methods are categorized as case studies (Creswell, 2003). Although there is great overlap, the distinction we see between life history methods (as making meaning of symbol and text) and the universal tradition (case study) is with intention: Are you using the method to describe a bounded system in which you plan to use various data sources to understand the context and activities of a case? Or are you interested in using the method to reflect solely on the process of meaning making via language or another symbol (e.g., social phenomena)?

This research tradition has been used in various disciplines such as literature, anthropology, history, sociology, and psychology. It was first introduced in sociology by Thomas and Znaniecki (1927), when they used personal letters and autobiographies to examine the relationship between Polish peasants' native culture and community disunion. Life histories gained significance in the 1930s with works of Chicago School researchers (Shaw, 1930, 1938; Sutherland, 1937), which explored criminality via criminal careers, and in the 1940s with works such as Allport and his colleagues' study of the life histories of refugees in Nazi Germany (Allport, Bruner, & Jandorf, 1941). Furthermore, research by theorists such as Levinson (1978) and Erikson (1963), in their efforts to understand developmental stages, demonstrated that this method could be a viable means for understanding psychological processes. Recent examples of the life history method that could be applied to counseling and education include the works of Sommers and Baskin (2006), who collected life histories of 205 methamphetamine abusers to understand violent behavior, and Powell (2006), who interviewed 10 adults who had repeated a grade in elementary school to examine factors related to grade retention.

Hermeneutics

Hermeneutics is an approach that originated from scriptural interpretations and has been applied to other fields, including counseling and education. It is the art of interpreting "sacred" texts, such as religious documents, mythology, history, art, and politics. With hermeneutics, the assumption is that texts are recorded expressions of human experience. Recording expressions of experience may be a subjective representation of lived experience to be used to consider current phenomena. Thus, the text comes alive for the qualitative researcher. It is a form of "cultural inquiry that seeks to construct a historical understanding of the experience and realities of other persons" (McLeod, 2001, p. 26). Practitioners interpret something based on the cultural context they are in as well as the cultural context in which the text was created (Patton, 2002). Thus, the reader must have information not only on the cultural and historical aspects of the text but also on the researcher's life.

Qualitative researchers move back and forth between parts of a text and the whole text to gain understanding while extending the meaning of the text to apply to phenomena in counseling and education. Through this process, both researcher and text are changed (McLeod, 2001). One historical figure in counseling that has served as the subject of this approach is Sigmund Freud. Bonomi (2005) reviewed a recent text that comments on one of Freud's essays related to self-analysis. Bonomi examined how Freud's original essay sparked commentaries among a new wave of psychoanalysts in the 1960s. The cultural and historical contexts of both when the original essay and text were written are discussed. Also, Bonomi emphasized that Freud's essay and resulting commentary heavily influenced the psychoanalytic community.

Narratology

Similar to the hermeneutic and life history approaches, **narratology** or narrative analysis seeks to understand what stories or narratives reveal about an individual. With origins in social sciences and literature, it extends the hermeneutic approach by examining data sources such as interview transcripts, life history and other historical narratives, and creative nonfiction (Patton, 2002). Just as in other approaches in this cluster, recorded data are seen as revealing cultural and personal information about an individual with potential applicability to a larger context. Individuals communicate their sense of their worlds through stories.

There are additional key assumptions underlying narratology. First, individuals speak in narrative form, connecting events over time through stories. In a sense, our stories are not random sentences but constructed in a personally and often culturally meaningful manner. Second, individuals' identities are shaped by the stories they recount and share with others. Finally, narratives change depending on the narrator, audience, and context. What is deemed important often depends on these three dimensions. A narrative thus is not just text but a sequential and causal account of events, people, and processes that expresses how individuals make sense of their worlds (Murray, 2003).

Narratology is concerned with the plot structures, contents, and story purposes we exchange in social interactions. Through narratives, a sense of order can be established to help understand larger phenomena (Polkinghorne, 1988). Stories are thus viewed as primary data that may be examined as a whole, by specific events and processes, or by the ways in which they are communicated (McLeod, 2001).

Narratology may be a natural research tradition for counseling, particularly for those in the field who subscribe to a narrative therapy or a postmodern approach. In narrative therapy counselors search for dominant plot lines, "restorying" opportunities, story linkages, and breaks in sequences (White & Epston, 1990). Similarly, the qualitative researcher examines how individuals tell about their lives through personal narratives. Although themes are important, researchers often focus more on plot structure and process (Murray, 2003). These narratives provide information about the personal meanings of various phenomena to a participant (Hays & Newsome, 2008). Additionally, a narrative may illuminate multiple voices for a current or historical event or process and provide information about the temporal nature of human existence. For instance, Freud's study of his patients' stories greatly influenced the development of psychoanalytic theory (Murray, 2003).

Narratives can be analyzed by various methods, including examining the poetic features of a story, particularly how specific language is used (Gee, 1991); comparing various narratives (Ruth & Öberg, 1996); and focusing on the interpersonal context of a particular narrative and how it might be shaped by a larger context (Mishler, 1997).

ACTIVITY 2.7. Applying the Meaning of Symbol and Text Cluster

Consider a study in your discipline focused on how children's literature has communicated information about gender roles. How might each of the traditions described in this cluster address this research topic?

TABLE 2.3. The Study of Dual-Career Families across Traditions

Research tradition	Focus	Research study example[a]
Cluster 1: The universal tradition		
Case study	Case description and comparison	A researcher is interested in conflict among partners in dual-career families. With "dual-career family" as the case, the researcher studies the individuals, activities, events, and processes of several families (i.e., *collective or multiple case study*) to uncover ways that family and career are balanced for the cases (*instrumental case studies*).
Cluster 2: Experience and theory formulation		
Grounded theory	Theory development	To develop a local theory to describe and explain how conflict impacts dual-career families, a researcher uses an *inductive approach* and *theoretical sampling* to understand sequences, processes, conditions, and actions associated with this phenomenon. The researcher remains close to the data and seeks a *core category* or central idea that unites other constructs and accounts for variation in conflict effects.
Phenomenology	Essence of direct experience	A researcher is interested in interviewing dual-career family members who have directly experienced conflict due to career–family balance concerns. After bracketing his or her experiences with, and assumptions about, conflict, the researcher seeks to fully describe the collective and individual experiences of the phenomenon.
Heuristic inquiry	Integration of personal experience for intense phenomena	Similarly to the phenomenology example above, the researcher interviews dual-career families who have had difficulty balancing career–family roles. However, the researcher integrates personal experience throughout the research process.
Consensual qualitative research	Use of consensus and shared power to describe experience and develop theory	To understand how families negotiate whether both partners will work outside the home, a researcher collaborating closely with participants and team members may arrive at consensus of a local theory that includes in-depth participant experiences of this process.

(cont.)

TABLE 2.3. *(cont.)*

Research tradition	Focus	Research study example[a]
Cluster 3: The meaning of symbol and text		
Semiotics	Search and interpretation of codes; rules for code acquisition	A researcher focuses on rules that guide how dual-career families learn to label themselves as such.
Life history	Individual narratives of social experience	A researcher conducts personal interviews with partners on their process of both deciding to enter the workforce, and then reflects how this relates to the larger society.
Symbolic interaction	Personal and shared meanings of language	A researcher explores the context that provides indicators of meanings in dual-career families (*context symbols*) that lead to label identification, and reflects back to a context to identify personal and shared meanings for dual-career families (*identity in context*).
Hermeneutics	Sacred text applied to present time	To assess the rise of dual-career families, a researcher may analyze several historical political documents and report their influence on past and present-day contexts.
Narratology	Plot structure, content, and purpose of narratives	A researcher examines contemporary books and magazines to explore themes related to attitudes toward dual-career families, reviews themes with participants, and solicits potential "re-storied" personal narratives.
Cluster 4: Cultural expressions of process and experience		
Ethnography	Social, behavioral, and linguistic group patterns and norms	To explore the attitudes and practices of dual-career African American families living in a small community, a researcher builds a relationship over time, engaging in fieldwork that involves participant observation and interviews.
Ethnomethodology	Social order and "everydayness" of behavior	A researcher examines shifts in social patterns after a sudden, nontraditional shift in breadwinner roles for a heterosexual couple.
Autoethnography	Researcher as group member; self-reflexivity in report writing	Using his or her personal experience as a dual-career family member, a researcher explores other group members' attitudes toward resources for dual-career families. The researcher then synthesizes data from self and others to understand a greater social need.
Cluster 5: Research as a change agent		
Participatory action research	Emancipation and transformation; research as a vehicle for specific change	A researcher works with dual-career families who need assistance with child care policies at a particular work setting. He or she critically reflects on his or her power as a researcher, as well as ways in which he or she can equitably include participants in the research process, and works collaboratively with them to collect data to enact policy changes.

[a]A general research topic has been altered based on the research tradition used to orient the design.

CULTURAL EXPRESSIONS OF PROCESS AND EXPERIENCE: ETHNOGRAPHY, ETHNOMETHODOLOGY, AND AUTOETHNOGRAPHY

The fourth cluster, cultural expressions of process and experience, includes the essential feature of a culture-sharing group. That is, examining social and cultural norms is a significant aspect of ethnography, ethnomethodology, and autoethnography. No matter the tradition in this cluster, researchers share the following in common: (1) knowledge and understanding of cultural anthropological terms and concepts, (2) prolonged engagement with the culture studied, (3) manuscripts that are narrative and literary in style about the cultural group, and (4) challenges in fieldwork (e.g., "going native," whereby the researcher is unable to continue the study due to absorption by the culture studied or compromised data; Creswell, 2006). Ethnographic research also shares an acknowledgment that the research process is recursive, demanding flexibility on the part of the researcher and attention to the contextual realities involved in conducting fieldwork. Activity 2.8 provides an opportunity to apply these traditions to a research topic of your choice.

Ethnography

Ethnography is a research paradigm in which the researcher describes and provides interpretations about the culture of a group or system (MacDonald, 2001). A data collection method common to ethnography, **participant observation**, is often utilized by the researcher and involves **prolonged engagement** over a significant period of time with the group studied, in order to describe the process and experience of its culture (Lincoln & Guba, 1995). Ethnographic research has its intellectual roots in anthropology (e.g., Bronislaw, Malinowski, M. Mead), whose researchers examined comparative cultures (Pollner & Emerson, 2001). These early scholars were dedicated to ethnographic research that provided a firsthand account of a group's culture, and their research was typically reported in the form of a monograph that resulted from long-term participant observation (MacDonald, 2001). Fieldwork is a critical aspect of ethnography in that the researcher becomes immersed in the context of the group (e.g., daily life activities of members) in order to understand the culture of the group (Stanley, 2001).

Ethnographic research first emerged from the British and French social anthropologists in the 1920s and 1930s who studied "exotic" cultural groups that were typically living in colonized regimes (MacDonald, 2001). These early researchers separated themselves from the more traditional research methods of anthropological sciences in that they were interested in studying the cultural norms (e.g., language, behavior) of various cultural groups. Soon after European ethnographic researchers began producing monographs and detailed texts of these cultural groups, ethnography was used in the United States by sociologists at the University of Chicago in what came to be called the culture and personality school of American anthropology (James, 2001). The American school of scholars expanded the focus of ethnography to the "use of childhood and the study of children as the location for the study of broader social values ... and a method for observing their inculcation in children through daily life"

(p. 247). As a primary way to examine socialization processes, ethnographies continue to be utilized in the social sciences.

Ethnographic approaches are valuable to the counseling field, in that counselors typically have prolonged engagement with cultural groups and systems, as well as with individuals. Quimby (2006) advocated for the utilization of ethnography for research and practice in mental health. He underscored the utility of ethnographic methods, such as fieldwork and prolonged engagement, as a way to effectively gather, describe, interpret, and understand the cultural identities of informants. In advocating for qualitative approaches such as ethnography, he has focused on clients who are female and of African American heritage as a group that is typically invisible in large, quantitative research methods in mental health. Recognizing the ways in which African American women face challenges in receiving culturally appropriate treatment, in addition to being underrepresented and understudied in research, Quimby asserts that ethnography is a way to rectify their absence in the counseling literature and inform more effective practice. Ultimately, ethnographic research serves as an important research tradition for counseling researchers who seek to conceptualize, build hypotheses, and test outcome data for groups that typically are marginalized in society.

Ethnomethodology

Ethnomethodology is similar to ethnography in that both are inductive approaches that examine the lives of their participants in a structured manner, while having a strong sense of respect for the informants in the group studied (Pollner & Emerson, 2001). This research tradition, first used in the 1950s in the sociological sciences, seeks to study social orders and patterns (Heritage, 1994). The focus of study in ethnomethodology is on the informants' perspectives of social order, assessments, and explanations. Similarly to ethnography, researchers are expected to remain close to participants as they gain details of their social and cultural lives.

Ethnomethodologists are most interested in studying the everydayness of social behaviors, and research is usually a product of intentional or unintentional social changes. In order to study everyday "normal" social activities, qualitative researchers may opt to "shake things up" and do something outside a cultural norm to assess how people respond to conditions that differ from what they normally expect. For example, let's say a teacher, instead of standing in front of the classroom to teach, decides to move to the back of the classroom, or maybe even sits among the students. An educator might observe and conduct interviews of students to better understand their perceptions of this change in classroom behavior and structure.

Autoethnography

While ethnography and ethnomethodology both face epistemological challenges in "getting close" to their informants, **autoethnography** resolves this challenge by being a first-person account of events, interactions, and relationships (Murphy & Dingwall, 2001). Autoethnographers use their own thoughts, feelings, documentation of fieldnotes, and other personal experiences they have in response to their ethnographic examination of a culture as data (Ellis, 1991). For example, one autoethnography documented the researcher's experience growing up as the child of a mother who lives with a mental illness (Ronai, 1996).

There are two types of autoethnography. The first type, *evocative autoethnography*, involves primarily description of what goes on in an individual's life or social environment and seeks to evoke emotion from the reader. This description is presented in relation to how it is influenced by and influences a culture-sharing group specifically. For more information on evocative ethnography, we refer the reader to Denzin (2006). The second type, *analytic autoethnography*, has been argued to move "beyond" description of social structure to generalize data to larger social phenomena (Anderson, 2006; Atkinson, 2006). Furthermore, Anderson (2006) argued that analytic autoethnography is more aligned with traditional ethnography, yet allows for greater self-reflexivity in ethnographic research, which he argues is more aligned with postmodern paradigms.

Anderson (2006) noted several key features of analytic autoethnography:

- The researcher is a complete member of the social world being researched (i.e., complete member researcher status, CMR), with group membership commonly preceding the research process.

- There is greater attention to the researcher's impact on the research context, and vice versa, to allow for mutual understanding.

- The researcher is visible in the text, accounting for important data.

- The researcher is actively involved with others to ensure representation in findings. (Vryan, 2006, noted that a representative sample of a social group is not a necessity.)

- There is a focus on actively gathering empirical data to understand a broader social phenomenon than that provided by data themselves, connecting biography with social structure.

Autoethnography has its beginnings in the Chicago School (discussed in Chapter 1), when researchers gave greater attention to research in a context—both participants and researchers. Later generations of Chicago School researchers used more explicit self-reflexivity in reporting findings. There came an increasing realization that there was difficulty in "keeping the researcher out" of the process and thus greater autobiographical connection in research reports (Anderson, 2006).

A major benefit of autoethnography is the accessibility of data. Qualitative researchers have a vantage point that allows often for more flexible, unrestricted data (Anderson, 2006; Vryan, 2006). There is an opportunity to switch between being a member and being a researcher, to have an "engaged dialogue" rather than a "detached discovery." This benefit is also a potential drawback if not carefully monitored: a risk of "self-absorbed digression" (Anderson, 2006). Atkinson (2006) describes this critique further:

> There is the elevation of the autobiographical to such a degree that the ethnographer becomes more memorable than the ethnography, the self more absorbing than other social actors. ... This in turn reflects a wider problem in that the methodological has been transposed onto the plane of personal experience, while the value of sociological or anthropological fieldwork has been translated into a quest for personal fulfillment on the part of the researcher. (pp. 402–403)

Thus, qualitative researchers are cognizant of not using this tradition as a springboard for documenting personal information or simply providing an insider's perspective.

**ACTIVITY 2.8. Applying the Cultural Expressions
of the Process and Experience Cluster**

Select a topic of interest in your profession. Consider how each of the traditions in this cluster would influence how you would study the research topic.

RESEARCH AS A CHANGE AGENT:
PARTICIPATORY ACTION RESEARCH

Participatory action research (PAR) is a tradition that focuses on facilitating change in the participants and the researcher in the process of the examination (Nastasi, 1998). Essentially, the goals of PAR are emancipation and transformation, and the researcher is required to critically reflect on the power of research as a change agent (Chiu, 2006). Furthermore, participants and researchers share power, and participants are a part of planning research and implementing its findings.

PAR emerged from the applied anthropological inquiry and is recursive in nature because it seeks to align research with both practice and theory in order to encourage change in a culture and society (Schensul, 1998). Researchers in school psychology have a long tradition of utilizing action research, where the data collection and analysis process drive decisions about practice and intervention (Graham, 1998). PAR involves a collaborative approach to problem solving between the researcher and other key stakeholders (e.g., parents, teachers, school administrators) to guide interventions and practice with one or more students (Nastasi, Moore, & Varjas, 2004).

Theory, previous research, and collaborative interaction between the researchers and stakeholders provide the foundation for PAR inquiry and guide formulation of research questions. Nastasi and colleagues (2004) describe PAR as using this foundation to generate a culture or context-specific theory that applies to the examination, which will then guide the development of the culture- or context-specific intervention or practice. Ongoing evaluation of the research process is a critical way in which the researcher adapts the intervention or practice in the course of the inquiry, and ultimately provides the field with additional theory that is both general and culture-specific. Theoretical information that is generated, in turn, changes researcher and participants, thus continuing the recursive process of the examination.

Previous to initiating PAR, **critical reflection** is demanded of the researcher. Critical reflection is derived from Friere's (1972) work, which provided a critical analysis of power holders as a way to generate social and systemic change. PAR integrates critical reflection previous to and throughout the research process as a validity check and as a way to ensure that the focus is not merely a discovery of knowledge, but is a collaborative creation of knowledge that will promote systemic change (Chiu, 2006). Thus, critical reflection is an active process that does not merely focus on the outcomes of change in PAR, but also on the research processes so that readers may learn how to initiate change in a similar manner.

Consider a study of exploring bullying intervention methods for lesbian, gay, bisexual, and transgender (LGBT) adolescents in schools (Varjas et al., 2006). Varjas and her colleagues interviewed 16 community and school service providers to better understand how they respond to LGBT bullying as well as how they perceive school barriers, resources, and existing bullying interventions influencing changes to meet the needs of these youth. For this study, critical reflection not only involved the reflections of the researcher on the informants (third-person reflection) but also incorporated an analysis of the researcher of him- or herself (first-person reflection) in addition to the researcher *and* the informants (second-person reflection). In this example, the critical reflection on all three levels provided a more authentic way to document and promote change during the research process because the reflection was not limited to, and situated in, the researcher alone.

PAR is a useful research tradition to employ in the field of counseling, especially as the social justice movement in counseling continues to grow. Social justice has been named the fifth force in counseling, and it urges counselors to move beyond acquiring multicultural awareness, knowledge, and skills to advocacy on behalf of clients (Ratts, D'Andrea, & Arredondo, 2004). PAR is a research paradigm that traditionally has been utilized more in school psychology research. However, the recent focus on social justice in counseling may urge counseling scholars to consider using PAR as the inquiry of choice when seeking to promote change in a community through the research process.

Stoecker (2005) advises researchers to answer three questions when selecting participatory methods. First, he suggests that the researcher ask: Who is the community? For instance, in a study of homeless individuals who were being displaced by the 1996 Olympics in Atlanta, an organization called Project South used participatory research methods, including challenging government policies, to collaboratively change the living situations of these individuals (Project South, 1996). In this study the community was identified as comprising the homeless individuals, the organization and members of Project South, government agencies, and the Atlanta community at large, and the community was the sources of data collection and analysis (e.g., interviews, archival data, community meetings). A second question to ask: Is conflict or cooperation involved in the situation that the researcher is interested in examining? This is an especially important question because the researcher will want to be aware of how conflict or cooperation may shape the research process from collaborative research question design to evaluation. A third question to ask: Is the PAR approach biased in terms of voices that are present and absent in the collaborative process of research? A subset of questions may include attention to who the stakeholders are and which groups hold more or less power in the focus of inquiry.

In the course of the PAR examination, traditional data collection methods are used, such as semistructured interviews, artifacts and archival data, focus groups, and participant observation, among others (Lincoln & Guba, 1995). Nastasi and her colleagues (2004) described using PAR methods to initiate a mental health services plan for schools that met certain required criteria. Six phases were used to create a collaborative and recursive research process: (1) examining existing theory, research, and practice (exploring personal theory); (2) learning the culture; (3) forming partnerships; (4) identifying goal or problem; (5) conducting the formative research; and (6) conceptualizing a culture-specific theory or model. They also used a similar approach to an HIV/AIDS prevention project with adolescents in Sri Lanka (Nastasi, Varjas, Sarkar, & Jayasena, 1998), where initial theories and existing information generated data about alcoholism as a stressor for the adolescents, and social stressors (e.g., intimate partner violence, cultural norms of shame) were revealed to impact the transmission of HIV/AIDS. This information was gathered through semistructured interviews with individuals, in addition to community focus group interviews, which were also methods of building collaboration and stakeholder identification for the next stages of the PAR inquiry.

In sum, PAR is a tradition that focuses on a specific setting in counseling and education and seeks to readily apply research findings to real-world problems. To apply these findings, researchers are charged with working actively with participants on solutions. Complete Activity 2.9 to practice applying the PAR tradition.

 ACTIVITY 2.9. Applying the PAR Tradition

Select a topic of interest in your profession. Consider how each of the research clusters would influence how you would study the research topic.

 ACTIVITY 2.10. Qualitative Article Review

Select an article in your specific profession. Determine which research paradigms and traditions the authors chose. To what degree did they discuss these? How are the paradigms and traditions reflected in the methodology and findings sections of the article?

PROPOSAL DEVELOPMENT 2.2. Selecting a Research Tradition

Which research traditions(s) resonate(s) most with you? Why? Which seems least appropriate for you? Why? (Remember, your final choice for a research tradition will likely change once you select a proposal topic.)

CHAPTER SUMMARY

Your research orientation is an important foundation in constructing a qualitative study. This orientation is influenced by how you envision scientific pursuit in your profession, which impacts the various research paradigms and traditions you select. The five core philosophies of science are ontology, epistemology, axiology, rhetoric, and methodology. Brainstorming and addressing questions that correspond to each of these philosophies is an important first step in constructing your research design.

Philosophies of science are related to research paradigms such as positivism, post-positivism, social constructivism, critical theory, feminism, and queer theory. Research paradigms are belief systems upon which you may rely to investigate a research problem. With the increased focus on culture and context in counseling and education research, qualitative researchers are adhering to social constructivist paradigms.

Selecting your research tradition helps solidify the foundation for your research inquiry. There are five major clusters presented in this chapter: (1) the universal tradition (case study); (2) experience and theory formulation (grounded theory, phenomenology, heuristic inquiry, and consensual qualitative research); (3) the meaning of symbol and text (symbolic interaction, semiotics, hermeneutics, narratology, and life history); (4) cultural expressions of process and experience (ethnography, ethnomethodology, and autoethnography); and (5) research as a change agent (PAR).

RECOMMENDED READINGS

Clarke, A. E. (2005). *Situational analysis: Grounded theory after the postmodern turn.* Thousand Oaks, CA: Sage.

Guba, E. G., & Lincoln, Y. S. (2005). Paradigmatic controversies, contradictions, and emerging confluences. In N. K. Denzin & Y. S. Lincoln (Eds.), *The Sage handbook of qualitative research* (3rd ed., pp. 191–215). Thousand Oaks, CA: Sage.

Ponterotto, J. G. (2005). Qualitative research in counseling psychology: A primer on research paradigms and philosophies of science. *Journal of Counseling Psychology, 52,* 126–136.

CHAPTER 3

Ethical Issues in Qualitative Research

CHAPTER PREVIEW

Research ethics, the final foundational topic addressed in this section, is multilayered and ever evolving, particularly as researchers increasingly engage in qualitative research. Using select ethics codes from clinical and educational disciplines, we present several key ethical constructs, dilemmas, and considerations that apply to all aspects of the research process. Figure 3.1 on the next page illustrates the interconnection of these constructs with qualitative research design.

A CASE FOR ETHICS IN QUALITATIVE INQUIRY

Ethics is part of our human world. Whether we are acting in the role of practitioner, educator, peer, researcher, or concerned citizen, ethical dilemmas and decisions surround us. When we are conducting qualitative inquiry, often these roles become blurred, and we must justify the benefits and costs of research for all involved. And, the emergent nature of qualitative research creates unique ethical dilemmas and often political choices. The feature (and sometimes "flaw") in qualitative research from an ethical perspective is the openness of the design, the changing views of what is deemed important to ask, observe, collect, and report.

First and foremost, it is *ethically* imperative that practitioners who conduct research contribute to the knowledge base and improve clients' lives. For example, the Introduction of the American Counseling Association (2005) Code of Ethics (Section G) articulates this value:

> Counselors who conduct research are encouraged to contribute to the knowledge base of the profession and promote a clearer understanding of the conditions that lead to a healthy and more just society. Counselors support efforts of researchers by participating fully and willingly whenever possible. Counselors minimize bias and respect diversity in designing and implementing research programs.

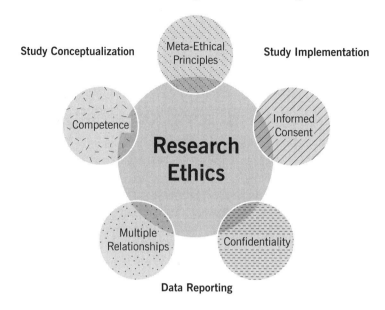

FIGURE 3.1. Ethical constructs and qualitative research design.

So, what is ethical research practice in general? And how is it unique in qualitative inquiry? The question is not, *do* we need to engage in qualitative research, but *how* do we do it in an ethical way.

Let's first define ethics. Overall, **ethics** can be considered a set of guidelines established within a professional discipline to guide thinking and behavior. These standards and principles are quite similar across disciplines, although subcomponents may be emphasized more so than others depending on the discipline. And, professionals within the same discipline may interpret guidelines very differently. Thus, making sound ethical decisions involves understanding various ways to think about ethics, and blending them as appropriate (see Activity 3.1). An important note before we go further: Although it is beyond the scope of this chapter to differentiate ethics from other terms such as *morals, values, laws*, and *mores*, it is important to mention that qualitative researchers likely assume that these concepts are interdependent and, based on their views, vary greatly depending on what they determine as ethical.

The rubric of *ethics* has been parsed into several subcategories. Two subcategories considered more traditional are principle and utilitarian ethics. **Principle ethics** encompasses minimal acts or choices that focus heavily on morality and obligations in relation to stated ethics codes. What should I do, based on the outlined standards of my profession (Corey, Corey, & Callanan, 2003)? Similarly, **utilitarian ethics** assumes a universal set of moral rules that determine what we ought to do. This value-free notion of moral behavior has implications for ethics in clinical and educational settings: Codes of ethics can guide research in an almost linear manner (Christians, 2003). In essence, these types of ethics suggest that a more value-free approach to research is more ethical.

Traditionally, research ethics indicated that research was conducted for the benefit of society as whole (with assurance that the costs of conducting research did not outweigh its benefits). Rowan (2000) noted: "Most of the ethical codes which have been drawn up are based on the empirical paradigm, where the researcher is the one in charge, keeping his distance, and using the subjects for his convenience" (p. 103). However, Lather (1991) noted that with qualitative inquiry there is an increased focus on individual benefits, including self-empowerment and social advocacy. These benefits are assumed to result from research relationships and from participating in the research process (Haverkamp, 2005). In sum, we have to stop thinking of the "expert" and "objective" researcher as the most ethical.

Based on this conceptualization of ethics—participants should experience/receive maximum benefit and relationships are valuable—several other types of ethics should be considered. **Virtue ethics** covers "being a good person." That is, virtue ethics relate to nonobligatory ideals and personal characteristics of the researcher and participants. Am I doing what's best for those involved, given the context (Meara, Schmidt, & Day, 1996)?

Since the late 1980s to the present, there has been increased challenge to the value-free, linear perspective of utilitarian ethics. Gillies and Alldred (2002) noted: "The research we produce and the values we promote are inevitably grounded in partial, invested viewpoints" (p. 48). *Social ethics* views the moral judgments involved in research as a complex issue wherein neutral espoused principles cannot be easily applied. The premise is that decisions should be made in terms of ever-changing human relationships and social structures. Carol Gilligan wrote of an *ethic of care*, wherein conflict resolution (in this case, in terms of ethical dilemmas) involves fostering relationships and nurturance as opposed to simply avoiding harm and liability. Determining ethics is to be viewed as a more fluid process, without the assumptions of impartiality and formality (Christians, 2003).

We would like to spend some time on an emerging framework for ethics that is particularly relevant for qualitative research: communitarian ethics. In general, communitarianism is a social philosophy that emphasizes the need to balance individual rights and interests with those of the community, with a greater focus on collective goals. Individuals absorb social values in their own individual identities. When we assess benefit, then, we assess increasingly in terms of community benefit, and individual benefits and rights are minimized. There is a commitment to a core of shared values, norms, and meanings, as well as collective history and identity (i.e., moral culture; Etziono, 2009). Since qualitative research often focuses on social context and participants as experts and often co-researchers, communitarian ethics seems congruent and important to examine.

Communitarian ethics, also referred to as *feminist communitarianism* (Denzin, 1997), extends the ethic of care idea and challenges the mission of research to be on building community among researchers and participants, involving them in ethical decisions and research design. It emphasizes both process–outcome and community participation and includes the following characteristics (Denzin, 2003; Malone, Yerger, McGruder, & Froelicher, 2006):

- The community is the unit of identity.
- There is a focus on community strengths.
- Research is a collaborative process among academic researchers, community organizations, community members, and others.

- Participants have a voice in how and when research is conducted and whether findings are relevant and accurate.
- All partners work together as co-learners.
- Researchers value empowerment, solidarity, community, and shared governance.
- Knowledge based in local and cultural experiences is disseminated to all partners because it benefits all.

Communitarian ethics is sometimes at odds with traditional perspectives of research ethics that use a biomedical model and focus on individual rights and institutional protection. Later in this chapter we discuss challenges from those who espouse communitarian ethics to the Institutional Review Board's criteria for determining ethical practices.

Finally, to complicate matters, there is another way to examine ethics in qualitative research: ethics about the research design itself (**micro-level ethics**) and ethics about how knowledge is used (**macro-level ethics**; Gillies & Aldred, 2002). As you can see from the following excerpt, these types may conflict with aspects of communitarian ethics:

> It is indeed important to obtain the subjects' consent to participate in the research, to secure their confidentiality, to inform them about the character of the research and of their right to withdraw at any time, to avoid harmful consequences for the subjects, and to consider the researcher's role. But it is also important to consider how the knowledge produced will circulate in the wider culture and affect humans and society. (Brinkmann & Kvale, 2005, p. 167)

Questions of micro- and macro-level ethics in research might include: To what degree are participants protected during the research process? (micro) Are worthwhile societal goals being met? (macro) How does politics shape the way data are interpreted and presented for a sampling frame (micro) as well as for the larger community of knowledge (macro)?

There can be ethical behavior at a micro level, but unethical at a macro level, and vice versa, as the experiments in Table 3.1 demonstrate. The rub comes when we try to balance wanting to collect as much information as possible with respecting the integrity of the individual.

 ACTIVITY 3.1. Conceptualizing Ethics

Review the following research topic in dyads and respond to the questions that follow.

You are required to develop a qualitative proposal for your qualitative research course. One topic that has intrigued you for quite some time is the role of sponsors in Alcoholics Anonymous (AA). You would like to conduct interviews with sponsors with varying durations of sobriety on their experience supporting individuals with addictions. Given the difficulty of obtaining participants, you consider approaching sponsors at several AA meetings and soliciting their participation.

- Based on the various ways to conceptualize ethics, develop an argument for how this plan for participant recruitment is *both* ethical and unethical.
  - Principle
  - Utilitarian
  - Virtue
  - Social
  - Communitarian
- What are some micro-level ethical considerations?
- What are some macro-level ethical considerations?
- Which ways of viewing ethics seems most comfortable for you?

In this chapter, we discuss the foundational nature of ethics in qualitative inquiry. Beginning with some historical information and key meta-ethical principles, we then move to specific ethical considerations and how they apply to qualitative research.

A BRIEF HISTORY OF RESEARCH ETHICS

The history of research ethics reflects quite a bumpy road to the development and application of ethical codes and legal statutes and research compliance. In fact, the evolution of ethical standards and legal protection resulted from reactions to atrocities against participants. Wester (2009) reminds us that although it may seem intuitive to protect participants from harm, a history of unethical practice corrects our assumption. Table 3.1 outlines some of the major examples of ethical malpractice across disciplines.

The **Nuremberg Code** was the first legal attempt to deal with research-related controversies, specifically those of the Nazi medical experiments. Established in 1947, the Nuremberg Code was an initial effort to put forth guidelines for social, medical, and behavioral research, with particular emphasis on the importance of informed consent.

In response to continued ethical violations and a need for more comprehensive standards, the National Research Act of 1974 was passed and mandated that a commission be developed to identify the primary ethical principles with which researchers should comply to protect human subjects. The National Commission for the Protection of Human Subjects in Biomedical and Behavioral Research was established in 1978 to develop the **Belmont Report**.

The commission in the Belmont Report (1979) defined research as a structured, premeditated method with the primary purpose of testing hypotheses and generating theory (National Commission for the Protection of Human Subjects of Biomedical and Behavioral Research, 1979). Although there is some attention in the document to the integration of research and practice, the authors emphasize that research is most likely to occur in conjunction with practice when there is a significant departure from a standard or accepted practice. One can readily see how qualitative research, with its emphasis on the continual infusion of research and practice, and its lack of "testing hypotheses" and valuing generalizability, could create ethical dilemmas in terms of the commission's definition of research in this report!

The Belmont Report identified what were considered at the time the three moral standards of researchers: respect for persons, beneficence, and justice. *Respect for persons*

TABLE 3.1. Key Research Studies Demonstrating Ethics Violations

Nazi medical experiments (1940s)	Experiments conducted on Nazi prisoners involving exposure to high altitude, freezing, malaria, sterilization, sea water, poison, and mustard gas led to the eventual illness and death of thousands. These experiments were reportedly designed to assess physiological changes to various conditions; however, *participants were never provided with the opportunity of informed consent.*
Tuskegee syphilis experiment (1932–1972)	With a purpose of understanding the natural course of syphilis in black men, and trying to justify treatment programs for them, the U.S. government intentionally withheld life-saving, well-accepted medical treatment (i.e., penicillin) as symptoms worsened. Participants had been told that they would receive free medical treatment for their condition, although they were not informed of what that condition was, and they were deceived about the treatment they were receiving (i.e., a placebo). *This case highlights the improper use of deception in research.*
Milgram blind obedience experiment (1960s)	Stanley Milgram and his associates investigated participants' responses to demands from an authority, in an effort to assess the construct of *blind obedience*. Most participants obeyed the researcher's request to deliver "shock treatment" for incorrect answers, resulting in severe distress for them. *The researchers did not tell participants of the true research purpose, nor did they debrief them at the end of the study.*
Jewish chronic disease hospital study (1963)	Patients of various health statuses were injected with live cancer cells so that researchers could evaluate the body's reaction to cancer cells based on the health status of the patient. *Patients never knew that they were injected with these cells and thus did not give consent.*
Willowbrook study (1960s)	Using a school for children with mental disabilities as a controlled setting in which to examine the effects of hepatitis, researchers injected all admitted children with the virus. Informed consent was obtained from parents; however, *there was no indication in the document that participation was voluntary and that a child's admittance was not based on the decision to participate or not.*
Tearoom trade study (1970)	Laud Humphreys researched the prevalence of male–male sexual activity in restrooms, then followed up with "participants" at their homes from contact information he obtained through license plate numbers. Although the intention of this dissertation was to better understand the lives of these men, Humphreys did not get his participants' consent. *Participants were not aware of the nature of the study, nor were they debriefed after data were collected.*

Source: Based on Wester (2009).

was primarily an informed consent issue, whereby potential participants were notified of relevant information about a study and the researcher, as well as the voluntariness of their participation in that project. *Beneficence* in this report combined elements of this meta-ethical principle as well as nonmaleficence (see below), whereby researchers were to avoid harm whenever possible and, at the very least, ensure that the participant benefits were maximized and harm was minimized. *Justice* refers to fair representation; specifically, individuals of dominant groups should not be overrepresented in a research design (nor should those individuals benefit unsystematically from its findings). Collectively, these principles indicate prominent ethical notions of autonomy, a thoughtful benefits–risks analysis for participants, and fairness in involving individuals of various groups and demographics (Christians, 2003).

The commission set forth regulations that helped to operationalize the Belmont Report. These regulations, known as 45 CFR 46 (Code of Federal Regulations, 2001), called for protection of human subjects for research that was federally funded in some manner (known as the Common Rule). As part of 45 CFR 46, **institutional review**

boards (IRBs) were created to review research applications and monitor federal compliance with aspects of the Belmont Report. In 1989, with the formation of the Commission on Research Integrity, IRBs also focused on issues of data fabrication and plagiarism (Christians, 2003).

Today it is common practice to have all research involving human subjects reviewed by an IRB, even though it may not be a federally funded study. In fact, many ethical codes require IRB approval of a project prior to collecting data (e.g., B.7.a. Institutional Approval of the ACA [2005] Code of Ethics).

What is an IRB? Although IRBs help to protect an institution (e.g., university, hospital, federal agency) from liability, their primary purpose is to protect human subjects. An IRB is composed of five members from an institution; these members should come from various disciplines and possess expertise in research, and there should also be a nonscientist and community member. Depending on whether a project crosses the minimal risk threshold (i.e., a study involves more than minimal risks for participants), a project can be exempt from review or need an expedited or full exemption from the board.

IRBs often carry a utilitarian agenda in terms of scope, procedures, and assumptions (i.e., research is seen as value-free). Adhering to a communitarian ethics approach to evaluating qualitative research practice, Denzin (2003) critiqued IRBs based on their primary adoption of the Belmont Report and its general disallowance of collaborative and participatory research designs. That is, the current IRB model assumes that all research fits into the Belmont criteria of beneficence, respect, and justice, which, despite their grand meanings, actually establish minimal guidelines. Denzin notes:

> Belmont principles, which focus almost exclusively on the problems associated with betrayal, deception, and harm, ... call for a collaborative social science research model that makes the researcher responsible not to a removed discipline (or institution), but to those he or she studies. [The feminist communitarian ethics model] stresses personal accountability, caring, the value of individual expressiveness, the capacity for empathy, and the sharing of emotionality ... [and it] implements collaborative, participatory, performative inquiry. It forcefully aligns the ethics of research with a politics of the oppressed. (p. 258)

Some of Denzin's arguments include the following:

- The current definition of research contends that a design is created to test a hypothesis, researchers are value-neutral, and human participants are turned into research subjects, which removes the essence of what it means to be human.

- Research is seen as event-based rather than process-based.

- The IRB often fails to see humans (participants and researchers) as social and complex creatures that are not value-neutral, anonymous subjects.

- Because beneficence is impossible to quantify, it is difficult to determine minimal risk.

- Respect for persons should go beyond the informed consent to include caring for, honoring, and treating the person with dignity.

- Justice extends beyond equal selection and benefits to society to include care, love, kindness, shared responsibility, honesty, balance, and truth.

- It is difficult or sometimes inappropriate to maintain participant anonymity, given the goals of qualitative research.

- IRB staff reject or are unaware of several qualitative research traditions.

- IRBs do not typically address research with indigenous people, espouse universal human rights, or regulate inappropriate conduct in the field (which should include a grievance process for participants).

With their more complex view of ethical practice (e.g., social ethics, communitarianism), qualitative researchers may come into conflict with what IRBs have traditionally viewed as ethical research. Waldrop (2004) added some concerns IRBs might have about qualitative inquiry based on traditional criteria. IRBs might contend that:

- Emotional expression during data collection can create unexpected psychological harm for participants.

- The fluid nature of qualitative research may pressure individuals who are selected to participate to feel coerced to continue participation, even when they perceive an intrusion of their privacy.

- The thick description of data collection and analysis compromises participant confidentiality.

- There can never be any real guarantee of the depth and scope of the project, including specific data collection and analysis procedures.

As qualitative inquiry gains prominence in clinical and education settings, researchers must remind IRB members that traditional ethical principles must be reconsidered, given the complexities of qualitative inquiry. This is particularly salient when you consider the conflict among ethics types (see Table 3.2 for a case example of communitarian ethics).

ETHICAL GUIDELINES IN CLINICAL
AND EDUCATIONAL DISCIPLINES

With the primary goal of promoting the welfare of others, ethical codes serve three key roles: (1) to establish ideal methods of practice and educate individuals within a discipline about sound ethical behavior, (2) to serve as an apparatus for accountability in situations where an individual has deviated significantly from an agreed-upon standard of practice, and (3) to guide improvements in practice (Corey et al., 2003). Even with the legislation, ethics codes, and IRB monitoring, ethical issues still occur, though to a lesser extent (Christians, 2003). As we increase qualitative inquiry, special challenges to utilitarian ethics are bound to occur.

There are many associations within clinical and educational settings, each having various specialty areas within that organization. With each division and subdivision of disciplines, codes for ethical practice abound. We highlight five codes of ethical conduct in this chapter, pertaining to counseling, psychology, social work, couple and family therapy, and education. In our discussion, we focus attention to codes that focus

TABLE 3.2. The PHAT Project: Ethical Tensions in Community-Based Research

The following material describes issues arising with an IRB for a participatory research project funded by the California Tobacco-Related Disease Research Program, the Protecting the 'Hood against Tobacco (PHAT) project (Malone et al., 2006):

The PHAT project was initiated in 2002 to address tobacco usage for two predominantly African American neighborhoods in San Francisco, based on community survey data indicating that approximately half of residents were smokers with half who believed that health and illness were beyond their control. The researchers wanted to engage in a project wherein participants were considered community partners who could assist in reducing the limits of single-cigarette sales at convenience stores. (State law prohibited sales of single cigarettes, and the availability of single-cigarette sales in these communities served as an obstacle to smoking cessation.)

The PHAT project began as exploratory focus groups among community members to assess their responses to tobacco industry marketing of cigarettes to African Americans. Based on their focus group participation, several African Americans agreed to serve as community partners and assist in designing the project further. Based on community surveys that confirmed the availability of single-cigarette sales and their connection to relapse, PHAT researchers and community partners were committed to assessing the proportion of convenience stores in their community that sold cigarettes in violation of state law.

IRB approval for an observational study was obtained; however, researchers and partners noted the impracticability of collecting data this way and resubmitted the proposal. The revised proposal outlined a procedure wherein the partners would approach a clerk to purchase a single cigarette. In the modified proposal, the researchers guaranteed that clerk confidentiality would be maintained at all stages of the research process.

The IRB at the researchers' institution did not approve the application, citing that the research partners were not viewed as co-researchers, and that they were placing store owners and managers in potential entrapment situations. In their appeal, the researchers defended the use of community partners and cited that store owners and clerks had a right to refuse sale of single cigarettes (an illegal activity). The appeal was reviewed by the university's risk management and legal departments, and the legal department stated that it could not approve any university "involvement in illegal activity" (the researchers pointed out that the sale, not purchase, of single cigarettes was illegal, and the university was not liable). The legal department determined that the IRB had final approval. A third request for IRB approval was denied, even though the researchers argued, with support of the state attorney's written opinion, that there was no risk of entrapment and that it was important for the university to respect the community's knowledge and skills in this type of research.

Interestingly, the community partners conducted the study without the assistance (and research expertise) of the university researchers. Unfortunately, the knowledge gained from the process could not be published or presented as an aspect of the PHAT project: The IRB holds the power for dissemination of research related to this project.

Source: Based on Malone, Yerger, McGruder, and Froelicher (2006).

specifically on research and publication issues, although other areas are mentioned as they relate to the practice of qualitative research.

Although there are parallels across codes, it is important to review the codes and standards for your particular discipline if it is not covered here. In addition, examine specialty areas and their ethical guidelines in relation to a broader discipline (e.g., American School Counseling Association guidelines within the American Counseling Association). Ford (2006) mentions two additional considerations when reviewing and adhering to ethical codes. First, codes present very general and often vague guidance on key ethical issues. Second, many codes and standards present several interrelated issues, such as informed consent and confidentiality, as if they were independent issues that can be solved simply by "looking up rules" for a particular issue. Finally, judgment of ethics is situation-specific, and thus codes of practice in counseling and education only frame these discussions. At best, standards of ethical practices for effective research are a work in progress. Thus, we believe it is important to think critically about ethical issues and review thoroughly codes across sections (and specialty areas) to formulate a more ethical and effective response.

American Counseling Association

The American Counseling Association (ACA) first published its code in 1961. After five revisions the current version of the *ACA Code of Ethics* was published in 2005. The code is organized in this manner: preamble and purpose, followed by eight sections (i.e., The Counseling Relationship; Confidentiality, Privileged Communication, and Privacy; Professional Responsibility; Relationships with Other Professionals; Evaluation, Assessment, and Interpretation; Supervision, Training, and Teaching; Research and Publication; and Resolving Ethical Issues). Ford (2006) noted that the ACA code provides more concrete guidance on practice issues. The ACA Code of Ethics can be found at *www.counseling.org/Resources/CodeOfEthics/TP/Home/CT2.aspx*.

American Psychological Association

The American Psychological Association (APA) was the first professional association to develop an ethical code. The first version, *Ethical Standards of Psychologists*, was published in 1953 and resulted from 15 years of committee discussions. The document has been revised six times, with the most updated (revised in 2002) one entitled *Ethical Principles of Psychologists and Code of Conduct*. The 2002 code is outlined as follows: preamble, five general principles, and 10 general ethical standards (i.e., Resolving Ethical Standards; Competence; Human Relations; Privacy and Confidentiality; Advertising and Other Public Statements; Record Keeping and Fees; Education and Training; Research and Publication; Assessment; and Therapy). The APA Ethical Principles can be found at *www.apa.org/ethics/code/index.aspx*.

National Association of Social Workers

Since its first published code in 1960, the National Association of Social Workers (NASW) has revised the code five times, although the 2008 revision reflects minimal changes to the 1999 code. The *Code of Ethics of the NASW* was developed on the foundational concept of altruism (Ford, 2006) and is presently organized in this manner: preamble; six general principles, including service, social justice, dignity and worth of a person, importance of human relationships, integrity, and competence; and six ethical standards. These ethical standards speak to social workers' responsibilities to clients, colleagues, and other professionals; settings and organizations in which they practice; themselves as professionals; the social work profession; and society in general. The NASW code of ethics can be found at *www.socialworkers.org/pubs/code/default.asp.*

American Association for Marriage and Family Therapy

The 2001 American Association for Marriage and Family Therapy (AAMFT) Code of Ethics includes eight ethical principles: responsibility to clients; confidentiality; professional competence and integrity; responsibility to students and supervisees; responsibility to research participants; responsibility to the profession; financial arrangements; and advertising. The AAMFT code of ethics can be found at *www.aamft.org/resources/ LRM_Plan/Ethics/ethicscode2001.asp.*

American Education Research Association

The American Education Research Association (AERA) put forth a code of ethics to guide the work of those conducting research in education settings, emphasizing the connection between research and education. The *Ethical Standards of the AERA* were first adopted in 1992, with a second and most recent revision in 2006. The code is divided into seven principles: Responsibility to Clients, Confidentiality, Professional Competence and Integrity, Responsibility to Students and Supervisees, Responsibility to Research Participants, Responsibility to the Profession, and Financial Arrangements.

KEY ETHICAL CONCEPTS IN QUALITATIVE RESEARCH

No matter the discipline, certain basic principles govern research with human subjects. In this section we describe six meta-ethical principles: autonomy, nonmaleficence, beneficence, justice, fidelity, and veracity. These principles lay the groundwork for several important components of ethical practice: informed consent, confidentiality, multiple relationships, and researcher competence. After reviewing the key concepts outlined in this section, see Case Example 3.1 on page 89.

Meta-Ethical Principles

Kitchener (1984) and Meara and colleagues (1996) identified six principles that have guided the development and revision of ethical codes for several disciplines (see Table 3.3 for a listing of these as well as communitarian ethics considerations). We briefly define the principles here and highlight ways in which they might apply to qualitative research. As you review these principles, you will likely believe it is important to apply them all, and apply them all well. Unfortunately, though, when we start to apply them at the same level in research design, conflicts arise. Each principle has its own "agenda," and thus ethical dilemmas, it could be argued, result when there is conflict in trying to

TABLE 3.3. Meta-Ethical Principles and Selected Ethical Codes and Standards

	ACA Code of Ethics (ACA, 2005)	APA Principles of Psychologists and Code of Conduct (APA, 2002)	NASW Code of Ethics (NASW, 1996/2008)	AAMFT Code of Ethics (AAMFT, 2001)	AERA Ethical Standards (AERA, 2006)
Autonomy	G.2.c. Student/Supervisee Participation G.2.d. Client Participation G.2.f. Persons Not Capable of Giving Informed Consent	Principle E 8.02 8.03	5.02 Evaluation and Research (g) Value: Dignity and Worth of a Person	5.3	Standard 5 (II)
Nonmaleficence	A.4.a. Avoiding Harm A.4.b. Personal Values G.1.d. Precautions to Avoid Injury G.1.f. Minimal Interference	Principle A Standard 3.04	5.02 Evaluation and Research (d, j)	3.9 5.1	Standards 6, 7, 8 (II)
Beneficence	A.1.a. Primary Responsibility	Principle A	1.01 Commitment to Clients 5.02 Evaluation and Research (i) 6.01 Social Welfare Value: Service	3.5	Standard 9 (II)
Justice	G.1.g. Multicultural/Diversity Considerations in Research G.4.a. Accurate Results	Principle D	6.04 Social and Political Action Value: Social Justice	3.12	Standard 7 (I) Standards 6, 7, 8 (II)
Fidelity	G.2.g. Commitments to Participants	Principle B	Value: Importance of Human Relationships	3.5 5.3	Standards 1, 2, 3, 4, 11 (II)
Veracity	G.2.b. Deception G.2.h. Explanations after Data Collection	Principle C	Value: Integrity	5.2	Standard 3 (II)
Communitarian ethics considerations	Introduction, Section G: "Counselors who conduct research are encouraged to contribute to the knowledge base of the profession and promote a clearer understanding of the conditions that lead to a healthy and more just society."	Principle E	Preamble Core values: service, social justice, importance of human relationships Ethical Standard Part 6	6.6 6.7	Standards 8, 9, 10 (II)

Note. ACA, American Counseling Association; APA, American Psychological Association; NASW, National Association of Social Workers; AAMFT, American Association for Marriage and Family Therapy; AERA, American Educational Research Association.

adhere to these moral principles in an equal manner. To complicate matters, ethical dilemmas (or conflict among these principles) arise in different ways depending on the topic, population, and setting. Thus, we believe that researchers must weigh for themselves the degree to which each principle "matters" in research design and process, given contextual information and personal and professional values.

Autonomy

Autonomy refers to the right of individuals to choose. In qualitative research, autonomy relates to participants' awareness of the voluntariness of research and thus their right to withdraw from participation without penalty. To operate fully autonomously, a participant must also be completely informed about the research request (and understand the implications of the information and his or her decision). It is difficult to facilitate individual agency, though, in cases of covert observational research, for example. Covert research, by definition, violates participants' right to autonomy (Murphy & Dingwall, 2001).

Nonmaleficence

Nonmaleficence is avoidance of harm, or "do no harm." In qualitative inquiry, researchers limit or prevent situations wherein participants experience undue harm during, or as a result of, the research process. Furthermore, James and Busher (2007) stated that researchers should engage in an *ethic of respect*, keeping individual participants from harm while engaging in research that is intended to benefit a larger community. Risks for harm are prominent in qualitative research: We immerse ourselves in participants' settings, invading their privacy and potentially inducing reactions such as anxiety, stress, or sadness. We ask much of their time and energy. We analyze data and present findings that often have been analyzed only by a research team. The list goes on. Given the often intense relationship in qualitative research, it is important to constantly monitor participant reactions and to refrain from allowing unnecessary risks for the sake of research.

The concept of minimal risk is the primary indication of nonmaleficence. What is minimal risk? According to the Code of Federal Regulations Title 45, part 46 (CFR, 2001), it "means that the probability and magnitude of harm or discomfort anticipated in the research are not greater in and of themselves than those ordinarily encountered in daily life" (Section §46.102, i). Where risk of harm exceeds this minimal level, the risk must be weighed against potential benefits of the research (Smythe & Murray, 2000). One can easily see how there can be tension between micro- and macro-ethics for this principle alone!

Beneficence

Beneficence means "doing good" for others. In qualitative inquiry, researchers are to maximize the benefits to individuals who participate in research. At the same time, qualitative researchers are to ensure that participants, and possibly the community at large, gain something valuable from the findings. Fisher (2000) extended Gilligan's work to research and describe an *ethic of care* as the accountability of a qualitative researcher to participants' needs in relation to interactions that occur during the re-search process. We as qualitative researchers, then, engage in work that "gives some-thing back" in a significant way.

Justice

Justice as an ethical principle promotes good equally for individuals from various groups, circumstances, and statuses. In essence, the principle of justice addresses voice and representation. Whose perspective do we privilege? The principle of justice urges us beyond simply maximizing benefits to include an intentional focus on the possi-bility of any risk that individuals of certain backgrounds are being left out, or even objectified, by a research design. Additionally, justice involves ensuring that findings derived from a disproportionate or unfair sampling process are not misapplied to cer-tain groups.

Fidelity

Fidelity refers to being honest, being trustworthy, and acting with integrity toward in-dividuals with whom we are working, whether in a practitioner or researcher role. It involves creating a trusting relationship. It is the extent to which we honor participants during research in a manner that maximizes trustworthiness (Haverkamp, 2005). In many cases, researchers hold greater power due to the dynamics of the research pro-cess. Haverkamp stated: "We must consider how we, as researchers, assume a fiduciary role in reference to our research participants. A fiduciary relationship is one of trust, in which one party with greater power or influence accepts responsibility to act in the other's interest" (2005, p. 151).

Veracity

The final meta-ethical principle discussed here, *veracity*, involves being truthful to indi-viduals we encounter, holding the relationship as a top priority. Veracity may be viewed as overlapping or as a precursor to fidelity: We cannot build a strong, trusting research-er relationship if we are not truthful with participants.

Informed Consent

Traditionally, **informed consent** has been viewed as a cornerstone of research whereby a researcher seeks permission from participants to collect data from them. In the discus-sion, the researcher describes the purpose of the research study and provides informa-tion about the researcher, the extent of participation, limits of confidentiality, and any foreseeable risks and benefits of participation and nonparticipation, and emphasizes the voluntariness of participation (see ACA Section 6.2, APA Principle 8.02 and 8.03, NASW Section 5.02.e, AAMFT 5.2, AERA II, B1). Furthermore, qualitative research-ers indicate in informed consent how and what data will be accessed and presented. Informed consent is an important ethical and legal concept that clearly identifies and outlines research activity and the rights and responsibilities of all parties involved.

We believe that there two elements of an effective informed consent process. First, the terms *capacity* and *comprehension* refer to having the functional cognitive ability to acknowledge one's rights and responsibilities as a research participant and to consider these as one makes and communicates choices to participate in a study, and understanding content-specific information of the document, respectively. ACA (2005) noted in their code:

> When a person is not capable of giving informed consent, counselors provide an appropriate explanation to, obtain agreement for participation from, and obtain the appropriate consent of a legally authorized person. (Section G.2.f)

NASW (1996/2008) added:

> When evaluation or research participants are incapable of giving informed consent, social workers should provide an appropriate explanation to the participants, obtain the participants' assent to the extent they are able, and obtain written consent from an appropriate proxy. (Section 5.02.f)

The second element, *collaboration*, refers to the ongoing process of informed consent, wherein the researcher and participant partner to discuss and negotiate the research relationship and process. Smythe and Murray (2000) recommended that qualitative researchers use **process consent**, whereby informed consent is viewed as an ongoing, mutually negotiated and developed activity. If used, specific procedures for process consent need to be outlined at the outset of the research.

There are several special considerations in qualitative inquiry related to the informed consent process. (After reviewing these, see Activity 3.2.) First, the research process is emergent; the design unfolds and changes based on changing directions of the study purpose or other design reflections. In quantitative research, there is often an assumption that informed consent is obtained at the outset of a study that is well planned with a definite conclusion. In qualitative inquiry, however, the beginning, end, and everything in between are nebulous at best. And, the degree of involvement is often unknown and more often quite involved. Due to the interactive and emergent nature of qualitative inquiry, individuals who agree to participate in interviewing cannot be guaranteed that a certain type of content will be discussed, or the length of time data collection may take. This nebulous quality can cause difficulty when presenting informed consent to participants, as well as addressing review committees (Van den Hoonaard, 2001).

The process of qualitative inquiry as egalitarian and in-depth also asks for a greater contribution from participants, often creating situations in which participants do not know to what they are consenting specifically (Miller & Bell, 2002). Haverkamp (2005) raises an important question of consent, given the emergent nature of qualitative inquiry: "How does one offer informed consent . . . in which the content cannot be specified beforehand?" (p. 148).

A second related issue is the potentially coercive nature of qualitative inquiry, given the often unknown course of the process. No matter the type of research, the process of obtaining informed consent is inherently hierarchical. Consent must be reviewed throughout the research process, particularly for individuals from vulnerable populations. Qualitative researchers take special care to note communication indicators of withdrawal of consent. Qualitative researchers continually reflect: Is coercion "worth it" to collect necessary data?

Covert research—data collection without the knowledge of the participant—is a third concern related to the informed consent process. Covert research is likely an aspect of observational research, particularly in naturalistic settings. If we told participants that we were watching for behavioral problems within the classroom, or disclosed that we were assessing the degree to which they discussed multicultural issues in an introductory counseling course, we would likely have very different and biased results! According to 45 CFR 46 (CFR, 2001), informed consent can be waived, or some aspects can be adapted or omitted, if "the research could not practicably be carried out without the waiver or alteration" (§46.116, c). APA, in Principle 8.05, noted that psychologists can dispense with informed consent if "only anonymous questionnaires, naturalistic observations, or archival research for which disclosure of responses would not place participants at risk of criminal or civil liability or damage their financial standing, employability, or reputation, and confidentiality is protected." NASW (1996/2008, Section 5.02.g) cautioned:

> Social workers should never design or conduct evaluation or research that does not use consent procedures, such as certain forms of naturalistic observation and archival research, unless rigorous and responsible review of the research has found it to be justified because of its prospective scientific, educational, or applied value and unless equally effective alternative procedures that do not involve waiver of consent are not feasible.

The final consideration relates to participant characteristics. Why do some agree to participate? Are there specific participant characteristics, and do these carry ethical concerns? Threats in participant selection are a concern no matter the research design; however, given the intensive nature of qualitative inquiry, you have to consider why individuals would commit to such involvement. Do they feel coerced? Do they want to put forth a certain agenda? Are they similar to others in the sampling frame?

Participant characteristics are also important relative to marginalized populations, as well as to those obtained through a gatekeeper or key informant. Miller and Bell (2002) noted that marginalized populations may be less likely to give formal consent. In addition, written consent can jeopardize relationships. Why do we identify certain individuals as key informants? Are certain, more powerful gatekeepers "volunteering" less powerful groups? Who is actually giving consent? Are gatekeepers excluding certain individuals?

 ACTIVITY 3.2. Who Is Consenting to What?

Murphy and Dingwall (2001) remind us that the rights of participants aren't protected simply because they signed an informed consent document. In fact, these documents probably more often protect the researcher.

Examining the four considerations of informed consent described in this section, debate both sides of this argument.

Use of Deception

A major issue related to informed consent is the use of deception. What constitutes deception can range from omitting minor information about the purpose of a research study to failing to disclose that research is being conducted at all. Deception may be warranted if there are provisions in the informed consent that allow the researcher to withhold information, assuming that the benefits of the research outweigh participant risks (Pettinger, 2003). In general, participants should not be deceived about aspects of research that would significantly influence their decision to participate (Smythe & Murray, 2000). ACA (2005, Section G.2.b) states:

> Counselors do not conduct research involving deception unless alternative procedures are not feasible and the prospective value of the research justifies the deception. If such deception has the potential to cause physical or emotional harm to research participants, the research is not conducted, regardless of the prospective value. When the methodological requirements of a study do necessitate concealment or deception, the investigator explains the reasons for this action as soon as possible during the debriefing.

APA (2002, Section 8.07) echoes these guidelines:

> Psychologists do not conduct a study involving deception unless they have determined that the use of deceptive techniques is justified by the study's significant prospective scientific, educational, or applied value and that effective nondeceptive alternative procedures are not feasible. Psychologists do not deceive prospective participants about research that is reasonably expected to cause physical pain or severe emotional distress

Should you decide to deceive your participants for the benefits of research, you will need to discuss the deception as soon as possible—usually during debriefing procedures (e.g., ACA, G.2.h; APA Section 8.08). Debriefing is especially important because it provides participants with an opportunity to withdraw data if they so choose. In covert research, the use of deception, and debriefing, is obviously trickier.

PROPOSAL DEVELOPMENT 3.1. Developing Informed Consent

If warranted, construct an informed consent document for your proposal, using the 45 CFR 46 guidelines (CFR, 2001). After completing a draft, reflect on the following items:

- Did I include all the necessary components of informed consent? If I have omitted certain elements, what is my rationale?
- To what degree are procedures for ongoing consent addressed?
- To what degree is deception a part of my study? How do I, if at all, deal with debriefing procedures?
- Who is protected by the document or informed consent process? Participants? The larger community? The institution?

Confidentiality

Confidentiality is linked to the informed consent process and relates to the client's right to privacy in the research relationship. Laws recognize the necessity of keeping personal and medical records confidential, and researchers are to keep these laws in mind as they conduct qualitative inquiry. For example, the **Privacy Rule** is a federal law that protects participants' health information and limits who can receive that information (Department of Health and Human Services, 1996).

The Code of Federal Regulations (1991) indicates that the only record that can connect participant identity to a research study is the informed consent document (see 45 CFR 46), and that great care must be taken to prevent a breach of confidentiality. To further protect participants' confidentiality, researchers may not need to offer a consent form to be signed, but rather review the form with participants, seek verbal consent, and note in the transcript that verbal permission was obtained. Then the researcher could provide participants with a copy of the informed consent document.

When our roles as practitioners and researchers become blurred, several constructs may be pertinent. Let's review some other terms related to safeguarding participant information:

• **Privacy.** Privacy refers to the basic human right of protecting an individual's worth, dignity, and self-determination. Individuals should not feel intruded upon by the research process. If a participant agrees to the research process, researchers must ensure participant comfort with, and safety in, the process.

• **Anonymity.** Research is truly anonymous only when participant identity is concealed from the researcher. Since researchers are primarily interviewing and observing participants directly, anonymity is seldom possible. And, given the nature of qualitative reporting, true anonymity is indeed a difficult task, given the depth and detail of reports. Confidentiality is often confused with anonymity; confidentiality refers to protecting an individual's identifying information (known to the researcher) from disclosure, and it must be maintained even if anonymity is not.

• **Privileged communication.** This term refers to the notion that confidential communication is protected within a judicial system, unless that right is waived by the individual. Depending on the state, you may have judicial protection should details of a research study be subpoenaed.

ACA (Section G.2.e) indicates that information obtained about research participants during the course of an investigation is confidential. Some cited exceptions include when there is danger to self or others (B.2.a and B.2.b) and court-ordered disclosure unless otherwise protected (B.2.c). Other relevant codes in disciplines pertaining to confidentiality include:

> Psychologists have a primary obligation and take reasonable precautions to protect confidential information obtained through or stored in any medium, recognizing that the extent and limits of confidentiality may be regulated by law or established by institutional rules or professional or scientific relationship. (APA, 2002, Section 4.01)

Social workers engaged in evaluation or research should ensure the anonymity or confidentiality of participants and of the data obtained from them. Social workers should inform participants of any limits of confidentiality, the measures that will be taken to ensure confidentiality, and when any records containing research data will be destroyed. Social workers who report evaluation and research results should protect participants' confidentiality by omitting identifying information unless proper consent has been obtained authorizing disclosure. (NASW, 1999/2008, Section 5.02, l, m)

Marriage and family therapists use client and/or clinical materials in teaching, writing, consulting, research, and public presentations only if a written waiver has been obtained in accordance with Subprinciple 2.2, or when appropriate steps have been taken to protect client identity and confidentiality.

Marriage and family therapists, when consulting with colleagues or referral sources, do not share confidential information that could reasonably lead to the identification of a client, research participant, supervisee, or other person with whom they have a confidential relationship unless they have obtained the prior written consent of the client, research participant, supervisee, or other person with whom they have a confidential relationship. Information may be shared only to the extent necessary to achieve the purposes of the consultation.

Information obtained about a research participant during the course of an investigation is confidential unless there is a waiver previously obtained in writing. When the possibility exists that others, including family members, may obtain access to such information, this possibility, together with the plan for protecting confidentiality, is explained as part of the procedure for obtaining informed consent (AAMFT, 2001, 2.3., 2.6, and 5.4).

Researchers are responsible for taking appropriate cautions to protect the confidentiality of both participants and data to the full extent provided by law. Participants in research should be made aware of the limits on the protections that can be provided. … Anonymity should not be promised to participants when only confidentiality is intended. … It should also be clear to informants and participants that despite every effort made to preserve it, anonymity may be compromised. Secondary researchers should respect and maintain the anonymity established by research participants. (AERA, 2006, II, B2 and B11)

Maintaining confidentiality in qualitative inquiry may be difficult in several instances. First, confidentiality becomes an ethical concern in qualitative data collection, management, and analysis. The nature of collecting depth and detail of personal stories places "risks" in breaching confidentiality. As Waldrop (2004) reported, "Qualitative data are, however, 'live,' encompassing tapes and transcripts of interviews as well as the researchers' notebooks and journals, all filled with purposefully thick and rich descriptions. Coding does not always remove identifying information" (p. 244).

There are several additional potential breaches of confidentiality. First, on-site research methods such as observations and interviews often complicate protection of participant confidentiality since there are often few, quite visible, individuals in a setting. Second, transcriptions provide another ethical concern when individuals external to the process are involved.

A second issue involves third parties. Examples of third parties might include counselors, teachers, administrators, parents, peers, gatekeepers, and key informants. Third parties in qualitative research are more likely to know that someone is participating in research given the intensive engagement involved. Qualitative researchers are charged with keeping information confidential, particularly from those whose interests conflict with the participants (DiCicco-Bloom & Crabtree, 2006). At the extreme, this may mean adapting the report to change particular site or demographic characteristics.

Third parties can also be harmed or have their privacy violated during data collection. When we interview participants, observe them in a setting, or even review documents and use other unobtrusive methods, it is quite likely that others will be mentioned in some manner. At times individuals may mention identifiable information about a third party in connection with sensitive issues. And, while we often ensure participant confidentiality on consent forms, we seldom include third parties (Hadjistavropoulos & Smythe, 2001). Haverkamp (2005) noted that third parties mentioned in transcripts, involved in observations, etc., are least likely to have their confidentiality protected because they are not direct research participants. It is imperative that qualitative researchers remember to mask their identities, even though they have not provided formal consent.

A final consideration related to confidentiality in qualitative research concerns researchers' duty to warn and protect in research settings when child or elder abuse or neglect is occurring. **Duty to warn and protect** is the ethical and legal responsibility to warn identifiable victims and protect others from dangerous individuals, or in some instances, from danger to themselves. All states have legal mandates for child abuse and neglect reporting, with several similar protections for elders (Williams & Ellison, 2009). In instances where researchers are serving multiple roles concurrently, such as a counselor or educator, they should follow state mandating laws as well as adhere to ethical standards of their profession (e.g., ACA, APA, Association for Specialists in Group Work, AAMFT, AERA). Although there are several articles that discuss duty to warn and protect in practice, there is minimal coverage of this topic in research settings. Additionally, major ethical standards do not specifically address the issue of duty to warn and protect in research settings.

Resnik and Zeldin (2008) provided some guidance for medical researchers serving solely in the role of researcher, which can be applied to practitioners. The researchers highlighted a controversial Maryland case finding in favor of families whose children were exposed to high levels of lead as a result of participating in a study of the effects of lead abatement in their housing complex. Resnik and Zeldin noted that the Maryland case highlighted the need for researchers to warn participants about residual effects related to the subject under study. Furthermore, they proposed the following ethical and legal guidelines when deciding on duty-to-warn procedures: (1) as health care professionals, researchers must report suspected abuse and neglect of children and other vulnerable adults living in the home; and (2) health researchers are not required to report "spouse abuse, domestic violence, recreational drug use, gambling or illegal immigrants in the home" (p. 215) unless they directly harm children or other vulnerable adults in living in the home.

Multiple Relationships

Practitioners who engage in qualitative research often do so because they want to collaboratively explore a phenomenon or they want to provide an opportunity for individuals who are typically "left out" of the research process. The term **multiple relationships** refers to having (1) more than one role with the same individual, (2) a role with an individual as well as with someone who is closely associated to that individual, or (3) a role with an individual with the intention of having a future role with that same individual or someone closely associated with that individual (APA, 2002). Multiple relationships in research involve blurring boundaries and roles to meet several goals: to improve practice, to better understand an individual, to expand knowledge, to empower an individual, to advocate and create political or institutional change—and the list goes on. The issue of multiple relationships is particularly important with culturally diverse groups. No matter our good intentions, though, there will be power issues related to possessing multiple roles and agendas. Conflicts of interest due to multiple relationships are nearly unavoidable because most qualitative inquiry occurs in naturalistic settings (Smythe & Murray, 2000).

In quantitative research, researchers are deemed ethical to the extent to which they protect participants by maintaining objectivity and clear boundaries, and by keeping researcher values out of the research process. ACA (2005, Section G.3.a) indicates that nonprofessional multiple relationships should be avoided. And, APA (2002, Section 3.5) asserts, "A psychologist refrains from entering into a multiple relationship if the multiple relationship could reasonably be expected to impair the psychologist's objectivity, competence, or effectiveness in performing his or her functions as a psychologist, or otherwise risks exploitation or harm to that person with whom the professional relationship exists." AAMFT (2001, 5.3) asserts: "Marriage and family therapists … make every effort to avoid multiple relationships with research participants that could impair professional judgment or increase risk of exploitation." NASW (1999/2008, Section 5.2, o) noted: "Social workers engaged in evaluation or research should be alert to and avoid conflicts of interest and dual relationships with participants, should inform participants when a real or potential conflict of interest arises, and should take steps to resolve the issue in a manner that makes participants' interests primary." Davison (2004) adds that carrying out practitioner and researcher roles is not mutually exclusive or facilitative, and that too much self-disclosure in the context of other roles can damage the integrity of the research design. Yet, isn't a feature of qualitative inquiry to collaborate and engage with a participant, sometimes disclosing information to establish rapport and gather a thick description of a phenomenon? How do we negotiate the functions of qualitative research with these ethical codes? With qualitative data collection, a great challenge for the researcher is to maintain the role of "ethical researcher" in the quantitative sense when qualitative inquiry typically requires establishing rapport and personal disclosure (Haverkamp, 2005).

An initial response may be that we cannot often avoid multiple relationships in qualitative inquiry. We have to manage them well. We provide some strategies for managing multiple relationships in Table 3.4 on the next page.

TABLE 3.4. Strategies for Managing Multiple Relationships in Qualitative Inquiry

- Discuss the nature of your roles with participants during the informed consent process.
- Document the reasons you believe that multiple roles are beneficial to research participants and the study itself. Continually reflect in a journal on these benefits in the context of minimal risk issues.
- Anticipate potential consequences of the multiple relationships and brainstorm ways you will work to minimize and/or remediate those consequences.
- Consult with colleagues should you or a participant be concerned about negative consequences.
- Consider the short- and long-term impact of being an insider, or studying your own group, as applicable.
- Assess any alternatives to engaging in multiple relationships for your study.

Researcher Competence

To be passionate about and to take on a research idea is an exciting adventure. To be competent to address the topic or engage in qualitative research in general can be an ethical dilemma. **Competence** refers to having the necessary training, skills, professional experience, and education to work with a population of interest in some capacity. When conducting research, practitioners need to determine if they have taken into account any special issues of the population and the corresponding necessary competencies, including training and specialty training (Hadjistavropoulos & Smythe, 2001). Various codes speak to the issues of acknowledging and expanding boundaries of competence:

> Counselors practice only within the boundaries of their competence, based on their education, training, supervised experience, state and national professional credentials, and appropriate professional experience. Counselors gain knowledge, personal awareness, sensitivity, and skills pertinent to working with a diverse client population. ... Counselors recognize their need for continuing education to acquire and maintain a reasonable level of awareness of current scientific and professional information in their fields of activity. (ACA, 2005, C.2.a and C.2.f)

> Psychologists provide services, teach, and conduct research with populations and in areas only within the boundaries of their competence, based on their education, training, supervised experience, consultation, study, or professional experience. ... Psychologists planning to provide services, teach, or conduct research involving populations, areas, techniques, or technologies new to them undertake relevant education, training, supervised experience, consultation, or study. (APA, 2002, Standard 2.01)

> Social workers should educate themselves, their students, and their colleagues about responsible research practices. (NASW, 1999/2009, Section 4.01)

> Marriage and family therapists, as presenters, teachers, supervisors, consultants, and researchers, are dedicated to high standards of scholarship, present accurate information, and disclose potential conflicts of interest (AAMFT, 2001, Section 3.5).

REFLEXIVE ACTIVITY 3.1.
Determining Your Research Competence

Consider the following:

- In what areas of qualitative research do I feel most competent?

- In what areas of qualitative research do I feel least competent?

- What clinical issues or phenomena do I have an interest in pursuing as a research agenda? To what degree to I feel competent to address that research topic?

- In what ways can I build my competency as a researcher for my research proposal?

- How will I manage times when my competence may be impaired during the research process (e.g., consultation)?

At times, practitioners may be harmed in some manner by the research process. Perhaps negative emotional reactions result from interacting with participants and hearing or observing their experiences. If so, it is important to reflect on this impairment and consider how it is impacting the research process and ultimately the participants involved.

CASE EXAMPLE 3.1. Katherine

Katherine is considering a multiple case study of the experiences of families with children involved in special education in a local school district. She has been a school counselor in the school district for 12 years and has worked with several special education students in her current school. In working with these children and their families, she noted that parents and guardians seemed to not be involved in the classroom. Katherine plans to conduct several interviews with the children and their family members to better understand their relationship with the school system. She hopes that her findings will provide insight into ways by which to increase family involvement.

- To what extent do you apply each of the six meta-ethical principles? How might they conflict with one another?
- What are some issues related to developing and securing informed consent?
- How might confidentiality be a concern?
- Does Katherine have multiple roles? To what extent do any multiple relationships conflict with one another?
- What areas of competence are important for Katherine to possess?

ADDITIONAL ETHICAL CONSIDERATIONS IN QUALITATIVE INQUIRY

This section highlights some additional ethical issues related to the above ethical concepts in designing, implementing, and reporting a qualitative study. Specifically, we address pertinent ethical issues in conceptualizing the study (e.g., research paradigms and traditions, research goals, and the role of the researcher), implementing the study (i.e., qualitative interviewing, Internet and online research, and working with vulnerable and marginalized populations), and reporting qualitative data. Furthermore, other parts of this text introduce other aspects of qualitative inquiry with ethical and professional implications. In Chapter 7 we introduce the term *ethical validation*, which refers to considering the qualitative research process as a moral and ethical issue (Angen, 2000). Every task in qualitative inquiry, from planning the study, to entering the field, to building relationships, to collecting and analyzing data, should be considered in the context of how it benefits individuals at the micro- and macro-level.

Conceptualizing the Qualitative Study

Several foundational and design aspects of qualitative inquiry—research paradigms and traditions, research goals, and the research relationship—are discussed here. These concepts are presented more fully in Chapter 2 and Part II of this volume.

Research Paradigms and Traditions

Participants should not be exposed to a design that is not sound because the benefits of the information obtained will never likely outweigh the risks to participants (Hadjistavropoulos & Smythe, 2001). A sound design involves selecting research paradigms and traditions that are suitable for the research purpose. The reasoning is that, if the design is not congruent with research goals, then the design may not be working in the best interest of those involved because participants may be placed at unnecessary risk during data collection and reporting.

There are ethical concerns working within any research paradigm, and researchers are to consider how the assumptions inherent in a paradigm could harm participants. Gillies and Alldred (2002) note a paradigmatic danger in claiming that there is an objective truth. Any claim to know an objective truth creates issues about knowledge and power, with an assumption that any generated knowledge that is labeled as universal is oppressive. Conceptualizing knowledge as a subjective construction between researcher and each participant (i.e., postmodernism) can highlight power imbalances in knowledge that may be implicit in positivistic and postpositivistic approaches. Brinkman and Kvale (2005) stated: "Qualitative researchers may nevertheless fail to be objective—ethically and scientifically—if they fail to situate their means of knowledge production in power relations and the wider cultural situation" (p. 165). However, as some argue, focusing too much on idiosyncratic findings may mask commonalities in experiences for typically marginalized groups (Gillies & Alldred, 2002). In addition to concerns with selecting a research paradigm, qualitative researchers should reflect upon how each research tradition and its assumptions create ethical dilemmas.

Research Goals

In Chapter 4 we present three types of research goals and discuss their role in topic selection and the development of a conceptual framework. Each goal has an agenda, and there are usually multiple goals in qualitative inquiry. Unfortunately, these goals relate to competing agendas among participants, researchers, funders, and the community at large. Although we make compromises given competing personal, scholarly, and funder goals, we as qualitative researchers as charged with doing what is best for participants. A researcher may then be faced with conflicting interests.

The goals or intentions of our research need to be readily acknowledged, given embedded political assumptions (Gillies & Alldred, 2002). Political views at the micro- and macro-level are to be acknowledged by all stakeholders involved in qualitative inquiry: It cannot be assumed that even those who share identities share similar political beliefs and intentions. Researchers need to carefully identify both policies and issues of particular, personal concern in their own research agenda and those in the community (Ebbs, 1996).

The Role of the Researcher

We see two key ethical issues with the researcher's role: researcher as instrument and researcher as a person who develops and maintains an appropriate researcher relationship relative to the research purpose. As Corbin and Strauss (2008) asserted, we cannot separate who we are from what we do in qualitative research. Haverkamp (2005) expanded on this report: "The researcher's values, personal history, and 'position' on characteristics such as gender, culture, class, and age are inescapable elements of this inquiry" (p. 147). Furthermore, "the researcher is continuously and simultaneously an observer and a subject in the research process. There is a constant awareness that the central research instrument in this context is a fallible, real, sensitive, fearful, fearing, anxious *person*" (Soobrayan, 2003, p. 118). The researcher as instrument may have both positive and negative ethical implications for the qualitative inquiry, and these implications all need to be considered when conceptualizing a research study.

In qualitative research the researcher relationship is the major conduit for collecting quality data as well as for understanding the study context. From an ethical standpoint, this is both a feature and a flaw: The more we create connections and thus stronger relationships, the more likely power comes into play. Both researcher subjectivity and neutrality can create ethical dilemmas.

Researchers observe and interpret data, often from their own frames of reference. Thus, researchers should constantly evaluate why particular participants, topics, or methods were selected, and how these might relate to personal interests. These reflections can indicate important data as well as help researchers avoid harming participants (Halbrook & Ginsberg, 1997). A hallmark of qualitative researchers is their ongoing reflections on how they as individuals influence the process and outcome of qualitative inquiry, and how research relationships reflect their professional selves (Haverkamp, 2005).

Power imbalances in research relationships are inevitable. Ebbs (1996) emphasized a necessary research bargain: Researchers create a reciprocal interaction wherein participants are very much a part of design decisions and how data are interpreted and reported. When we treat participants as great contributors to theory in education and social sciences, listening to and valuing their perspectives regarding a phenomenon, we are only beginning to address power imbalances.

Implementing the Qualitative Study

In this section we discuss ethical considerations in interviewing, conducting Internet and other online research, and working with vulnerable and marginalized populations. (Additional information about data collection methods can be found in Part III of this volume.) Table 3.5 at the end of this section provides key strategies to deal with many ethical considerations in this section.

Interviewing

When does interviewing, and often accompanying observations, become too intrusive? The interview process can involve an immersion in intense and difficult experiences—and thus often unforeseen emotional experiences—that may create psychological harm for participants (DiCicco-Bloom & Crabtree, 2006; Hadjistavropoulos & Smythe, 2001; Waldrop, 2004). Furthermore, Davison (2004) argues that the qualitative interview is even more intense than a clinical interview. Given this intensity, Hadjistavropoulos and Smythe (2001) recommended that researchers should screen potential participants as much as possible for specific vulnerabilities and be prepared to exclude those who might have significant difficulty with the interview process.

There are power imbalances inherent in interviewing, although interactive interviewing helps with this (see Chapter 8). Kvale (2004; as cited in Brinkmann & Kvale, 2005) presented some additional ethical challenges in the qualitative interview related to power imbalances:

- There is an asymmetrical power relation in the interview. The qualitative researcher defines, initiates, and dictates the interview. There is a research agenda as well as research goals. Even when the goal is to hear participant voices, researchers still dictate that focus.

- Interviewing is not a bidirectional process—interviewees don't typically ask questions.

- The interview is a means to an end. It is a tool to gather data according to a researcher's interests, not a goal in itself.

- It can be a manipulative dialogue, with hidden agendas on the part of the researcher or the participant.

- The researcher is privileged as the interpreter and reporter.

In addition to these considerations related to power, James and Busher (2007) add that generated information is often highly personal and creates situations that rely heavily on researcher veracity and competence.

Internet and Online Research

In Chapter 9 we discuss the use of the Internet and online data collection methods, and argue that the use of these methods often helps to improve access and data collection. In an effort to participate in research that reaches a variety of often underrepresented participants and transfers findings to the greatest number (i.e., transferability, see Chapter 7), researchers should consider the feasibility of traditional data collection methods and examine alternative methods such as the Internet and online research. Yet, how might the use of technology complicate individuals' right to privacy?

With the use of online methods, several ethical implications surrounding privacy and confidentiality ensue. Here are some issues with privacy and confidentiality that may result from online research:

- Anonymity of the Internet may also make it difficult to verify who is participating in research.
- E-mail correspondence can easily be forwarded or copied, unknown to the writer, to those outside a study.
- E-mail addresses often contain all or part of participant names.
- Individuals often are unknowingly a part of e-mail lists that a particular site or organization provides to researchers who pay for these lists, leading to unsolicited contacts and potential coercion to participate.
- "Lurking" can occur (participants observe but do not participate) and, although beneficial for covert observation, may be viewed as invasive.

It is important to note that there is great debate as to whether a sender of electronic data, or one who opts to join an online group, is considered to have a "right" to privacy, given the public nature of various online communications. Pettinger (2003) asks, are all online communities essentially public, or are there certain ones that warrant greater privacy? He argues that using the Internet and joining online communities are common occurrences with which many people are familiar, and that an individual could easily maintain his or her anonymity by using a pseudonym.

One way to address this question is to distinguish between data collected from private (e.g., e-mails, closed chat rooms) and those from nonprivate (e.g., bulletin boards) venues (Brownlow & O'Dell, 2002). However, these forums differ in degree of privacy. One way to consider if a participant is entitled to privacy is to look at the process by which he or she joined a list or online community. If the process involved less screening and few barriers to entry, there is likely less expectation of privacy. Conversely, if there are more requirements for participation and other confidentiality requests, you can assume that members might have more expectations for privacy.

Aside from issues of privacy and confidentiality, a challenge in online research involves the degree to which participants are able to engage in a mutual research process, including member checking. In face-to-face research when data collection is not anonymous, a downside may be the very social interactions that facilitate data could also pressure participants to distort their views in a socially desirable manner. Unlike face-to-face data collection (or at least methods that allow for verbal and nonverbal exchanges), participants completing research through digital means may not receive confirmation or affirmation that their responses are relevant or thorough responses (James & Busher, 2007). The lack of communication signals may greatly impact the depth, quality, and accuracy of data. James and Busher noted that webcams can be useful tools to maximize authentic and meaningful research interactions. Additionally, Sharf (1999) provided guidelines for researching online groups:

1. Consider whether the research purpose is in conflict with that of the group.

2. Reflect on whether the research will benefit the group.

3. Identify oneself, including role and intention, to potential participants.

4. Make an effort to contact directly those participants you plan to quote in a qualitative report.

5. Seek continual feedback from participants about the research study.

6. Be sensitive to boundaries, vulnerabilities, and privacy of individual members, as well as of the virtual community.

7. Consider those who may not have access to online methods and thus are not represented fairly.

Vulnerable and Marginalized Populations

Chapter 1 outlines a brief history of qualitative research. In the review we highlight several eras of history where qualitative researchers studied the "other," those with less power and representation, and fit findings into a dominant schema. When researching vulnerable or marginalized populations, it might be easy to reinforce a power imbalance and repeat history. *Vulnerable populations* include minors, prisoners, pregnant women, and those with mental retardation or mental disabilities (CFR, 2001). In this section we will highlight relevant literature for minors as well as for a marginalized group: families of lower socioeconomic statuses.

A significant aspect of researching vulnerable and marginalized populations is getting a handle on the outsider–insider debate. Loutzenheiser (2007) cited DuBois's concept of *double consciousness*, which assumes that a researcher who is a member of an underrepresented or vulnerable group (i.e., an "insider") can conceptualize a perspective from his or her own as well as from a dominant ideology and thus better represent it than a member of a dominant group (i.e., the "outsider"). Feminist researchers often attempt to represent experiences of oppression to challenge the status quo of women, and as such, there is question whether those outside a marginalized group can represent well groups with less power and influence (Gillies & Alldred, 2002).

Others (e.g., Narayan, 1993) note that whether you are an insider or outsider, there is no better perspective with which to conduct research. From a moral perspective, we cannot rely solely on those with less power and voice to speak on behalf of themselves (Gillies & Alldred, 2002); researchers of dominant statuses have an important role in taking what is co-constructed with those of nondominant statuses and helping them address social injustice. The key, according to Loutzenheiser (2007), is to critically analyze how one's power position relates to views of normalcy. Gillies and Aldred (2002) add:

First, the overall intention of specific representational research needs to be acknowledged and clarified in terms of what might be achieved by speaking for or about "others." Secondly, the researcher's position in relation to those whom she is representing
needs to be thoroughly explored, in terms of her own social, political, and personal
interests, and the assumptions she brings to her understanding of those she is researching. ... Thirdly, there needs to be careful consideration of the likely impact of
the "knowledge" produced, to ensure that it could not work against the interests of
those it seeks to represent, or against another group. (p. 42)

RESEARCHING MINORS

Voices of marginalized youth are underrepresented in research in general. It is important not only to engage in dialogue with this population for the sake of interactions, but
also to assume that minors are experts of their own experiences and thus have something of value to say to add to theory in education and social sciences (Loutzenheiser,
2007). Ireland and Holloway (1996) and Nelson and Quintana (2005) outline several
key ethical issues related to conducting research with minors:

- Children may be difficult to access.
- The research relationship is likely influenced by the context and setting sur-
  rounding the individual, which is largely outside the child's control.
- Children may feel powerless and consent to research when they are not alto-
  gether comfortable.
- Developmental issues, such as language development and attention span, can
  impact a child's power to be a part of the research.
- Developmental factors may inhibit the data collection process.
- The use of particular measures (interviewing, projective techniques, observations) can further intrude upon children's privacy.

Minors do not and cannot consent to research. Parents or guardians give proxy
consent for children. However, an ethical dilemma arises when the parent's consent is
not in the best interest of the child, or the child cannot understand in what he or she
is participating (Ireland & Holloway, 1996). An IRB will determine the methods for
obtaining assent if it is determined that minors are capable of providing assent, given
developmental, psychological, and other factors (45 CFR 46; CFR, 2001). In addition,
practitioners are to be cognizant of avoiding penalty for minors who withdraw from
research. For example, APA (2002, Section 8.04) notes: "When psychologists conduct
research with clients/patients, students, or subordinates as participants, psychologists
take steps to protect the prospective participants from adverse consequences of declin-
ing or withdrawing from participation."

The content of data collected from minors may also place them at risk. Such content can include illegal drug use, unsafe sex practices, and criminal behavior, to name
a few. It is imperative that qualitative researchers are careful to protect their young participants by ensuring that the data shared do not harm them. Sometimes this may mean
leaving out "great stories" that could reinforce negative stereotypes and/or jeopardize
their confidentiality (Loutzenheiser, 2007).

FAMILIES OF LOWER SOCIOECONOMIC STATUSES

Families of lower socioeconomic statuses have received little attention in the literature. Gorin, Hooper, Dyson, and Cabral (2008) identified several ethical issues when interviewing vulnerable families. These included use of insensitive language, lack of privacy, and intrusive data collection from families with traumatic histories. When families have experienced trauma, for instance, the qualitative researcher is to be prudent about using language that pathologizes their recovery or retraumatizes individuals (e.g., using the phrase *being safe* rather than *abuse* or *harm*). We have to be careful to not objectify the oppressed; we then become oppressive and thus research becomes harmful (Davison, 2004).

Gorin and colleagues (2008) also noted the importance, when interviewing vulnerable families, of attending closely to nonverbal cues that might indicate that participants were no longer interested in sharing data or, alternatively, when they were more motivated to share their stories. Furthermore, it is important to redress power imbalances between researchers and this population. This may be done by reminding participants that they are experts of their own experiences, as well as by giving them opportunities to shape the research process.

TABLE 3.5. Strategies for Minimizing Ethical Dilemmas in Qualitative Data Collection

- Maintain an ongoing informed consent process.
- Discuss in advance with members of the target group any issues that are sensitive and relevant to the consent process, to minimize the hierarchical nature of providing informed consent.
- Spend time learning about the populations and settings you are studying, particularly when research involves vulnerable populations (Waldrop, 2004).
- Form partnerships with community organizations and share power positions in research design decisions. As Waldrop (2004) states, "Be a good guest."
- Anticipate and plan, to the extent possible, potential participant reactions to content and process during data collection. For example, Waldrop recommended making a list of community resources available to participants.
- Combine both online and offline data collection methods to allow for depth, privacy, and authenticity of data. For example, consider using the Internet and online communities to recruit participants, but collect data offline.
- Whether using online or offline methods, create a process, whenever possible, in which participants can return data responses in an anonymous manner. Consider use of pseudonyms.
- Use trustworthiness strategies (Chapter 7) to assist in managing ethical dilemmas (e.g., reflexive journaling, member checking, triangulation of investigators, peer debriefing).
- Strike a balance between personalizing and distancing yourself from the research topic and setting.
- Remember to "give back" to participants. DiCicco-Bloom and Crabtree (2006) remind researchers to not exploit the participant for personal gain of data or access.
- Provide adequate protections for participants and third parties with respect to confidentiality.
- Do not approach participants by presenting a study as a method for them to gain self-awareness of the injustices they face, as this may be taken as patronizing and damaging and leave them feeling more vulnerable.
- Be aware of any previous experiences participants may have had with researchers. Whether negative or positive, seek to understand and value their experiences.

Reporting Qualitative Data

There is power in the qualitative report; it speaks volumes as to what is most important and from whose perspective (Brinkmann & Kvale, 2005; Soobrayan, 2003). Who gets to say what goes in it—or who has control of what and how data are presented (i.e., **narrative ownership**)? Well, usually the qualitative researcher does. Ethics codes only begin this conversation by indicating that, in general, researchers are to report findings "accurately":

> Counselors plan, conduct, and report research accurately. They provide thorough discussions of the limitations of their data and alternative hypotheses. Counselors do not engage in misleading or fraudulent research, distort data, misrepresent data, or deliberately bias their results. They explicitly mention all variables and conditions known to the investigator that may have affected the outcome of a study or the interpretation of data. They describe the extent to which results are applicable for diverse populations. (ACA, 2005, G.4.a)

> Psychologists do not fabricate data. ... Psychologists do not present portions of another's work or data as their own, even if the other work or data source is cited occasionally. (APA, 2002, Sections 8.10 and 8.11)

> Social workers should report evaluation and research findings accurately. They should not fabricate or falsify results and should take steps to correct any errors later found in published data using standard publication methods. (NASW, 1999/2008, Section 5.02, m)

> Educational researchers must not fabricate, falsify, or misrepresent authorship, evidence, data, findings, or conclusions. ... Educational researchers should attempt to report their findings to all relevant stakeholders, and should refrain from keeping secret or selectively communicating their findings. ... Educational researchers shoul communicate their findings and the practical significance of the research in clear, straightforward, and appropriate language to relevant research populations, institutional representatives, and other stakeholders. (AERA, 2002, I, B2, B6; II, B10)

A couple of issues arise: How do researchers know if a report is comprehensive? What constitutes accurate data? First, let's consider the comprehensiveness issue.

Should all or only parts of a report be shown to participants for their approval? There are several ways to negotiate what gets included in the report, and the degree to which participants will be involved in interpreting and selecting "meaningful" data. These decisions may be based on the research design itself, on the strategies for trustworthiness that are in place (see Chapter 7), and on the resources available to conduct the project. No matter what you decide, participants need to be informed at the outset that their narratives, even told from their perspective, will ultimately be presented through the researcher's perspective (Hadjistavropoulos & Smythe, 2001). Remember, the published report may affect relationships with your participants as well as a community, so this is a delicate issue. For example: "When researcher and participant are at odds in their narrative accounts of a given life experience, whose account is to be considered the more credible and on what grounds?" (Smythe & Murray, 2000, p. 326).

Murphy and Dingwall (2001) note: "Research participants may be wounded not only by what is contained in a report, but also by what has been left out: this may seem to treat as trivial or unimportant something which has great significance for them" (p. 341). How do qualitative researchers negotiate these risks to participants to present data in an authentic and rigorous, yet concise, manner? Sometimes the best we can do is tell the whole, rich truth, even if parts of the report contradict each other.

Another issue in ethical behavior involves data accuracy. Ethical issues in this arena involve data fabrication, use of fraudulent materials, omissions, and either intentional or unintentional false interpretation and reporting of findings (Christians, 2003). There are a couple of clear ways in which qualitative researchers may interpret and report data falsely (intentionally or not). First, we risk misinterpretation when we don't check data with participants (i.e., member checking) or other investigators (i.e., triangulation; see Chapter 7). Second, we act unethically when we fail to report our process through an audit trail. Since a qualitative report is often limited in scope by journal restrictions, the audit trail is an ideal place to "show your work" to participants, peers, and others in the community.

CHAPTER SUMMARY

This chapter outlined several key ethical constructs and issues in qualitative inquiry. Like many research ethics chapters, it covers some but not all dilemmas and raises many questions with few definitive answers. We have defined ethics and outlined several ethical concepts, including meta-ethical principles, informed consent, confidentiality, multiple relationships, and researcher competence. Furthermore, we have explored ethical dilemmas in conceptualizing, implementing, and reporting qualitative data.

We hope you will consider each of these areas and reflect on their interconnections in qualitative inquiry (see Proposal Development 3.2). Ethical issues and salient concepts should not be considered from a top-down approach, whereby the qualitative researcher simply examines material in this chapter in a compartmentalized fashion. Rather, it should be experiential and inductive, whereby the researcher continually reflects on ethical concerns with self and team, as well as with those being studied (van den Hoonaard, 2001).

RECOMMENDED READINGS

Christians, C. G. (2003). Ethics and politics in qualitative research. In N. K. Denzin & Y. S. Lincoln (Eds.), *The Sage handbook of qualitative research* (2nd ed., pp. 139–164). Thousand Oaks, CA: Sage.

Denzin, N. K. (2003). *Performance ethnography: Critical pedagogy and the politics of culture.* Thousand Oaks, CA: Sage.

Mauthner, M., Birch, M., Jessop, J., & Miller, T. (2002). *Ethics in qualitative research.* Thousand Oaks, CA: Sage.

Maxwell, J. A. (2005). *Qualitative research design: An interactive approach* (2nd ed.). Thousand Oaks, CA: Sage.

PROPOSAL DEVELOPMENT 3.2. Considering Ethical Dilemmas for Your Study

In the first column reflect on each ethical consideration for your study. How do you anticipate addressing each in your study? Next, consider how you think about and what you plan to do in your study in the context of the meta-ethical principles listed in the column headings. Which are in conflict with one another? In what ways? Which areas of your project present greater ethical dilemmas?

	Autonomy	Nonmaleficence	Beneficence	Justice	Fidelity	Veracity
Informed consent						
Confidentiality						
Multiple relationships						

	Autonomy	Nonmaleficence	Beneficence	Justice	Fidelity	Veracity
Competence						
Conceptualization/establishing research agenda						
Implementation						
Reporting data						

PART II

QUALITATIVE RESEARCH DESIGN

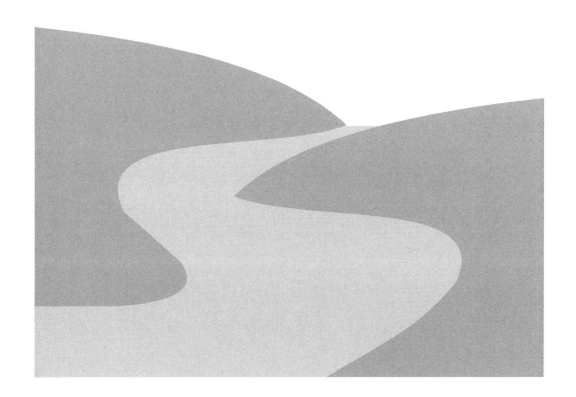

CHAPTER 4

Selecting a Topic

CHAPTER PREVIEW

Building on the discussion of research paradigms and traditions in Chapter 2, this chapter addresses the many interdependent considerations of selecting a topic in qualitative inquiry. These include (1) establishing research goals, (2) developing a conceptual framework, (3) writing a purpose statement, (4) determining a research question or questions, and (5) deciding if a mixed methods approach is more suitable (see Figure 4.1). Each consideration is addressed in major sections of this chapter. Topics such as case and unit of analysis, research purpose, literature review, and concept mapping are explored with respect to the five major considerations.

SELECTING A TOPIC

Ideas or research topics are *everywhere.* Selecting a general research topic is as natural as considering why you chose this career path. We have had experiences and interests that have led us to choose to become a counselor, an administrator, a special educator, and so forth. One student described choosing to become a high school administrator after, in his role as a high school teacher, noticing greater teacher attrition in predominantly urban schools. A natural research topic for him involved teacher retention. Thus, on a broad scale, your general topic can relate directly to your discipline itself. A good question to ask is, *What are you passionate about that led you to your profession?*

Sometimes it may be a combination of previous or current personal experiences that creates general areas of interests. As humans, we have a natural curiosity to understand things more clearly, particularly if we have a personal connection to a topic. For example, several colleagues have investigated the effects of trauma on social and academic performance after working with the American Red Cross with children in the aftermath of Hurricanes Katrina and Rita in 2005. Another colleague studies the longitudinal impact of autism in an effort to understand better the experiences of a family member.

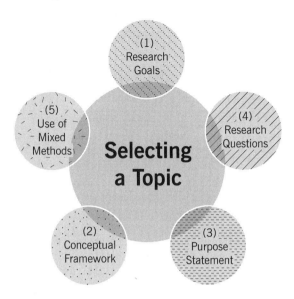

FIGURE 4.1. Considerations in research topic selection.

What may be obvious in selecting a general area of interest or research topic—whether personal or professional—is that *selecting a topic is not a neutral process.* There are likely personal and/or professional motivations underlying our interests, often based on our social interactions. We have assumptions about what *the* problem is and who might likely be influenced by it. It is important, then, to reflect on our interests and their origins. Ongoing analysis of a selected topic paves the way for a more rigorous qualitative research process. Perspectives 4.1 provides examples of how students selected their research topics for qualitative inquiry.

Once you have some idea of a general research topic, it is imperative that you refine your topic to make it more manageable. That is, what aspect of a larger issue can you tackle effectively in one study? The following are some general strategies for refining a research topic:

- What do you already know about the topic? Reflect on what you already know *personally* about a general topic. You may have some personal connection to a topic that can direct you to more specific areas of inquiry.

- Additionally, think about what you already know *professionally* about a general topic. What does previous research tell you about the topic? Conducting a thorough literature review is important to uncover areas or perspectives that could and should be explored.

- Brainstorm potential research questions from your general topic and consider how each question will be answered. Also, what do you think the answers might be? What specific audience perspective might be most informative for a specific question? Often, how you answer these questions is heavily influenced by your research tradition—a point to note.

- Creswell (2008) suggested drafting a brief or working title, or alternatively developing a brief question, for a study topic. He contends that this strategy, done early in the research process, serves as a road map for the research design process. We agree that this may be helpful as an initial step in determining research goals, conducting a literature review, and developing a sound conceptual framework.

- As you become more specific about your topic, consider if it can be researched. For instance, do you have the necessary resources to investigate the refined topic? Qualitative researchers need to consider how time, financial, and social resources impact their topic. How much time is necessary to collect and analyze data? How much money is necessary to complete the research, considering things such as travel and supply expenses? To what degree does access to the research population influence the quality of obtained data?

- Consider if the research topic is feasible. Even if you have ample resources, there may be ethical or professional barriers that inhibit a specific investigation. What might be some ethical and professional considerations related to your specific topic?

These strategies are discussed more fully throughout this chapter and other sections of this volume. Remember, whatever topic you select for qualitative inquiry will stay with you throughout the life of the study and beyond, so choose wisely. There is a significant time and energy (scholarly and otherwise) commitment to the selected topic. In the remainder of this chapter, we discuss these key considerations in topic selection: (1) determining research goals, (2) developing a conceptual framework, and (3) outlining quality research questions. Although these components are presented independently, they often co-occur in qualitative design because decisions in one area typically impact another.

●•

Perspectives 4.1. Selecting a Topic

"I have been interested in LGBTQ [lesbian, gay, bisexual, transgender, and questioning] issues in adolescents in the school system for quite some time, particularly in how these students are being supported and counseled. In my master's program, I did work on this topic and wanted to expand my own knowledge while discovering new ideas and offering information to the field. Narrowing the topic to a research project that was doable was the major struggle. I decided to focus on schools in a particular area and on the perceptions of school counselors—as it was more feasible to discuss the topic with adults than with minors in the school."

—Counseling Student

"As a special educator, my interest lay in the area of teaching functional academic skills to students with severe and profound disabilities. As I began to conduct a preliminary literature review on that topic, I was able to locate dozens of quantitative studies, which documented progress and/or compared effective intervention strategies. However, I was unable to locate any research that conveyed the educator's views on teaching these students academic content. Therefore, I decided the best way to approach this subject would be to conduct a qualitative study. The research study would involve

conducting a series of interviews with educators and administrators in order to ascertain their opinions regarding providing educational programming, based on an academic curriculum, to students with severe disabilities."

—Curriculum and Instruction Student

"I worked for 3 years in a university career center and provided career counseling to many international students. I noticed that they had different career needs than domestic students. For example, most international students are limited by their visa status as to where they can work, both during and after completing their education. I also noticed that the career development process of international students was different than many domestic students. For example, many international students did not go through a career exploration and decision-making process, but rather followed their family's expectations for their career. Because their experience of career development and needs were very different from domestic learners, career services did not seem to offer helpful/beneficial services to international students. I was tired of not being able to help this population when they came to my office. I selected a research topic of identifying vocational and psychological needs of U.S. international students from varying academic programs and student statuses. Some of the challenges of this inquiry include access to the population due to cultural barriers (e.g., language, unfamiliarity with social research or my research purpose in particular)."

—Counseling Student

"I had initially wanted to compare test scores for seventh-grade students in schools in two adjacent cities in which one city's students received comprehensive sex education and the other city's students received abstinence-only sex education. I became interested in the topic through my volunteerism with Planned Parenthood. I ended up having to switch topics, though, because a school district administrator who approves outside research would not give me approval. He said that the principals could speak to me if they wished but that the project would not have official approval. Yeah, right! When I called the principal in one of the cities to ask for an interview, he said that he "chose to forgo this opportunity." It definitely taught me to check accessibility issues BEFORE committing to a project—especially in qualitative studies where you can't just download spreadsheets but really have to get in there and talk to people who are getting told NOT to talk to you! I believe it was political, due to the controversial topic, because another student in our class got the go-ahead from the same administrator for another study she wanted to do."

—Urban Studies and Public Administration Student

"I want to study the experiences, expectations, and reactions of students in a graduate-level multicultural class. I have been personally and professionally connected to the topic as a multiculturally aware counselor. I value studies that support the influence of culture and diversity in our counselor education as a significant competence for counselors. I sense that we are still finding our way in teaching multicultural competence and therefore this subject is important to me on those levels. I have faced many challenges—finding research that relates to the experiences of students in a classroom, arguing or defending why I think their voice is one we as educators should listen to, as well as why I am approaching this study from a qualitative research approach rather than a traditional quantitative approach. I am currently struggling to identify whose voice and context I should focus on: instructor, student, those of minority or majority status, one or several university settings, current students or alumni, doctoral or master's-level students, and so forth."

—Counseling Student

RESEARCH GOALS

In Chapter 2, we considered 14 qualitative research traditions commonly used in counseling and education. Even in collapsing them into five clusters, the decision of which tradition (or traditions) to frame your study can be cumbersome! To help with that decision, sometimes it is helpful to consider the research goals. A research goal is a *broad plan for achieving a desired result that considers what data need to be obtained, based on the needs of all those involved in the qualitative inquiry.* Maxwell (2005) noted that there are three kinds of research goals—personal, practical, and scholarly—and it is imperative to reflect on what motivates you personally to conduct a qualitative study, what need or objective you want to meet, and what intellectual understanding you want to obtain about a topic, respectively. Your research topic can address any of these three goals, although the latter two are often deemed more justifiable in qualitative inquiry and thus more germane to the task of developing research questions (discussed later in this chapter). Maxwell noted five scholarly goals (Items 1–5) that can benefit three practical goals (Items 6–8):

1. Understand the *meaning*, for participants in the study, of the events, situations, experiences, and actions in which they are involved or engaged.

2. Understand the particular *context* within which the participants act, and the influence that this context has on their actions.

3. Identify *unanticipated* phenomena and influences, and generate new, "grounded" theories about the latter.

4. Understand the *process* by which events and actions take place.

5. Develop *causal explanations*.

6. Generate results and theories that are understandable and experientially credible, both to the people you are studying and to others.

7. Conduct formative evaluations that are intended to improve existing practice rather than simply assess the value of the program or product being evaluated.

8. Engage in collaborative or action research with practitioners or research participants. (pp. 22–24)

With an understanding of the three primary goals for research goals, let's move on to additional aspects to consider in developing these goals. Key questions in determining research goals are:

- What is the case to be investigated?
- What is the purpose of the inquiry?
- What type of information is sought?

What Is the Case?

Think about the case in which you are interested. A **case** is the focus of our study and can be an individual or individuals, setting, process, or event (Miles & Huberman,

1994). In addition, cases have boundaries around them in that they can be explored as a unique and independent entity. Although a case could be potentially classified as all four of these types (i.e., individual, setting, process, and event), it is likely that one form of case best exemplifies an area of inquiry. In determining a case, it is helpful to ask: What or whom am I spotlighting? How do decisions I make in my qualitative research design affect (and are affected by) that case?

An *individual* case is specifically focused on one or a few informants with a distinct purpose of gaining information about them personally. An individual case may be a particular person, group, couple, or family, for instance. A *setting* case would attend to characteristics of a site, such as an agency or a classroom. A researcher may be interested in an individual or individuals within that setting to inform the study, yet the primary goal is to learn about that setting. Researchers exploring *process* cases are primarily interested in phenomena and the content and dynamics surrounding those phenomena. Finally, an event may be viewed as significant by qualitative researchers in counseling and education disciplines. Thus, an *event* case would isolate an event and study it from multiple angles and perspectives. Individuals, settings, and processes inform our knowledge of the event. Table 4.1 provides examples of each of the four case types.

The term *unit of analysis* is often used interchangeably with case; however, it has a slightly different meaning. As mentioned in the previous two paragraphs, a case can take on several forms: individual (e.g., person, group, couple, family), setting, process, and event. A unit of analysis is the "angle" or perspective toward a case. Qualitative researchers can use various units of analysis to study a case. VanWynsberghe and Khan (2007) likened the relationship between unit of analysis and case to that between a

TABLE 4.1 Examples of Types of Cases in Qualitative Inquiry

Case type	Study reference	Study description
Individual	Palmer, K., & Shepard, B. (2008). An art inquiry into the experiences of a family of a child living with a chronic pain condition. *Canadian Journal of Counselling, 42,* 7–23.	The purpose of the study was to examine the experiences of the chronic pain sufferer and her family members through art making. The case was one family (father, mother, two children) with one 6-year-old child with chronic pain. Within six 60–90-minute in-home sessions, family members were interviewed and asked to complete art images.
Setting	Wolkomir, M., & Powers, J. (2007). Helping women and protecting the self: The challenge of emotional labor in an abortion clinic. *Qualitative Sociology, 30,* 153–169.	This study focused on difficulties with balancing personal and professional needs for abortion clinic workers in a particular clinic. The setting was the abortion clinic.
Process	Jones, R. E. J., & Cooke, L. (2006). A window into learning: Case studies of online group communication and collaboration. *Research in Learning Technology, 14,* 261–274.	The purpose of this study was to explore how collaborative communication tools could be used to understand student learning. The process studied was that of how students learned, and their online discussions were analyzed to uncover learning methods as they communicated with one another.
Event	Daud, R., & Caruthers, C. (2008). Outcome study of an after-school program for youth in a high-risk environment. *Journal of Park and Recreation Administration, 26,* 95–114.	The purpose of this study was to evaluate which components of an after-school program promoted positive social and academic outcomes in youth from high-risk environments. The event was the program itself.

defense lawyer and the perspective he or she presents (unit of analysis) to a jury during a trial (case):

> A defense lawyer could choose a variety of types of evidence in defending his or her client, including the life history of the accused, the mental state of the accused at the time of the crime, the circumstances of the crime, the networks and associations of the accused, and even specific cultural aspects of his or her life. … As evidence continues to be gathered in the construction of this case, the unit of analysis is further delineated, and the case becomes more refined. (p. 7)

What Is the Purpose of the Inquiry?

Now that you have an idea of what type of case you are interested in exploring, consider what type of information is most important to you. One of the first steps in the research process is getting clear about the research purpose. That is, in what types of outcome are you most interested? Identifying the purpose of your inquiry early in a proposal will facilitate the development of meaningful research questions (Haverkamp & Young, 2007; Patton, 2002). There are four major types of research you can pursue, each with a different purpose. These four can be considered to fall on a continuum, with theory development on one end and social action on the other end. Most often, research begins with more general findings and is eventually applied to specific populations and problems.

The first type, **basic research**, serves to expand the scope and depth of knowledge of a case for the sake of contributing knowledge to a particular discipline. **Applied research** often builds upon collective findings of basic research and seeks specialized knowledge about a specific problem in order to intervene in it. For example, basic research endeavors may yield a clearer understanding of the etiology of eating disorders, whereas applied research may use that knowledge as a foundation to study how to treat African American females with eating disorders. The third type, **evaluative research**, assesses the effectiveness of a program or intervention throughout its course. There are two common forms of evaluative research: *formative evaluation*, which examines the practices used throughout a program or intervention in an effort to improve and shape it, and *summative evaluation*, which assesses the outcomes at the end of the program or intervention. Using the eating disorders topic as an example, let's say that a 4-week psychoeducational program was employed in a school of predominantly African American students to educate females about the prevalence and potential causes of eating disorders. Examples of formative evaluations might include interviewing females after each week to explore their knowledge of the topic and administering screening tools to assess for the presence of correlates of eating disorders (e.g., depression, anxiety). Based on these weekly data, program effectiveness would be monitored and changes to the program would be made to address the needs of the students accordingly. A summative evaluation might involve administering a posttest to assess knowledge, attitudes, and behaviors related to eating disorder symptoms. The fourth type of research, **action research**, seeks to engage individuals in solving specific problems. That is, the researcher focuses on a specific site, collaborates with individuals who have a connection to the topic, and works to resolve key issues to improve the lives of those at the site. As one can surmise, evaluative research could be an important component of action research,

---

TABLE 4.2. Four Purposes of Research

Basic research

- Gain knowledge for the sake of knowing
- Build theory and test existing theory
- Publish findings in scholarly journals and books
- Attend to the rigor of the study (validity, accuracy, and integrity of the results)

Applied research

- Investigate generalizability of the results
- Apply knowledge gained to human/societal problems
- Use knowledge to intervene
- Share findings with policymakers, directors of human service organizations, and those working with the problem
- Limit results to a specific time, setting, and condition/problem

Evaluation research

- Evaluate the effectiveness of solutions and interventions to human/societal problems
- In formative research: improve a specific program while it is in progress
- In summative research: investigate the effectiveness of the program after it has been completed

Action research

- Seeks to solve specific community, program, or organizational problems
- Investigates problems specific to a particular group, setting, and time
- Focuses on fostering change
- Actively involves participants in research
- Mirrors researcher's social values

Sources: Haverkamp and Young (2007) and Patton (2002).

---

specifically if the evaluative methods are geared to a particular site or problem. Table 4.2 highlights key points regarding each of the four purposes in research.

Some of the research traditions discussed in Chapter 2 correspond to particular types of research. For example, if you are interested in action research, a PAR tradition may be congruent with your research goals. A grounded theory tradition may be suitable for basic research, whereas an ethnographic or phenomenological tradition may be appropriate for applied research, and so on. As you decide on a tradition and related paradigms most suited to your research topic, be sure that they are congruent with your research goals, and vice versa.

In determining your research purpose, it may be helpful to reflect on *who your audience is*, or *who will be most impacted by your findings*. What outcomes are you most interested in, and for whose benefit? Those who are most affected would be considered your *primary audience* (e.g., students, clients). In basic research the primary audience may be other professionals in your discipline, whereas in action research the primary audience may be individual clients, students, or teachers, to name a few possibilities. As we move along the continuum from theory to action, the primary audience tends to become more specific. If you are interested in theory development, you are more likely interested in a group rather than specific cases such as in action research.

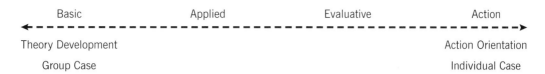

FIGURE 4.2. Determining your research purpose.

There may be others who hold interest in your study and who need to be considered in selecting a research topic. These who are indirectly affected by specific findings would be considered a *secondary audience* (e.g., prospective students, family members of clients). This type of audience varies depending on the purpose of your research and needs to be addressed in some manner in all aspects of the research process. Figure 4.2 shows the relationship between type of research and audience type.

What Type of Information Is Sought?

Another consideration in conjunction with the purpose of the research is the *depth* and *scope* of your research topic. Are you interested in studying a topic, such as eating disorders, intensely for a specific subpopulation (depth)? Or are you interested in studying the topic at a broader level, such as across various populations (scope)? Obviously, there is a trade-off of resources here. Researchers have to choose how they want to use their time and financial resources when studying a topic in more detail. The greater the degree to which you intend to study a topic in depth, the less likely you are to cover the scope or breadth of the topic. Therefore, it is important to consider whether your interests and resources for completing a research study lean more toward depth or scope and what the limitations of that bias may be for your overall findings.

PROPOSAL DEVELOPMENT 4.1. Topic Selection

1. Write down two to three general research topics that you would be interested to investigate as a qualitative inquiry.

2. For each general topic, brainstorm subtopics that would be interesting. What do you already know, personally and professionally, about each subtopic?

3. Consider each subtopic and its initial supporting evidence. (*Note:* You may find that your initial topic needs to be tweaked as you develop a conceptual framework, discussed below.) What research goals do you intend to address for each subtopic? What case will you investigate for each subtopic? What is the purpose of each subtopic? In what outcomes are you most interested and for whose benefit?

4. Outline the benefits and challenges of each subtopic in relation to the feasibility of your study. What are the necessary resources and participants needed to study each subtopic?

5. Discuss your general research topic and subtopics with your peers.

6. Decide on a tentative research topic for the qualitative proposal.

CONCEPTUAL FRAMEWORK

In addition to identifying research goals and selecting a general research topic, another component is developing and revising a conceptual framework throughout the research process, also referred to as a *theoretical framework* or *idea context*. Establishing a detailed conceptual framework will assist you in refining your research topic and in creating a clear purpose statement and sound research questions.

Maxwell (2005) described a **conceptual framework** as a network of concepts, theories, personal and professional assumptions, exploratory studies, and alternative explanations that collectively inform your research topic. He identifies four major sources of a conceptual framework:

- *Experiential knowledge.* This component is composed of the qualitative researchers' assumptions, expectations, and biases regarding the research topic in general and the interconnections among concepts more specifically. Experiential knowledge, also known as *researcher bias* (Maxwell, 2005; Patton, 2002), *critical subjectivity* (Reason, 1994), and *reflexivity* (Corbin & Strauss, 2008), is discussed further in Chapter 6. Corbin and Strauss also use the term *sensitivity* to refer to an "ability to pick up on subtle nuances and cues in the data that infer or point to meaning" (p. 19). Sensitivity, then, is the skill of using our insight—informed by previous knowledge and experience—to become more "tuned in" to the data and arrive at an understanding of what the data are telling us. "Background, knowledge, and experience not only enable us to be more sensitive to concepts in data, they also enable us to see connections between concepts" (p. 34). In sum, experiential knowledge may be positive or negative and must be carefully reflected upon when we are developing and revising a conceptual framework.

- *Prior theory and research.* This component, also referred to as the *literature review*, typically comprises the preponderance of the conceptual framework. However, when there is little theory or research available for a topic, this may be a very minor component of the conceptual framework. The literature review is described more fully in the following major section of this chapter.

- *Pilot and exploratory studies.* In preparing a conceptual framework, some concepts may be derived from pilot and exploratory studies you have conducted on the research topic. The purpose of these types of studies is to develop an understanding of the concepts and theories held by the individuals you are investigating, also referred to as **in vivo codes** (Corbin & Strauss, 2008). Pilot and exploratory (or open-ended) studies are a good idea for developing an accurate picture of the "middle range" theory of your research topic. A *middle range theory* refers to one that is firmly situated in the data, rather than a "grand theory," which might purport an interpretation of the data that is universal. These concepts can be added to the initial conceptual framework. You may want to differentiate the concepts from pilot and exploratory studies from those of previous theory and research in your conceptual framework.

- *Thought experiments, "waving the red flag," and the "flip-flop" technique.* Corbin and Strauss (2008) discuss using these techniques as useful for developing theoretical sensitivity during grounded theory analysis. However, we believe that these three techniques can be used to help you develop your conceptual framework as well. Thought experiments can inform developing a conceptual framework. After articulating their conceptual frameworks, it is imperative that qualitative researchers rely on research team members and/or colleagues outside the inquiry to critically analyze their work. A thought experiment is a strategy that you can use to test or develop your and others' ideas about alternative ways that concepts and assumptions can be connected to describe your research topic. It is imperative to think of several possibilities that explain and relate concepts other than the initial conceptual framework or model. "Waving the red flag" refers to the process of identifying researcher biases and assumptions and how these influence interaction with the phenomenon of the research. Using this technique in developing a conceptual framework would translate to identifying how your research assumptions are shaping the framework of your study. Using the "flip-flop technique" in developing a conceptual framework involves comparing opposites or extremes in order to identify salient aspects of the framework that may not be readily apparent.

As you can gather from this description, developing a conceptual framework goes beyond simply conducting a literature review. Doing only the literature review may leave invaluable personal and professional resources untouched. Qualitative researchers have several unique personal and professional experiences that provide assumptions and hunches about concepts that may be related to their overall topic. In addition, we often work in research teams to strengthen the research process, and additional team members provide divergent views on the research topic.

It is important to note that a conceptual framework for a qualitative inquiry is tentative and may change throughout the process of data collection and analysis. That is, qualitative inquiry is, in its very nature, interactive and is influenced by changes in the research questions, access to specific data sources, selection of data collection methods, and views of various research team members and participants. Case Example 4.1 demonstrates a conceptual framework of a study examining cultural issues in clinical supervision (McLeod, Chang, Hays, Orr, & Uwah, 2011).

CASE EXAMPLE 4.1. Conceptual Framework: Attention to Cultural Issues in Clinical Supervision

McLeod, A. L., Chang, C. Y., Hays, D. G., Orr, J. J., & Uwah, C. J. (2011). *Attention to cultural issues in multicultural supervision: Supervisors' and supervisees' perspectives.* Manuscript under review.

The following material outlines important components that created a conceptual framework that led to assessing the following research question using a phenomenological tradition: How is attention to cultural issues experienced in supervision?

Experiential Knowledge

- The researchers were licensed professional counselors, and all had completed coursework and attended numerous workshops related to achieving competency in multicultural counseling.
- All researchers had completed didactic coursework in counselor supervision and had provided counselor supervision for 1–4 years.

- Some of the researchers' assumptions regarding the role of attention to cultural issues in supervision included the following: (1) the definition of culture should be expanded beyond race and ethnicity; (2) it is important to be active in addressing cultural issues when serving as counseling supervisors; (3) constructive attention to cultural issues will benefit the supervisory relationship and the supervisee's level of multicultural competence; (4) supervisors and supervisees will perceive attention to cultural issues in supervision differently; and (5) supervisors of color and female supervisors may be more attentive to cultural issues in supervision.

- This component was continually reflected upon as researchers continuously monitored their expectations and assumptions through regularly scheduled research team meetings and independent journaling.

Prior Theory and Research

This component comprised several areas of prior literature:

- Importance of giving attention to multicultural competence in counseling in general and supervision more specifically
- Definition of multicultural supervision
- Review of available empirical research on multicultural supervision, which included two broad categories of research: (1) investigating supervisor multicultural competence and (2) presenting supervisors' and supervisees' perspectives of positive and negative experiences regarding attention to cultural issues in supervision and the impact of these experiences on supervisory relationships and outcomes.
- The researchers found several limitations of prior research in their review: (1) Only one study assessed both supervisor and supervisee experiences with multicultural supervision; (2) most studies focused solely on race and ethnicity as cultural issues to be addressed in supervision; and (3) participants often received mailed questionnaires for assessing retrospective accounts of supervisory experiences.

Pilot and Exploratory Studies

There were no pilot or exploratory studies conducted for this research. Thus, this component was not included in the conceptual framework.

Thought Experiments

- The research team analyzed the data and then met to discuss their independent findings. In these meetings team members presented alternative models to challenge the assumptions of the findings initially identified. An auditor external to the study also challenged emerging models and theoretical frameworks to strengthen the final presentation of findings.
- Throughout this process the research team identified biases and compared salient components of the selected model.

Literature Review

A literature review presents "what we already know" about a topic. It involves gathering, reading, and synthesizing prior research on a particular topic (Moore & Murphy,

2005). It provides a snapshot of what studies in a general topic area have been found, summarizing key findings and highlighting major limitations or "holes" in the literature most related to your research topic. That is, a review of the literature sets the proposed research in context, frames it within what has already been done, and provides a rationale for the current investigation. There are some qualitative approaches (e.g., grounded theory) for which a literature review may not be necessary in advance of the study.

Wiersma and Jurs (2009) articulated the value of performing a literature review. Specifically, it (1) limits and identifies the research problem and the expectations of findings, (2) informs the researcher about what has been done, (3) provides possible research designs and methods, (4) suggests possible modifications to avoid unanticipated results, (5) identifies research gaps, and (6) provides a backdrop for interpreting research results. We diverge from Wiersma and Jurs's opinion that there may not be a need, in qualitative research, to "avoid unanticipated results," since qualitative research findings often offer the researcher unexpected results to integrate with identified themes. This unexpected aspect is a natural part of qualitative inquiry, in our view.

Conducting a literature review also provides two other main advantages. First, a sound literature review helps to justify the need for your specific study. Second, it can be source of data that builds or tests theory related to your topic. Qualitative researchers should be cautious, though, in two areas: (1) relying too much on existing theory without critical analysis of it or (2) not using existing theory enough to inform their topics. For example, McLeod and colleagues (2011; see Case Example 4.1 on pages 113–114) conducted a thorough literature review of available empirical research on multicultural supervision since 1988. In their review, they carefully analyzed each study's findings and noted methodological limitations in order to identify a preliminary theory of multicultural supervision.

Qualitative inquiry poses unique considerations when conducting a literature review. Due to the nature of qualitative research as exploratory and emphasizing missing voices in the literature, qualitative researchers may find that there are limited studies available on a particular topic. This may be quite different from quantitative approaches for which many studies are available and are suited for hypothesis testing and more deductive approaches in general.

Second, there must be great thought given to the depth to which a literature review is to be done prior to conducting a qualitative inquiry. On one hand, conducting a comprehensive literature review allows us to identify more confidently the gaps in research as well as collective limitations of previous research. On the other hand, having this knowledge from a comprehensive literature review risks confounding the data analysis. That is, the more we know about what already has been found, the more likely we are to "see" phenomena in a similar manner. We recommend that you begin with some review of previous research as well as consult the literature on an ongoing basis as you identify themes for your study.

Third, how a literature review is conducted is often influenced by the selected qualitative research tradition. For example, the more a tradition relies on experience and theory formulation (e.g., grounded theory, phenomenology), the less likely previous literature will guide the study. Because these traditions are primarily inductive and refer to generating theory for often unexplored topics, it makes sense that there may be little previous literature to frame the study. For those traditions that rely on symbols, text, or cultural context (e.g., narratology, ethnography, symbolic interaction), you will likely provide a more thorough literature review to help familiarize the reader with some background of a particular text or culture.

The qualitative research tradition also influences when previous literature is presented in a qualitative report or proposal. In preparing a qualitative report, Creswell (2008) identified three uses of a literature review. The first use involves relying on it to establish a rationale for a particular topic; available literature is presented in the beginning of a report with a primary emphasis on demonstrating why a topic needs to be investigated. The second use of literature is the traditional review, or use of a separate section of the report to discuss in-depth the various factors or constructs associated with a research topic. This use is common in positivist or post-positivist approaches. The third usage presents the literature at the end of a report to couch present qualitative findings. With this final method, the literature typically does not direct the qualitative inquiry, a characteristic common of more inductive approaches.

Speaking to research goals in general, the three components of establishing research goals discussed earlier in the chapter (i.e., case type, purpose, type of information sought) have specific implications for the role of previous literature. Table 4.3 presents a guideline indicating degree of reliance on previous literature based on research goals.

Moore and Murphy (2005, p. 120) cite questions to help you shape and determine the scope of the literature review needed for a particular study:

- What knowledge does the current research contain, and who are the leading authors, recognized experts, and researchers in this area of study?
- What different definitions, concepts, and issues are relevant to this topic?
- What changes have been made in the subject's research over the past few years?
- What are the different and sometimes conflicting theories in this topic area?
- What are the key points of disagreement in the existing literature?
- What are the unanswered problems in the literature, and what attempts have been made to address them?
- Where is the future research on your topic headed?
- What is your own research's place in the field?

TABLE 4.3. Research Goals and the Use of Previous Literature				
	Increasing reliance on previous literature			
Case type	Individual	Process	Event	Setting
Purpose	Action	Evaluative	Applied	Basic
Information	Depth			Scope

We present these questions to stimulate you to think broadly about your literature review—especially because we know that beginning qualitative researchers may or may not have acquired this learning. However, we also want to remind you as the reader that these are initial suggestions and that ultimately one must be flexible in determining your degree of reliance on previous literature and the bodies of knowledge you select to review, which we discuss further below.

Strategies for Conducting a Literature Review

There are two major steps involved in conducting a literature review: selecting specific pieces of literature to include in the review and the actual writing of it (Wiersma & Jurs, 2009). Various strategies are associated with these two steps, and the following material is not intended to be exhaustive. A study idea examining dating violence attitudes among adolescent and young adult females is used to elaborate on several of these strategies.

First, create a list of keywords for your general research topic. Use this list to help you narrow the scope of what you are researching. Specifically, what areas related to your research topic do you *really* want to address in the literature review?

Where do you go for information? Your library is an important resource for you in obtaining data sources, either in person or through virtual means. Most libraries provide orientation workshops and written materials describing their services as well as how a researcher could go about locating specific data sources. It is also important to know your library's resources online and how to gain access to them. Familiarize yourself with library databases. Search engines such as EBSCO Host, First Search, ProQuest, and Cambridge provide several electronic research databases with access to abstracts and often full-text articles, books, papers, and monographs. Table 4.4 lists some of the more common electronic databases used in counseling and education. This list provides access to initial data sources related to your research topic. Also, it is important to expand your search beyond databases specific to your discipline.

Individuals in your discipline are also an invaluable resource for locating data sources. Make time to speak with your peers, colleagues, professors, and others you trust to guide you to pertinent literature. As you are locating literature, they may also be helpful in guiding you in gathering data that may be most relevant to your research topic. Requesting references for books, papers, and articles within the past 5–7 years, as well as original, seminal works, is most beneficial.

The Internet can be an important resource, although you should use it with caution. Because there is a vast amount of information available, often from noncredible websites, you should carefully review the legitimacy of any online document and seek outside opinion. Your librarian, professor, or colleague can provide you with lists of important and credible websites related to your research topic. Some Internet sources that we recommend, depending on your research topic, are listed in Table 4.5.

There may be useful data sources that do not immediately come to mind for you. For example, it may be helpful to begin with secondary sources when you are less familiar with a general topic. Examples of secondary sources include textbooks and encyclopedias. Secondary sources are invaluable for citing seminal articles or works and primary sources. Another data source is dissertations and theses. Graduate students

TABLE 4.4. Electronic Databases

Academic Search Complete	1887–present; provides a multidisciplinary database with selected full-text articles for approximately 1,000 journals.
Dissertation Abstracts	1861–present; author, title, and subject information for most U.S. dissertations. Some information about theses since 1962 is available.
Dissertations and Theses	1861–present; contains a comprehensive database for dissertations and theses. Selected full-text sources.
Education Research Complete	1984–present; references for all levels of education and all educational specialties. Selected full test is provided for over 900 journals and 100 books, monographs, and conference papers.
Education: A Sage Full-Text Collection	1982–present; although coverage varies by journal; contains over 5,000 articles in education, assessment, counseling, and school counseling published in Sage journals.
ERIC	1966–present; Internet-based digital library of educational research by the Institute of Education Sciences.
Medline	1965–present; provides medical information for various health care disciplines. The database was created by the National Library of Medicine.
Mental Measurements Yearbook	1985–present; reviews English-language assessments covering educational skills, personality, career, psychology, and other related areas.
PsycARTICLES	1894–present; contains full-text articles from the American Psychological Association journals.
Psychology: A Sage Full-Text Collection	1982–present; provides psychology-related articles from approximately 30 journals published by Sage Publications.
Psychology and Behavioral Sciences Collection	1965–present; contains selected full-text articles covering topics such as psychiatry and psychology, mental processes, anthropology, emotional and behavioral characteristics, and observational and experimental methods.
PsycINFO	1887–present; contains selected full-text articles from psychology and other related disciplines.
Social Sciences Citation Index	1956–present; indexes journals and specific articles across social science disciplines.
Social Services Abstracts	1979–present; provides abstracts of research in social work, human services, and related areas.
Tests in Print	Current; contains test information for commercially available tests in the English language.

TABLE 4.5. Internet Sources for Research	
American Counseling Association	*www.counseling.org*
American Educational Research Association	*www.aera.org*
American Psychological Association	*www.apa.org*
Bureau of Labor Statistics	*www.bls.gov*
Centers for Disease Control and Prevention	*www.cdc.gov*
FedStats	*www.fedstats.gov*
Library of Congress	*www.loc.gov*
National Institutes of Health	*www.nih.gov*
Substance Abuse and Mental Health Services Administration	*www.samhsa.gov*
U.S. Bureau of the Census	*www.census.gov*
U.S. Department of Education	*www.doe.gov*
U.S. Department of Justice	*www.usdoj.gov*

write countless dissertations and theses to fulfill degree requirements, yet may not publish these manuscripts in journals or other resources.

Organization is key as you collect pertinent literature. First, summarize individual empirical and conceptual works that relate to your topic in a detailed and organized manner. Then, develop an organized system for recording the important information about each data source. This creates a reference system that can be used in the future to expand upon and refine your conceptual framework.

For each data source that you include, be sure to write down a complete reference in addition to specific notes and the significance of the study. A complete reference includes the title of the data source, author name(s), publisher and publication date, page numbers, journal title, and volume and issue numbers if applicable. Software programs such as EndNote®, RefManage® (Thomson Reuters, n.d.), and Refworks® may be helpful in creating an electronic reference system. Table 4.6 provides an example of a reference system for a study examining clinical diagnosis.

After you collect several data sources, Creswell (2008) recommends constructing a **literature map**—a figure, table, or flowchart, perhaps—that visually organizes themes of prior literature. The primary purposes of the literature map are to help you remain organized and to give you new ideas about the literature itself or future research directions. This graphic can be considered a variation of the concept map, discussed below. There are three proposed models for literature maps. The first model, a hierarchical structure, funnels prior literature from most general to most specific with a primary goal of a top-down presentation, ending with a specific rationale and proposed study.

TABLE 4.6. Reference System for an Empirical Article

The following case study was included in a literature review of diagnostic strategies among mental health practitioners. Following the citation, an example for developing a reference system is provided.

O'Byrne, K. R., & Goodyear, R. K. (1997). Client assessment by novice and expert psychologists: A comparison of strategies. *Educational Psychology Review, 9*(3), 267–278.

Type of data source:	Empirical article (qualitative case study)
Keywords:	*Counseling* and *assessment*; *expertise*; *counseling psychology*
Rationale:	To examine cognitive processes used by expert and novice psychologists during a diagnostic task, how they each select and employ case features to formulate clinical impressions. (Do they differ in the amount and type of client information they seek?) Novices are more likely to place greater than necessary emphasis on superficial aspects of a particular problem and mistakenly interpret irrelevant aspects of the problem (i.e., focusing on initial vs. deeper/covert presentations of a problem).
Method:	14 clinical and counseling psychology students early in their doctoral studies (novices) and 14 PhDs working at counseling centers (peer-nominated as experts). Participants were presented individually with an incomplete case of a hypothetical client and asked what additional information they would like to elicit from the client. Their questions were matched to 1 of 39 questions developed during a pilot (with flexibility to develop new categories of questions).
Results:	Participants' expertise level affects both the amount and type of information they seek. Novices focused more on "crisis-oriented" aspects of the case. There was no difference between the two groups in their confidence in their assessments.
Implications:	Additional research is needed to examine how the clinical judgment process may interact with expertise.

Figure 4.3 presents an example of a hierarchical literature map. The second model, a flowchart, might present prior literature along a timeline, with more recent studies toward the right side of the chart. The third model, similar to a Venn diagram, displays areas of research represented by distinct circles. The circles might intersect, indicating future research directions. Figure 4.4 presents an example of this third model.

In addition to the strategies for conducting the literature review, there are several general strategies associated with the actual writing of it. No matter what type of data sources you use to when conducting a literature review, it is important to avoid plagiarism as well as to limit the use of direct quotes. The *Publication Manual of the American Psychological Association* (APA, 2010) warns about these two issues explicitly. To balance these two requirements, consider if you are able to rephrase the article or book content in a unique way. If you are unable to paraphrase the content, be sure to limit the word count of direct quotes. Perspectives 4.2 on pages 122–123 provides our approaches to writing the literature review.

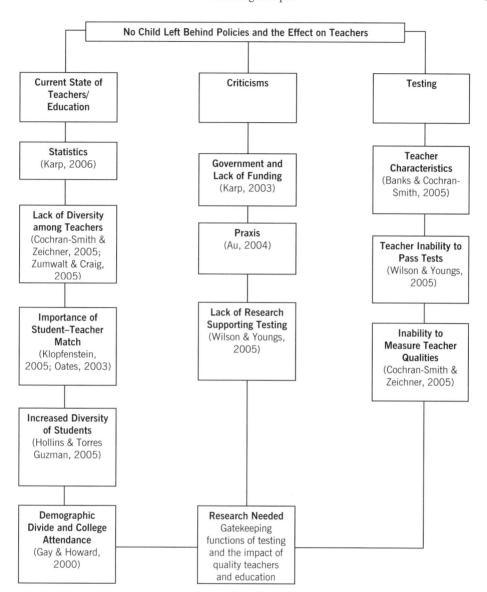

FIGURE 4.3. Literature map example: Hierarchical literature map. This literature map depicts Selwyn (2007), a conceptual article that examines the impact of No Child Left Behind (NCLB) policies on teacher education programs and the impact of testing on the teacher workforce.

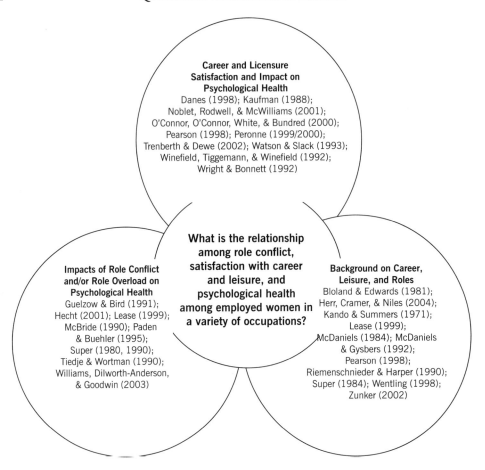

FIGURE 4.4. Literature map example: Venn diagram. This literature map is a Venn diagram of Pearson's (2008) empirical investigation of role overload, job satisfaction, leisure satisfaction, and psychological health among employed women. The primary research question is located in the center of the diagram.

Perspectives 4.2. *Writing the Literature Review*

"Having an organized reference system really helps me look at a snapshot of each data source related to my research topic. With these snapshots I collapse the literature into broad themes, setting literature aside that no longer seems relevant to my research topic. Then, I create a detailed outline of how the literature review will funnel into a sound rationale for a study. Once I have this outline, I can set writing goals and deadlines.

"I primarily write for a couple of hours per day, usually at the same time each day. My writing goals typically involve working on one section of my outline at a time. After completing an initial draft of my literature review, I create a literature map to assess visually how the literature flows from broader concepts to a more detailed rationale that frames my research questions and research paradigm and tradition. I then compare this literature map with my evolving conceptual framework and integrate the two into a more final draft of the introduction of an article."

—*DGH*

"Once I have identified an area of research, such as resilience and child sexual abuse, I conduct a literature search and identify articles that will be necessary for my literature review. I spend a good amount of time reading each article and summarizing the authors' main points, in addition to my own reactions to the article in terms of what I see as its unique contributions and/or limitations. I then create a literature map of the introduction to my study, which becomes a more solid outline for the manuscript. If I am working with a strict page limit, I may even include the number of pages I will allot to each section of my outline in order to keep the manuscript concisely written.

"Similarly to Danica, I write regularly at the same time each day. I write best in the late morning, so I try my best to make sure I do not schedule meetings or other appointments during this time period. My mantra for writing is: 'If I say "yes" to this appointment, then I am saying "no" to my writing!' This helps me set and maintain boundaries around my writing. Now, I look forward to my writing time—especially since I know it is a time I have all to myself without distractions."

—AAS

••

Concept Maps

Concept maps can be quite useful in displaying the components of a conceptual framework graphically. A **concept map** is a visual display of an evolving theory, or at least your assumptions, about an area of inquiry. The idea is that your concept map shapes how you collect data and changes as you analyze data. Concept maps are used in qualitative research because they are useful in displaying a large amount of information in a simpler way; they can be presented linearly or systemically. Researchers typically design concept maps to be read top-down. Qualitative researchers often develop maps with different colors to differentiate among conceptual framework components.

In general, concept maps can be categorized as variance or process maps (Maxwell, 2005). **Variance maps** depict causal links or relationships between particular constructs or variables. **Process maps** are context-specific and tell a story about specific events or situations rather than variables. In many cases the most important component of concept maps is the use and direction of arrows, which typically are used to connect nodes (or circles) to describe a process or sequence that is part of a research topic.

Maxwell (2005) and Miles and Huberman (1994) described concept maps as representing any of the following: (1) an abstract framework, (2) a flowchart of states and/or events, (3) a causal network of variables, (4) a tree-like diagram, or (5) a Venn diagram presenting concepts as overlapping circles. An abstract framework is a graph that presents the relationship between concepts. Figure 4.5 on the next page presents an example of an abstract framework of the common components of assessment tools measuring intimate partner violence (see Hays & Emelianchik, 2009, for more information on this qualitative study).

A flowchart can be helpful to show sequence of events or processes in education and clinical settings. Figure 4.6 on page 125 demonstrates a flowchart of how the contents of this textbook are presented.

Concept maps can also represent causal networks, or links among variables and influences. Causal networks involve significant independent and dependent variables or constructs and include directional plots (Miles & Huberman, 1994). Figure 4.7 on page

125 presents an example of a causal network of the influence of a mentoring program for graduate students in education disciplines.

A tree-like diagram has a vertical display of nodes starting with a broad concept with "branches" representing subconcepts. Figure 4.8 on page 126 provides an example of a treelike diagram. Additionally, the literature map in Figure 4.3 on page 121 provides a variation of a tree diagram.

Researchers represent the final type of concept map, a Venn diagram, by using overlapping nodes or circles. The degree of overlap among the circles indicates the relative strength of the relationship among the concepts. Figure 4.4 on page 122 presents an example of a Venn diagram.

Concepts maps have several advantages. First, they can structure your literature review, as in the case of literature maps described in the previous section. Second, they can help you make decisions about other aspects of your research design. That is, examining what existing literature and any exploratory studies have done in the way of research design can help you select data collection sources (e.g., interviews, documents) as well as help you identify what type of sampling method and how many informants would be useful for your study. You can also gain information about previous studies' limitations and validity issues, helping you make better decisions about your design. Third, concept maps help you visually see any assumptions you may have about

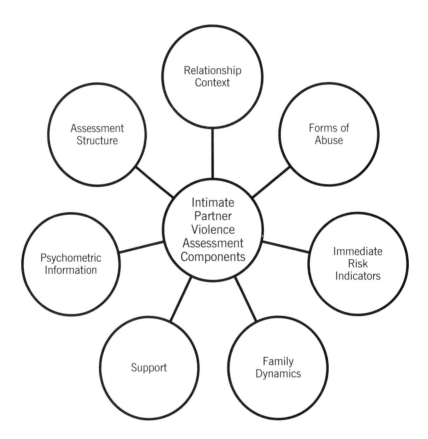

FIGURE 4.5. Abstract framework of assessment tools measuring intimate partner violence.

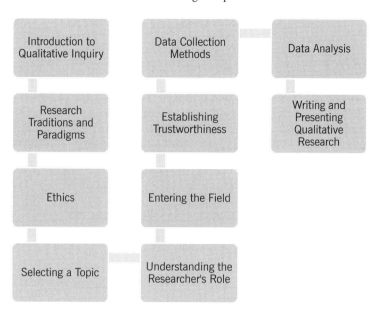

FIGURE 4.6. Flowchart of *Qualitative Inquiry in Clinical and Educational Settings.*

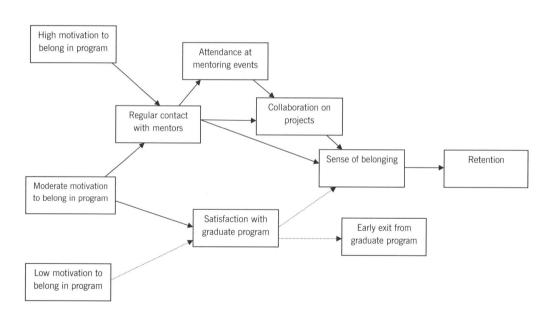

Note. (——▶) Direct causal relationship; (┈┈┈▶) Inverse causal relationship

FIGURE 4.7. Causal network.

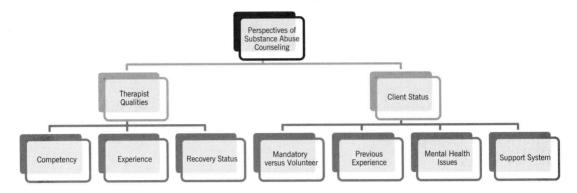

FIGURE 4.8. Tree-like diagram.

the research topic in general. By including your experiential knowledge as a component of the conceptual framework and thus the concept map, you are able to see the proportion of your "theory" regarding a topic that is based on experience only and thus needs empirical support.

Finally, concept maps are very useful for depicting an emerging theory as data are collected. Many qualitative researchers develop an initial concept map and further revise it as they collect more literature as well as gather data. You may find that it is helpful to construct a concept map before data collection and analysis begin, develop independent concept maps based on independent informant perspectives, and then integrate informant perspectives and the initial conceptual framework as one concept map. This final map would indicate a more defined theory related to your research topic.

PROPOSAL DEVELOPMENT 4.2. Developing an Initial Concept Map

This exercise has been adapted from Maxwell (2005) with permission from Sage Publications.

1. Write your preliminary research topic on a blank sheet of paper.

2. What are the keywords related to this topic? This list of keywords may come from the literature, personal experiences, professional experiences, or all of these.

3. For each keyword, brainstorm all the things that might be related to it. You may want to place an asterisk next to terms that are derived from experiences but perhaps not yet researched.

4. Review your list of keywords and related terms. Are any of the terms overlapping and perhaps could be collapsed as one new term? What are some connections you see between the keywords? What are some concrete examples of these connections?

5. Draw a concept map using different colors to indicate what is research-based and what is from experiential knowledge.

6. Examine how nodes (circles) are connected, such as the types of arrows that connect them.

7. Have your peers review your initial concept map and challenge your connections (i.e., thought experiments).

PURPOSE STATEMENT

Once your research topic has been refined, it is time to develop a purpose statement for your qualitative inquiry. The point of a purpose statement is to anchor the proposal or study; it is where the conceptual framework and research design meet. Creswell (2003) notes that the "purpose sets the objectives, the intent, and the major idea of a proposal or a study. This idea builds on a need (the problem) and is refined into specific questions (the research questions)" (p. 88). Sometimes beginning researchers confuse the purpose of research with the research questions. A well-constructed research purpose statement should situate your *interest* in the topic or phenomenon, whereas your research questions situate the *actions* you will take regarding your research purpose. Hopefully you can see that although your research purpose and research questions are separate concepts, both should complement and inform each other.

Although purpose statements obviously vary in the literature, there are some common components and guidelines that frame them (see Creswell, 2008). (See Proposal Development 4.3 on the next page to practice developing a purpose statement.) First, purpose statements are best displayed in a separate paragraph following the conceptual framework. Second, provide as much information about the selected research paradigms and traditions as possible. This will allow readers to better understand the values and assumptions upon which you, as the researcher, relied to structure the research topic and overall research design. Some examples in which the terminology of the purpose statement corresponds to the research tradition are (Haverkamp & Young, 2007): "to explore underlying processes" (grounded theory), "to describe the lived experiences" (phenomenology), "to uncover the plots within stories" (narratology), "to describe beliefs, values, and practices of a group" (ethnograhy), or "to learn about a problem to affect change in that problem." If you are using a mixed methods approach (discussed later in this chapter), be sure to note if the design is sequential, concurrent, or transformative.

Third, focus on one phenomenon in your statement and keep the statement open, without suggestion of a particular outcome. For example, the following purpose statement would be neutral: "The purpose of this case study is to explore the expectations of third-grade mathematics teachers for male and female students." Finally, operationalize words in the purpose statement based on those definitions derived from the literature. In the previous sentence, the concepts "expectations," "third-grade mathematics teachers," and "students" need to be operationalized. Case Example 4.2 provides an example of a former student's purpose statement, a reminder that you should keep in mind the context in which research purpose statements are written. For instance, if you were writing a qualitative research purpose statement for a grant committee, you would not use words such as *ontologically* or *epistemologically*, as are used in the Case Example 4.2.

CASE EXAMPLE 4.2. Purpose Statement Example

The research will aim to develop understanding of the psychological factors, environmental factors, and relative differences of American and British culture that significantly influence expatriates' acculturation strategies. The study will employ a phenomenological research tradition, which will reveal the "essence" of the lived experience of the phenomenon of acculturation by examining individual and collective meanings. These meanings can be amalgamated to explain the essence of a shared experience (Patton, 2002). The paradigm for the research will be social constructivism. Ontologically, it is assumed that culture exists only as an individually perceived phenomenon, and therefore there is no objective reality or "truth" of acculturation and perception of American culture by participants. Epistemologically, it is assumed that the uniformly known meaning "out there" of one particular culture is socially constructed; therefore, the study's method of gaining knowledge will be through an iterative construction of meaning and experience by participant–researcher interaction.

The understanding and experience of acculturation is an extremely personal and reflexive phenomenon. Because the axiology of social constructivism states that researcher values cannot be excluded and should not be excluded, sharing of participant and researcher values will be emphasized for the purposes of developing a shared understanding. In this sense, the researcher will also be considered a participant. A primary reason for the appropriateness of the social constructivist paradigm is the assumption that the participants—including the researcher—will have a limited understanding of their own experiences with respect to the research questions. The study will therefore be idiographic and the findings will be emic in character (Ponterotto, 2005). A hermeneutic dialectical method can therefore be adopted (Guba & Lincoln, 1989) as the primary mechanism of constructing "lived experiences," the first part of which is determination of life experiences using traditional phenomenological interviewing on an individual basis. A key assumption underlying the social constructivist paradigm, when it is employed in phenomenological research, is that the participant cannot fully understand his or her individual lived experiences without engaging first in a dialogue about the experience.

Reflect on the following:

- What do you notice about this purpose statement?
- How does the student attend to research paradigms and traditions?
- To what degree is the purpose statement neutral?
- To what degree are the key terms defined in the statement?
- How would you approach this purpose statement differently?

PROPOSAL DEVELOPMENT 4.3. Writing a Purpose Statement

In one to two paragraphs, develop a purpose statement for your refined research topic. Attend to the following components:

- Discussion of research paradigm(s) and related philosophical influences (i.e., ontology, epistemology, axiology, rhetoric, methodology)
- Description of research tradition(s)
- Neutrality
- Operationalization of key terms
- Attention to a single phenomenon

Review your purpose statement with a peer.

RESEARCH QUESTIONS

In the qualitative proposal, a research question or questions are located close to the purpose statement. According to Maxwell (2005), your research questions should take into account your research goals, research paradigms and traditions, and conceptual framework. That is, a research question for a phenomenological study will differ from one for a narratological study. For a study involving the phenomenon of loss, an example of a phenomenological research question might be: *How do recent immigrants experience loss associated with acculturation?* A narratological research question might be: *How is loss communicated in the plot and structure of 20th-century children's books?* Readers are cautioned not to confuse research questions with interview questions: There may be a couple of broad research questions that help to frame the research design, whereas there are several or many questions tied to qualitative interviewing that serve to elicit pertinent data.

Qualitative research questions differ from quantitative research questions in many ways. Quantitative research questions tend to be very specific in nature and are developed prior to the study. That is, quantitative researchers use a deductive approach that often relies on existing theory and previous knowledge to conceptualize specific research problems. Quantitative designs are also fairly linear, determined prior to beginning data collection, and do not usually change (Frankel & Devers, 2000; Haverkamp & Young, 2007). Maxwell (2005) added quantitative researchers "tend to ask what extent *variance* in *x* causes variance in *y*" (p. 23).

Researchers using qualitative research questions seek to discover, explore a process, or describe experiences. That is, they typically attempt to obtain insights into particular processes that exist within a specific context. This type of research tends to address "what" and "how" questions. These questions may be causal questions such as "how *x* plays a role in causing *y*" (Maxwell, 2005, p. 23). Although comparative research questions could be specified before the qualitative inquiry begins, most often, these questions emerge at some point during the study (Frankel & Devers, 2000; Haverkamp & Young, 2007). Remember, mixed methods studies (discussed later in this chapter) contain both qualitative and quantitative research questions.

Because qualitative research is a nonlinear and emerging process—and data collection and analysis occur simultaneously—findings may suggest that the original research question be modified. Thus, qualitative research questions need to be designed to strike a balance between being refined enough to delimit the study but general enough to allow for an emerging design that is open to change as data are collected and analyzed. As Haverkamp and Young (2007) noted, "with each version of the purpose or question, it is helpful to cycle back and forth between one's rationale and one's anticipated outcomes, asking whether the question provides sufficient focus to achieve one's purpose" (p. 281).

Developing Research Questions

Qualitative researchers need to consider three broad areas when developing sound research questions: content, coherence, and structure. **Content** refers to the facts and information related to the specific interest area of the research topic; ideally, the content should be presented in a clear and concise manner. **Coherence** involves clearly bringing together the philosophical and theoretical assumptions that underlie the study; a good research question reflects the underlying research paradigm(s) and tradition(s) (Mantzoukas, 2008). (The next subsection provides examples of coherence.) **Structure** refers to the branches of information about the study topic, participants, context, time, and the way the study is conducted (Mantzoukas, 2008). Morrison (2002) suggested that the structure of the research question should address the who, what, when, where, how, and why of the study. Wild Card 4.1 presents some cautions when writing research questions.

Related to the content component of research questions, qualitative research questions should be framed by the research goal components: case, research purpose, and type of information sought. Thus, information related to these components should be included either implicitly or explicitly in the research questions. With respect to a case, an individual, process, setting, or event should be mentioned in the research question(s). Some examples include:

- How do first-generation Filipino Americans experience government programs? (individual)
- What are the pedagogical practices of history teachers? (process)
- What are the benefits of an after-school program at Newbury Middle School? (setting)
- How did state budget cuts in 2009 impact educational planning? (event)

Qualitative researchers should also integrate the research purpose into their selected research questions. This involves shaping the research questions so that readers can ascertain the degree to which knowledge obtained from the study will be applied to a specific context (i.e., basic, applied, evaluative, or action research). Additionally, research questions should be framed in a manner that allows readers to determine who the primary audience is. Frankel and Devers (2000) suggest that a primary research audience can be determined by reflecting on the research goal. For example, if the research purpose is basic research, then the primary audience is most likely other researchers.

Finally, qualitative researchers must attend to the depth and scope when developing research questions. That is, how specific should attention to the case be? How broad should the research purpose be? Given that one of the strengths of qualitative research is describing phenomena in depth, researchers should take advantage of this when formulating questions (Haverkamp & Young, 2007).

⚠ WILD CARD 4.1. PITFALLS IN DEVELOPING RESEARCH QUESTIONS

Attention to the following pitfalls will minimize your risk of later realizing that your question is neither answerable nor feasible. (This list is not exhaustive.)

- Do not be concerned with the effect magnitude of a construct. Research questions that include terms such as *best*, *worst*, or *most* should be avoided.
- Defined variables are not included in the question, only the intent to describe the

variables during the inquiry. This may be intuitive since one of the key purposes of qualitative research is to explore an understudied phenomenon or construct.

- Avoid positivist terms in your research questions, such as *significant, test, universal, predict,* or *hypothesize.* Consider using these nonpositivist terms: *interpret, explore, construct, describe, view,* and *perspective,* to name a few.

- Do not be afraid to refine your research questions if your research design needs to be changed due to access or data collection issues.

- Debate sufficiently the merits of whether to review the literature before developing research questions or to identify the research question after research is under way in order to potentially minimize researcher bias and/or to give participants increased voice in the inquiry.

Research Questions by Research Tradition Clusters

Research questions need to be congruent with the selected research tradition, and vice versa. The following are sample research questions by cluster derived from the counseling and education literature to help you design a research question in consideration of a selected research tradition or traditions.

Cluster 1: The Universal Tradition

- Case study: How did one school counselor respond before and after a school hostage incident? (Daniels et al., 2007)

- Case study: What are the affective states in the counseling session? (Melton, Nofzinger-Collins, Wynne, & Susman, 2005)

Cluster 2: Experience and Theory Formulation

- Grounded theory: How does instructional leadership for special education occur in elementary schools? (Bays & Crockett, 2007)

- Phenomenology: What are the disclosure processes and effects of child sexual abuse on both female and male survivors? (Alaggia & Millington, 2008)

- Phenomenology: What are teachers' perspectives of children's mental health service needs in urban elementary schools? (Williams, Horvath, Wei, Dorn, & Jonson-Reid, 2007)

- Heuristic inquiry: What is the effect of conducting reflexive research on the development of the researcher? (Etherington, 2004)

- CQR: What themes are present in college students' descriptions of their career decision making? (Bubany, 2008)

Cluster 3: The Meaning of Symbol and Text

- Symbolic interaction: How do self-injurers use the Internet to form subcultural and collegial relationships? (Adler & Adler, 2008)

- Life history: How do aspiring teachers relate to literacy and to older forms of technology once used for reading and writing? (Johnson, 2007)

- Hermeneutics: What are older Korean graduate students' experiences in American higher education? (Seo & Koro-Ljungberg, 2005)

Cluster 4: Cultural Expressions of Process and Experience

- Ethnography: How effective is a drop-in program for homeless and marginally housed women in San Francisco's mission district? (Magee & Huriaux, 2008)

- Ethnography: What are the reproductive histories of adolescent married women in Bangladesh? (Rashid, 2007)

- Ethnomethodology: Are cross-cultural comparison of norms on death anxiety valid? (Beshai, 2008)

Cluster 5: Research as a Change Agent

- PAR: What are the experiences of three undergraduate students who engaged in a project with a group of preadolescent Latina girls attending a public school in Boston? (McIntyre, Chatzipoulos, Politi, & Roz, 2007)

 ACTIVITY 4.1. Moving from "Flawed" to "Better" Research Questions

A "bad" research question leads to a poor qualitative design. Before developing your research questions, consider the following "bad" research questions. After noting the limitations of all questions, discuss how they could be revised to become "good" research questions. Also, articulate how each research question could be rephrased to fit within each research tradition cluster.

1. What is the most effective method for implementing preservice learning?
2. How can teachers strategize to improve children's social interactions?
3. How do addicts experience substance abuse treatment?

4. What are the latest interventions used with people who have schizophrenia?
5. In what ways has technology harmed instruction?

PROPOSAL DEVELOPMENT 4.4. Developing Your Research Questions

Refer back to your purpose statement and develop an initial draft of your research question(s). Use the following checklist as discussion points to determine if each of your research questions is suitable for your purpose. This is a beginning checklist, and additional considerations will be offered in other parts of this section.

✓ I have available necessary resources (e.g., personnel, equipment, supplies, travel).

✓ I have an adequate timeline for data collection and analysis.

✓ I can articulate needed participant resources.

✓ The research question is interesting.

✓ The study is feasible.

✓ The research question is worth pursuing.

✓ I am considering various participants' perspectives.

✓ My question attends to content, coherence, and structure considerations.

IS A MIXED METHODS APPROACH SUITABLE?

Considering a **mixed methods** approach is important when determining if your research question is "answerable." Typically, mixed methods approaches involve "mixing" qualitative and quantitative methods in one study (or among several studies) to best address a research question or questions. As a researcher, if you decide to mix qualitative and quantitative methods, it is important that you have some conceptual knowledge of statistics and quantitative data analysis—even if this means hiring or consulting with a quantitative statistical expert to bolster your knowledge. The term *mixed method approaches* can also refer to purely qualitative designs, where the mixed methods that are used in research combine, for example, discourse analysis, interviewing, and direct participant observation. In this section, we focus on the mixing of qualitative and quantitative methods.

Because research questions drive methods, a mixed methods approach may be more suitable for several reasons. First, this approach can offset some of the limitations of qualitative and quantitative methods, allowing an expansion of the findings with a more comprehensive picture. Second, it may triangulate data from one method to another. Finally, this approach may confirm findings from a qualitative or quantitative investigation. Case Example 4.3 highlights examples of a mixed methods approach.

CASE EXAMPLE 4.3. Mixed Methods Studies

Ames, G. M., & Grube, J. W. (1999). Alcohol availability and workplace drinking: Mixed method analyses. *Journal of Studies on Alcohol, 60*(3), 383–393.

The authors examined the correlation between the amount of workplace drinking that takes place at a large factory and the workers' perception of actual alcohol availability and social availability. That is, is there alcohol physically around, and is it perceived to be socially acceptable to drink on the job? The researchers obtained their results via qualitative and quantitative methods using a sequential exploratory strategy. First, researchers participated in naturalistic observation, interviews, and archival data collection over a 3-year period. They looked at the culture of the job, interactions among employees, and different stressors. This initial process led to the development of a quantitative survey that examined the following factors: frequency of alcohol consumption, employees' perceptions of how often they thought coworkers drank right before or during work, perceptions of how much they thought fellow employees/friends would approve or disapprove of workplace drinking, thoughts about how easy/hard it would be to get a drink at work or to drink at work, and demographic information (i.e., race, religiosity, years of education, gender, marital status, work shift, and employee type).

Waldrop, D. P. (2007). Caregiver grief in terminal illness and bereavement: A mixed methods study. *Health and Social Work*, 32(3), 197–206.

This study used a concurrent triangulation method to examine caregiver grief during the bereavement period in addition to during the actual care process. The participants were interviewed twice, first during the caregiver process and then approximately a year following the death of the care recipient. Both interviews used open-ended questions designed to encourage caregivers to process their experience of caregiving and mourning, from the actual care of the patient to the patient's subsequent death. The authors used two quantitative measures to assess grief and loss symptoms.

A thorough defining and outlining of the various mixed methods approaches is beyond the scope of this text. However, the reader is encouraged to review the recommended readings at the end of the chapter (see Recommended Readings).

There are several ways to determine how a mixed methods approach can be implemented depending on how and when each individual method takes precedence in a research design. Creswell, Plano Clark, Gutmann, and Hanson (2003) highlighted four interdependent domains about which decisions must be made when selecting a particular mixed methods strategy (see Figure 4.9).

First, researchers must decide on when each method is introduced into the research design, or the *implementation* procedure. Will you gather quantitative and quali-

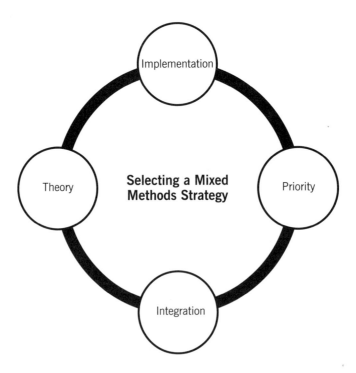

FIGURE 4.9. Domains to consider in selecting a mixed methods approach.

tative data at the same time (concurrent) or at different phases of a research project (sequential)? In **concurrent designs** qualitative and quantitative data collection processes are implemented at the same time. In **sequential designs**, researchers can collect either quantitative or qualitative data first depending on the research purpose and question(s). Researchers might collect qualitative data first to explore a topic from a small group's perspective and then survey a larger, more representative sample. When researchers employ qualitative strategies first, the design is referred to as an *exploratory* design. When they introduce a study with quantitative measures, the design is referred to as an *explanatory* design. Creswell and colleagues (2003) identified six mixed methods strategies based on when qualitative and quantitative data are introduced in a research design (see Table 4.7).

A second decision when selecting a mixed methods strategy is how much *priority* each method should be given in a research design. One assumption is that the method that is more prioritized by the researcher carries more weight in a design and is thus introduced first and used more often. In concurrent designs both methods tend to receive equal priority. In sequential designs the method introduced first tends to be more highly valued.

A third decision involves when each method will be *integrated* within a study. In concurrent studies quantitative and qualitative data are integrated after a single data collection phase. In sequential studies researchers may analyze data from each method independently (the order depends on whether it is an exploratory or explanatory design). Then, findings from each method are integrated for a broader interpretation.

A final decision involves the *theoretical perspective* used in the mixed methods study. There are various ways that theories can guide research design. Depending on the degree to which theory guides a mixed methods design (whether it is implicit or explicit in a study), a researcher may select a particular strategy over another. For example, if a researcher takes an advocacy stance regarding a research topic, emphasizing par-

TABLE 4.7. Mixed Methods Strategies

Strategy	Description
Sequential exploratory	Qualitative data collection and analysis followed by quantitative data collection and analysis to explore an emerging phenomenon with a larger sample
Sequential explanatory	Quantitative data collection and analysis followed by qualitative data collection and analysis to interpret more thoroughly broader findings
Sequential transformative	Quantitative or qualitative data collection and analysis may occur first in a design, depending heavily on a guiding theoretical perspective and/or available resources to conduct the study
Concurrent triangulation	The most common strategy whereby both methods are used simultaneously to confirm or converge findings in a single study
Concurrent nested	A similar strategy to the concurrent triangulation strategy, except that the less dominant method is nested within a more dominant method
Concurrent transformative	Simultaneous qualitative and quantitative data collection depending heavily on a guiding theoretical perspective and/or available resources to conduct the study; data collection may be triangulated or nested

ticipant empowerment and highlighting missing voices or perspectives, he or she may make a theory more explicit in a design as well as prioritize qualitative approaches.

 ACTIVITY 4.2. Dissecting the Mixed Methods Strategies

Review the six mixed methods strategies in Table 4.7 in small groups. How does each strategy relate to the four decisions proposed by Creswell and colleagues (2003)? Identify potential advantages and disadvantages of each. Brainstorm research examples of each.

CHAPTER SUMMARY

This chapter reviewed the five major considerations or components of selecting a topic in research inquiry. Chapter 2 presented 14 research traditions that could also shape topic selection, although decisions about traditions should not be made in isolation. Although the components discussed in this chapter influence each other, they are presented separately to highlight some of the key aspects of each.

The first consideration, *research goals*, refers to examining the unit of analysis of a case of interest. In addition, researchers need to consider the overall purpose of their research (i.e., basic, applied, evaluative, action) as well as the type of information sought (depth vs. scope) and by whom (primary and secondary audiences). The second consideration, *conceptual framework*, involves four components: experiential knowledge, prior theory and research (i.e., literature review), pilot and exploratory studies, and thought experiments. Guidelines for conducting a thorough literature review were discussed, as well as the various types of concept maps.

The third and fourth considerations, *purpose statement* and *research questions*, tend to form as the general research topic becomes more refined. The chapter offers suggestions and cautionary statements for writing both of these. Finally, since a research topic can be addressed by multiple research designs and can include quantitative features, mixed methods strategies are discussed in this chapter.

RECOMMENDED READINGS

Creswell, J. W. (2008). *Research design: Qualitative, quantitative and mixed methods approaches* (3rd ed.). Thousand Oaks, CA: Sage.

Haverkamp, B. E., & Young, R. A. (2007). Paradigms, purpose, and the role of the literature: Formulating a rationale for qualitative investigations. *The Counseling Psychologist, 35*, 265–294.

Mantzoukas, S. (2008). Facilitating research students in formulating qualitative research questions. *Nurse Education Today, 28*, 371–377.

Tashakkori, A., & Teddlie, C. (Eds.). (2003). *Handbook of mixed methods in the social and behavioral sciences.* Thousand Oaks, CA: Sage.

Wiersma, W., & Jurs, S. G. (2009). *Research methods in education* (9th ed.). Boston: Pearson.

CHAPTER 5

Understanding the Researcher's Role

CHAPTER PREVIEW

You should not underestimate the importance of the role you, as the researcher, have in qualitative inquiry. This chapter reviews the researcher's role as it relates to the influence of reflexivity and subjectivity in the course of a study. We explore the challenges of faithfully representing a phenomenon of inquiry, with emphasis on honoring the "voice" of participants in qualitative research. A component of the researcher's role—whether to work as a part of a research team or not—and the use of peer debriefers are also explored. We discuss the steps involved in building a research team, reviewing strategies such as peer debriefing. Figure 5.1 illustrates these five primary components of the researcher's role in qualitative inquiry.

RESEARCHER REFLEXIVITY

Researcher reflexivity is defined as the active self-reflection of an investigator on the research process (Hammersley & Atkinson, 2007). Reflexive processes allow a researcher's audience to grasp not only the phenomenon of inquiry, but also the development of the research itself (Watt, 2007). Because the thoughts and feelings of the researcher, including his or her reactions to and interpretations of the data, are part of the research process, reflexivity of the researcher becomes a lens into the research process itself (Stake, 1995). Therefore, it is not surprising that researcher reflexivity becomes one of the benchmarks for how credible and trustworthy a qualitative research design is for its audience (see Chapter 7 for an in-depth discussion of these topics). Indeed, reflexivity is one of the major distinguishing factors between quantitative and qualitative research; it is viewed as being a critical researcher role to self-reflect throughout the research process (Morrow, 2005). However, reflexivity is one of the most challenging concepts to understand *and* to put into action while conducting qualitative inquiry. Therefore, we discuss the foundations of reflexivity and provide examples as well.

We can turn to the field of psychology for some hints as to how a researcher can more fully grasp the foundations underlying reflexivity. Carl Rogers, a well-known psy-

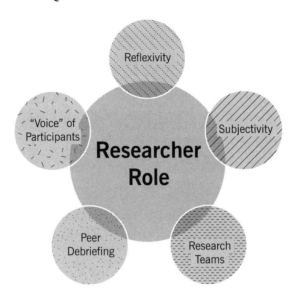

FIGURE 5.1. Considerations for the role of the researcher.

chologist, inspired the humanistic movement in psychology with his book, *On Becoming a Person* (1961). In this book, he made the case for a new paradigm of psychotherapy and counseling that moved away from one previously focused on behavior change. In this model, counselors strove to provide three core conditions in their counseling work: authenticity, unconditional positive regard, and empathy. So, you ask, what does a humanist have to do with a qualitative researcher? Rogers's core conditions provide a guideline—or a "gut" check—for your own use of reflexivity in your research. Without these three conditions, your reflexive processes may be too easily coopted by negative, unconstructive criticalness.

Rogers defined *authenticity* as the congruence between the inner and outer world. As a qualitative researcher, authenticity becomes a mirror through which to interpret data. For instance, consider the example of conducting a qualitative inquiry of teachers and their thoughts on the educational policy implications of the No Child Left Behind Act (2001). It is very likely that you have strong thoughts and opinions about the act—or at the very least are aware of the debate within education on the benefits and challenges of this legislation. Using your reflexive abilities, you would identify your authentic thoughts and feelings about the legislation prior to engaging in the research process.

Rogers discussed *unconditional positive regard* as creating a space of acceptance for a client's true thoughts and feelings, without judgment. Unconditional positive regard can assist qualitative researchers in delving deeply into their expectations and convictions about their research topic, which may be controversial or previously not acknowledged. An example would be a researcher who examines perpetrators of intimate partner violence, who in the middle of his study discovers he is developing strong thoughts and feelings of doubt about the rehabilitation potential of these perpetrators. Unconditional positive regard, as part of his reflexive process, would allow this researcher to welcome these reactions during the research process, in addition to being accountable for how these shape his interpretation of the data.

Finally, Rogers described *empathy* as the counselor's ability to accurately identify the thoughts and feelings of the client. For the qualitative researcher, empathy generates more meaningful and in-depth reflexivity. Let's say a qualitative researcher is studying teacher–parent interactions in a rural elementary school setting. She begins coding the first interview transcription she conducted with a teacher–parent pair, and she notices that she asked leading prompts that were not on the interview protocol. Generating empathy for herself will provide the road she needs to examine the "why" and the "how" of her departure from the interview protocol. This researcher can use these reflections to anticipate the urge to use leading prompts in her next interviews, as opposed to discovering this impact on the research process at a later date. Although it is certainly true that qualitative research is *not* counseling, you can use Rogers's core conditions to assist you in becoming a better, more reflexive researcher. See Table 5.1 for an expanded list of questions to guide you before, during, and after the completion of your study.

Especially when first learning about reflexivity, it is easy to feel lost in how to "do" it, since there are not many examples provided in the literature. To begin to address this lacuna, Watt (2007) wrote about her process of keeping a reflexive journal during her qualitative study on home education. Her reflexive process began in advance of the study, when she reflected on her motivations and interests in this line of inquiry. As a parent who home-schooled her children, Watt had intimate experience of the phenomenon at hand. She wrote questions in her reflexive journal asking how these experiences would shape her expectations of participants and of the data, in addition to how she would manage hearing information that contradicted her experiences. The journal was also a method of considering how she would react to more challenging aspects of qualitative research. Consider her following journal entry, written prior to a pilot interview with her first participants:

Do I have the courage to be totally honest no matter what I might find? I know my participants and would never want to hurt them. However, it wouldn't matter who the participants were, I would not wish to paint anyone in a negative light. This issue has led me to question whether I am cut out to be a qualitative researcher. Why would any-

TABLE 5.1. Using Rogers's Core Conditions in Researcher Reflexivity

Core condition	Reflexive questions
Authenticity	• What are my *thoughts* about my research topic? • How do I *feel* about my research topic in terms of quality and degree of feeling (positive, negative, neutral)? • What do I expect to find in the data from my participants? • How will these expectations shape how I interpret the data?
Unconditional positive regard	• Are my reactions about my topic area and/or what I am discovering about my participants surprising me? • What judgments do I have about my participants and/or topic area?
Empathy	• Am I having reactions to my study that I am not identifying or not wanting to accept or acknowledge? • Am I "seeing" the data in my study in ways that are either aligned or not aligned with what participants actually said in their own words?

one participate in a research project if they thought I might write something negative about them anyways? (Journal entry, November 1, 2003) (Watt, 2007, p. 87)

Interestingly, Watt's journal entries over a month's time are about similar concerns: How would she negotiate identifying data or writing about "negative" aspects of her participants or about her study? How would she manage the tensions of being both a researcher and a person who was intimately connected to her phenomenon of inquiry? Her journal entry a week later sheds some light on this tension:

What will I do if my participants and I don't agree on some aspect of the "findings"? You certainly can't misrepresent your participants. At the same time, you are more familiar with the literature, and as a researcher have your own expertise/perspectives. It is my research. These issues are complex, and frankly, more than a little scary. ... It seems that qualitative researchers are constantly engaged in a fine balancing act on a number of levels. (Journal entry, November 7, 2003) (Watt, 2007, p. 88)

It is clear that Watt's reflexive journaling becomes a strategy of accountability, honesty, and trust, which allows her to document her internal processes as a researcher and understand her influence on the research process itself.

Watt discusses several values of maintaining her reflexive journal in advance of her study, during the data collection and analysis, and after the study's completion. Indeed, she notes, "If I had not kept a journal much would have been lost, both during and now after the project" (Watt, 2007, p. 98). She also notes the advantage of being able to understand the connections between the theory of qualitative research and the practice of it. Finally, Watt recognizes her reflexivity as being a goal without an end point: "Becoming a qualitative researcher is a never-ending process indeed" (p. 98). In this manner, Watt identifies her reflexive journal as being one of the key ingredients in her becoming a stronger qualitative researcher and actually *seeing* herself in this light as well.

Because the concept of reflexivity is complex, Hellawell (2006) wrote about a heuristic device he uses with graduate students beginning qualitative studies to assist them in thinking about their role as a reflexive researcher. When mentoring students in qualitative designs, Hellawell first describes the notions of "insider" and "outsider" research to stimulate students to consider what position they may have. He cited Merton's (1972) definition of **insider research**—research where the investigator is not necessarily part of an organization and/or the phenomenon of inquiry, but rather has knowledge of the organization and/or phenomenon prior to the study's commencement. He then described **outsider research** as studies where the investigator has no prior intimate experience with the participants or topic area of interest. Hellawell (2006, p. 488) then asked the following five heuristic questions of students regarding their qualitative studies:

1. How many of you consider you're doing insider research?
2. How many of you think you're doing outsider research?
3. How many think you're doing both?
4. How many think you're doing neither insider now outsider research?
5. How many of you simply don't know where your research fits into this debate?

Interestingly, Hellawell (2006) noted that students often respond that they fit into the second possibility listed above—they identify as outsider researchers. He then provided an example of graduate students in education who believe that they are outsider researchers because they are examining school settings of which they are not a part. Hellawell challenged these students to consider their perceived outsider status in these educational organizations by asking the following question: "Would you not be much more of an outsider were you to be researching into the perceptions of, for example, workers on a car assembly track in the motor manufacturing industry?" (p. 489). Locating your position as a researcher as an insider or outsider is an important component of developing your skills as a reflexive investigator.

While Hellawell encouraged students to identify their location as a qualitative researcher, Fawcett and Hearn (2004) insisted that investigators must think of the concepts of insider and outsider not merely in terms of organizations and phenomena, but also in terms of researchers' social locations (e.g., gender, race/ethnicity, disability). The authors asked questions such as: "Can men research women, white people, people of color, or vice versa?" (p. 201). These questions demand a discussion of the "otherness" of participants and the role of the researcher in relation to participants. Fawcett and Hearn identified four types of **otherness** that interact with one another: epistemological, societal, practical, and local otherness. *Epistemological* and *practical* otherness refer to the distance between the researcher and the participant within the research context, whereas *societal* and *local* otherness refer to the social context that privileges or diminishes people—researchers and participants alike—in terms of social power. The authors suggested that otherness does not eradicate understanding or invalidate the potential of examining a phenomenon in a faithful manner. Rather, Fawcett and Hearn argued that "it is how the research project is conducted, how the participants are involved, how attention is paid to ethical issues, and the extent of critical reflexivity, that have to be regarded as key factors … [and] need to be subject to ongoing critical appraisal at each stage of the research" (p. 216). They provided the following areas for reflection for addressing issues of otherness in qualitative research:

- Consider the historical and sociopolitical contexts.
- Conduct researcher self-reflexivity.
- Foster awareness of the social locations of researcher, participants, and phenomenon of inquiry.
- Give attention to how knowledge is socially constructed.
- Align with empirical inquiry, while refraining from asserting or speculating about participants or the phenomenon of inquiry. (p. 418)

When reflecting on the position of self as an insider or outsider researcher and considering the construct of "otherness" in research, Tinker and Armstrong (2008) challenged qualitative researchers not to paint their positions as dichotomous. They deem these types of conclusions as simplistic and not helpful to qualitative inquiry. Since qualitative investigators often hold multiple insider and outsider research characteristics, it is best to view it as a continuum. Possessing qualities that speak to an insider status (i.e., falling closer to the insider research side of the continuum) allows researchers access to specific knowledge about the topic or setting. Tinker and Armstrong noted that possessing more status as an outsider also has its benefits. They urge qualitative investigators to embrace their positions when they rest toward the outsider end of the continuum: "Being from a different ethnic or religious group [than] one's respondents can in fact have potential benefits, for the research process. It can enable the researcher to elicit detailed responses, ask comprehensive interview questions, minimize the respondent's fear of being judged, and maintain criticality in data analysis" (p. 58).

The authors use examples from their own qualitative research, where they held positions as white, young, British, and nonreligious, which were different from their participants, to illustrate this point. In a study of the controversy surrounding British state funding of Muslim schools, Tinker (2006, as cited in Tinker & Armstrong, 2008) interviewed key stakeholders: religious leaders, parents, teachers, and politicians. Tinker used her "cultural ignorance" of Islam to encourage "less confident interviewees into a position of authority ... talk[ing] more freely, thereby eliciting more detailed and in-depth accounts" (p. 56). In Armstrong's (2005) study of women's awareness of cervical screening procedures in a British-sponsored program, she sought to understand how ethnicity and religious views influenced participants' awareness. Armstrong did not hide or mask her researcher position as more outsider to this group; rather, she highlighted this difference between herself and her participants. This commonly took the form of saying something along the lines of, "It seems that X is important in how you think about this, but I'm afraid I don't know much about it. Can you please explain it to me and say why it is important?" Armstrong asserts that this question stimulated the participants to share more deeply about their awareness of cervical screening, including tapping into some of their assumptions and worldviews that might not have been as apparent if she had not taken the approach of highlighting the differences between herself and her research participants.

Tinker and Armstrong (2008) acknowledged situations where outsider positionality as a researcher may become a challenge in other ways to qualitative approaches. Participants may experience hesitation or fear about sharing their experiences of a phenomenon with researchers who hold vastly different social locations from them. Tinker and Armstrong provide a valuable reminder that thinking with complexity about issues of difference in researcher and participant location and positionality is important for qualitative inquiry.

 ACTIVITY 5.1. Identifying and Understanding Researcher Reflexivity

Select a qualitative journal article and identify the reflexivity of the author(s). Consider the following questions in your review:

- Is researcher reflexivity explicitly or implicitly shared?
- How could the researcher(s) be more forthcoming about his or her reflexivity?
- Is (Are) the author(s) an outsider or insider researcher(s)?

- If you were writing this article, how would you approach researcher reflexivity? How would you convey your reflexivity to your audience in a similar article?

Another strategy of incorporating reflexivity into the research process is to work on a research team and use *peer debriefing* techniques (Lincoln & Guba, 1985). We discuss peer debriefing in-depth in the last section of this chapter as well as in Chapter 7. For now, see Perspectives 5.1 for our narratives on actively using reflexivity in qualitative approaches.

• •

Perspectives 5.1. Reflexivity in Action

"Reflexivity is complicated, but it's simple at the same time. The first time I heard of reflexivity, I thought it meant I had to be transparent about my every thought and feeling with each participant, my research team, and my audience. As I have grown as a qualitative researcher, reflexivity is now just something I constantly do all the time—I don't have to think about it much. Right when I first begin thinking about a project, say, the topic area is school counselors and social justice, I open up a Word document and title it 'Reflexive Journal School Counselors and Social Justice.' I always put the date and time of my entry, in addition to the 'task' on which I am reflecting (in this case, it would be a brainstorming session). I allow myself to write whatever I am thinking and feeling at the moment.

"I like having two approaches to maintaining a reflexive journal. First, a structured approach is making sure that I journal each time I interact with my data and/or participants. That means having my laptop available before and after I interview a participant or conduct a focus group, since I keep my reflexive journals electronically. In a pinch, I will use a notepad and transcribe my notes into my electronic journal file later. The second approach I use is an unstructured one. If I am driving and a thought comes to me about the data or a focus group I just conducted, I will write that down in my reflexive journal as soon as I can. Then, my reflexive journal documents my process as a researcher throughout a study without my having to think too hard. There are all my thoughts and feelings about my study that then become important data to consider and acknowledge when it comes time to interpret the data."

—AAS

"Reflexivity begins for me in topic selection, when I challenge myself to think about how I am an 'insider' to the research. What is it about a topic that intrigues me? Am I concerned with a topic for my own interests? What about others' interests? Even at the initial research design stages, I note feelings and thoughts I have about the literature I search as well as the scholarship I opt to not review. During data collection and analysis, I use a spiral notebook to jot down my attitudes about the participants I encounter, those to whom I do not have access, the process of entering a site, as well as the fit between the data I am obtaining and the data I expected to find when I began the study.

"Reflexivity reminds me of keeping a diary, except you have to be aware that anyone can and should access it at any time. Just as we want our participants to be authentic and collaborative in our studies, we have to be authentic to them as well. Reflexivity (and subjectivity, for that matter) helps us remain more honest to our study as well as be more open to ourselves, participants, and readers."

—DGH

• •

PROPOSAL DEVELOPMENT 5.1. Being an Insider and Outsider

Tinker and Armstrong (2008) introduced the concept of being both an insider and an outsider researcher. For your research study, consider how you are both an insider and outsider to the study. In brainstorming, consider both personal and professional characteristics.

	Insider	Outsider
Research topic		
Research goal(s)		
Research question(s)		
Sample		
Access to research site		
Research team		

Now, review your characteristics with peers. What are their reactions? Do they have anything to add?

SUBJECTIVITY IN QUALITATIVE INQUIRY

While reflexivity in qualitative designs assists the researcher in self-reflection on the research process, the concept of subjectivity is just as important. **Subjectivity** is defined as the qualitative researcher's internal understandings of the phenomenon (Schneider, 1999). Subjectivity, similar to reflexivity, is an important concept that distinguishes qualitative from quantitative research. Whereas quantitative studies discuss issues of validity and controlling variables, qualitative researchers discuss researcher subjectivity as a factor either to minimize or to embrace. Qualitative researchers who seek to minimize subjectivity in their studies tend to advocate, for example, that data from participants be analyzed only on the basis of the transcribed text from their interviews (Muchielli, 1979, as cited by Drapeau, 2002). More recent trends in qualitative research have criticized this approach, asserting that attempting to minimize subjectivity aligns qualitative approaches too closely with quantitative paradigms of "objective" science. Instead, they advocate for researchers to view their subjectivity as a way to be closer to their study. Subjectivity then becomes a way to understand the phenomenon more intimately, rather than keeping one's distance from the topic (Patton, 2002; Schneider, 1999). We agree with this perspective, believing that researcher subjectivity is an integral aspect of qualitative researcher that should be not only acknowledged, but also viewed in a positive light.

Peshkin (1988) used the phrase of "virtuous subjectivity" to convey the idea that researcher subjectivity should be embraced. He discusses the importance of both individual and multiple subjectivities involved in qualitative research. Peshkin disclosed his own subjectivity as well. Peshkin, a Jewish man with a liberal political perspective, conducted research on a high school community founded on fundamentalist Christian values. Acknowledging his subjectivity, Peshkin struggled with the tension between his values and the values espoused by his subject matter. He ultimately reasoned that he was able to write a more nuanced account of his subject matter because he experienced this tension and struggle, acknowledged its impact on the research, and sought to share with his audience how his subjectivity influenced his interpretation of his topic. Yet, Peshkin also acknowledged that a researcher with different values—say, a fundamentalist Christian—would have produced a very different data set and interpretation of the same topic area. He believed that this perspective would be just as valid as his own study's findings. It becomes clear, then, that a researcher's subjectivity paves the road for a study's outcome. This is all the more reason to see subjectivity in qualitative inquiry as "virtuous"—not something to be overamplified or even overindulged, but rather as a critical role of the researcher that becomes the framework for a study's process.

Discussion surrounding the role of subjectivity in the research process intensified within the qualitative research field in the mid-1980s (Denzin & Lincoln, 2000). Particularly, researchers in the field began to explore the opportunities, limits, and challenges they encountered as they sought to understand the lived experiences of participants. During this discussion, a "crisis of representation" emerged (Schwandt, 2001). Because of the subjective nature of truth, how could researchers ever accurately portray the lives of their participants? In terms of accuracy, was this even a realistic goal for qualitative inquiry? If accurate portrayal of participants was not a realistic goal, then what was the goal of qualitative designs? These questions undergirded the crisis of representation, demanding that researchers acknowledge their inability to ever truly document the participants' lived experiences of a phenomenon. In doing so, the complexity of qualitative research was deepened. The discussion of the crisis of representation continues to this day.

The opportunity for the student researcher, in becoming aware of the crisis of representation, is to learn the inseparability of researcher and participant. Remembering this inseparability, researchers can search for ways to more faithfully represent their participants as experts in the phenomenon of inquiry. Morrow (2005) noted that "taking the stand of naïve inquirer … [is] particularly important when the interviewer is an 'insider' with respect to the culture being investigated or when she or he is very familiar with the phenomenon of inquiry" (p. 254). Another strategy she identifies as important is to conduct participant surveys, wherein the researcher shares his or her interpretations and findings with participants to gauge how aligned they are with participants' lived experiences. The strategies of being a naive inquirer and proactively engaging in participant checks both build the trustworthiness of a qualitative study (termed *validity* and *reliability* in quantitative research). We list a few other strategies summarized by Drapeau (2002) in Table 5.2 to give you a glimpse into how qualitative researchers typically have addressed subjectivity. We have an expanded discussion of these strategies in Chapter 7 when we discuss approaches to establishing trustworthiness. For now, it is important to understand that the need to establish trustworthiness emerges from both the role and the tension that concepts such as reflexivity and subjectivity play in qualitative inquiry.

TABLE 5.2. Strategies to Address Subjectivity in Qualitative Research

- Approach your study leading with your curiosity, rather than with your "expertise" as expert researcher. Leading with curiosity entails asking questions, questioning your assumptions about your study, and even developing rival hypotheses that might counteract your previous analyses.

- Use participant checks throughout your study to determine the alignment of your interpretation of the meaning of the data with your participants' lived experiences of the phenomenon of inquiry.

- Have experts in the field of your phenomenon of inquiry review your findings, in addition to having them provide feedback on how your findings relate to findings of other similar studies.

- Build a research team to conduct data analysis and come to consensus on the interpretation of the findings.

- Triangulate data collection techniques and other research processes to build trustworthiness.

- Use a discussant or peer debriefer during the data collection and analysis process. You may consider adding a peer who does not have an investment in the process or outcome of the study.

- Actively counteract "groupthink" and acknowledge research team member "roles" in the study. With any group, there is bound to be some version of groupthink that emerges. Stay on top of this by having healthy dialogues and debates—endeavoring to have divergent views of the data explored and analyzed. Also, are all the voices of your research team contributing to the analysis—or are some heard or valued more than others? Seek to value every team member's contribution in a consistent manner.

- "Waving the red flag" (Corbin & Strauss, 2008) involves noting any time you and/or your co-researchers—and even your participants—use words such as *never* or *always* and questioning these instances. Corbin and Strauss also encourage researchers to explore the instance when the word *sometimes* is used, as it is typically a rich information source of participants' experiences.

- Consider checking in with your participants during the data collection and analysis in order to ensure that your research interpretations are consistent with their interpretations and understandings of their own data.

Sources: Drapeau (2002); Morrow (2005); and Lincoln and Guba (1985).

PROPOSAL DEVELOPMENT 5.2. Reflecting on Subjectivity in Your Study

Write one to two paragraphs exploring your thoughts on your subjectivity as a researcher in your topic area. Respond to the following questions:

- What are your thoughts on "virtuous subjectivity"?
- How will you "embrace" subjectivity in your role as a researcher?
- What are your thoughts about how the "crisis of representation" will influence your study?
- How will you seek to faithfully represent the participants in your study?
- How will you enact your role as a researcher so that it aligns with the role of "naive inquirer" in your study?

Ahern (1999) identified a "Top 10" list of tips for addressing your role as a researcher. We elaborate on each of Ahern's points below by providing examples:

1. Identify some of the personal and professional issues that you might take for granted in undertaking this research (e.g., gaining access, cultural variables, power). For instance, if you have never worked with children before and your study involves middle school students, you will need to take some time to reflect on how your lack of experience will affect your interactions. You may also have differences with your participants in terms of race/ethnicity, gender, educational attainment, sexual orientation, socioeconomic status, disability status, etc. These differences influence how we act both personally and professionally. Note how any such differences might influence your interaction with your study.

2. Clarify your personal value systems and acknowledge areas in which you know you are subjective. One might argue that values and subjectivity are involved in everything we do as researchers—from the data we collect to how we approach analysis and write up our studies. Related to our discussion in #1 above, how do these variables influence the "lens" you use to view your study?

3. Describe areas of possible role conflict. There may be times your role as a researcher intersects with your study. In one qualitative study I (Singh) conducted on LGBTQ bullying, one of the students selected for the study by the school counselor was an adolescent who cut my grass monthly. You may have conflicts that are more serious than this example. Regardless, you should describe these to yourself *and* to others.

4. Identify gatekeepers' interests and consider the extent to which they are disposed favorably toward the project. An example might be a case study of a rural mental health center where there are limited resources and/or high investment in being understood and/or portrayed in a certain light. This stance could definitely influence your study's findings.

5. Recognize feelings that could indicate a lack of neutrality. It is more than likely that you will be moved by what participants share with you during your research.

You shouldn't feign objectivity, but you should also not let your study be driven by your emotions.

6. Is anything new or surprising in your data collection and analysis? Research can and should be about discovery! What aspects of your study are unexpected, that you didn't account for, and possibly that you cannot describe? These aspects will ultimately enrich your study.

7. When blocks occur in the research process, reframe them. How could you change your methods and view the blocks as an opportunity? Obstacles can and will arise during research. Make sure your decisions about how to address them are guided by the spirit of your research tradition. If you are unable to conduct a focus group due to difficulty recruiting participants, how might your research tradition, in tandem with your research question, guide you to find another source of data? You might examine the secondary data collection methods we discuss in Chapter 9.

8. Even when you have completed your analysis, reflect on how to write up your account. You have spent time and energy in the data collection and analysis process. Use the same care and attention in representing this research process in your ultimate final description of the study's participants.

9. Consider whether the supporting evidence in the literature is really supporting your analysis or if it is just expressing the same cultural background as yourself. This really translates into challenging yourself along the road of your research study. Revisit the literature in your discipline often. Ask yourself if you are resonating with, or not connecting with, various aspects of this literature and consider how this response may affect your study.

10. Counteract analytic blindness. Asking the question of how you, as a researcher, may be either masking or avoiding addressing an aspect of your data collection and analysis is the process of counteracting analytic blindness. (We actually prefer to use the word *masked* to refrain from using ableist language.) Overall, good reflexivity assumes that there will be masked aspects of your study of which you are not aware. Your job as a researcher then becomes to develop a plan to actively address these areas. For instance, in a qualitative study of how families interact with school personnel in after-school programs, you could plan to actively generate questions as a researcher about how you are defining what constitutes a "family" throughout the research process.

"VOICE" OF PARTICIPANTS IN QUALITATIVE RESEARCH

A major researcher role is to seek to understand the meaning of "voice" in qualitative research. When considering participants' voice, you should address issues of accuracy, completeness, and emotional content. In terms of accuracy, you will make decisions about transcription of the actual words spoken by participants. For instance, if there is a section of a transcript that is difficult to understand, as a researcher it might be important enough to revisit the participant and ask about it. This is a form of member checking, which we discuss further in Chapter 7. In terms of completeness, as a researcher you must decide how complete the voice of your participants is. The issues involved in this determination range from the comfort level of participants in talking about their experiences to whether enough time was allowed to capture participants' sharing on the research phenomenon. With regard to emotional content, the emotions expressed by participants about their experiences of a phenomenon are an important aspect of their voice. Because emotional content may be conveyed nonverbally, capturing this content may include observing the emotions, asking specifically about the emotions, and ensuring that this content is included in data analysis.

Faithfully representing participants' voices will become an important endeavor for you as you engage in qualitative studies. You will likely feel pressure to "get it right" in terms of your interpretation of what your participants share with you—as Watt's (2007) musing in her reflexive journal, discussed earlier, certainly illustrates. Mazzei and Jackson (2009) edited an entire book on voice in qualitative research, compiling the various views on this topic in the field. Indeed, it is no simple feat to manage the task of representing the voices of your participants.

The challenges and seeming impossibility of representing participant voices "accurately" led to the "crisis of representation" in qualitative research (Lincoln & Guba, 1985). As this dialogue continued, qualitative researchers began to take approaches such as including participants' text of transcribed interviews, even documenting paralinguistic cues (e.g., pauses, silences, starts) as integral to an audience understanding their participants' voice. Documenting in this manner became a focus of ethnomethodology techniques, where the goal was to understand the meanings revealed by language structures. For instance, Garfinkel (1967), who deeply influenced the field of ethnomethodology, studied a transsexual woman and the multiple processes in which she engaged to be able to "pass" as a woman in society. The language she used, the pauses in her transcripts, and the inclusions and omissions of words were all identified by Garfinkel to make meaning of her experience. Another example is Freebody's (2001) study of the practical reading practices used in homes and schools through examining reading session transcripts, where the communication patterns and learning process of students with both teachers and parents were the study's focus. Other researchers have responded to the crisis of representation by "recogniz[ing] the dangerous assumptions in trying to represent a single truth (seemingly articulated by a single voice) and have therefore pluralized voice, intending to highlight the polyvocal and multiple nature of voice within contexts that are themselves messy and constrained" (Mazzei & Jackson, 2009, p. 1).

Mazzei and Jackson (2009) acknowledged these responses to the crisis of representation. However, the authors also suggest that these responses do not address the core problem with seeking to represent participants' voice. They attempt to interrupt this notion that voice is "there to search for, retrieve, and liberate" (p. 2). Importantly, they asserted that even if the raw data of a transcription are provided to an audience, it does not acknowledge the influence of the researcher on that particular piece of participant text or voice. The authors cited Lather's (2007) encouragement that qualitative researchers not seek out a simplistic path to the issue of voice, but rather seek to "trouble" traditional notions of voice in qualitative inquiry that claim to represent a single and/or accurate voice of participants.

So, how will you address the complex issue of voice in your study? Mazzei (2009) guides the researcher to interact with participant texts in multiple ways: "First ... I am bound to the text ... as where the voice resides. ... I relisten. ... I turn a focus not on what is evident ... producing a listening that can no longer be ignored" (p. 55). Mazzei shares a transcript of an interview with a teacher in her study, with probes that she might have used to understand the aspects of the participant's voice that were not as evident:

> Anne: I never really saw myself as prejudiced, but then I never really had to deal with any "other people." [**Other people? Who do you mean by** *other people*?]. So I was raised this way and now I've come to a *very, very, very* liberal, *very* open-minded understanding as far as my friends. [**When you say** *liberal*, **you mean** ... ?] I'm also a single mother, as far as people who I go out on dates with, political views, everything and it's very, *very* conflicting with my parents. [**How is that conflict lived out in your relationship with them?**] (pp. 55–56)

Mazzei's transcript provides a good example of embracing the challenges and opportunities that voice brings to a study in qualitative research. Had she asked the bracketed questions in bold font as probes, the less evident aspects of the teacher's voice would emerge. We hope that this example encourages you to reflect on what your role as a researcher is in portraying the voice of the participants in your study.

In addition to attending to participants' voice during qualitative inquiry, presenting that voice in the qualitative report is another consideration. Once you have obtained authentic participant data, you can decide the degree to which verbatim data are presented. For example, some researchers may present participant voice by providing individual narratives for participants. Other researchers may provide several direct participant quotes to more thickly describe a theme or code. Still other researchers may limit or avoid use of participant quotes or attention to individual participants yet still provide voice. Your decision of how to present voice may be based on your research tradition, restrictions on page limitations by journal editors, complexity of research topic, and sample size, to name a few considerations.

PROPOSAL DEVELOPMENT 5.3. Your Role as a Researcher

Write one to two paragraphs discussing your role as a researcher in your study. Answer the following questions in your discussion:

- What will your role be in your proposed study?

- What are your thoughts, feelings, and expectations about your topic? Do you think these will change throughout the research process, and if so, how?

- What are your perspectives on reflexivity, subjectivity, and voice in your topic area?

- What have been the perspectives of previous researchers on your topic in terms of reflexivity, subjectivity, and voice?

- To what degree will your presence, interests, and motivation for conducting a study in your area of interest play out in your role as a researcher?

USE OF PEER DEBRIEFERS

As a researcher, it is helpful to integrate peer debriefing into your research process. *Peer debriefing* is defined as a reflexive technique whereby research team members "serve as a mirror, reflecting the investigator's responses to the research process … serv[ing] as devil's advocates, proposing alternative interpretations to those of the investigator" (Morrow, 2005, p. 254). Lincoln and Guba (1985) assert that peer debriefing can strengthen a qualitative study's credibility (a construct we discuss further in Chapter 7). The authors suggest that the researcher view him- or herself as an "instrument" of any qualitative endeavor. Peer debriefing provides essential accountability in the effort to recognize and understand the influence of the researcher on the interpretation of the data. We agree with this view of the researcher as instrument, and we encourage you to identify ways in which you may incorporate this strategy throughout your study.

Spall (1998) explored the use of peer debriefing sessions by graduate students in education who used peer debriefing in their dissertations, and found three key ingredients to the process. First, participants described trust not only as being an important aspect of selecting a peer debriefer, but also as playing an important role in the interpersonal interactions involved in peer debriefing (e.g., trust that peer debriefing was a collaborative dialogue rather than a debate). Second, participants reported that both the researcher and the peer debriefer focused on the study's methodology in their debriefing sessions. For instance, if the peer debriefer was playing the role of devil's advocate in relation to the researcher's interpretation of findings, both turned to the methodology of the study to guide them in the session (e.g., if a grounded theory study, considering the goals of the tradition as they related to the peer debriefing session). Third, the graduate students described peer debriefing as vital to further developing their research skills in the course of a study.

Spall (1998) also found that the sessions varied in terms of how many people were involved (in pairs or small groups) and the length of time they met. Some peer debriefing groups met from the beginning to the end of the research process, whereas others met only at certain stages—such as after interviewing participants or analyzing findings. Spall also discussed the challenges of documenting the proceedings of peer debriefing sessions. In many cases, the participants reported that they did not take notes to document their discussions, instead relying on memory to incorporate the process and outcome of the peer debriefing sessions. Because peer debriefing is such an important reflexive strategy, we recommend that you keep Spall's findings in mind as you consider the roles your research team members may have in your study. From our experience, we suggest that you attempt to anticipate questions important for peer debriefing, such as the size, timing, and purpose in using this strategy in your study. We also encourage you to be flexible; there may be opportunities to use peer debriefing in your study that you could not anticipate, but that make sense according to your study's needs.

A real benefit of peer debriefing that one might not anticipate is the emotional support that the sessions can provide during the course of your study. Rager (2005) identified peer debriefing as not only strengthening the credibility of a qualitative study, but also, importantly, providing the qualitative researcher with the support needed to manage "compassion stress." She defines *compassion stress* as the feelings of empathy researchers experience—especially when researching a phenomenon and/or participants from marginalized backgrounds (e.g., Rager studied breast cancer survivors). Rager goes so far as to equate peer debriefing as an essential "self-care" strategy that should be central to the research process.

In a similar vein, Lalor, Begley, and Devane (2006) wrote about the influence of painful experiences on research team members conducting qualitative studies. Although the authors analyzed two reflexive journals and an interview with a supervisor of a qualitative study on a mother who had received a diagnosis of fetal abnormality, we believe their findings strengthen the case for peer debriefing in qualitative research. Underneath a large theme of "connecting with the data," the authors identified three categories in which research team members experienced painful emotions interacting with the data: "bearing to watch, bearing to listen, and bearing to support" (p. 209). In reflecting on their findings, Lalor and colleagues suggested that it is not appropriate to use an objectivist perspective when managing emotionally laden data. Rather, they recommended seeking to understand this affect as an integral aspect of the data collection and analysis process. We agree and see this function as an additional value of using peer debriefing in a qualitative study.

Because it can be challenging to understand how exactly to conduct peer debriefing, Spillett (2003) provided the following prompts to use:

- "What do you mean by .... ?"
- "What is important (or not) about this to you?"
- "Let's brainstorm some alternatives."
- "Why do you think this is true?"
- "What were you thinking at that point?"
- "What would happen if ... ?"
- "What are the benefits or risks of that approach?"
- "How does that relate to ... ?"
- "What areas do you feel uncertain about?"

These questions go to the heart of the purpose of debriefing: to understand the influence of the researcher on a study. Maxwell (2005) advised paying specific attention to the outcome of peer debriefing. In this light, documenting the peer debriefing process though note taking or audiotaping becomes an important way to assess the results from peer debriefing. What specifically was noted in the sessions? How did the sessions specifically alter and/or influence the decisions of the researcher(s) at critical points of the study, such as data collection and interpretation of findings?

TO USE A RESEARCH TEAM—OR NOT?

It can also seem like a luxury to think about building a research team for your qualitative study. Your decision of whether to use a research team or not is less a function of your researcher role and more a matter of the focus, goals, and needs of your research.

However, we wanted to discuss the use of research teams in this chapter exploring the researcher's role because we view the decision that you will make regarding the use of research teams as closely related to your role as a researcher. For instance, if you decide that your qualitative study of how long-term couples manage conflict in their relationships requires multiple members of a research team in order to make the data collection feasible over a short period of time, the needs of your research should drive you to build a research team. Once you make that decision to have a research team, then there are additional decisions you must make in your role as a researcher—such as whether the research team solely collects data or meets regularly throughout the research process, for instance.

We want to note that a research team is not a prerequisite to strengthening the trustworthiness of your study; however, when it "makes sense" for your study and you decide to use a research team, it has the potential to become an additional method of trustworthiness (as we discuss further in Chapter 7)—for instance, a research team to manage the amount of data generated by a qualitative study. Research teams are also a good strategy to address issues such as researcher reflexivity and subjectivity in the course of your study. Using research teams, also referred to as *triangulation of investigators* (also discussed in Chapter 7), is thus an important component of establishing rigor in qualitative research.

There may be instances where you would like to use a research team, but you are absolutely unable to build one or to accomplish each of the steps in organizing one (which we discuss below). In these situations, you can adapt your approach to data collection and analysis accordingly. One example of such a situation is a study I (Singh) worked on, where a colleague had expedited IRB approval and the opportunity to collect data about the sexual orientation identity development of female-to-male transsexuals at a U.S. conference. My colleague collected the data in a 1-day period by interviewing each participant (nine in total) one time each. However, he solicited the help of another colleague and myself (who had expertise in transgender research and qualitative designs) in order to analyze the data as peer debriefers. In another situation, you might not have the luxury of having another set of eyes on your data collection and analysis, so you will be unable to build a research team. However, there might be a way to involve others to help you with specific aspects of the project. Often, we find students are willing to support one another in "swapping" data analysis duties with one another's projects.

Remember that using a research team should be a decision based on the study's context and purpose—and your decision in this regard does not determine whether of not your research is "good." For some areas of inquiry, there simple may not be the need for a research team. An example would be if you were conducting an autoethnography of your own experiences as a person going through a divorce. For other researchers who are working outside academic settings and/or in academic/community collaborations, decisions may be made about the people involved in the research that most closely match the study's goal. An example might be a grant-funded study of Native American families and their children's experiences in middle school. If the requirements of the grant and/or the access to participants would be best facilitated by the primary researcher who also shares the same tribal heritage as the participants, then a research team would not be a "need" of this particular study.

Using a Research Team

We believe that a good first step to building your research team is doing some self-reflection on group dynamics—how groups function as a unit, how a research team is a group of people with different personalities and perspectives. It can be important to reflect on how you have functioned in groups in the past. For example, have you had predominantly negative experiences in groups, or have your group experiences been mostly positive? If you have had negative experiences on group projects, what have been the typical issues? Have you typically been a leader or a follower when you have worked in groups? Does the idea of participating in a group project—in a class, for example—excite you because of the multiple perspectives and shared workload, or does the prospect bring up concerns about who will get "stuck" doing most of the work? Your answers to these questions can provide good information as to what you may want to do in the process of building your research team. We provide these questions not to prescribe what your answers should be, but rather to support you in developing your awareness of how you work in groups and to help you anticipate what it will be like to work within a group for a potentially significant period of time. Additionally, theories of group dynamics remind us that there are discrete and predictable stages of how a working group functions (Gladding, 2008). So, your self-reflection on group dynamics should also include how you see your research team forming, working, and ending the study.

A second step in building your research team is a concrete one: Identify potential team members for your study. You can consider several strategies in this step. Ideally, your research team members will be interested in your study, able to meet in person during the research process, and able to participate in the study through its completion. However, you may only be able to realistically identify research team members who fit a few of these important categories. When identifying potential team members, as a student, think about who in your cohort and/or research network would be a good fit for your study. In these situations, there may be a way you can collaborate. For example, a fellow student in your cohort may be on your research team, while you offer to be a team member on his or her study in exchange. Another strategy could be talking with your research mentor or advisor—would he or she be willing to be a team member? Are there people who share an interest in your topic who would make sense to invite into your study? These people may or may not be located in the same city as you. If the person is not in your city, how will you manage the distance factor in the research process? Finally, you will want to think about how many team members you would like to have. Although there is no set or ideal number of people on a qualitative research team, it is important to consider how many people would make sense, considering the scope and needs of your topic of inquiry. In our experience, research teams average between two and five people.

Once you have identified and established your research team, a third step is to discuss the roles you and your team members will play in the course of a study. We cannot overestimate the importance of having discussions about the roles of you, as the leader, and the members of your research team. Typically, when group experiences go badly, there has been role confusion ("Who is the leader?"), a lack of attention to the kind of structure that groups need to function well, and/or inattention to the strengths and challenges each person brings to a group project. Having an initial meeting with your team members, wherein you clarify each team member's role, will be important. Below are some questions to consider as you discuss roles in your research team:

- What is the role of the leader in your team?
- What are the various roles members will play on the team?
- How often, and over what length of time, will the group meet?
- What are the anticipated challenges the group members and leader may face? How does the team want to anticipate and address these challenges?

Again, we provide these questions as a general guide to what you may want to explore. You may decide to use all of these questions, or only some, and/or generate your own. The idea is not to develop an authoritarian structure of how your research team will function, but instead to provide opportunities for your research team members to build a strong foundation upon which to support and challenge one another during the research process. After you have discussed the roles of the leader and members, a fourth step in building your research team is to institute regular check-ins on the team's functioning. How will you know if your research team is functioning well? How will you alter the functioning of the research team, should unavoidable challenges arise? How often will you assess the functioning of the team? Will it be at each team meeting, monthly, or on another schedule? Figure 5.2 provides a summary of the steps involved in building a research team.

· ·

Perspectives 5.2. Working on a Research Team

"A lot of times when I am doing the formative research—conducting focus groups and key informant interviews and doing literature reviews—for my studies in HIV/AIDS, I definitely want to work with a research team. We have about five of us who work together, and we are a mix of qualitative and quantitative researchers. I think one of our strengths is that we come from a variety of backgrounds when researching HIV/AIDS. We have folks with backgrounds in social work, public health, and even business! Some of us have worked in the HIV/AIDS community, and others really have never been out of academia and worked "on the ground." The variety of these perspectives on the research team is invaluable. There are so many contextual factors influencing risky behaviors that lead to HIV/AIDS infections, and it is important to not stigmatize these individuals. We have quantitative researchers who look at the numbers and run mathematical models of behaviors that can be measured, and then our qualitative designs allow us to examine the contextual factors that you could never measure.

"We need that mixed methods approach in our line of inquiry. The most important part of working on a research team is taking your own agenda and ego out of it—it's not about you. Your expertise is valuable. But realizing that you are just one person on the team is important too—that helps create the space for many quality perspectives and direction for the research. A challenge in working on research teams is to really keep your goal in mind, or those different perspectives can have you heading off in a scatterbrained way—or worse, head in the direction of only one person's perspectives on the team. One more point: Be open to learning new things. That's the best part of being on a research team."

—*VEL S. MCKLEROY*

· ·

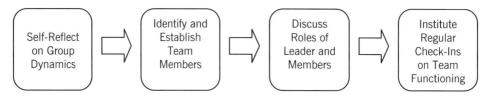

FIGURE 5.2. Steps to building your research team.

   ACTIVITY 5.2. Building Your Research Team

Identify peers and/or colleagues who will be involved in your study and discuss the following with them:

- What do you and your research team members see as your potential role and influence in the study?
- To what degree do you and your research team members see yourselves as being involved in data collection and analysis?
- How will you and your research team members address researcher reflexivity and subjectivity?
- How often and for how long will your research team meet?

Perspectives 5.3. Researcher Role

"I was interested in how school counselors became leaders in their schools. As a school counselor myself, I had worked on leadership issues practically the entire time in the school system. So, I think about my role in my study as a researcher similarly to the topic I was researching—I was leading this study, so I better think carefully about how I was going to influence participants. I also knew I had big opinions on how I felt about school counselors being increasingly pulled away from counseling students to more administrative tasks, and I am a social justice advocate. I thought a long time about how these biases would influence my study. This was a good thing because if I had not done this, I know the study would have been more about me and my experience of leadership and schools than it was about the participants in the study. What I love about qualitative research is that it gives you the freedom to acknowledge who you are as a researcher—from your experiences and interests to your biases—instead of ignoring them or pretending they aren't there."

—COUNSELING STUDENT

"I never realized how important my role as a researcher was until after my study was complete. I investigated how students of color from impoverished backgrounds in urban settings were being 'lost' in the educational system around late-middle school. I started keeping a reflexive journal because my professor had recommended it. I was hesitant at first because I had never journaled before and really didn't like the thought of writing long journal entries. Then I realized I didn't have to write full sentences in the journal. I just wrote words, phrases, and brief thoughts. It wasn't as difficult as I thought it would be, and it worked for me to have a paper journal since I was in the schools so much. Unfortunately, I didn't consider the journal as data as much as I thought of it as my own comfort zone as a researcher. I could write anything I wanted in there! After I completed my research, I went

back and looked at the journal, and there were several key themes that I could have explored further if I'd had my research team code my journal. My advice is to keep a reflexive journal and analyze it along the way in your study!"

—EDUCATIONAL POLICY STUDENT

"There are so many things to consider about your role as a researcher in qualitative studies. I studied the experiences of microaggressions by lesbian, gay, and bisexual people. I am straight, so I thought long and hard about why the research was important to me and the reactions people might have to me along the way. I was glad to have a research team of both heterosexual and lesbian women. We were able to check in with one another whenever we had questions, felt lost, or just overwhelmed. It was important for me as a heterosexual person to consistently check in with myself about how I was learning and growing as a person doing this study. I didn't feel like I had anti-gay biases when I started the study, but my research team was able to help me see things that I just couldn't see without them—from LGBT slang to LGBT experiences I just never had been exposed to before as a straight person. I was really motivated to give participants a 'voice' after spending so much time with them. I discussed this desire with my team, and they pointed out that I was seeing the participants as more vulnerable and helpless than for who they were. Then I started peer debriefing after my interviews, and I realized that my enthusiasm to give them a voice made me ask more questions and not listen as much. I don't know what I would have done without my research team."

—COUNSELING PSYCHOLOGY STUDENT

⚠ WILD CARD 5.1. PITFALLS TO AVOID IN YOUR RESEARCHER ROLE

There are many important considerations regarding your researcher role in qualitative studies. Review the following list to ensure that you are paying close attention to how your role can influence your study:

- Understand, reflect, and be able to articulate how you will build reflexivity into your study.

- Do not assume a reflexive journal will provide adequate attention to reflexivity in your study. Also incorporate peer debriefing pairs and/or groups throughout your study.

- Address subjectivity in your research. From the researcher-as-instrument perspective, how are you influencing the research process?

- Consider where your position as a researcher falls along the insider–outsider continuum. Do not assume that you are an outsider researcher just because you are not involved in a certain organization or topic of inquiry.

- Make sure to address contextual factors and social locations of privilege and oppression as you seek to understand the relationships between yourself and your participants.

- Do not assume that you, as the researcher, are "giving voice" to participants. Understand the problematic notions of this assumption, and seek to interrupt any tendency you or your research team members have to view participants in this light.

- Plan ahead to use peer debriefing in your study, and be open to the opportunities that arise throughout the research process to further incorporate peer debriefing sessions in your study.

- Be sure to document how the peer debriefing sessions influenced the process of your research.

- If it is feasible for you to build a research team and you elect to work with one, think carefully about building a research team. Put considerable thought into your working style in groups, the role of team members, and the length and frequency your team will meet. If you are conducting qualitative research without a team, have a strong rationale as to how and why this single-person format is important, in addition to addressing your researcher reflexivity and subjectivity.

CHAPTER SUMMARY

This chapter has addressed five key researcher roles that are part of qualitative inquiry. First, researcher reflexivity was reviewed, including its influence on the research process and using reflexive journals to document your reflections throughout the study. Second, we discussed the importance of embracing the role that researcher subjectivity plays in a qualitative study, and how to seek to understand your position along the insider–outsider continuum and its impact on your study. Third, we explored the problematic issue of voice in qualitative inquiry, encouraging you to seek to interrupt notions that your role as a researcher allows you to portray a singular truth of participants' voices. Fourth, we discussed strategies for using peer debriefers and/or building a well-functioning research team, including considerations of how group dynamics and your previous experiences in groups may influence your research process. We also discussed strategies you may use if you elect to not use a research team or are unable to do so because you do not have access to fellow researchers. Finally, we reviewed how you may use a research team to further build reflexivity into your study's design by holding peer debriefing sessions.

RECOMMENDED READINGS

Jackson, A. Y., & Mazzei, L. A. (2009). *Voice in qualitative inquiry: Challenging conventional, interpretative, and critical conceptions in qualitative research.* New York: Routledge.

Peshkin, A. (1988). Virtuous subjectivity: In the participant observer's I's. In D. Berg & K. Smith (Eds.), *The self in social inquiry: Researching methods* (pp. 267–281). Newbury Park, CA: Sage.

Schwandt, T. (2001). *Dictionary of qualitative inquiry* (2nd ed.). Thousand Oaks, CA: Sage.

Watt, D. (2007). On becoming a qualitative researcher: The value of reflexivity. *Qualitative Report, 12*(1), 82–101.

CHAPTER 6

Entering the Field

CHAPTER PREVIEW

Once you have selected a topic in qualitative inquiry, it becomes important to consider how you, as a researcher, will enter the field. These considerations include choosing a sampling method; identifying sample size; selecting and entering a field site; building rapport with gatekeepers, stakeholders, and key informants in the field; and exiting the field. Figure 6.1 summarizes the main topics of this chapter.

ENTERING THE FIELD

Entering the field is one of the most critical aspects of qualitative inquiry. There are numerous ways to enter the field in terms of methods you use to gain access and the degree of interaction you intend to have with participants. We do not provide a comprehensive list of the wide variety of ways you can enter the field. In this section, rather, we introduce some of the common aspects of entering the field across research traditions. Once you select a research tradition, we encourage you to delve into the literature within your discipline to consider additional aspects important to entering the field. Although we discuss some of the ethical issues involved with entering the field, please refer to Chapter 3 for additional information on ethical issues.

Setting aside time and effort to intentionally consider how you, as a researcher, will enter the field is a necessary step after you have selected your topic of inquiry. Considering how you will enter the field is an important first step across all the research traditions because this is really the time in the process of your research where the "rubber meets the road." We use the word *field* to designate the context in which your study takes place. The field might be the Internet if you are conducting qualitative research online (see Chapter 9 for more information about online research), for instance. The field could also be a nonprofit agency where you have secured a confidential office space to

159

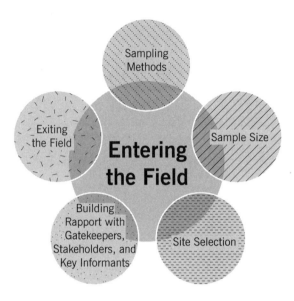

FIGURE 6.1. Considerations when entering the field.

interview participants for a study. The field can also be the focus of your study itself—such as a case study or ethnographic design. The field may also involve several locations and/or be selected by participants. For instance, in one of our studies, we interviewed child sexual abuse survivors in locations of their choice because we decided it was important for participants to be able to select the spaces in which they felt comfortable being interviewed. Thus, for this study, our "field" involved numerous locations—from participants' homes and office spaces to coffee shops and outdoor parks. The field is not, however, only a setting. The field you enter is populated by people and the relationships and interactions they have within the settings in which they work, in addition to the larger context that encapsulates those settings, people, relationships, and interactions. We encourage you to think about the field broadly in terms of the spaces in which your activities will take place in your study.

When you selected a topic, you spent a good deal of energy in identifying research goals, considering the use of mixed methods, designing research question(s), developing a purpose statement, and identifying a conceptual framework. Now it is time to bring all your hard work to life in the real world. Because the real world—or the field—is often an unpredictable place, being deliberate and purposeful about how you enter this arena will help you anticipate potential challenges and capitalize on potential opportunities as your study unfolds.

Entering the field can often seem overwhelming—especially to those conducting their first qualitative study. In order to enter the field in an effective and ethical manner, we must actively assess *ourselves* as researchers. If we do not take the time to do this type of self-assessment, we may risk damaging our relationship with research participants and research sites. When we do take this time, we easily identify ways to build trusting relationships with our research participants and the associated sites. Thinking about both our interpersonal skills (how we relate to others) and our intrapersonal skills (how we relate to ourselves) is a good first step. It is important to consider even the most basic aspects of our personality as we assess our personal strengths and "growing edges"—areas in which we could continue to learn skills—as researchers. Before we discuss the sampling methods most relevant for your study, take a moment to ask yourself the following questions as a self-assessment:

- What previous knowledge do you have of your sample?
- What knowledge do you need to acquire about your sample?
- What strengths in interpersonal/intrapersonal skills do you typically have in building relationships?
- What are your growing edges in interpersonal/intrapersonal skills in building relationships?

Below, I (Singh) note the importance of self-assessment when conducting research:

"When I initiated a line of research with transgender people about their resilience processes, I had personal knowledge of this group through my friendships and community activism. This personal knowledge informed me about the importance of using accurate pronouns and correct names (chosen names as opposed to names assigned at birth) with these individuals. I also had intimate knowledge of some of the struggles transgender people experience through witnessing friends and community members experience transphobia in their daily lives—from receiving poor health care to being discriminated against at work. However, I did not have personal or professional knowledge about other stressors transgender people experience, such as career discrimination and health care concerns. Obtaining this knowledge prior to entering the field not only provided me with additional information about my topic of study, but also importantly allowed me to use this knowledge to build trusting relationships with transgender people in my study. In terms of building relationships, I have often been told my strengths are having a warm and inviting personality that makes it relatively easy for people to relate to me (Danica says I will 'speak to anyone'—not true!). However, I have also received feedback that one of my growing edges can be that I talk really fast and sometimes it is hard to keep up with what I am saying. Reflecting on both my strengths and growing edges in building relationships gave me the tools I needed to create trusting relationships with the transgender participants in my study."

CHOOSING A SAMPLING METHOD

There are many sampling methods from which to choose, and the best sampling methods in qualitative inquiry are aligned closely with the aim of your research. In other words, what sampling methods will best help you answer your research question(s)?

The good news and the challenging news about selecting a sampling method is that there are no strict rules dictating these decisions. Although there are no "right" or "wrong" answers to these questions, it is important to critically consider which sampling method is most appropriate for your study. This may feel like strange territory if you have primarily engaged in quantitative research. However, remembering that quantitative research is interested in answering "what" questions and that the focus of qualitative inquiry is answering the "how" and "why" questions will help you in thinking about selecting a sampling method for your study.

A good starting point in sampling decisions is to consider the attributes most important to the focus of your study. Answering the following questions will guide you in the first step toward identifying your sampling method:

- *What is the unit of analysis in which you are most interested with your study?* In Chapter 4 we discussed four types of cases or units of analysis: individual, setting, process, and event. Additionally, Patton (2002) describes these four units of analysis: (1) perspective/world-based (e.g., culture-sharing groups), (2) geography-focused (e.g., neighborhood, state, region), (3) activity-focused (e.g., critical event, period of time), and (4) time-based (e.g., season of the year, academic semester). He also noted that there may be overlap among the four categories.

- *Are there demographic factors important to your research question?* Demographic factors that may be important to your study include gender, race/ethnicity, socioeconomic status, ability status, and religious/spiritual affiliation.

- *Do participants have institutional roles that are essential to your study* (LeCompte & Preissle, 1993)? For instance, if you are studying student bullying in schools, are you interested in students, teachers, counselors, and/or other school personnel?

- *Are you interested in creating a diverse sample?* There has been much debate within the field of qualitative research as how to most effectively attend to multicultural issues, so it is important to decide how you will address issues of diversity within your sample (Jones, 2002). Including one woman in a qualitative study of chemical engineers does not necessarily attend to diversity issues. However, because sample sizes (discussed shortly) are often small in qualitative work, it is also not necessary or realistic for you to include participants from every identity group. Most important is that you are able to answer the question of how you have attended to multicultural issues in your study. Even better is when you can link this answer to your research tradition(s) and research question(s).

These are some general reflections to get you thinking about sampling in qualitative research. Read about students' perspectives on their approach to sampling methods, depending on their stage of research, in Perspectives 6.1.

● ●

Perspectives 6.1. Entering the Field

"I knew it was going to be tough to find the group I wanted to study. My first career was teaching sixth grade. I taught sixth grade in a suburban area, and the students were mostly white. I always noticed how bullying would start to go up in sixth grade. I saw these students struggle and not want to come to school. But there were some students who seemed to just deal with the bullying in a different way. When I started my Ph.D., I knew I wanted to study the perspectives of the students who seemed to cope better. Fortunately, I know what it's like in the school system! There are many gatekeepers I need on my side for this study—namely, the principal, students, and parents. I am thinking about building a relationship with the school counselor at one suburban school because the school is known for having problems with bullying. I am hoping this relationship will help me establish a relationship then with the principal and a few teachers. Then, when I put my IRB [application] through for the county, the principal may be more likely to approve my study because she knows me."

—EARLY CHILDHOOD EDUCATION STUDENT

"I decided to study sexual identity development of female-to-male transgender people who identify as gay men. I attend a yearly transgender health conference, and I had an opportunity to complete an IRB [application] before I went to the conference. I didn't have a lot of time to think about sampling—it was a rare chance to have several transgender men in the same place who identified as gay men so I had to go for it! I used purposeful and convenience sampling—I had a booth in which to interview folks. I knew I would use snowball sampling too because I had asked participants to tell their friends and people in their community about the study. Only thing is, when my research team started to take a look at the data from the interviews, it was difficult because there were so many other questions that arose and that I wanted to follow up with participants. But it was too late because I had no way to contact many of the participants. They truly wanted to be anonymous and would only agree to be in the study if I interviewed them that one time. Although I would ideally go back and interview one person at a time, it wasn't realistic for this population. I used purposeful sampling. I think it was the best way to answer my research question: How do transgender men who identify as gay describe their sexual identity development? We got a lot of rich data in the end. I think this study will be a real contribution to the field."

—COUNSELING PSYCHOLOGY STUDENT

"I study reading and multicultural education. Most recently I decided to use critical race theory to examine the counter-stories of struggling readers in middle school who are from families that are from rural, poor, and agricultural backgrounds. In critical race theory counter-stories are the narratives from people who have been marginalized—and, boy, have these struggling readers been robbed of some important resources in their education. These kids get stigmatized early on in their education, but I have noticed that they nevertheless succeed in environments where they get to read about what goes on in their daily lives—like the places in which they live and where they see their parents work— so I have been most interested in what their 'funds of knowledge' are. I decided to use multiple sites in my study so I could access more students and get a larger sample size. I had a relationship with one of the schools. A teacher there introduced me to another teacher in a neighboring school—so I also used a convenience sampling method. I needed a larger sample size. I knew the larger size would help me

present more convincing data in talking with legislators about resources these kids need to succeed. I did classroom observations and focus groups with the kids and ended up with 50 participants at four different sites in three counties."

—LITERACY EDUCATION AND READING STUDENT

"I want to understand how indigenous practices of healing are addressed in counseling. There is a lot of information out there about what indigenous practices are, but we know so little about how these healing methods are used in the counseling office. I am not even sure if there has ever been a qualitative study on this before because I have only seen conceptual work in the field. After I finish my lit review, I want to identify which indigenous group in the United States is most underrepresented in the literature. I have planned a year for my fieldwork—which I know is rare for a doctoral student— but I have good contacts in the southwestern U.S., mostly anthropologist friends who work in reservation settings. I want to use a phenomenological approach, so that means I won't predetermine a sample size, but will still aim for about 10–15 participants and interview them several times each. I have a place to live with friends during my study, so now I just need to identify what and whom I want to study. That will guide me to the site I go to—and because counseling centers on reservations are so rare, I am already preparing myself to think about using more than one site. I will not have a car, and public transportation is not so great on many reservations, so I definitely need to keep that in mind. I am excited to get started, but it will also be a bit stressful being so far away from my advisor, who is on the East Coast. I am planning monthly phone calls with her so I stay on track and focused. I am also thinking it might be hard to come back home after being in the field so long, but this is really what I want to do. I am interested in an academic position after I graduate and want to teach qualitative research, so my dissertation is not only of interest to me—it also will help me get a job later hopefully."

—COUNSELING STUDENT

• •

PURPOSEFUL SAMPLING METHODS

In the current field of clinical and educational research, purposeful sampling has come to exemplify building rigor into your sampling strategy. **Purposeful sampling**— sometimes called *judgment sampling*—requires that you develop specific criteria for the sample of your study prior to entering the field (Patton, 2002). You may see this same strategy described as *purposive sampling* (Denzin & Lincoln, 2000). Both terms refer to establishing criteria to obtain information-rich cases of your phenomenon before you sample your population. This may sound like a simple—and commonsense—way to go. However, many students have embarked on qualitative studies without giving intentional thought to the criteria for their sample. This lack of deliberate planning never pays off in a solid (or ethical) qualitative study—so beware and pay close attention to this section. Using our previous example of sampling with South Asian American survivors of child sexual abuse, the purposive sampling of our study included the following criteria: above 18 years old, having an experience of sexual abuse between the ages of 5 and 18 years old, and being of South Asian American heritage.

Miles and Huberman (1994) discuss 16 types of purposeful sampling methods. We organized these 16 sampling types into three different categories to help you think

> **TABLE 6.1. Three Categories of Purposeful Sampling Methods**
>
> Representativeness of sample
>
> - Convenience—relatively easy access to a sample; least representative
> - Homogeneous—participants who share many similarities to one another
> - Maximum variation—participants who share many differences from one another
> - Stratified purposeful—unique features of subgroups (or strata) of a phenomenon
> - Purposeful random—randomly selecting from a purposeful sample to increase sample variation
> - Comprehensive—selecting an entire group of people by established criteria; most representative
>
> Description/presentation of phenomenon
>
> - Typical case—average example of the focus of your study
> - Intensity—cases that intensely demonstrate a phenomenon of inquiry
> - Critical case—"benchmark" cases for other participants because of irregularity or richness
> - Politically important—cases that draw political attention to the phenomenon
> - Extreme or deviant—participants with the most positive or most negative experiences
>
> Theory development and verification
>
> - Snowball, chain, or network sampling—participants who "know" one another
> - Opportunistic—appearance of new potential samples as research evolves
> - Criterion—meet an important, predetermined criterion of the phenomenon
> - Theoretical—evolving theory of data collection guides sampling strategy
> - Confirming and disconfirming—during theoretical sampling researcher searches for cases to support and refute findings

about the best fit for your study: (1) representativeness of sample, (2) description and presentation of the phenomenon, and (3) theory development and verification. See Table 6.1 for a list of purposeful sampling methods within these three categories.

Representativeness of Sample

In the first category of purposeful sampling methods, representativeness of sample, the main goal guiding your selection of participants is representing individuals themselves. We discuss six subcategories of purposeful sampling: (1) convenience, (2) homogeneous, (3) maximum variation, (4) stratified purposeful, (5) purposeful random, and (6) comprehensive.

Of these subcategories, **convenience sampling** is the least representative strategy of the six. Convenience sampling is a method based on the researcher's relatively easy access to a population (Schwandt, 2001). For instance, a counselor working in a community mental health center may decide to study the population using their mental health services—this is a convenient sample. The advantages of using convenience samples center on resources of the researcher. Convenience samples are easy to access because you use the sample available to you (Hood, 2006). So if you, as a researcher, are short on money, time, or energy, this can be a helpful sampling approach. In our example of sampling South Asian American survivors of child sexual abuse, convenience sampling translated to focusing on gaining access to participants within a South Asian nonprofit that served survivors of various types of violence.

However, carefully consider your decision to use convenience sampling because there are significant disadvantages as well to this method. Because convenience samples are so readily accessible, there are drawbacks to the type of information you can gather if you used a more rigorous approach. One of the key drawbacks is that obtaining data from a readily accessible sample likely results in a nonrepresentative sample with flawed findings and at best a gross estimate for a population. Werle's (2004) study of the responses of eighth-grade students to the use of storytelling in violence prevention is a good example of when a researcher may choose to use a convenience sample. The author had convenient access to a health education class in a public middle school— so she studied the responses of 13 students to storytelling methods about aggression. This study generated important exploratory information about how this convenience sample responded to violence prevention techniques—namely, the positive response of students to storytelling tools when learning about aggression—and future research may build on these findings to use a more rigorous sampling approach. Because of this sacrifice of quality in the sampling process, many researchers will combine convenience sampling with another sampling approach.

When establishing criteria for your sample, you should consider whether you want to identify a homogeneous or heterogeneous sample (Miles & Huberman, 1994). **Homogeneous sampling** involves including participants who share many similarities to one another. You would select a purposeful homogeneous sampling method if you were interested in gaining comprehensive information about one specific subgroup. An example of a homogeneous sample would be sampling a group of nontraditional black college students over the age of 50—from a larger, more diverse student sample—to understand their use of technology in mathematics courses. On the other hand, you may be more interested in a heterogeneous purposeful sampling strategy. Heterogeneity seeks to have **maximum variation** of characteristics within a sample. Using the previous example, maybe an important aspect of your research question is to understand generally the experience of nontraditional college students—not using race/ethnicity as a characteristic—and their use of technology in undergraduate mathematics courses. In this case, you are talking about a potentially huge sample! The idea of maximum variation turns what could be challenging about this type of sample into strengths: The themes you identify across a group that has maximum variation of characteristics importantly illustrate the central aspects of your research topic (Patton, 2002). When you decide to use heterogeneous sampling, it is important that your data collection and analysis illustrate how this sampling technique impacts your findings. We discuss maximum variation further in Part III of this volume when we discuss data analysis and collection. With the example of sampling South Asian American survivors of child sexual abuse, we sampled a homogeneous group culturally, yet we had variation within our sample in terms of the age the abuse occurred and current age, and participants varied in terms of the ages they immigrated to the United States and/or being second- or third-generation Americans.

Within purposeful sampling, you may decide to use a random or stratified technique. You may decide to use **random purposeful sampling** to increase the variation of cases within your study. Random purposeful sampling literally means randomly selecting from a purposeful sample. For instance, in a study of coping resources of white women who are in recovery from alcoholism, you may decide that your potential sample is too sizeable to manage realistically. In this case, random sampling not only helps you manage potentially large samples, but also gives you more credibility in your study because you reduce what Patton (2002) calls "suspicion about why certain cases were selected for study" (p. 241). One of the common misconceptions of random purposeful sampling is that it is representative and thus that its findings are generalizable. Although it does help to minimize any bias associated with hand-picking cases, random purposeful sampling does not guarantee that these were "random" cases, as in quantitative research.

Stratified purposeful sampling allows you to demonstrate the distinguishing features of subgroups (or strata) of a phenomenon in which you are interested. As a result, these unique features also allow a comparison of different subgroups, if that is an important aspect of answering your research question. We return to the phrase *maximum variation of a sample with stratification* because your aim is to identify a broad range of unique qualities specific to certain subgroups—and then you may choose to compare subgroups to illustrate their differences. As an example of stratified purposeful sampling, suppose you are interested in instructional strategies at the high school level. Your strata could include the various instructional strategies, whereas selected participants would represent each stratum (e.g., teachers are selected based on their instructional strategy). With our example of South Asian American survivors of child sexual abuse, stratified purposeful sampling would have allowed us to examine the distinct meaning of participants' experiences according to the type of abuse and/or age when the abuse occurred. Because the focus of our study was on the resilience of survivors of child sexual abuse and the meaning they made of their resilience and abuse experiences, we elected not to use purposive stratified sampling.

Finally, the **comprehensive sampling** method is the most representative of the six in this category. In this sampling strategy, the researcher selects an entire group of people by an established set of criteria. An example would be if the focus of research is an examination of a multicultural counseling class to understand students' experiences of racial identity development within the classroom. In this case, your sample is the entire group—students in a multicultural course. The main criterion for the participants in this study would simply be that they were a graduate student in a multicultural counseling course. Typically, comprehensive sampling methods are most appropriate when the population is small. To revisit our example of South Asian American survivors of child sexual abuse, if we had selected to study a support group geared to this population, we might have selected to use comprehensive sampling. Also, if we were studying a training group of counselors or educators seeking cultural competence in working with this group of people, we might have used a comprehensive sampling method for the study.

Description/Presentation of the Phenomenon

For some qualitative studies, as a researcher your sampling decisions will be guided by the goals of describing or presenting the phenomenon of your investigation. For instance, in a study of a culture-sharing group, such as Korean American first-generation families, perhaps the focus of your study is describing their experiences of acculturation processes. In this example, a presentation of participants' acculturative stressors would be critical, and you would want to use a sampling method that allows you to describe and present this focus. We group together five subcategories in this section: (1) typical case, (2) intensity, (3) critical case, (4) politically important, and (5) extreme or deviant.

If you select a case study, life history, or biography research tradition, you may decide to use the first subcategory as your sampling method. A **typical case sampling** strategy represents an average example of the focus of your study (Miles & Huberman, 1994). Similar to convenience and snowball sampling, critiques of using a typical case rely on the lack of heterogeneity in the sample. However, an advantage to using typical case sampling is that the researcher can study a complex phenomenon on a more individual basis. Sampling a typical case may also be helpful when a field of inquiry is relatively new and qualitative investigations are rare. In a study of play therapy, Snow, Hudspeth, Blake, and Seale (2007) decided to use a typical case sampling method to examine the therapeutic environment and play themes and behaviors of children over a time period of 6 weeks. The researchers honed in on two typical cases for their study, acknowledging "the shortcomings of the method ... nevertheless, the case study ... allows for the presentation of information which should never go unnoticed in a field of study as new and complex as that of child psychology" (p. 148). Focusing on typical cases for two 6-year-old children allowed the researchers to identify in-depth findings rich in information about the complex interactions within a play therapy context.

Whereas typical case sampling identifies an average case for a study, the second subcategory of **intensity sampling** refers to identifying cases that demonstrate a phenomenon of inquiry involving strong affect. It is important to note that these are not cases that are extreme in nature—those types of cases would misrepresent the phenomenon and are not intense cases. An example of an intense case would be a qualitative examination of the grief and loss of parents who have lost a child. In this instance, every participant in your sample will likely be an intense case. But you would potentially decide to not interview parents who had lost multiple family members (i.e., extreme) in the study to avoid the potential distortion of the phenomenon.

In the third subcategory of **critical case sampling**, the researcher is looking for experiences that are particularly significant because of their irregularity in order to serve as a benchmark of "cutoff score" for other participants (e.g., "If it happens here, it can happen anywhere"). Critical case samples can be conceptualized as a variation of intensity sample; they involve cases with strong affect, yet these cases occur in unexpected ways. The cases are selected because the researcher believes that they can be used to illustrate a point particularly well and provide the most knowledge about the phenomenon of interest. For example, consider a historical analysis of hate crimes against transgender individuals. A researcher may want to select a particular incident that was intense (e.g., murder and sexual assault of Brandon Teena, a transgender female to male) and analyze documents and interview participants who were associated with the event in some manner.

The fourth subcategory of description/presentation of phenomenon emphasizes significant experiences; a **politically important sampling** strategy is a type of critical case that draws political attention to the phenomenon. To understand this sampling strategy, think of typical news stories that "grab" your attention. There are usually several political components to this type of story, and you may have several political reactions to these components. However, don't be fooled by the word *political*—it may or may not refer to issues of politics on the main stage of the United States or world. Really, a politically important case may be one that especially demonstrates a political issue, potentially motivating others to take action as a result.

The final subcategory in this section is the **extreme or deviant case sampling**. The purpose of this form of sampling is to select participants whose experiences were the most positive or most negative, thereby helping researchers to discover the "boundaries of differences within an experience" (Polkinghorne, 2005, p. 141). You can investigate either or both of the extremes, looking for illuminative cases. For example, suppose that you want to evaluate a training seminar on counseling racial/ethnic minorities. You might seek out participants who rated the experience high (i.e., seminar was extremely helpful) as well as those who rated it low (i.e., seminar was not helpful at all) and interview them in depth to understand the boundaries of the experience. Unusual conditions or extreme outcomes (i.e., looking at outliers on a normal curve) can be relevant particularly in program evaluations. From which cases can you learn the most? One weakness of this sampling approach is that it lacks generalizability.

In each of the examples provided to illustrate these sampling strategies, it is important that the novice qualitative researcher reflect on the empathy he or she would need for participants in such a study. For instance, in extreme or deviant sampling, as a researcher you are literally on the "outskirts" of a sample, which likely will involve participants who have had intense experiences of a phenomenon; therefore, researcher empathy will be an important component of this sampling strategy. It can be helpful to integrate interactive interviewing—wherein the researcher provides opportunities for the participant to ask the researcher questions—into these sampling strategies (see Chapter 8). In addition, researcher ethics and integrity are always important, but especially so when your sampling strategy involves seeking to understand intense experiences of participants.

Theory Development and Verification

This final section of purposeful sampling focuses on the development and verification of theory. We organize five subcategories in this section: (1) snowball, (2) opportunistic, (3) criterion, (4) theoretical, and (5) confirming and disconfirming cases.

The first category of **snowball sampling**—also called *chain* or *network sampling*—is often a natural fit for a convenience sampling strategy. As the name implies, once you find a typical case for your study, you then ask if the individual knows other people who are also typical cases. This sampling method goes on and on, having a "snowball" or "chain" effect because you are using people's relationships with one another to identify your sample. This method can give you quick access to a population of study—a main advantage. Also, similar to convenience samples, if you are studying a vulnerable group of people—such as people who have survived violence—snowball sampling may be a good choice for your investigation. You should also address questions of whether a more diversified sample may have captured different information. Although it was previously thought that the main disadvantage of using snowball sampling in qualitative research is that you would not have a heterogeneous sample (or maximum variation, discussed above), it is possible to use snowball sampling to *sequentially* build variation into your sample (Polit & Beck, 2003). For instance, you could use snowball sampling as a method to reach several different types of participants. In this case, rather than following the snowball sample within just one group, you would initiate the snowball sample within several different groups of potential participants. With both convenience and snowball sampling, it is important that you select participants who are information-rich cases, meaning that they exemplify the phenomenon in which you are interested.

The second subcategory, **opportunistic sampling**, is sometimes called *emergent sampling* because it seeks to capitalize on the appearance of new potential samples as the research process evolves. This sampling method may seem to focus more on how to build advantages into your sampling strategy for your study. However, there is a deeper purpose for this sampling approach. Because so much of qualitative research involves aspects one cannot predict ahead of time, opportunistic sampling allows the researcher to address when *both* barriers and opportunities in the sampling process occur. This sampling strategy reminds researchers of the creativity inherent in qualitative inquiry.

The third subcategory of **criterion sampling** refers to when researchers sample participants who are selected because they meet an important, predetermined criterion. The purpose is to review all cases that meet a criterion. For example, a researcher studying the experiences of racial identity development among counselor education students who have taken a multicultural counseling course would select only participants who had completed the course. Criterion sampling is typically used when program evaluation is an important aspect of your study.

Whereas purposeful sampling generally establishes criteria for finding your participants prior to beginning your study, the fourth subcategory of **theoretical sampling** proposes that the evolving theory from your data collection should guide your sampling strategy (Strauss, 1987). Theoretical sampling is an obvious match for grounded theory designs because of the emphasis on having a systematic process in which you sample your population of inquiry. Theoretical sampling begins with criteria for the anticipated sample, similar to process involved in purposive sampling. For instance, if you are studying the impact of the achievement gap on Latino(a) students in elementary school, your sample—in both purposive and theoretical sampling—may begin with the following criteria: (1) identify as Latino(a) and (2) attend elementary school. As we discussed, the criteria of the purposive sampling would guide the selection of each of your participants. However, the process of theoretical sampling guides the researcher to systematically collect data in discrete steps—taking one step at a time. At the completion of one step, the researcher then revisits the previously collected data and analyzes if "saturation" (explained shortly) has occurred. It is important to be aware that unlike other sampling methods we discuss, theoretical sampling is often more linked to your data collection and analysis process than to the initial participant selection.

To use the example of a research question about Latino elementary schools and the achievement gap, to answer this question, perhaps you find that you also need to include the perspectives of teachers, parents, and other key informants because they are able to provide critical information on systemic barriers the students identified.

One of the advantages of using a theoretical sampling method is that you will strengthen the rigor of your study if your aim is to generate a grounded theory of your phenomenon of inquiry. Another advantage is that the systematic method provides some structure to the process that may guide you through some of the challenges of the qualitative research process. Often during your sampling, you may be confronted with challenge of two key questions: "Have I collected enough data?" and "Am I missing important information for this study?" Theoretical sampling is clearly linked to a grounded theory research design and reminds you to use theory and your research questions to answer these challenges. The disadvantages of theoretical sampling are similar to its inherent strengths—your study's focus may not require as much structure throughout each step of the sampling process to answer your research question. For instance, if your research question is "What are the experiences of white, rural high school students with their school counselors as they prepare for college?" and if you are most interested in the students' perspectives, purposive sampling is a better fit for your line of inquiry. Because theoretical sampling demands a systematic process, it may require resources (e.g., time, money) that are beyond the reach of the investigator. Remember that although theoretical sampling is a type of purposeful sampling, it is distinguished from other types of purposeful sampling "because the theoretical categories that guide the sampling are the result of the previous stages of analysis and are analytical rather than simply demographic categories" (Hood, 2006, p. 217).

The final subcategory of this section is the **confirming and disconfirming sampling** method. This is a strategy that is often conducted as part of theoretical sampling. As patterns emerge, the researcher looks for confirming cases to add depth to the study *and* seeks disconfirming cases to look for "exceptions that prove the rule" or exceptions that disconfirm the pattern. An important reminder is that whereas theoretical sampling involves selecting cases in an exploratory, inductive manner as concepts emerge, the confirming–disconfirming strategy is selected to verify emerging theory.

Now that you have learned more about sampling methods, it is helpful to discuss their different merits with qualitative scholars. See Activity 6.1 for guidelines in conducting an informational interview about sampling methods. Additionally, it is important to consider how your proposal might use the various sampling methods (see Proposal Development 6.1).

 ACTIVITY 6.1. Interviewing a Qualitative Researcher about Sampling Methods

Before you enter the field and make decisions about the best sampling method to help you answer your research question, it is helpful to talk to other qualitative researchers about their experiences in this area. Set an appointment for an informational interview with one of the qualitative scholars in your department, college, or university. When you meet, start your informational interview with the following questions:

- "How do you think about sampling methods in qualitative research?"
- "What are the typical challenges and successes you have faced when using sampling methods?"
- "In your most recent study, how did you choose a specific group to sample?"
- "How has your perspective on sampling methods changed since you first began conducting qualitative research?"

Keep a journal during and after this interview to track your interviewee's responses. Make a list of insights about sampling for your study.

PROPOSAL DEVELOPMENT 6.1. Selecting a Sampling Method

After you have selected a topic for your qualitative proposal, it is time to weigh the various purposeful sampling methods to consider the most optimal way to address your research question(s). Consider the following:

- What is your research topic?
- What are your research goals?
- What is (are) your research question(s)?
- What general category of purposeful sampling methods do you perceive as most appropriate for your study? Why?
- For each method within that category, consider what your sample would look like.
- Are there sampling methods outside your primary category that might be suitable to integrate in your sampling plan? How would you do so?

SAMPLE SIZE

It is quite probable that as soon as you decided to conduct a qualitative study, you began to think about sample size! It is interesting how this question immediately lands the beginning qualitative researcher in the quantitative land of numbers. It makes sense that numbers would be a concern, actually. For graduate students, there are concerns about the time, scope, and focus of research projects—in addition to questions of whether you can complete your study in time to graduate. Although sample size concerns are normal, we suggest that you shelve the potential to obsess about number of participants and return to what got you started on a qualitative study in the first place—your research question.

Sample size is perhaps one of the most hotly contested issues within both the qualitative and quantitative fields (Jones, 2002). Merriam (2002) best addresses the need to consider the function of qualitative inquiry as compared to other approaches: "To begin with, since you are not interested in 'how much' or 'how often,' random sampling makes little sense. Since qualitative inquiry seeks to understand the meaning of a phenomenon for the perspectives of the participants, it is important from which [participants] most can be learned" (p. 12). Therefore, sample size in qualitative inquiry depends largely on the degree to which the research purpose is met.

Unfortunately, some purely quantitative researchers may critique qualitative research for having typically smaller sample sizes. Indeed, a well-established quantitative scholar in counseling psychology loves to deride qualitative research, asking, "What is the difference between journalists and qualitative researchers?" Of course, there are many significant differences—namely the rigorous standards of quality demanded by qualitative designs and the focus on in-depth understandings of phenomena. By the time you finish reading this book, you will have a well-nuanced answer to this type of critique.

For now, we encourage you to remember that your decisions about sample sizes—even when samples are small—tend to be one of the strengths of qualitative research. As we discussed in Chapter 4, the goal of qualitative inquiry is to gain a depth of understanding about a topic area, rather than the breadth that is often the goal of quantitative research. Qualitative methodologists agree that the sample size should be consistent with the minimum number of participants you need to adequately represent the phenomenon of inquiry—a number that is guided by the study's purpose (Hood, 2006; Miles & Huberman, 1994; Patton, 2002). A good example of determining sample size for a study investigating a complex phenomenon with a vulnerable population is the research by Yeh, Inman, Kim, and Okubo (2006), which investigated the collectivistic coping strategies used by Asian American families after losing a loved one in the 9/11 attacks on the World Trade Center. In this study, researchers used purposeful sampling to identify information-rich cases of the phenomenon. Initially, the researchers worked on outreach with multiple community organizations to identify 28 potential families that met the study's criteria; however, the sample size was reduced to 16 scheduled interviews and resulted in a final sample size of 11 Asian American participants. The purposeful sampling method (e.g., Asian American, loss of a family member during 9/11), combined with researcher intentions to capture as many participants as possible, yielded in-depth findings for the study and a strong rationale for their sample size of 11 participants.

Creswell (2006) and Morse (1995) provide general guidelines for sample size according to several research traditions. With case studies, Creswell suggests using three to five participants, and for phenomenology, he suggests a sample of up to 10 people. In ethnographic research, Morse encourages conducting interviews with between 30 and 50 participants, whereas in grounded theory, Creswell recommends a sample size between 20 and 30 people. It is important to begin thinking about sample size by understanding these general guidelines for your selected research tradition. Sandelowski (1995) illustrated this point: "A sample size of 10 may be judged adequate for certain kinds of homogeneous or critical case sampling, too small to achieve maximum variation of a complex phenomenon or to develop theory—or too large for certain kinds of narrative analysis" (p. 179).

For those using a grounded theory tradition, saturation becomes an important goal of participant sampling. **Saturation** of the data generally refers to the point in data collection and analysis where the researcher does not identify any ideas, themes, or large constructs as new data are collected (Corbin & Strauss, 2008). At this point as a researcher, you are recognizing all the new incoming information as confirming what previous participants have shared. This saturation of the data is closely aligned with your research question: Are the new data giving the same "answer" to your research question that your previous sample has shared? The idea of saturation is the point at which theoretical sampling diverges from its common beginning with purposive sampling.

Saturation may sound like a simple concept, but there is complexity in identifying when it has occurred. Recognizing saturation of the data is a qualitative skill that is similar to filling up your gas tank and topping it off—it is a point where you know there is no more "theoretical room" for more information. The skill of detecting saturation of the data is more than what Corbin and Strauss call "no new categories or themes emerging. It also denotes a development of categories in terms of their properties and dimensions, including variation, and possible relationships to other concepts. ... It is to tell us something about those categories" (2008, p. 148).

A note on language: You will often see qualitative methodologists and researchers refer to concepts as "emerging" from the data. We encourage you to *not* use this term as you learn about, conduct, and write up your qualitative work. *Emerging* is a word that masks the researcher's role, skills, and power in the interpretation of the data. Being clear about these areas is part of our accountability as researchers; we endeavor to convey respect for our participants and field sites *and* we fully own that we are the people interpreting the data. If we don't "own" this researcher role, we are letting ourselves off the proverbial hook in terms of our responsibility as qualitative scholars. Although we discuss saturation briefly here because it is closely linked to discussions of sample size, look for a more in-depth further discussion in Part III of this volume.

Your sampling decisions will likely involve attention to the degree of depth and breadth in your sample. Sampling strategies aiming for a smaller sampling typically desire more depth, whereas sampling strategies seeking larger sizes tend to build more breadth into the sample. For instance, if you are seeking to gain an in-depth understanding of the meaning of a reading intervention for elementary school students, a smaller sample size of eight will perhaps allow you to interview the students multiple times and/ or analyze their data for more distilled themes. In this sample research topic, sampling a larger size of 25–40 participants would ultimately give a researcher the opportunity to examine the meaning of the reading intervention from many more perspectives. Thus, your decisions about the depth and breadth of your sample should be guided by the research goals. Revisit Chapter 4 for our discussion of determining research goals.

It is important to have some flexibility in how you think about your sample size— you may begin collecting data (discussed further in Chapter 8) and decide you will need fewer or more participants in order to answer your research question. Because we find that it is easy to get lost in the qualitative world of sample size, we believe it is important to attend to the following questions in order to build a strong rationale for your study's sample size:

- What are the research paradigm(s) and tradition(s) for your study, and are there suggestions for sample size? Asking this question importantly grounds you in the underlying theoretical constructs of your research paradigm. This way, you aren't picking a sample size out of the air. You are firmly situating your sample size decisions in your research tradition. We think it is helpful to look at the most recent qualitative studies examining your phenomenon of inquiry or the nearest area of inquiry to your phenomenon. There is also a strong line of scholarship on qualitative sampling approaches related to sample size and other components of sampling strategies that continues to evolve. You can find these discussions in journals such as *Qualitative Inquiry, Qualitative Research*, and *The Qualitative Report*. For a comprehensive list of field-specific and multidisciplinary qualitative journals, visit *www.slu.edu/organizations/qrc/QRjournals.html*, a website that was developed based on resources listed by Dr. Judith Preissle and Dr. Linda Wark.

- Is saturation of the data an important aspect of your research tradition? If yes, then you may decide to stop sampling when you see a recurrence of the same themes and do not identify any new themes with the most recent participants.

- What are the dangers and opportunities of sampling too many or too few participants for your specific study?

See Figure 6.2 for a flowchart to help you think about issues of sample size for your study.

Perspectives 6.2. Bringing Sample Size Concerns to Life

"I have resisted concerns about sample size for the majority of my studies because they have been primarily phenomenological studies where I was more concerned about capturing the lived experiences of a phenomenon for participants. In these examinations, I used purposeful sampling methods with convenience and snowball sampling. Now that I am moving into using more grounded theory research designs, sample size is on my mind much more from the beginning of a study. I review the grounded theory studies in counseling, and the 'golden number' is typically somewhere between 15 and 20, but definitely more than 10 participants. Although I am looking for saturation of the data, I still remind myself that sample sizes—no matter how much we try—cannot be set in stone in advance of a study. Rather, we can establish general guidelines for our sample size and pay attention to what our data are telling us the sample size should be."

—AAS

"Some of the biggest concerns with selecting a sample size involve two phrases commonly heard among educators, students, and researchers in general:

"1. Saturation indicates validity. *Not exactly. Remember, saturation has to do with testing for redundancy of themes when the end goal is ensuring that all themes are identified thoroughly. Although researchers may be interested in achieving saturation in traditions such as grounded theory or ethnography, it makes little sense (and is antithetical) for other traditions such as phenomenology and life history.*

"2. You need about 10 participants in your sample. *Students are often trained by instructors (who were trained by their instructors) to obtain 'about 10 participants' for their study, particularly when they are conducting individual interviews. I am unsure where this magic number of 10 originated, but the 'magic number' (or at least the initial sample size) derives from general guidelines of the research tradition and/or sampling method."*

—DGH

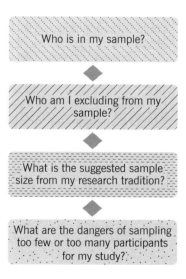

FIGURE 6.2. Flowchart for thinking about sample size.

CASE EXAMPLE 6.1. Three Different Rationales for Sample Size in Qualitative Design: Ethnography, Hermeneutics, and Grounded Theory

Ethnography

Jones, S. (2006). *Girls, social class, and literacy: What teachers can do to make a difference.* Portsmouth, NH: Heinemann.

"For me, the site was the most important factor in my sampling decision. I wanted to be in a neighborhood and a school that was mostly a high-poverty context, but not with a majority–minority population. The site needed to be either a racially diverse context with high poverty, or if a white context, it had to be high poverty. I ended up with a white and high-poverty context because there were still significant enclaves of poverty from Appalachian areas where folks had migrated into the city, but were still poor. Particularly in education, there is a dearth of research about white, high-poverty contexts—usually the field talks about African American students and recent immigrants.

"Once I was at the site, I was introduced to a teacher who was willing to work with me. She said, 'Sure, you can come in whenever you want during class.' That's when participant selection started for my study—from a small elementary school class. In the beginning, I invited all students to participate, and all their families agreed. So, I had a total sample of 18, with 9–10 girls and 8–9 boys. However, I realized over the first year of my 3-year ethnographic study that there were very different things working across the gender domains. I then decided, since this was my dissertation research, I could not focus on both girls and boys. I decided to focus on the girls because I found more theoretical help in the international field of gender in education literature for my study. There just was not as much information on the boys—so I guess I decided to not be a pioneer in that area and to go with the paths that had been paved relatively well in the literature. I ended up with eight focal participants and their families."

Hermeneutics

Graff, J. M. (2007). *The literary lives of marginalized readers: Preadolescent girls' rationale for book choice and experiences with self-selected books.* Gainesville: University of Florida.

"I used purposeful sampling, convenience sampling, and snowball sampling because I was interested in a specific demographic group. I had three criteria for my sample: preadolescent girls who (1) were considered marginalized by two school indicators—(a) socioeconomic status, as measured by students who were eligible for free or reduced meals in their schools, and (b) race/ethnicity, which was marginalized within the school system; (2) were struggling readers who were placed in remedial classes based on their latest performance on their standardized reading assessment test; and (3) expressed extreme dislike or apathy toward reading, which was identified through formal surveys and conversations with teachers. I established these criteria because I wanted a lot of depth in the study, and I realized to do this I needed a smaller number of individuals. I originally decided to start off with 8 participants, but then increased to 10 because there was a large possibility that girls would drop out of the study, and I did not want attrition to negatively influence the research. Also, because I was using a hermeneutical research paradigm, when I looked at previous research the hermeneutics literature suggested sampling anywhere between 2 and 12 participants."

Grounded Theory

Burnes, T. R. (2006). Opening the door of a bigger closet: An analysis of sexual orientation identity development for lesbian, bisexual, and queer college women of color. *Dissertation Abstracts International* (DAI-B 67/07).

"I knew from the beginning of my dissertation process that I wanted to do a grounded theory design, so the biggest factor for me in terms of sample size was the saturation of the data. From my qualitative research classes, I had been exposed to several types of designs. But for my study—understanding the sexual identity development of lesbian, bisexual, and queer college women of color—I thought grounded theory was the best fit. I knew I would need to interview upwards of 25–30 people based on the literature. At the same time, I knew I would never finish my dissertation if I collected that much data! In the end, I decided to make my dissertation an exploratory study using grounded theory, so I sampled 15 people. Later, after I had graduated and when I was a first-year faculty member, I decided to write a grant offered through my professional association that would support me with the time and resources I needed to interview 30 participants as a follow-up grounded theory study. That's the best part about qualitative research, I think. The way you think about sample size doesn't have to be restricted to one certain number in one certain study. Who knows how many participants I will have by the time I finish this next project?—but I do know that I will be looking to the data to let me know when I have reached saturation. I am also thinking about conducting a similar study with gay and bisexual men of color."

SELECTING AND ENTERING A SITE

Just as researchers select a sampling method that is a good fit for their research question(s), their selection and entering of a site should also be guided by the major focus of investigation. This is a decision that should take some time and effort. You may immediately have a site that comes to mind. For instance, if you are conducting an ethnography of community-based organizations (CBOs) serving queer (i.e., gay) youth, you have an obvious site of study. However, the site for your study may not be as obvious. Perhaps, for this same example, you are interested in queer youth who live with depression. You may have greater success with a CBO that provides counseling services for queer youth. Either way, a careful process is involved. We discuss five steps for selecting and entering a site: (1) identify a site, (2) gain access to site, (3) plan site activities, (4) consider length of time at site, and (5) consider potential pitfalls of site. See Figure 6.3 for a flowchart of these steps.

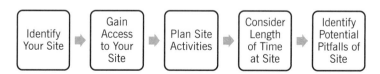

FIGURE 6.3. Selecting and entering a site flowchart.

Identify a Site

The first step, identifying a site, may be the most difficult one in the process. Several factors will guide your site selection, including your sampling method and accessibility of the site. An essential question to ask is, "Where will I find my targeted sample?" If you are studying children and adolescents, schools and other youth-oriented settings may be ideal sites. If you are investigating how urban policy around low-income housing impacts the lives of children and adolescents, community centers with after-school care may be a better fit. When discussing site selection, we often forget to think about our comfort level with a particular site. However, comfort is an important factor, especially because you could be in the field for a significant period of time collecting data. Of course, we want to assess our "discomfort" level with potential sites as well. If you feel uncomfortable about a specific site, is that about your lack of skills, knowledge, and experience—and if so, how can you, as the researcher, plan to develop these skills? All of these factors are important in selecting a site appropriate for your study. At this stage, you may also realize that to gain an adequate sample, you will need to work with multiple sites. Especially if your research tradition guides you toward a large sample size, you may need to identify and work with several sites in your study.

Gain Access to Your Site

We discuss the second step, gaining access to your site of interest, in further detail in the next section because it relates to gatekeepers, stakeholders, and key informants. For this section, we discuss potential issues that may make accessing your site challenging. Are there certain time periods when you have access to the site, and other times when you do not? How will this access impact data collection and analysis while you are in the field? Do you have the resources you will need (e.g., transportation, other equipment) to gain entry to the site? For example, one community mental health center we visited required two forms of photo identification and a security escort to access the area where counseling services took place. Once you have identified a site in the previous step, planning exactly how you will access the site paves the way for the third step—planning site activities.

Plan Site Activities

By the time you are ready to plan site activities, you have already developed a general idea of what research components you would like to conduct at your site. Most likely, you identified these activities in your IRB application, but you also may have determined new site activities that are important to your study based on another review of the literature or on your sampling method. Regardless, during this third step of selecting and entering a site, you methodically lay out the specific activities you will be conducting at a site. On one of my (Singh) recent studies on reducing bullying in a seventh-grade cohort in middle school, as soon as I identified the middle school with which I wanted to work and gained access and permission to be at the site, I conducted a few visits to ensure that my planned activities "made sense" based on the physical building and classrooms of the school. For this study, I had art activities planned as part of the data collection, but on a site visit I noticed that the art classroom was in a different wing of the building from where I was granted permission to conduct the study. Between this site visit and the commencement of the study, I was able to gain permission to conduct the study in these areas. When planning site activities, make sure to also plan a site visit to cover all your bases so that your research gets off to a smooth start.

Consider Length of Time at Site

In the fourth step you carefully consider the length of time you will be at the site. Counseling and educational research sites tend to carry immense demands on time and resources. Preparing in advance of your study for how long you will be at the site—from the length of the entire study to the length of your time needed with participants—will help you communicate with your site personnel. In qualitative research, we know that plans for data collection may change while in the field. However, if you have previously planned the length of time for your study and communicate that information to the staff at your site, you additionally build trust with the key players there. Then, if there are changes in length of time that your study requires as it commences, the site staff may be more flexible in responding to your needs based on this trusting relationship.

Identify Potential Pitfalls

Finally, it is essential to identify the potential pitfalls of a site. These pitfalls can be small or large challenges that, if not addressed, can derail your study. When seeking to foresee these pitfalls, brainstorm broadly. From people and time to resources and the site's unique strengths and challenges, make a list of any possible barriers at the site. Then address each barrier, one by one, to ensure that you are adequately prepared in the event that you encounter one of these pitfalls. We conducted a phenomenological study on the resilience of transgender people. The individual interviews went extremely well; however, site challenges arose when conducting the focus group. I (Singh) had taken each of the steps systematically as I selected and entered the site—a community-based organization serving transgender people. However, on the night the final focus group was scheduled, 16 participants showed up to attend the focus group. We had expected and planned for six to eight participants. Why were so many participants in attendance? Hurricane Katrina had just broken the levees in New Orleans in 2005, and a group of transgender people had just been evacuated from the city. Our study gave out gift cards as participant incentives, so the focus group was a mighty fine place to be from the perspectives of participants! Fortunately, we had brought more than enough informed consent forms, gift cards, and equipment to accommodate participants.

At the same time, there were serious issues of researcher ethics and integrity for us to address in this situation as well. How would participant incentives influence what participants shared? We asked this question directly in the beginning and end of the focus group. Notice we did not make the assumption that there would be no influence. Instead, we worked with the assumption that participant incentives influence participants, so our goal as researchers was to identify the "how" of this. If we had not asked these questions directly, the ramifications for our research might have been dire. For instance, participants might have felt they "had" to share certain things we as researchers "wanted to hear." An additional ramification might have been that only those participants who were in need of financial assistance came to the focus group. Our direct questions allowed us to identify these issues and influences right away, in addition to ensuring that we, as researchers, reminded participants that the incentive did not mean that they had to share in a certain manner or about a certain topic. We took serious efforts to provide ongoing informed consent and remind participants that they could end their participation in the study at any time. In the end, we collected some wonderfully rich data. The lesson of the story is that when it comes to working in the field, always plan for the unexpected and keep your researcher ethics and integrity "hats" on at all times.

Now that we have discussed sampling methods, issues of sample size, and selecting a site, answer the questions in Proposal Development 6.2 to integrate what you have learned into your own study proposal.

PROPOSAL DEVELOPMENT 6.2. Developing Criteria for Selecting and Entering Your Site(s)

Write one to two paragraphs discussing guidelines and criteria for entering your site. Include the following components:

- What are the site(s) where you will find your participants?
- How will you gain access to your site? What permissions do you need?
- What potential pitfalls might you encounter as you enter the site(s)?
- What are your planned activities at the site(s)? Should you make a site visit?
- What is the length of time you will be at your site(s)?
- How will you prepare yourself as a researcher to relate to your participants?
- Who are the important gatekeepers, stakeholders, and key informants with whom you will interact at the site(s)?
- How will you conclude your research at the site(s)?
- Will you provide participant incentives? If so, how will these influence the sharing of your participants?
- Are there other considerations for entering your site(s)?

Share and review these criteria with a peer and/or a research team.

BUILDING RAPPORT WITH GATEKEEPERS, STAKEHOLDERS, AND KEY INFORMANTS

A study's success or failure can depend on how well you identify the important players in your field of inquiry. We call these critical connections the *gatekeepers, stakeholders,* and *key informants* who can either help you access your sample or, in the worst-case scenarios, establish barriers so that you cannot access the sample you need for your study. **Gatekeepers** are those people who hold access to your participants and/or site of study.

For instance, if you are investigating how a prekindergarten program prepares students for learning, the gatekeepers would be the school administrators who are in charge of granting you access to your participants. **Stakeholders** are described as people or groups who have an investment—or "stake"—in the findings of your study (Stoecker, 2005). For example, stakeholders in an evaluation of a math tutoring program might include students, parents, teachers, and school administrators.

Key informants have some important distinctions from gatekeepers and stakeholders, although we include a discussion of key informants here because we view all three groups as ones with which you will potentially interact in significant ways during your research process. Key informants include people who serve as important contacts for your study and who often provide important information that may shape your study. The strengths of working with key informants is that they can potentially give you critical information, and they can be participants in your study whose data elucidate the phenomenon you are studying. At the same time, there are challenges involved in the very nature of what a key informant represents—a one-person perspective that is inherently biased in one manner or another. Therefore, a good strategy in working with key informants is to keep both the strengths and challenges involved in their perspectives in mind as a researcher. In one of my (Singh) recent studies, a key informant was the security guard at the middle school at which I was conducting a study on bullying. He would update me when participants were going to be late to focus groups. One person may have some overlap in two or three roles. For instance, your gatekeeper may also have a stake in your study's outcome, as well as be an important person with whom to talk in designing your study.

However, merely identifying these important players is often not sufficient; building rapport with them can sometimes make or break your study. In addition, there is often a brief time period during which you not only meet with participants for the first time, but you also negotiate the way that the participants experience you and the impression you leave with them (Pitts, 2007). In essence, building rapport is about building trust. We appreciate Pitts's (2007) study of 16 qualitative researchers and how each built rapport with his or her participants. The findings of this study identified five rapport-building stages that we believe are useful to be aware of as a researcher. We include these five stages in Table 6.2.

TABLE 6.2. Pitts's (2007) Stage Model of Participant–Researcher Relationships in Fieldwork

Pattern	Question elucidating pattern
Other orientation	*How can I help you feel comfortable participating in this research?*
Self-in-relation-to-other	*Who am I (as researcher) to you (as participant)?*
Self-and-other linking	*Who are we to each other as knowledgeable persons?*
Interpersonal connection	*Where is the line between participating in research and friendship?*
Partnership	*How does our relationship enhance the research in which we are mutually invested?*

It is also true that, depending on your study's focus and goals, the mere topic you are attempting to investigate may put you at odds, as a researcher, with the goal of building rapport and trust with your participants. For instance, I (Singh) research gay bullying in middle school settings. Often, participants—whether they be school counselors and teachers or students and parents—are hesitant to discuss their experiences of gay bullying behaviors or their perpetration of such behaviors for fear of "getting in trouble" or of what the findings may "say" about their school setting. In such instances, you may be unable to enact the rapport-building stages discussed by Pitts (2007). However, we encourage you to attempt to build whatever trust you can with participants— even if that entails a simple acknowledgment of the difficulty participants may have in discussing a certain topic with you as the researcher.

Along with the importance of rapport building, there are also issues of access and cooperation when working with the important players involved in your gaining access to your site and participants. Of course, you hope that you get good access to a site loaded with participants, and then full cooperation from participants when you enter that site. However, remember there are important differences between these two terms— *access* and *cooperation*—and just because a gatekeeper grants us access to a site does not translating into the full cooperation of participants at that site! There are subtle and not-so-subtle complexities involved in identifying gatekeepers, and we believe that Wanat's (2008) questions are important to answer in this endeavor:

- Who grants access and cooperation?
- What are the differences between *access* and *cooperation*?
- How do perceived benefits or threats influence the granting of access and cooperation?
- How do gatekeepers and participants withhold cooperation when access has been granted?

See Case Example 6.2 regarding how you might think about both the expected and unexpected issues that may arise in working with gatekeepers, stakeholders, and key informants in the field.

CASE EXAMPLE 6.2. Working with Gatekeepers, Stakeholders, and Key Informants

Williams, S. M. (2007). The dynamics of adolescent friendships: An investigation of school, classrooms, and peer groups—implications for educational policy. *Dissertation Abstracts International, A, 68/04.*

Dr. Sheneka Williams's qualitative dissertation examined adolescent cross-racial friendships within a desegregated school setting. She was interested in whether desegregation policy had reached the individual student level, and she used cross-racial friendships as a lens to examine policy implementation. Her investigation was a spin-off of her advisor's study on how African American parents made choices among magnet schools. The main gatekeepers were the parents, because Williams was interested in how the parents interacted across racial lines within those schools. Dr. Williams shared:

"If the parents said I could not interview the child, then I would have lost that potential participant. My advisor was another gatekeeper in many ways, because she had the prior information for the parents and children. My advisor was really the main conduit for all of this to happen. During her own study, my advisor asked the participants she interviewed if I could later follow up with them and talk to their children. In many ways, this helped me have an established prior relationship with the parents on which to build rapport with them. Interestingly, my advisor had a book deal with a publisher for the study. The publisher has said that the only way the book would get published was if we had the voices of the students. So, in a way, the publisher became a key stakeholder in the process as well.

"For my study, there was a series of building relationships—first, with my advisor, then with the parents on my advisor's study, and then with the children. A lot of times you can get through the 'gate' if some of the gatekeepers feel like they can trust you. This is true especially in the case of the parents and children with whom I worked. As long as they knew I wouldn't harm them or their children, I could get through the gate to them. Also, racial/ethnic identity became a gatekeeper of sorts—with the Black families especially. It was who I was as a person and how I presented myself that allowed me entry through the gate. I was just an African American student at Vanderbilt University, but to share these identities with the African American parents—that was golden. They wanted their children to see this African American doctoral student, which meant they wanted their children to see me. I represented something that their children didn't see that often. So, the interviews would often go beyond the focus of my study. The parents and children would ask me about my career path and life experiences. Really, who I was in terms of my identities and all I represented to them gave me the credentials to get through the gate."

Using a Mind Map Strategy

It is helpful to use a mind map (Buzan & Buzan, 1996) to brainstorm and identify the gatekeepers, stakeholders, and key informants in your study. **Mind maps** are visual diagrams that organize your thinking about this area, allow you to think broadly about the important players in the field, and document potential challenges and opportunities while you are in the field. Mind maps are particularly useful if you are a more visual person who needs to "see" on paper what the brainstorming process of identifying important players in your study "looks like." In addition to utility, your research study might benefit from the use of a mind map if you are having difficulty identifying key players who can help you gain access to participants or if you want to ensure that you have examined a multitude of potential people to contact for your study. Mind maps can be a fun way to free your mind to think more creatively about how you will enter the field and relate to people. They are easy to create, can be done alone or with others on your research team, and require simple tools—a large chalkboard, a large piece of paper, or even your notebook.

To create a mind map, start by placing your topic—for instance, your field site—in the middle of the page. You then brainstorm any important considerations that "branch" off from this central idea. Each branch may lead to other important sub-branches that also will require important consideration. For instance, if your research inquiry is investigating African American female students' experiences in historically black colleges and universities (HBCUs), and you intend to use purposive sampling of participants, the key word in the middle of your mind map for entering the field might be *HBCUs*. As you brainstorm the important considerations in identifying gatekeepers in these sites, the branches radiating out of the central idea may be certain people you know or need to identify through other relationships you have. Perhaps a branch represents a relationship you have with a president, dean, or faculty member at one of these institutions. From this branch emerge important considerations in working with these people—from a president's busy schedule to the best way to contact her and other people she may know. See Figure 6.4 for an example of a mind map of this topic.

As you can see, mind maps "keep going" and end only when you can brainstorm no further. The most important approach to developing a mind map is that you commit to using the more creative aspects of yourself: Don't think too hard, access your intuitive abilities, and if you get stuck, go to another part of the mind map. Mind maps also assist researchers in remembering critical connections and considerations for their study. So, in many ways, mind maps helps you identify new or previously untapped resources you may develop or have. By the time you complete your mind map, you will have a thorough picture of the important people and considerations involved in entering your research site. Next, see Reflexive Activity 6.1 (on page 187) to start a journal entry on how you see yourself entering the field for your study.

EXITING THE FIELD

You should put as much thought into exiting the field as you have placed into thinking how you entered your field of study. This is a step many beginning researchers forget, give little thought to—or worse, ignore. Actually, there is a real lack of information about exiting the field in educational research, so we offer four points we believe are important to consider: (1) review ethical practice, (2) evaluate researcher and participant relationship, (3) leave participants with research products, and (4) conduct researcher self-assessment.

The first area—reviewing ethical practice—involves revisiting how you as a researcher managed the previous stages of entering the field: selecting a sample method; thinking about sample size; selecting a site; and working with gatekeepers, stakeholders, and key informants. Have you made any missteps in ethical practice along the way? If you have, a good time to address this is *before* you exit the field. Obviously, no researcher plans to practice unethically. However, there are always challenges that appear along the research process that you should be assessing ethically, and exiting the field is a good time to review your ethical standards of research. Especially in working with vulnerable populations, such as children, this is also a good time to review your informed consent forms, your relationships with key players in your study, and even your IRB approval to ensure that you have followed the ethical research strategies you previously planned. Because there is no way to detail the unanticipated processes in qualitative inquiry, your IRB will probably seem woefully inadequate looking back on how your study was conducted. Good ethics questions to ask as you exit the field are: "How would I rewrite my IRB now that the study has concluded?" and "What implications do these revisions have for the protection of my participants?"

A long-time critique by feminist qualitative researchers has been that researchers rarely consider the impact of the researcher–participant relationship. This is the second important area of reflection as you exit the field. Huisman (2008) examines the

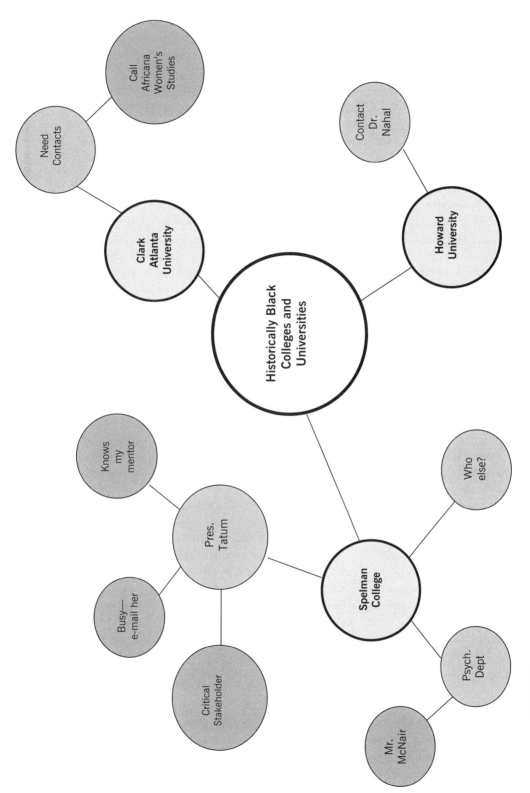

FIGURE 6.4. Mind-mapping gatekeepers for a study of women's experiences in historically black colleges and universities.

issues of reciprocity and positionality and how researchers can reflect on these areas to minimize exploitation of participants in qualitative research. **Reciprocity** is the idea that there is a relationship between researcher and participant wherein knowledge is constructed and shared, and new ideas are formed. **Positionality** refers to the social locations of the researcher and participants: What are the identities (e.g., gender, race/ethnicity, sexual orientation) of both? We believe it is important to discuss reciprocity and positionality in tandem so that the researcher can also reflect on how power is distributed in the researcher–participant relationship and recognize where there are power differentials (often with the researcher often holding more power than the participant). In Huisman's qualitative inquiry with Bosnian Muslim refugees, she "outlines three tensions she experienced and addresses how these tensions were related to her shifting and sometimes contradictory positionality as a woman, a researcher, a friend, a graduate student, and as a person who was straddled between two classes" (p. 372). She experienced these tensions within herself, with academia, and with the Bosnian community. We share this example to help you think about what tensions existed when you were in the field, which you are now preparing to exit. Once you identify these tensions, there may be actions you want and/or need to take before you leave the site of your study.

The third question to ask yourself as you exit the field is to what degree have you left your participants with the products of your research? Have you made promises to share your research findings with individual participants, field sites, or both? Prior to leaving the field, establish a timeline and gather contact information so that you can follow through with distributing research findings. It is easy to skip over this step; however, it is important for two reasons. Should you wish to return to the site to conduct further research, you would be able to build on a strong relationship you established during this first study. Doing what you said you would do in delivering the products of research will help strengthen those relationships. Additionally, providing those findings could positively impact the site and the participants with whom you worked, as well as give rise to new research questions, interesting community conversations, and the possibility of learning to use research in a multitude of manners (e.g., advocacy). Make sure that you have conversations with gatekeepers, key informants, and stakeholders—in addition to the participants—about the format in which they would most prefer to receive your research. They may request a PowerPoint presentation to other stakeholders at the site, creation of a brochure of your findings, or even a final copy of your study in a report or manuscript format. Leaving participants with the products of your research is typically most helpful when they are provided in a nonacademic, easily readable form.

A fourth consideration as you exit the field is to conduct a self-assessment of the researcher. At the point that you exit the field, you have spent a good deal of time on designing your study, reviewing appropriate literature, relationship building, interviewing participants, and a multitude of other tasks. You may even have been anxiously anticipating the end of your time in the field so that you could move on to the latter stages of the research process: data analysis, interpretation, writing, and publication. However, you may also be surprised by some of your reactions as you prepare to leave the field. Take some time to reflect on what your anticipated reactions may be as you leave your field of inquiry. Reflect on the ideas, thoughts, and feelings that come up as you exit the field. Consider Case Example 6.3, in which Dr. Corey Johnson reflects on her insights about her experience exiting the field.

CASE EXAMPLE 6.3. Exiting the Field

Johnson, C. W. (2008). "Don't call him a cowboy": Masculinity, cowboy drag, and a costume change. *Journal of Leisure Research, 40*(3), 385–403.

"This was an ethnographic study focused specifically on how a gay male country western bar's clientele used dress (e.g., saddlebags) as a marker of hegemonic masculinity and how bar patrons changed their dress, and consequently their masculinity, as they migrated to other bars in the city. My selection of dress was no accident; I consciously selected it for a variety of reasons. What I didn't consider, however, was the impact the people I met in the bar would have on my feelings, perceptions, and actions. My connections to these individuals have made it particularly hard as I move on. Since my data collection ended, I have frequently experienced withdrawal from my dress. There is something to be said about the comfort of familiarity. For me, this dress became familiar, and I grew to care about the people and the bar as an institution. Even now, 6 months after my data collection ended, I want to know information about these men's everyday lives. And, the truth is that I can't stay away. I miss these men, and I know they miss me. But I also know that all good things come to an end, and I have spent some time grieving for the loss of community I am currently experiencing. In leaving the field, I also thought about how I would share my research in a consumable manner, instead of merely in academic form. I repackaged my dissertation in a readable form, and the key informants placed it behind the bar—it lives there."

REFLEXIVE ACTIVITY 6.1. Journal Entry
on Entering the Field

Congratulations! You have spent a good deal of time learning about entering the field for qualitative research. Now it is time to reflect on some of what you have learned for your study. In your journal, write the answers to the following questions:

- What interpersonal and intrapersonal considerations/skills do you need to consider as you select and enter the site of your research?

- What are the potential challenges as you build trusting relationships with your participants in your study?

- Will you need multiple sites for your study? If so, how will you interact with these sites?

- What are the best ways for you to interact with the gatekeepers, stakeholders, and key informants in your study?

- How will you know you have "completed" your study?

- What steps do you plan to take as you exit the field?

If you have not selected a site, select a fictional site and respond to the above.

⚠ WILD CARD 6.1. PITFALLS TO AVOID IN THE FIELD

Pitfalls abound when entering the field! From selecting the sampling method; thinking about sample size; entering sites; working with gatekeepers, stakeholders, and key informants; and knowing when to conclude your sampling, pay attention to these reminders to enter the field in a strong, effective, and ethical manner:

- A solid sampling method is grounded in your research paradigm. Be able to deliver an "elevator speech"—20 seconds or less—of how your research tradition guides your sampling strategy.

- Do not select a sample simply because the possible participants would be easy to access. You might miss out on participants who would best answer your research question. Additionally, you might overlook the people who would most benefit from your research.

- Do not select too few people for your study. A good practice is to consider a sample size larger than the actual number of people you think you will need. You do not want sample attrition to negatively influence your study.

- Follow the criteria you have established for your sampling. You spent good time and energy identifying why these criteria were important! At the same time, you do not want to find yourself in the middle of your study only to realize that your sampling criteria have been too restrictive or too general to answer your research question. Stay flexible, but have a good rationale for why you might alter your sampling criteria during your research process.

- Reflect on why you selected criteria for the sample you want to study. Ask yourself if these are the criteria that are really important. If they are not, you might begin your study only to realize that you need other voices to answer your research questions.

- Remember that no one sampling method is "better" than another. You are looking for the best fit for your research question. Sometimes snowball sampling is the best way to go. Your sampling method may not be popular or en vogue at the time of your study. Still, it should be the most appropriate strategy for your study.

- Do not underestimate the importance of building trusting relationships with the gatekeepers, stakeholders, and key informants in your study. They can make or break your access to participants.

- Do take access issues with your site seriously; take time to plan how you will enter the site, conduct research, and exit the field.

- Do not forget to plan for the unexpected. You cannot anticipate everything in the field—but you can think wisely about the potential opportunities and challenges that may come your way.

CHAPTER SUMMARY

This chapter reviewed important aspects of entering the field to conduct qualitative research. First, we discussed the different types of purposeful sampling methods and both their advantages and disadvantages. Three categories of purposeful sampling methods were outlined and categorized based on research purpose: representativeness of sample, description/presentation of phenomenon, and theory development and verification. Second, we discussed the opportunities and challenges of deciding upon the sample size for your study, including issues of research tradition and access to participants. Third, we reviewed the different steps involved in selecting a site—specifically, considering issues of access, planning research activities, considering the length of time to be spent at a site, and addressing potential pitfalls of being in the field. Fourth, we reviewed how to best work with gatekeepers, stakeholders, and key informants in the field; in short, we build trusting relationships and minimize our demands on their resources so that we gain good access to our participants. Finally, we discussed how to conclude research and exit the field in an ethical manner, while considering the important researcher and participant relationship, leaving participants with research products, and conducting a researcher self-assessment of the research process.

RECOMMENDED READINGS

Buzan, T., & Buzan, B. (1996). *The mind map book: How to use radiant thinking to maximize your brain's untapped potential.* New York: Penguin Books.

Guest, G., Bunce, A., & Johnson, L. (2006). How many interviews are enough?: An experiment with data saturation and variability. *Field Methods, 181,* 59–82.

Huisman, K. (2008). "Does this mean you're not going to come visit me anymore?": An inquiry into an ethics of reciprocity and positionality in feminist ethnographic research. *Sociological Inquiry, 78*(3), 372–396.

Jones, S. R. (2002). (Re)Writing the word: Methodological strategies and issues in qualitative research. *Journal of College Student Development, 43*(4), 461–473.

Miles, M. B., & Huberman, A. M. (1994). *Qualitative data analysis: An expanded sourcebook* (2nd ed.). Thousand Oaks, CA: Sage.

Morse, J. M. (1995) The significance of saturation. *Qualitative Health Research, 5,* 147–149.

CHAPTER 7

Maximizing Trustworthiness

CHAPTER PREVIEW

How do we know if qualitative research is rigorous or not? Determining the quality of qualitative research is one of the most debated topics today in clinical and educational research today. This chapter presents important aspects of validity, or trustworthiness, to consider as you conduct, participate in, and review qualitative research. It begins with a review of three lenses for evaluating research in general, then moves on to specific features of evaluating qualitative research. Additionally, criteria and strategies for trustworthiness are presented. Finally, considerations for selecting criteria and strategies are discussed.

WHAT IS "GOOD" RESEARCH?

Many of you were likely exposed very early to the scientific method—most likely this occurred in elementary school. The **scientific method** describes, through the use of experimental approaches, how researchers move from asking a research question; to formulating findings based on observation, experimentation, and hypotheses testing; to generalizing any findings to a population of interest. You were taught that this strategy is the only legitimate way of arriving at "truth" or "good science." As elementary school students, engaging in good science seemed so easy to do! All you had to do was identify a problem, formulate a research question, construct a hypothesis, test that hypothesis by doing an experiment, analyze data, draw conclusions, and report findings. This basic process, you were taught, was the path to the "holy trinity" of "good" research: validity, reliability, and generalizability (Kvale & Brinkmann, 2009).

The other shoe drops when you start to apply what you know from practice to research areas of interest. As clinicians and educators, you quickly learn that you cannot conduct experiments all the time (or at all) where individuals are randomly assigned to a certain classroom experience, mental illness, or socioeconomic status, and so forth. The problem with the scientific method, you quickly surmise, is that there are very few instances where you can look at phenomena purely, outside of the context in which they occur. That is, the scientific method assumes a reality in which *everyone* and *everything* experiences whatever occurs similarly and objectively (Fossey, Harvey, McDermott, & Davidson, 2002).

As qualitative inquiry becomes more prevalent and useful in clinical and educational settings, ideas of what "good" science and thus "good" research are expanding. The discussion of this expansion somewhat parallels that of paradigms in Chapter 2. However, there are specific terminologies more closely relevant to these shifts in how we judge or evaluate research. Figure 7.1 illustrates the emerging continuum of evaluation lenses or criteria.

Traditionalism, also known as positivist realism and naive realism, represents a lens by which clinicians and educators verify a single truth for a phenomenon in science by using the five physical senses (Angen, 2000; Guba & Lincoln, 2005; Lincoln & Guba, 1985). If we cannot observe it or experience it directly, it does not exist. Through experimental methods and empirical verification, we look for rational, objective, and logical explanations to our research questions. Guba and Lincoln (2005) describe this lens as viewing reality as real and apprehensible. The traditionalism lens best captures the "holy trinity" described earlier. This lens for evaluating research is closely aligned with a positivist paradigm (see Chapter 2).

Realism, or subtle realism (Hammersley, 1995, 2004), pertains to the notion that we can know reality only from our own perspective. However, most realists argue that there is an underlying common or objective reality. For instance, Silverman (1993) suggested that clinicians and educators should use inductive analysis *and* quantify qualitative data to the extent possible to arrive at an approximate understanding of a common reality for the phenomenon of interest. To this end, there are always limitations to how we understand reality based on personal perspective. Subtle realists would assert that validity should be framed as confidence rather than certainty (as naive realists would argue). Also known as a **modernism** (Giddens, 1990), this lens for evaluating research is closely aligned with the post-positivist paradigm (see Chapter 2).

Interpretivism, viewed as the polar opposite of traditionalism, refers to the perspective that "everything is relative." Interpretivists believe that criteria for determining the value (or *valid*ness) of research are socially constructed, just like everything else (Angen, 2000). Polkinghorne (1988, 1989) labeled this lens as **postmodernism**. Interpretivists assert that validity should be reframed as *validation*, since "what we know is always negoti-

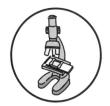

Tranditionalism Lens
(Positivism, Naive Realism)
Objectivity, Truth

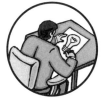

Realism Lens
(Subtle Realism)
Multiple truths but not equally valid

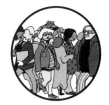

Interpretative Lens
Multiple truths equally valid,
relativity

"Good" Research

FIGURE 7.1. Three lenses for determining "good" research.

ated within the culturally informed relationships and experiences, the talk and text of our everyday lives … constant meaningful interactions with people and things" (pp. 384–385). This approach for evaluating research is most closely assigned with constructivist, critical theory, feminist, and queer theory paradigms (see Chapter 2).

These three lenses present various ways of evaluating research. Be cautioned that both poles may present distinctive threats to research as a whole: using positivist (primarily quantitative) criteria to judge qualitative research (traditionalism) and interpretivist (primarily qualitative) criteria to judge quantitative research may prove no research as helpful or valid. Each lens has an appropriate utility in research as a whole and can offer helpful criteria no matter the approach. We believe that qualitative inquiry is best judged by a blend of subtle realism and interpretivism.

VALIDITY AND QUALITATIVE RESEARCH

In quantitative research, **validity** is defined as evidence of authentic, believable findings for a phenomenon from research that results from a strict adherence to methodological rules and standards. Validity is further categorized as internal and external validity. **Internal validity** refers to the likelihood that there is a causal relationship between two variables without interference from other variables or threats. **External validity** refers to the degree to which a study's sample, research design, and findings may generalize to an outside population or setting. Both forms of validity are examples of the traditionalism lens for judging research.

Validity in qualitative research is known by many names: *truth, value*, and *credibility* (Lincoln & Guba, 1985), *trustworthiness* (Eisner, 1991), *rigor, authenticity* (Guba & Lincoln, 1989), and *goodness* (Emden & Sandelowski, 1998; Marshall, 1990), to name a few. (We refer primarily to the term *trustworthiness*.) In essence, the validity of your study is the truthfulness of your findings and conclusions based on maximum opportunity to hear participant voices in a particular context. In discussing the "truth value" (Lincoln & Guba, 1985) of the research process, it is imperative that clinicians and educators also think of establishing validity not only as demonstrating research strengths but also noting research limitations. Maxwell (2005) summed up criteria and strategies for trustworthiness best by asking readers to reflect upon why others should believe their findings, as well as how they might be wrong. Thus, to establish validity it is imperative that clinicians and educators find the "holes" in their research designs and findings even while locating study strengths.

In considering all three potential lenses, there are several possible positions to take to determine rules and standards appropriate for establishing theoretical and methodological rigor in qualitative inquiry. Reviewing the four positions listed below, we can see that *determining validity is based on the degree to which you think qualitative and quantitative research are similar as well as your desire to see qualitative research recognized as equally scientifically legitimate as quantitative research* (Tobin & Begley, 2004). The primary four positions are:

1. Use quantitative criteria such as validity, reliability, and generalizability.

2. Translate quantitative criteria to be more aligned with the goals of qualitative research.

3. Allow new evaluation criteria to emerge from qualitative inquiry; evaluation should be framed as interactive and inclusive of quantitative criteria, as appropriate.

4. Disregard quantitative criteria altogether, since "everything is relative"; that is, the judgment is based on the researcher, participant(s), and reader(s) in a particular context; there are no set criteria by which qualitative research can be evaluated.

The "Holy Trinity"

The first position is typically argued by the biggest critics of qualitative research. That is, qualitative research is "research" only to the extent that it looks like quantitative research. Those that adhere to this position assume that qualitative research is less used in clinical and educational settings, since they believe it lacks rigor (Chwalisz, Shah, & Hand, 2008). Furthermore, quantitative research evaluation criteria have become the "language" of research rather than that of only one research approach (Tobin & Begley, 2004). Because of these reasons, many researchers overall are hesitant to move away from the known and well-received quantitative standards and rules.

Daly and colleagues (2007) identified a hierarchy of four levels of qualitative research evidence that seems most congruent with this first position (see Figure 7.2). Level I research is characterized as generalizable and is the most important in the hierarchy; it includes qualitative studies that most mirror population representativeness in the quantitative sense. Level II, theory-driven research, incorporates studies that may not be most representative of a population but are conceptual pieces that inform theory in innovative ways. Level III, descriptive qualitative research studies, includes those that describe participant experiences and views, provide practical information for the practitioner, yet do not necessarily provide theoretical or generalizable findings. Level IV, considered the least weighty source of evidence, comprises what they refer to

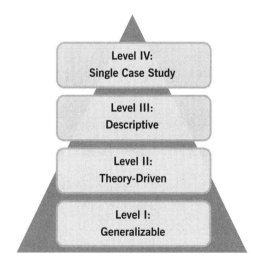

FIGURE 7.2. Hierarchy of qualitative research.

as the single case study. This type of research may involve a single or small sample of interviews with thick description of those interviews.

Translation of Quantitative Standards

Lincoln and Guba (1985) are major proponents of the second position. They identified four components of rigor in qualitative research by translating the quantitative concepts of validity and reliability into something more aligned with the goals of qualitative research. These components are credibility, transferability, dependability, and confirmability (see next section for further description). These terms or criteria have become the gold standard in judging trustworthiness in qualitative research, as some (e.g., Morse, Barrett, Mayan, Olson, & Spiers, 2002) argue that we can still use reliability and validity as criteria. Authenticity (Lincoln & Guba, 1985), described later in this chapter, was a fifth component added to possible criteria in an attempt to move beyond methodological issues.

It is important to note that although this position is predominant in evaluating qualitative rigor, it is considered biased because it translates quantitative criteria—and assumes that those criteria are valid. Whittemore, Chase, and Mandle (2001) warn that an exact translation of quantitative standards is inadequate and inappropriate. Morse and colleagues (2002) explained that introducing new terms that share the meanings of reliability and validity serves only to further marginalize qualitative inquiry from mainstream science. Thus, when siding with this second position, it is imperative that

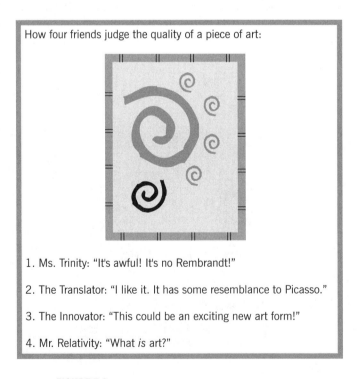

How four friends judge the quality of a piece of art:

1. Ms. Trinity: "It's awful! It's no Rembrandt!"

2. The Translator: "I like it. It has some resemblance to Picasso."

3. The Innovator: "This could be an exciting new art form!"

4. Mr. Relativity: "What *is* art?"

FIGURE 7.3. Validity is in the eye of the beholder.

we legitimize both qualitative and qualitative research as equally valid approaches. Figure 7.3 summarizes the four positions.

Emergence of Qualitative Criteria

The third stance for evaluating qualitative research involves honoring qualitative research as having its own universal set of criteria independent of quantitative research. Qualitative criteria can be thought of as having different evaluative components and processes, given the nature of qualitative research. Thus, Angen (2000) proposes the term *validation* over validity to more accurately describe the process of establishing rigor in qualitative research. Validation, she argues, speaks to the interactive and contextual nature of qualitative research findings and less to the deterministic view of validity. Rolfe (2006) agrees with being more flexible in judging rigor: We must remain open to various standards of rigor: "The real issue is not whether a universal standard for judging the validity of qualitative research has or has not been argued, but rather, why so many different positions should remain not only viable but also fiercely contested" (p. 306). Table 7.1 summarizes the evidentiary rigor required by each of the four positions.

Criteria as Relative and Changing

The fourth position, that there should be no set criteria since every study is couched in its unique context, is even more tentative when it comes to establishing trustworthiness. For example, Tobin and Begley (2004) raised the question: Do we really need consensus of criteria or just simply increased acceptance that criteria are emerging? However, this position is less popular overall among qualitative researchers. Several argue (e.g., Cutliffe & McKenna, 1999; Hammersley, 1992) that not working toward establishing criteria and strategies for trustworthiness could further devalue qualitative research as merely "fiction writing."

TABLE 7.1. Sample Evidence of Rigor for the Four Positions		
1. The Holy Trinity	Randomization, controlled designs, generalizability, reliability, validity	Using a representative, randomized group of homeless individuals and applying established data collection methods.
2. Translation of quantitative methods	Credibility, transferability, dependability, confirmability, authenticity	Including homeless individuals in your study to produce information-rich cases and working with the individuals and your research team to arrive at consensus regarding established qualitative criteria.
3. Emergence of qualitative criteria	Validation versus validity, openness to new and different criteria	Following similar study design as Position 2 and using the translated methods as a guide, yet being open to determining what rigor is as the context changes.
4. Criteria as relative and changing	Establishing criteria as unnecessary since criteria are contextual and always evolving	Focusing primarily on interviewing homeless individuals about their experiences and remaining open to criteria that fit for the participants and context. It may be determined that establishing criteria for rigor is unnecessary.

ACTIVITY 7.1. Positions Debate

What is the best method for evaluating qualitative research? Divide the class into four groups and assign each group one of the four positions listed earlier. Distribute a copy of an article of a qualitative study and have each group discuss evidence of rigor within the article based on its position. More specifically, address the following questions:

- How would your position view this study's rigor?
- What would your position argue are the limitations of other positions for this article?
- How could you strengthen the study's trustworthiness based on your position?

Who Determines What Quality Is?

In addition to the degree to which quantitative criteria in evaluating qualitative inquiry should be considered, clinicians and educators are faced with two additional challenges. Specifically, what components of qualitative inquiry should be attended to when determining rigor? And, who determines if a study is trustworthy? Very few have weighed in on these challenges.

Rolfe (2006) took on a more "outcome" view of determining trustworthiness: We can make judgments only on what a researcher reports, and readers determine rigor. "Judgments can only be made about the way the research is presented to the reader rather than directly about the research itself ... such judgments are predominantly aesthetic rather than epistemological" (p. 308). That is, the reader is inevitably the reviewer.

Porter (2007) agreed with Rolfe (2006) but also argued that the process cannot be separated from the outcome or product of qualitative inquiry: The research design shapes how we report the findings. So, by determining the rigor based on the qualitative report, we are in some ways making judgments about the quality of the research itself.

However, Morse and colleagues (2002) asserted that the responsibility of establishing trustworthiness relies solely with the researcher(s) rather than the reader(s): "The lack of responsiveness of the investigator at all stages of the research process is the greatest hidden threat to validity and one that is poorly detected using post hoc criteria of trustworthiness" (p. 11). That is, clinicians and educators have an ethical and moral obligation to design, carry out, and report findings in a rigorous manner, no matter how much the reviewer or consumer ultimately sees.

Clinicians and educators tend to judge trustworthiness after the research has been conducted and presented. Thus, trustworthiness is largely determined by the degree to which readers/consumers have confidence in the findings (based on what is presented in the qualitative report and other tangible forms of evidence). We believe that there are three interrelated components of the research process that need to be examined when judging the quality of qualitative research: (1) the research design, including researcher characteristics that influence a study; conceptual framework; contextual factors; use of research paradigms and traditions; research goals, purposes, and questions; and data sources and data collection methods; (2) data analysis and interpretation, which refers to the description of the coding process and collapsed themes in the context of the researcher's theoretical perspective and the context of the study; and (3) the qualitative report itself along with any related physical evidence (i.e., audit trail, see below for more information). Thus, quality judgments rest with the process *and* outcome of qualitative research. Additionally, the researcher, reader/consumer, and participant are responsible for determining rigor, with the researcher solely accountable to research design.

REFLEXIVE ACTIVITY 7.1.
Trustworthiness in Qualitative Research

How do you see trustworthiness as similar to reliability and validity issues in quantitative research? How is it different?

ROLE OF THE RESEARCHER, REVISITED

In Chapter 5 we explored how the researcher's role influences qualitative inquiry in both potentially positive and negative ways. The extent and quality of the research relationship have the potential to serve as a major threat in qualitative inquiry. (Don't worry—the research relationship also has plenty of benefits to combat this threat.) Because we are researchers *and humans*, our professional and personal selves are likely to intertwine in developing the research relationship. "Although some would criticize the subjectivity that is inherent in interpretivist work, no research is free of the biases, assumptions, and personality of the researcher. We cannot separate self from those activities in which we are intimately involved" (Sword, 1999, p. 277). Table 7.2 highlights a sampling of the potential researcher threats in qualitative inquiry.

TABLE 7.2. Examples of Researcher Threats

- Developing inappropriate or unattainable study goals (e.g., focusing predominantly on personal or funder goals)
- Selecting an inadequate sample (e.g., sample does not meet criteria; not enough participants to address research question)
- Conducting an insufficient literature search for your research tradition
- Disregarding researcher bias (e.g., not bracketing your assumptions)
- Creating unanswerable research questions
- Describing data inaccurately (e.g., failing to check data with participants; not providing thick description)
- Failing to use multiple data sources (e.g., participants) and methods (e.g., interviews, photographs)
- Not noting patterns among data (e.g., limiting coding process; see Chapters 9 and 10)
- Selectively observing a setting to "see what we want to see" (e.g., observer bias, confirmation bias)
- Creating a Hawthorne or novelty effect for participants where their reactions are based primarily on being observed (i.e., Hawthorne effect) or experiencing something new (i.e., novelty effect)
- Biasing interview responses based on order and type of questions
- Creating a false consensus among research team members during data collection (e.g., engaging in "groupthink")

Miles and Huberman (1994) argued that the development and characteristics of the research relationship are influenced both by the effects of the researcher on participants and by the effects of participants on the researcher. Maxwell (2005) defined this bidirectional influence as reactivity, which is also known as reflexivity (see Chapter 5): "Researcher bias, which may affect participants, refers to the ways in which the researcher's values, experiences, or beliefs influence the research" (p. 108). The effect of the participant is another important component that impacts the research relationship and thus may bias or threaten the research design. This potential impact involves personal characteristics of participants—attitudes and actions both within and outside the research design that change researchers in some manner. Perspectives 7.1 describes an example of this effect from one of our research studies (Singh, Hays, & Watson, 2011).

• •

Perspectives 7.1. The Participant Effect

"In preparing to conduct a qualitative study [Singh et al., 2011] examining child sexual abuse experiences for South Asian women and the resilience strategies they used to survive, we bracketed our assumptions and relationships with the topic and population. We could easily speak to our personal and professional experiences with the topic. We knew what to watch out for. Or, at least we thought we did. As we started reviewing their stories in the interview transcripts and analyzing the data, we were overcome with unexplained emotion. We weren't surprised by what they said, but we were surprised by how it impacted us. Very early on in this research, we worked collaboratively on establishing self-care practices for the remainder of the study as well as having an open and honest discussion of how participants were affecting us."

—AAS AND DGH

• •

It is important to examine the interplay of five major components when considering how validity threats impact your research design. Kline (2008) coined the term **procedural rigor** to describe how bias impacts all components of the research design. The components include:

1. *Goal(s).* As discussed in Chapter 4, establishing study goals involves determining the unit of analysis, research purpose, and type of information sought.

2. *Conceptual framework.* A conceptual framework is composed of experiential knowledge, prior theory and research, pilot and exploratory studies, and thought experiments (see Chapter 4).

3. *Research question(s).* Outlining research questions dovetails with the purpose statement and should contain content, coherence, and structure that are congruent with the case studied as well as the research tradition used (see Chapter 4).

4. *Role of researcher(s).* As discussed in Chapter 5, this component refers to the various roles we play in the research study itself as well as the overall relationship we have with participants.

5. *Methods.* The fifth component, discussed in Chapter 6 as well as in Chapters 8–11, involves activities such as entering the field, interviewing and observing participants, and managing and analyzing data.

Case Example 7.1 provides an example of how these components may create validity threats. The process of considering threats to trustworthiness should begin early in proposal development. Proposal Development 7.1 outlines an activity for considering these components for your study.

CASE EXAMPLE 7.1. Potential Threats in a Technology Study

Proposal Topic: An Assessment of Generational Differences in Technology Comfort Level at a Public 2-Year Institution

Research design component	Study examples	Potential threats
Goal(s)	Examine impact of generational status on students' comfort level with technology at a 2-year institution	Is age the main influence? Is this an appropriate setting for this study? Am I missing any technologies?
Conceptual framework	Experiential knowledge—interaction with students as faculty member. Thought experiments—various models to explain technology comfort. Pilot study	Preconceptions based on own experiences, stereotypes. Four generations—Silent, Baby Boomer, Gen X, and Gen Y. Missing literature?
Research question(s)	How do students at a 2-year institution view technology? How, if at all, does generational status impact technology comfort?	Assumes they think about technology. Assumes age/generational status is main factor
Role of researcher(s)	Faculty member. Investigator	Involved with students on daily basis. Access issues. Grading issues. Power dynamics
Methods	Individual interviews. Focus group interviews. Chat room observations	Students know me so will act differently. Social desirability. Hawthorne effect. Are interview questions leading?

PROPOSAL DEVELOPMENT 7.1. Threats to Trustworthiness Considerations

This activity is intended to assist you in thinking about how various threats play a role in your proposed study. Create a grid similar to that in Case Example 7.1. In the first column, list the five components of goal(s), conceptual framework, research question(s), role of researcher(s), and methods. In the second column, briefly describe how each component relates to your study. In the third column, discuss how the components specifically may threaten your design.

Review your grid with a peer and/or your research team. Revise based on any feedback you receive. Remember, your grid is a "work in progress," so revise as your research design emerges.

CRITERIA OF TRUSTWORTHINESS

Now that we are aware of many of the limitations of our research, largely based on what we as researchers assume, believe, design, and implement, we can discuss the qualities that make our designs stronger. Quality in qualitative research involves both theoretical and technical concerns; thus, criteria address both research design and implementation.

This section presents several criteria for trustworthiness that involve various aspects of qualitative inquiry, such as the overall research process/design, data analysis, and the qualitative report. These criteria include credibility, transferability, dependability, confirmability, authenticity, coherence, sampling adequacy, ethical validation, substantive validation, and creativity. Table 7.3 on page 203 provides an overview of these criteria. Criteria of trustworthiness are different from strategies of trustworthiness, which are discussed in a later section.

Credibility

Lincoln and Guba (1985) referred to **credibility** as the "believability" of a study. They intended for credibility to be somewhat analogous to internal validity in quantitative research. Credibility is one of the major criteria qualitative researchers use to determine if conclusions make sense for a qualitative study.

Transferability

Transferability is similar to external validity in quantitative research (Lincoln & Guba, 1985). You may recall from earlier in the chapter that *external validity* referred to the degree to which findings could generalize to a population. In qualitative research, however, generalizability in the quantitative sense is *not* a goal. Rather, the goal is for clinicians and educators to provide enough detailed description of the research process, including the participants, settings, and time frame, so that readers/consumers can make decisions about the degree to which any findings are applicable to individuals or settings in which they work. Johnson (1997) also suggests using "replication logic." That is, the more times a research finding is supported for various groups of individuals, the more confidence we can place in the findings generalizing beyond the people in the original research study. Transferability is also referred to as **naturalistic generalizability** (Stake, 1990).

 ACTIVITY 7.2. Generalizability in Qualitative Research

Respond in dyads to the following questions:

* If qualitative research isn't generalizable like quantitative research, what good is it?
* How can we trust findings that cannot be generalized?
* How can a study with a small sample be useful?

Dependability

Dependability refers to the consistency of study results over time and across researchers (Lincoln & Guba, 1985). This is similar to the concept of reliability in quantitative research. Dependability goes beyond credibility, in that clinicians and educators are charged with engaging in strategies to show that the similar findings extend to similar studies, and all research team members agree with the study's findings.

Confirmability

Confirmability refers to the degree to which findings of a study are genuine reflections of the participants investigated (Lincoln & Guba, 1985). This concept is most similar to objectivity and neutrality in quantitative research. Achieving confirmability means the degree to which interference from the researcher was prevented. To achieve this, clinicians and educators must "listen to data" and report them as directly as possible.

Authenticity

Authenticity is similar to confirmability in that clinicians and educators strive to represent participant perspectives authentically (Guba & Lincoln, 1989). The subtle difference between these criteria is that confirmability refers to methodological criteria and authenticity refers to theoretical criteria.

Coherence

The decision of selecting a research tradition appropriate to your study is an important one. "If a research design is inappropriate for the [research] question, regardless of how well done the study is, it may not be sufficient to answer the study question" (Elder & Miller, 1995, p. 282). To assist with this important decision, Chapter 2 provides information on 14 qualitative research traditions, categorized in a manner to more easily identify which traditions may be more suitable for a research design based on a study purpose and research question(s).

Kline (2008) defines **coherence** as the degree of consistency of an epistemological perspective throughout the research design—that is, how we and the research tradition(s) we select assume that the knowledge to be constructed in our study is to be addressed. Once an appropriate research tradition(s) is (are) selected, the researcher is responsible for infusing it throughout the research process and describing it thoroughly in the research report. The research question matches the method, which matches data analysis and interpretation. Related checks for coherence include these questions:

- Does the methodology fit the study purpose?
- Does the researcher use terminology to describe a design that is appropriate to a selected research tradition?
- How comprehensive are the data collection and analysis procedures?
- Are conclusions consistent with other parts of the research design?

Coherence is also referred to as *congruence* (Whittemore et al., 2001).

Sampling Adequacy

Sampling adequacy refers to using the appropriate sample composition and size based on the research question(s) and research tradition(s). More specifically, the term refers to using a sampling method that is congruent with a research design, collecting data from enough participants to represent the sampling method, and including those who have specific knowledge of the research topic. Who and how many you involve in a qualitative study will depend on the overall nature of the study. Thus, determining sampling adequacy largely depends on the overall research design.

Ethical Validation

Ethical validation refers to treating all aspects of the qualitative research process—from designing a study to presenting findings—as a moral and ethical undertaking (Angen, 2000). That is, we should only engage in research that provides insights to practical and meaningful real-world problems. Horsburgh (2003) reminds us that we need to evaluate the potential of a study and its actual relevance to current and future theory and practice. Furthermore, clinicians and educators are charged with being sensitive to the nature of human, cultural, and social contexts in conducting and presenting qualitative research.

As Angen (2000) argues, we need to engage in research that informs practice, generates new ideas for the field, and transforms practitioners' actions. "We have a human moral obligation to take up topics of practical value, and we must do everything in our power to do them justice" (p. 391). Porter (2007) further asserts that "it is the relationship between knowledge and practice that provides the key to judging research" (p. 83). Whether individuals review the process or product of your work, they should get a sense that it truly contributes to the profession in some way and sparks new questions.

Ethical validation is also demonstrated by maintaining ethical practices (Drisko, 1997)—that is, by using informed consent appropriately, depending on tradition (Fossey et al., 2002); empowering and liberating individuals (Lather, 1991); and reporting findings that are useful in policy decisions (Onwuegbuzie & Leech, 2007).

Substantive Validation

Substantive validation relates to the question: Do the research report and other products have "substance" (Angen, 2000)? Qualitative research is substantive to the degree to which it significantly contributes to a profession. This form of validation is also known as **relevance criterion** (Mays & Pope, 2000), whereby research either adds new knowledge or supports existing information about a phenomenon.

No matter what research tradition you select, or which methodology you employ, the final products should be rich with evidence that both confirms and potentially disconfirms your conceptualization of a phenomenon. Does your work have quality, in that it strongly argues (with evidence) a perspective (Roberts, 1996)? That is, are claims relevant and appropriate (Pawson, Boaz, Grayson, Long, & Barnes, 2003), and is the process of arriving at those claims transparent and open to scrutiny?

Creativity

Whittemore and colleagues (2001) identified creativity as one of the hallmark criteria for a trustworthy qualitative study. **Creativity** refers to implementing novel methodological designs, including imaginative ways of organizing, presenting, and analyzing data. Furthermore, showing flexibility in the overall research process is a sign of rigor.

TABLE 7.3. Criteria of Trustworthiness

Credibility	Overall "believability," internal validity
Transferability	Generalizability, external validity
Dependability	Consistency, reliability
Confirmability	Neutrality of researcher
Authenticity	Truthful to participants
Coherence	Consistency of research approach
Sampling adequacy	Appropriate sample size and composition for research purpose
Ethical validation	Engaging in research that informs practice
Substantive validation	Is the research "meaty" and a worthwhile contribution?
Creativity	Novelty and flexibility in research design

Perspectives 7.2. Establishing Trustworthiness

Students completing their first qualitative proposals as part of an introductory qualitative research course were asked to write what they considered to be the most important strategy for establishing trustworthiness.

"Engaging with my research team on a weekly basis, sometimes more, was essential to maintaining the integrity of my study."

—COUNSELING STUDENT

"Triangulation is the most important because it gives a variety of ways to collect data. I used interviews, focus groups, and an observation. Each gave me a different view of how my research questions could be interpreted."

—LITERACY LEADERSHIP STUDENT

"I used interviews as well as unobtrusive methods in my study. Collecting data in multiple ways that still reflect common themes renders data more trustworthy and inspires trust in the audience of the researcher."

—CURRICULUM AND INSTRUCTION STUDENT

"Triangulation from several sources minimizes researcher bias because you have a certain amount of power, and if precautions are not put into place to prevent abuse of power, a researcher could lead a project in the direction of his or her choice."

—OCCUPATIONAL AND TECHNICAL STUDIES STUDENT

"Since the data are collected from the participants, it is important to cross-check the results the researcher found with the participants. This helps with making interpretations and minimizing researcher bias."

—COUNSELING STUDENT

"Simultaneous data collection and analysis are very important to ensure accuracy of interpreting results. Waiting too long to analyze information can distort understanding and allow for misunderstanding. During data collection, analyzing the results helped to shape my interview questions for the next data collection."

—LITERACY LEADERSHIP STUDENT

"Peer debriefing was most helpful for me because I had some blind spots in data analysis. It was difficult for me to see some of the discrepancies or some of the more negative aspects of what was said."

—COUNSELING STUDENT

"An audit trail—if you have a good audit trail, then it would include all of the evidence that you have been making a consistent effort to maintain trustworthiness."

—EDUCATIONAL LEADERSHIP STUDENT

STRATEGIES OF TRUSTWORTHINESS

There are many strategies available for maximizing the above criteria for trustworthiness (see Table 7.4). It is important to use multiple strategies that address the research process, data interpretation, and report writing. However, the use of multiple strategies does not guarantee validity (Angen, 2000; Morse et al., 2002). That is, no matter how many strategies you use to maximize trustworthiness, you can never fully establish a study's rigor. Furthermore, select strategies that are most congruent for establishing trustworthiness that make sense for your research tradition(s).

Reflexive Journals, Field Notes, and Memos

Given that the role of the researcher is an integral part of qualitative inquiry, keeping adequate notes and reflections throughout the research process is imperative. The first method for doing so is keeping a reflexive journal. A **reflexive journal** includes thoughts about how the research process is impacting the researcher. The nature of qualitative inquiry creates several moments throughout the research process wherein researchers need to reflect upon how the participants, data collection, and data analysis are impacting them personally and professionally. Several types of entries can be kept in either an electronic or a paper journal. These might include reactions to participants and settings involved in the research, thoughts about data collection and analysis procedures within a research team, hunches about potential findings, and descriptions of how data method, source, and analysis plans may need to change. It is important to keep this journal as part of your audit trail; notes about how data were collected and analyzed will be helpful reminders as to why you talked to various stakeholders and key informants, coded themes in a particular way, and so on.

Field notes and **memos** are other researcher records kept to describe and analyze findings as they develop throughout a study. These are typically associated with specific data collection methods, such as interviews, documents, and observations. For example, in a life history of 10 preservice teachers regarding their ethics toward social justice teaching, Johnson (2007) constructed memos when analyzing interviews. One of the memos concerning an interviewed preservice teacher, Gretchen, reads as follows (p. 303):

Memo: Gretchen's early literacy learning

Gretchen grew up in a suburban neighborhood that has all the classical markers of a middle-class community. Few of Gretchen's neighbors were from non–European American backgrounds, and most of her classmates came from English-speaking families. Gretchen's parents engaged in typical middle-class childrearing practices: They read nightly to their children, using materials often found in grocery store aisles—Dr. Seuss and Berenstain Bears' books. Her parents were both elementary school teachers, and they played active and foundational roles in her literacy learning, providing Gretchen with the materials she needed to become literate and limiting her access to materials they saw as hindering her learning. Gretchen described how her parents hid some reading materials from her. ... Gretchen also described how her parents provided her with access to reading materials that she would eventually encounter in school, such as books written by Lois Lowry and Jerry Spinelli. Gretchen does not mention reading many books about families from diverse backgrounds. ... Is this because her parents as teachers did not value such texts because they knew they were not yet being integrated into school instruction?

Field notes and memos are discussed in more detail in Part III of this volume.

Member Checking

Member checking has been cited as the key strategy for establishing trustworthiness (Guba & Lincoln, 1989). It is the ongoing consultation with participants to test the "goodness of fit" of developing findings. It requires involving participants in the research process and striving to accurately portray their intended meanings when outlining overall themes. There is an assumption with this strategy that participants' accounts are treated as at least as equally valid as the researcher's. *Member checking is not just reviewing transcripts with participants; it is asking them how well the ongoing data analysis represents their experience.* Member checking can be done in many ways, including the following:

- Clarify participant responses via probes during data collection.
- Request that participants review interview transcripts and/or field notes to confirm authentic representation.
- Conduct follow-up data collections to expand participant voices in the findings.
- Facilitate a focus group interview to review the overall findings for a study.
- Distribute the qualitative report to participants for their input.

Member checking is also known as *respondent validation* (Mays & Pope, 2000), *interpretative validity* (Johnson, 1997), and **reciprocity** (Fossey et al., 2002).

Seo and Koro-Ljungberg (2005) conducted a hermeneutic study that assessed older Korean American students' experiences in higher education. As part of the member-checking process, researchers reviewed translated interview transcripts with the participants to determine the accuracy of the Korean–English translation.

Prolonged Engagement

Prolonged engagement is another strategy of trustworthiness. It involves "staying in the field" to build and sustain relationships with participants and settings to be able to accurately describe a phenomenon of interest. The more time a clinician or educator stays in a setting or engages with a participant, typically the more trustworthy the findings. While the time and energy necessary to establish prolonged engagement varies depending on a study's goals and research question(s), this strategy is usually met once the researcher perceives that he or she has established trust with participants and gained detailed, sufficient information about them, their culture, the setting, and the phenomenon of interest.

Two examples presented here may illuminate the nature of prolonged engagement. First, Brown, Rogers, Feuerhelm, and Chimblo (2007) conducted a phenomenological study to examine the lived experiences of a second-grade teacher and her students to more clearly describe the teaching process. Prolonged engagement was achieved as five researchers spent 9 months with the teacher and her students, observing, interviewing, and reviewing journal entries. A second example of prolonged engagement can be found in Amatea and Clark (2005), who conducted a grounded theory study over a 2-year period, examining the perspectives of 26 administrators pertaining to the role of the school counselor.

Persistent Observation

Persistent observation produces depth in data due to the intentional effort of seeking detail regarding various aspects of a phenomenon. Depth in data collection can be achieved by engaging in several data collections with a participant, refocusing the way data are mined to more clearly address a research question, soliciting theoretically opposing data as an attempt to disconfirm a theme, and so forth. Although persistent observation may arise as a result of prolonged engagement, this is not always necessary or true. Clinicians and educators could establish persistent observation by simply asking increasingly refined and detailed questions or conducting more complex observations to better address a research question.

An example of persistent observation can be found in Alaggia and Millington (2008). In this phenomenological study the researchers investigated the lived experiences of 14 adult males who were sexually abused in childhood. They used in-depth interviews to examine the males' experiences of sexual abuse in childhood, the process of retelling the trauma, the influence of the abuse on them as children and adults, and the meaning attached to these three experiences. Implications for social workers were derived based on detailed interview data.

Triangulation

Triangulation is a common strategy for ensuring trustworthiness that involves using multiple forms of evidence at various parts of qualitative inquiry to support and better describe findings. That is, we hope to strengthen evidence that a particular theme exists by looking for inconsistencies among these forms. It is important to note that using these multiple forms only provides evidence and does not guarantee trustworthiness. Tobin and Begley (2004) proposed that we should not triangulate but "crystallize"; they view this process as one of *completeness*, not confirmation. It is important to consider which forms of triangulation—data sources, investigators, units of analysis, data methods, and theoretical perspectives—are most relevant for establishing your study's rigor.

Triangulation of Data Sources

Triangulation of data sources involves including several perspectives or participant voices during qualitative inquiry. Once we select a sampling method or methods for a study (see Chapter 4), we triangulate this method by recruiting participants in a manner congruent with our research design. Triangulation of data sources might involve

TABLE 7.4. Criteria and Strategies of Trustworthiness

	Credibility	Transferability	Confirmability	Authenticity	Coherence	Sampling adequacy	Ethical validation	Substantive validation	Creativity
Reflexive journals	X						X		
Field notes/memos			X	X				X	
Member checking			X	X		X	X	X	
Prolonged engagement			X	X				X	
Persistent observation		X			X			X	
Triangulation	X	X	X	X		X		X	X
Theory development								X	
Peer debriefing							X		
Simultaneous data collection/analysis	X		X	X		X		X	
Negative case analysis	X		X	X				X	
Thick description	X	X	X	X	X			X	
Audit trail	X				X			X	X
Referential adequacy	X					X		X	

Note. X's indicate key strategies of trustworthiness per criterion.

several participants representing a similar perspective, having multiple roles within a setting, experiencing a phenomenon in various ways yet possessing similar characteristics, and so forth. This form of triangulation is also known as *fair dealing* (Mays & Pope, 2000).

Lambert's (2007) work represents an example of a triangulation of data sources. In a hermeneutic study investigating first-time consumers of counseling and the evolution of their perspectives of it over time, Lambert interviewed eight participants about their ideas regarding counseling before, during, and after their treatment. The eight participants represent multiple data sources.

Triangulation of Investigators

Triangulation of investigators refers to using multiple researchers or teams of researchers to collect and/or analyze data, write reports, and present findings. This strategy is also known as *stepwise replication* (Mays & Pope, 2000). This strategy may take many different forms, including the following:

- Use of a single team or revolving teams during data collection only
- Use of a single team or revolving teams during data analysis only
- Use of a single team or revolving teams during both data collection and analysis
- Use of one team (or one investigator) for data collection and a separate team (or investigator) for data analysis

No matter the approach you take, including other investigators in qualitative inquiry significantly strengthens the design and builds others' confidence in your findings. However, Cutliffe and McKenna (1999) warn: "It is unlikely that two people will interpret the data in the same way, form the same categories/themes or concepts and produce the same theoretical framework" (p. 376).

Another method to supplement this strategy is to use an **auditor** or auditors. An auditor is an individual who reviews the audit trail to determine the extent to which the researcher or research team(s) completed a comprehensive and rigorous study. Selecting auditors is similar to selecting members of your research team: They must have the expertise and interest in your study to assist you in developing a trustworthy study (see Proposal Development 7.2). However, an auditor differs in that he or she should be a disinterested party. That is, there is no conflict of interest pertaining to your study for the auditor (e.g., he or she has no authorship rights and thus can actively search for disconfirming evidence to refute overall themes). We believe that selecting someone to audit your research process is similar to having an Internal Revenue Service (IRS) agent audit your tax report: this person should be objective, fair to the data and the individuals it represents, and detail-oriented.

The auditor or auditors selected should have some expertise in your research topic and qualitative inquiry in general. For example, Westerlund and Barufaldi (1997) used an auditor in their heuristic inquiry to review biology teachers' perspectives of an end-of-course examination. An auditor who had expertise in Texas examination standards reviewed the raw data to confirm that the overall themes were present in the data.

PROPOSAL DEVELOPMENT 7.2. Selecting an Auditor

Selecting an auditor involves a consideration of many factors. Write a few sentences for each of the questions below as you finalize your selection:

1. What are the areas of expertise needed to review your qualitative inquiry? What type of content knowledge is needed with respect to the phenomenon of interest?

2. Who might best understand the participants proposed in your study? Who could ensure that their voices are most fairly represented? In what ways?

3. How can an auditor be most helpful to you during your proposal? Who would be willing to invest the time and energy needed to ensure a trustworthy study?

4. What, if any, are the power dynamics between you and a potential auditor? How might these dynamics impact the research process?

Triangulation of Unit of Analysis

Another form of triangulation is *triangulation of unit of analysis* (Kimchi, Polivka, & Stevenson, 1991). Recall from Chapter 4 that a case, or unit of analysis, refers to individuals, settings, events, and processes. Clinicians and educators may at times want to select more than one case per research question to illuminate the complexity of overall themes for a study. In the Westerlund and Barufaldi (1997) study, discussed above, two units of analysis were triangulated to highlight the complex nature of the impact of end-of-course examinations. Specifically, both individuals (i.e., Biology I teachers) and settings (i.e., two high schools) were used to present themes.

Triangulation of Data Methods

Triangulation of data methods refers to using multiple methods to illustrate themes. Data methods, described in more detail in Part III of this volume, include individual interviews, focus group interviews, observations, documents, records, art, media, and photography. Often, using multiple methods in qualitative inquiry yields various findings. The key is to understand to what degree findings systematically differ based on the method employed to obtain them. Thus, it is acceptable to obtain different data from individual and focus group interviews, as long as the differences stem from the fact that one method was selected over another.

Auxier, Hughes, and Kline (2003) demonstrated an example of triangulation of data methods. The authors conducted a grounded theory study to explore the professional identity development of master's-level counselor trainees by using individual and focus group interviews. The use of these two methods assisted the researchers in describing a theory wherein identity formation occurred intrapersonally and was solidified through experiential activities. Another example of this form of triangulation can be found in McBride (2008). In this phenomenological study, McBride examined the experiences and unmet needs of the homeless population by conducting individual interviews and using photographs to capture "the day in the life" in a homeless individual in southeastern Virginia urban area. Through interviews McBride found that participants most needed career development and job searching skills; the photographs showed the communal nature of this sample while depicting how they met some of their basic needs each day.

Triangulation of Theoretical Perspectives

Triangulation of theoretical perspectives can involve integrating theories at any stage of the research process, such as constructing the conceptual framework and analyzing data. This strategy illuminates the importance of conducting a literature review throughout qualitative inquiry, as discussed in Chapter 4. Essentially, this strategy relies on using multiple theories—at times across professional disciplines (Janesick, 1994)—to better conceptualize, describe, and explain a phenomenon. For example, Sanchez, Reyes, and Singh (2006) used education, family and social capital theories in a grounded theory study to conceptualize struggles of Mexican Americans in higher education.

Theory Development

Depending on your research tradition and overall study purpose, developing theory about a phenomenon related to your research topic may be a valuable strategy for establishing trustworthiness. Theory development, also referred to as *theoretical validity* (Johnson, 1997), refers to generating tenets from data to describe and explain how a phenomenon operates. Theories are a product of a specific time, place, and person; they are derived from the interaction of participants, research, data, and evaluator (Horsburgh, 2003).

The notion is that, as we collect and analyze data, we should be "thinking theoretically." This cognitive activity involves movement toward a larger, more global description and explanation of the phenomenon of interest. To do this, clinicians and educators are charged with acting like detectives of data, using available evidence to inch toward a larger explanation without making huge, unsupported leaps.

Peer Debriefing

Consulting with a peer, or **peer debriefing** (Patton, 2002), allows for another check outside of a designated research team. Peers can be interested colleagues, classmates, or individuals within the community in which the phenomenon is investigated. Peers should play the devil's advocate in that, while they are supportive of the clinician or educator's research efforts, they also serve as another vehicle to challenge the findings. Additional information about this strategy may be found in Chapter 5.

Simultaneous Data Collection and Analysis

Another strategy for ensuring trustworthiness involves collecting and analyzing data simultaneously. Because qualitative inquiry is an emergent design (Maxwell, 2005), it is likely that your research questions and data sources and methods will change as you conduct a study. So, don't wait to analyze data until after all of your data are collected! You might miss out on important questions you should have asked, other information-rich participants whom you should have interviewed, clarification opportunities for data already collected, and so forth.

Negative Case Analysis

Negative case analysis involves refining a developing theme as additional information becomes available (Lincoln & Guba, 1985; Maxwell, 2005; Patton, 2002). The concept behind negative case analysis is one of constantly searching for data that go against your current findings, or searching for cases that may be represented by the same findings yet differ from the population of interest. When we search for evidence that refutes what we think we will find, we help to minimize researcher bias and ultimately strengthen a study.

When searching for disconfirming data in interviews, clinicians and educators often design questions that address "what else could be going on." For example, when I (Hays) was conducting individual interviews to assess the training needs of practitioners have with respect to promoting healthy relationships in school settings, I included in the interview protocol some questions that assessed how their training had already addressed this issue. By including these probes, I was working to minimize my bias that training had been inadequate by allowing an opportunity for participants to explain how training *was* adequate.

With respect to negative case analysis through use of different cases, let's say we are interested in career barriers among Native Americans. We develop a study using a sample of Native Americans—those living on reservations as well as those living in urban areas. There are two ways (among many others) we could engage in negative case analysis:

1. Include probes that could help to elicit descriptions of career support for this population.
2. Examine if similar career barriers are found for populations other than Native Americans.

Thick Description

One strategy you can implement to strengthen your study is to provide a thick description of your findings (Maxwell, 2005). To understand thick description, we think it is important to understand what *thin* description is: A thin description provides inadequate details, precluding readers or other researchers from inferring meaning from that description. **Thick description**, also referred to as *vividness* (Whittemore et al., 2001), is a detailed account of your research process and outcome, usually evidenced in your qualitative report but also possibly included in an audit trail (see below). The emphasis is on description and interpretation of aspects of the research context and the research process that go beyond simply reporting details of the study (Geertz, 1973). Given its importance as a tool, several scholars (Agar, 2006; Geertz, 1973; Hammersley, 2008) note that thick description is more than a strategy of trustworthiness; it is a way of thinking about data interpretation and reporting.

It is important to note that thick description goes beyond providing details of participant accounts in several ways. While thick description was coined by philosopher Gilbert Ryle, Geertz (1973) used the term to refer to an account of the details of a study's form and process, and the situational-specific reflections that build on the account of these details. That is, it goes beyond the basics of facts, feelings, observations, and occurrences to include inferences into the meaning of present data. It is important to convey the meaning or message behind an act, expressed feeling, and so forth. Denzin (1989) noted four components of thick description: "(1) it gives context of an act; (2) it states the intentions and meanings that organize the action; (3) it traces the evolution and development of the act; [and] (4) it presents the action as a text that can then be interpreted" (p. 33). Furthermore, Morse (1999) added, qualitative research must "add something more to the participants' words for it to be considered a research contribution, whether it be a synthesis, interpretation, or development of a concept, model, or theory" (p. 163).

A study example might help illustrate thin versus thick description. Let's say you are investigating the degree of client participation in couple counseling. The following statements represent thin and thick descriptions during an observation:

> One partner folded his arms and crossed his legs. (thin description)
>
> One partner, who stated some doubt to the counselor that counseling would be effective, folded his arms and crossed his legs as soon as his partner mentioned she was disappointed in his behavior that previous week. The partner remained in that position for approximately 20 minutes and unfolded his arms and uncrossed his legs when the counselor solicited feedback on how his behavior was positive that previous week. (thick description)

Here is an example of thin and thick descriptions when describing your research design:

> The researcher used phenomenological data analysis to identify themes. (thin description)
>
> The data collection and analysis process consisted of six steps and was recursive in nature to strengthen verification procedures in the study:

1. The primary researcher interviewed the first participant three times, with a week between each interview;

2. The primary researcher and counselor educator independently used phenomenological analysis (e.g., horizontalization) to engage with the data and identify themes and subthemes for Participant 1's interviews;

3. Steps 1 and 2 were repeated for the next 4 participants, and final themes and subthemes were identified across all 5 participants;

4. The primary researcher conducted a focus group with 8 participants to confirm the final themes and subthemes of the 5 individual participants;

5. The research team collapsed the themes of the individual and focus group interviews; and

6. An audit of the data collection and analysis was conducted. (thick description) (from Singh, Hays, et al., 2010, p. 448)

Components of your report that can be thickly described include the following:

- Research paradigms and traditions and how and why they were selected;
- Research questions and purpose statement;
- Researcher bias;
- Participant recruitment;
- Data collection procedures;
- Data methods used;
- How sampling method matches research tradition;
- Data analysis steps;
- Coding challenges and how coding system developed;
- Participant verbatim quotes;
- Researcher notes;
- Professional, ethical, and cultural implications of findings; and
- Trustworthiness strategies.

Audit Trail

Maintaining an audit trail is a necessity in qualitative inquiry, particularly since published qualitative reports limit wordage. An **audit trail** provides physical evidence of systematic data collection and analysis procedures. Typically, an audit trail can be kept in a binder or a locked file cabinet.

Audit trails are kept because they provide a collection of evidence regarding the research process for an auditor or any other consumer to review. Just as with record keeping with our clients and students, we have an ethical and professional obligation to keep records of the research we conduct. Table 7.5 provides some examples of what might be included in an audit trail.

TABLE 7.5. Sample Contents of an Audit Trail

• Timeline of research activities	• All drafts of codebooks
• Participant contacts	• Data management tools (e.g., contact summary
• Informed consent forms	sheets, document summary forms, case displays)
• Demographic sheets	• Research team meeting notes
• Data collections	• Reflexive journal
• Observation rubrics	• Transcriptions
• Interview protocols	• Instrument development procedures
• Checklists	• Video recordings, DVDs, audio recordings
• Field notes	• Artwork
• Memos	• Photographs
• Reflexive journals	• Copies of Internet blogs

Referential Adequacy

Referential adequacy involves checking preliminary findings and interpretations against archived raw data, previous literature, and existing research to explore alternative explanations for findings as they emerge. This strategy can also lead to searching for rival hypotheses or different interpretations of findings based on existing knowledge regarding the phenomenon at hand.

Hays, Chang, and Dean (2004) used referential adequacy as a strategy for trustworthiness in their grounded theory study of white counselors' conceptualization of privilege and oppression issues. After a theoretical model was developed that outlined how privilege and oppression awareness changes over time, Hays and colleagues used archived data collected at varying points to test the model. In essence, the notion behind referential adequacy is that data on which a theory is derived should be represented by that theory.

PROPOSAL DEVELOPMENT 7.3. Selecting Strategies for Trustworthiness

1. List the criteria for trustworthiness discussed in this chapter.

2. For each criterion, list associated strategies for trustworthiness.

3. Review the criteria and strategies and circle those that you feel most relate to your research proposal at this point.

4. Write a memo about why you feel that these strategies may be valuable to your study as well as how they might be implemented in your research design.

REFLEXIVE ACTIVITY 7.2.
Trustworthiness Criteria and Strategies

- What criteria of trustworthiness seem most important to you? Why?

- What strategies do you think are most helpful overall in qualitative inquiry? How so?

CONSIDERATIONS IN ESTABLISHING TRUSTWORTHINESS

While several criteria and strategies have been described to help ensure the rigor of your study, several considerations remain before selecting them for your particular study. First, some strategies may be more "worthwhile than others," depending on the research tradition. How do we weigh criteria? Often, clinicians and educators decide which criteria and strategies to use based on their research tradition. "Criteria for evaluating qualitative research must fit within the philosophical/epistemological assumptions, purposes, and goals of the paradigm selected for the research" (Drisko, 1997, p. 6).

For example, you may decide for a grounded theory study that ethical and substantive validation and theory development, sampling adequacy, and keeping an audit trail are the more important criteria and strategies, respectively. Or, let's say you are considering a phenomenological approach. You might decide that authenticity, prolonged engagement, persistent observation, and member checking are most important. In essence, selecting criteria and strategies of trustworthiness is a major decision based on your research design. This decision should not be made in isolation, so consult with peers, research team members, or auditors.

Relatedly, strategies for trustworthiness are not supported similarly for all paradigms and research traditions (Cutliffe & McKenna, 1999; Whittemore et al., 2001). As we increase our understanding of research traditions in mental health and education settings, there may be a need to consider new or at least more specific evaluation criteria. However, it is important to note that while there are some differences in evaluation criteria and strategies based on research approach, there are also some universal ones (Horsburgh, 2003).

Finally, clinicians and educators need to remember that the proposed criteria and strategies of trustworthiness have evolved as a movement away from a traditionalist lens and thus from a positivistic view of research. It might be natural to deduce that the more criteria and strategies you use in your study—and the more intensely you use them—the more rigorous the design. Angen (2000), among others, cautions that this assumption might lead us back to trying to get at a static truth (i.e., positivism) rather than honoring the contributions of qualitative inquiry. Be careful not to continue positivism by trying to get at a static truth (Angen, 2000). Others have highlighted how specific criteria and strategies might be harmful to our overall goals in qualitative inquiry (see Wild Card 7.1).

⚠ WILD CARD 7.1. CAUTIONS WHEN ESTABLISHING TRUSTWORTHINESS

The literature on qualitative research methods provides several criticisms, often contradictory, of trustworthiness types and strategies. Reflect on the following cautionary statements:

- Triangulation of investigators may lead to positivistic conclusions (Cutliffe & McKenna, 1999).

- Dependability as a criterion can be a threat to validity: Repeatability of data is not essential or necessary since we are interested in participant voices (Sandelowski, 1993).

- Member checking with respect to having participants review and confirm the overall findings does not make sense, since "study results have been synthesized, decontextualized and abstracted from (and across) individual participants" (Morse et al., 2002, p. 7). Horsburgh (2003) adds, it is "inappropriate to expect that individual participants will have the ability to 'validate' the findings of the research as a whole" (p. 310).

- Triangulation of data sources is difficult to determine (Horsburgh, 2003): What guides sample size—a research question or the research tradition?

- As we collect and analyze data, categories or themes may emerge. However, categories may produce a rather misleading clear-cut account of the findings when, in reality, findings may not be discrete, self-sufficient entries (Horsburgh, 2003).

- Audit trails "do little to identify the quality of [research design] decisions, the rationale behind those decisions, or the responsiveness and sensitivity of the investigator to data" (Morse et al., 2002, p. 7).

These are just some of the cautions the literature provides in relation to research trustworthiness in clinical and educational settings. It is important to consider these in more detail when selecting your criteria and strategies of trustworthiness (see Activity 7.3).

 ACTIVITY 7.3. Establishing Trustworthiness Can Be Dangerous!

Work in small groups and discuss one of the cautions of establishing trustworthiness presented in this section. Debate both sides of the point and provide examples. Additionally, what other aspects of establishing trustworthiness, not presented here, does your group view as potentially problematic?
    Present your comments to the class as a whole.

CHAPTER SUMMARY

This chapter illuminated the complexities of establishing rigor in qualitative research. It traced our assumptions of what determines "good" research to an early introduction to the scientific method and subsequently presented alternate lenses for evaluating research. When considering which lens and approach to use when judging the rigor of qualitative research, we are presented with four primary positions: (1) use quantitative criteria such as validity, reliability, and generalizability; (2) translate quantitative criteria into concepts that are more aligned with the goals of qualitative research; (3) allow new evaluation criteria to emerge from qualitative inquiry—evaluation should be framed as interactive and inclusive of quantitative criteria as appropriate; and (4) disregard quantitative criteria altogether, since "everything is relative"— that is, the judgment is based on the researcher, participant(s), and reader(s) in a particular context, and there are no set criteria for which qualitative research can be evaluated.
    Validity, a common term used in quantitative research, goes by many names in qualitative inquiry, including *rigor, trustworthiness, credibility,* and *goodness*, to name a few. Using *trustworthiness* as a primary reference label, we provide several criteria and strategies for promoting it. Criteria include credibility, transferability, dependability, confirmability, authenticity, coherence, sampling adequacy, ethical validation, substantive validation, and creativity. Strategies of trustworthiness include use of reflexive journals, field notes and memos, member checking, prolonged engagement, persistent observation, triangulation, theory development, peer debriefing, simultaneous data collection and analysis, negative case analy-

sis, thick description, audit trail, and referential adequacy. When selecting criteria and strategies, it is important to consider the weight of each per research tradition as well as any risks each might pose to being viewed as promoting positivism.

RECOMMENDED READINGS

Angen, M. J. (2000). Evaluating interpretive inquiry: Reviewing the validity debate and opening the dialogue. *Qualitative Health Research, 10*(3), 378–395.

Drisko, J. W. (1997). Strengthening qualitative studies and reports: Standards to promote academic integrity. *Journal of Social Work Education, 33*(1), 185–197.

Eisner, E. (1991). *The enlightened eye: Qualitative inquiry and the enhancement of educational practices.* New York: Macmillan.

Guba, E. G., & Lincoln, Y. S. (1989). *Fourth-generation evaluation.* Newbury Park, CA: Sage.

Hammersley, M. (1995). Theory and evidence in qualitative research. *Quality and Quantity, 29,* 55–66.

Kline, W. B. (2008). Developing and submitting credible qualitative manuscripts. *Counselor Education and Supervision, 47*(4), 210–217.

Lincoln, Y. S., & Guba, E. A. (1985). *Naturalistic inquiry.* Beverly Hills, CA: Sage.

PART III

DATA COLLECTION AND ANALYSIS

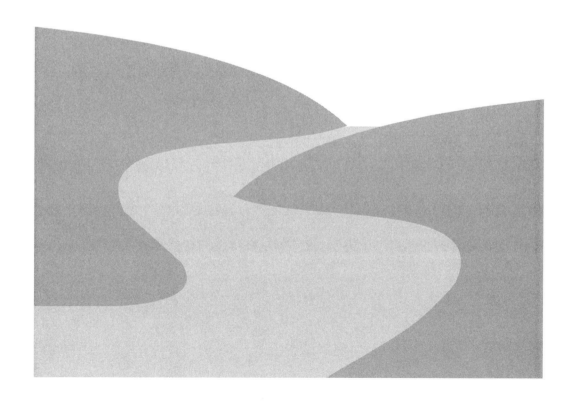

CHAPTER 8

Data Collection via Fieldwork, Interviewing, and Focus Groups

CHAPTER PREVIEW

Qualitative inquiry offers several strategies for collecting data. Decisions about data collection are influenced by and influence aspects discussed in Parts I and II of this volume, as well as data analysis (see Figure 8.1). This chapter reviews three of the primary forms of data collection: observations, individual interviews, and focus group interviews. In the discussion of each, information about the format, advantages and disadvantages, and strategies for successful data collection is presented. The chapter closes with additional data collection considerations, including data recording and initial management, data transcription, and member checking.

LINKING METHOD TO RESEARCH DESIGN

As noted in Part II of this volume, research designs can change, and thus qualitative researchers need to be open to variations in what and how data are collected. Several factors help determine the type and use of various data collection methods. These include (1) the nature of the study purpose (i.e., the more exploratory, the more open-ended the method); (2) the extensiveness of existing scholarship for a study topic; (3) available resources, such as researcher and participants' time, and the number of cases to be investigated; and (4) relationships with all stakeholders, including participants, gatekeepers, and funders (Devers & Frankel, 2000).

In essence, making a decision about data collection methods involves all the things we have discussed thus far in the text: selecting a topic and research question, distinguishing which research paradigms and traditions fit your topic, considering ethics, identifying your role in the research design, deciding the extent to which you will be engaged in a research setting, and including methods to maximize trustworthiness.

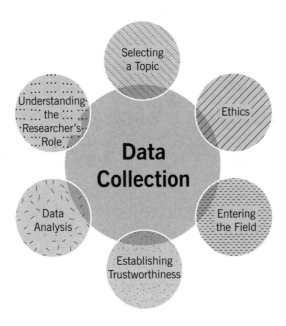

FIGURE 8.1. Design components influencing data collection.

REFLEXIVE ACTIVITY 8.1.
The Origins of Data Collection Methods

Do you believe that research questions drive methods or that methods drive research questions? Or, does data collection have more association with something else? Journal about where data collection methods originate.

We often hear of colleagues and students who want to conduct qualitative studies and, before considering all the necessary elements of research design, try to figure out *first* what methods they will use. Talking about methods before developing a solid research question and supporting materials is setting yourself up for failure: Without a proper foundation, what you do to collect (and analyze) data cannot be trusted.

Maxwell (2005) reminds us that research questions are a *guide* for data collection methods. That said, research questions cannot simply be translated into similar interview questions, observation protocols, or unobtrusive methods: Methods require flexibility and particular attention to issues of trustworthiness, research relationships, and so forth. Thus, we have to be careful to *not* select methods that will get the "data we want" at whatever costs.

Furthermore, qualitative data collection can serve as an intervention in itself for participants as well as the researcher. Be prepared to be changed by the research process as you uncover realities specific for participants and settings; your attitudes and behaviors related to a particular phenomenon may shift as you learn from your participants. Also, your motivation to continue to speak for those with limited or no voice in research will likely be strengthened. If you have interacted with someone in your role as a practitioner or educator, you are probably familiar with this change process. The social nature of qualitative inquiry generates new knowledge and affective understanding of phenomena: You start to think, feel, and respond in different ways as you become immersed in qualitative inquiry. Perspectives 8.1 offers some of our experiences with data collection as an intervention.

Whatever methods you select for your design (and we recommend using multiple methods), each method decision needs to be explained and justified in your qualitative proposal or report. Maxwell (2005) highlighted that describing the context or setting can help the reader understand why certain decisions were made.

The remainder of this chapter presents three primary data collection methods: observations, individual interviews, and focus group interviews. Toward the end of the chapter, data collection considerations are discussed.

• •

Perspectives 8.1. Data Collection as Intervention

"For a study on white counselors' conceptualization of privilege and oppression (Hays et al., 2004), I conducted individual interviews with the counselors and counselor trainees about their definitions and experiences with privilege and oppression. Although I perceived my interview protocol to be a straightforward, fact-finding endeavor, participants spoke to me several weeks after their interview, stating that the interview really made them think about things differently. They reported that talking about these issues had highlighted for them new ways of interacting with their clients as well as growing edges for themselves. I also learned a lot about myself, too."

—DGH

"At the outset of a study exploring the intersection of racial/ethnic and gender identities for transgender people of color who were survivors of trauma (Singh, 2010), I remember feeling really excited about the topic and working with participants. Then, as the interviews progressed, I heard numerous stories of severe victimization from participants. From severe beatings and hate crimes to intimate partner violence and child sexual abuse, these stories of violence all came back to transgender persons of color not being allowed to just grow, develop, and flourish in their identities. Fortunately, Hays and I had done a previous study with survivors of violence. From that experience, I remembered how we took care of ourselves as researchers and how we engaged in advocacy movements working to end violence."

—AAS

• •

OBSERVATIONS

Observations are a primary source of qualitative data; they can stand alone as their own method or supplement others. On the surface, observing something seems simple. It's just watching something and taking mental notes, right? People do this all the time! Wrong.

Try to describe this observation: You had dinner at a friend's home recently. What did the cookware and serving dishes look like? What was your friend wearing? What were the dinner topics of conversation? Can you remember some important quotes? Can you summarize the conversation? How long were you at your friend's house? How long did it take you to eat? Who initiated the welcome and goodbye? The questions about this dinner interaction can be difficult to answer, and they highlight the reality that witnessing and experiencing is not the same as *observing* something. Observing is so much more than watching or looking at something: It is training yourself to focus on relevant participant and setting characteristics and behaviors and examining these as you have never before.

Commonly referred to as **naturalistic observation**, this method has four guiding principles. First, there is typically noninterference on the part of the researcher. That is, one's impact should be as negligible as possible so as to not upset naturally occurring phenomena. A researcher can interact with participants, yet in most cases should not intrude so much as to change naturally occurring events. Second, the observation should involve invariants, or naturally occurring behaviors. Some of these behaviors might include hyperactivity, teamwork, client disclosure, group process, or meeting agendas. Third, observations should be used for exploratory purposes. Observations are quite beneficial when unexplored or underexplored phenomena are studied. Finally, the researcher should provide a thick description of the setting so that an outsider can imagine sensory and behavioral aspects, to fully experience it in great detail.

Why conduct observations? Why not just gather interview data or use some other method? Patton (2002) outlined several benefits to observational data: (1) observations allow the qualitative researcher to better capture and understand the context; (2) they involve more present moments during which a researcher can obtain setting details rather than relying on others' conceptualizations; (3) participants may not be willing to discuss certain things in an interview, and the researcher can obtain this information only by direct observation; and (4) participants being interviewed may not be aware of particular dynamics (e.g., political agendas, effects of their interactions with others), or they may have certain biases about a setting due to their subjective and active involvement. Furthermore, conducting observations involves ongoing and continual reflection on the setting, the participants, and your influence on both—and this need for reflection varies from interviewing or other forms of data collection.

 ACTIVITY 8.1. Developing an Observation Protocol

Reflect on the following in your research teams:

- How could observations be used in your study?
- What would you observe? How would you know you observed it?
- How do you envision your role in an observation?

- In your observations what degree of involvement do you believe would be appropriate for data collection?
- How might your presence influence participants? The setting?

Based on these reflections, develop an observation protocol that could be used in your study. Be sure to revisit your protocol after some data collection and consider ways in which it may need to be revised to better fit your research design.

Fieldwork

Fieldwork refers to research activities in which individuals engage when in a particular setting, whether it is a classroom, a counseling agency, a focus group session, and so on. The purpose of fieldwork is to gather a thick description of the context and provide a deeper understanding of a particular phenomenon. Qualitative researchers are trying to understand a research setting and participants and their behaviors and attitudes. So, if one is interested in the effectiveness of a grief group, conducting fieldwork (e.g., observations, focus group interviews, journal analysis) would involve thickly describing a setting in clear terms as well as providing information about participants in relation to that context. Although fieldwork as a term has been used primarily to describe observation, we believe that it can occur with other data collection methods, such as interviews and document analysis. Immersion in the field (i.e., prolonged engagement), no matter the data collections that follow, is important to "know" how participants think, see, feel, and experience their realities. Thus, the setting is an important window into participants' lives.

Fieldwork is harder than it may seem. As Glesne (2006) noted, doing good fieldwork involves making the strange familiar and the familiar strange. "You want to be open to exposing and rethinking that which you have taken for granted. Only then can you begin to expand on what you are capable of seeing and understanding" (p. 52). The notion of challenging all things familiar in a setting can be difficult: Imagine as a therapist conducting research in the hospital in which you work. You would have to look at all the people, places, and things that you are used to seeing in a manner that has come to be so natural and thus no longer readily visible and reexamine them as if encountering them for the first time.

Now, pretend that you have been invited to a party where you know very few people. Initially, being at that party is quite anxiety-provoking (especially for Hays, who is quite the introvert!). You try to observe everything about the party site, what people at that party are like, how they are dressed, how they interact, what they talk about, and so forth. Initially, you try to take it all in and observe everything that is happening. Eventually, you become more selective and specific regarding your focus. You've likely been to parties before, so you have some ideas of what is normative or not. You constantly reflect on what you are experiencing and integrate it into the information you have about those you do know at the party, those you just met, and your experiences of parties in general. Observations are a bit like attending this kind of party: You are constantly making detailed notes, whether mental or otherwise, about what you see and experience and how you feel about it. The key to observing well, though, is to assume you always have something to learn about a setting and the individuals or artifacts that comprise it.

A couple of other points. First, in Chapter 4 we discussed the importance of defining the unit of analysis, or your "spin" or perspective of a case to be studied (VanWynsberghe & Khan, 2007). This is particularly significant in observations. Let's take the grief group effectiveness example just presented. An *individual* case might lead you to observe more closely particular individuals and thus could involve observing those individuals in settings other than that grief group. Your unit of analysis may be those grieving who do not attend a group. A *setting* case could involve also making observations at that agency outside that group hour to learn about contextual dynamics that might relate to the effectiveness of that one group. The unit of analysis, for example, could be observing individualized interventions in that agency. A *process* case may focus more intently on group session dynamics, and a sample unit of analysis may involve remembrance and mourning. An *event* case could focus on something occurring within or outside the group (perhaps a group member's suicide attempt, i.e., unit of analysis) and observe various angles and perspectives to capture how that event shapes group effectiveness.

A second major point is that some study topics are more suitable to observations than others. As a general rule, if you are more interested in what people do rather than what they say they do, observations are more appropriate. If your research tradition lends itself more to creating change (e.g., PAR) or understanding process to generate theory (e.g., grounded theory), observations are more suitable as compared to capturing meaning ascribed to an experience (e.g., phenomenology, oral history).

The Observation Continuum

Observations do, for the most part, involve some degree of researcher participation. The observation continuum contains four points that range from little to no participant interaction to full participant interaction (e.g., "going native"; see Figure 8.2). The **observer role** refers to having minimal or no interactions with participants. In these cases, participants are often not aware that they are being observed. A study on secretly observing hand-washing behaviors in a public restroom might be an example of the observer role. Examining individuals through a one-way mirror is another example. Caldwell and Atwal (2005) noted that nonparticipant data collection (i.e., observer role) can also involve video recordings. If appropriately used, video recordings can enhance the credibility of an observation study by capturing and making permanent records of nonverbal and verbal communication. This permanence allows opportunities for independent researchers to review the data repeatedly. However, we caution that recording may make some participants even more unwilling to be observed, so taking care with the video recorder's presence is also an important consideration. In essence, the use of video recording needs to be justified as well as weighed against other forms of data collection, such as direct observation and audio recording.

The **observer as participant role** involves having a primary role as an observer with some interaction with study participants. An example of this role might be an education graduate student observing students from the back of a classroom with very few exchanges specific to the study. The **participant as observer role** can be considered the opposite of the observer as participant role: It involves becoming more a participant than an observer of others. Patton (2002) highlighted the paradox that as researchers participate more in a setting, they become less objective with respect to the study. However, researchers learn more as they participate more. Finally, the full **participant**

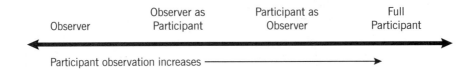

FIGURE 8.2. The observation continuum.

role refers to functioning both as a member of a community, classroom, or counseling agency under investigation and as an investigator. While "going native" is rare, it is most likely to occur with this role.

Participant observation refers to the researcher's active involvement in the setting and is best presented by the participant as observer and full participant roles. Participant observation, however, is much more than a point on one end of a continuum: It is often used in interviewing and other activities to negotiate tensions in a setting. It is a dance of participation, observation, and conversation that allows for deeper data collection, relationship building, and often stronger designs. Patton (2002) reminds researchers that playing an active role during data collection does not guarantee that you will be able to better understand participant experiences.

Where you begin on the observation continuum is influenced by many factors, including your selected research tradition(s), the context of your study, and your theoretical perspective. Furthermore, the degree of participation can change during the course of qualitative inquiry for several reasons. First, it can change based on research questions evolving or new ones emerging from data collection. As qualitative researchers collect observational data, it may become necessary to collect data more actively (i.e., involve participants directly) to answer a more refined research question. Or, observations may become more focused as you begin to search to confirm and disconfirm preliminary themes. Second, research relationships can dictate the qualitative researcher's involvement in observations. As relationships build, a researcher's participation in a setting may increase: Researchers communicate more with participants, engage in their daily activities, and observe them more intensely. Furthermore, researcher participation will likely lessen as a research study comes to a close and researchers leave the field or site.

No matter the course of participation throughout qualitative inquiry, it is important to figure out ahead of time what you might find, or expect to find, in a setting. These ideas are likely to come from your conceptual framework and the setting itself. Before conducting observations as a data collection method in itself or in conjunction with interviews, for example, it is prudent to jot down key behaviors or expressions that you expect to find. When studies are exploratory, enter the site with just these notes, if possible. At times, these "observation rubrics" become more focused (i.e., persistent observation) in cases where there is prolonged engagement in observing a setting or studying a phenomenon.

PROPOSAL DEVELOPMENT 8.1. Planning Your Participation

Construct a brief paragraph to provide a rationale and describe your planned participation using the questions below:

- What is the nature of your planned involvement at a site or sites?

- How much will be revealed to people in the setting about the study purpose?

- How much will they know about you?

- How intensively will you be present? Why?

- How might your personality characteristics (e.g., sense of humor, degree of introversion) impact your observation?

- How focused will participation be? Why?

- How does your participation relate to your research questions?

- What are some key components you might find in your site? From where do these components originate?

Field Notes

Field notes are written records developed within an observational period (when possible) and continually expanded and revised after the observation has occurred. Sometimes referred to as *observational records* (Marshall & Rossman, 1999), the primary purpose of field notes is to create an accurate and thorough written record of field activities. Additionally, data collections (especially observation) are assumed to be a representation of purposeful behavior and actual expressions of feelings, and field notes are assumed to be salient records of that information. They are an important data management and analysis tool that we think is pertinent to address in this chapter due to their use in real-time data collection.

Although we provide some examples of what to include as field notes and in what format, you, as an emerging qualitative researcher, need to develop a method that feels natural for you. Table 8.1 outlines some possible components of field notes. We recommend that you review Emerson, Fretz, and Shaw's (1995) work on writing up field notes for more specific components. Furthermore, Figures 8.3 and 8.4 on pages 230 and 231 provide field note templates you might consider adapting for your own use. These templates are useful for developing preliminary thick descriptions of your observation. They may be used in whatever format is most comfortable to you, whether it be a spiral notebook, index cards, a binder of loose-leaf papers, notepads, or computer programs.

While they are quite useful with observations, field notes can also supplement other methods. For example, field notes taken during an interview session can serve as supplemental evidence of a recorded one.

Bogdan and Biklen (2003) described two types of field notes: descriptive and reflective. Both of these types are important because you want to record objective facts and details as well as your responses and reactions to them. **Descriptive field notes** capture details of what occurred in a setting, providing behavioral descriptions of behaviors that are often abstract, such as teaching and counseling. With descriptive field notes, qualitative researchers are able to provide detailed depictions of participants and the physical setting; thick descriptions of specific events; and paraphrases, summaries, or verbatim quotations from participant conversations. Additionally, Bogdan and Biklen recommend that qualitative researchers should make field notes on *their* dress, actions, and conversations with participants.

Reflective field notes record subjective aspects of data collection such as assumptions, impressions, attitudes, and ideas (Bogdan & Biklen, 2003). These brief notes should be infused throughout your descriptive field notes. You are likely to initiate reflective field notes for a particular data collection before it occurs. For example, these reflective field notes might include comments about your worldview and/or your per-

> **TABLE 8.1. Components of Field Notes**
>
> - Descriptions of physical setting (e.g., physical space, décor, signs/postings, ratios of people based on various categorizations and roles)
> - Spatial or physical arrangement of people or things
> - Participant information (e.g., dress, demographic information)
> - Sensory impressions (what you see, smell, taste, hear, and feel)
> - Daily routines and patterns of individuals and subgroups
> - Transitions between activities
> - Special events within a setting
> - Important quotes
> - Summaries and paraphrases of conversations
> - Communication patterns (both verbal and nonverbal) and interactions among individuals based on various categorizations and roles
> - Diagrams and sketches of physical setting
> - Different participant perspectives
> - Comments about potential key informants to provide additional data
> - Data obtained unobtrusively during the data collection period
> - Your thoughts, feelings, and reflections regarding the setting
> - Notes about the participants' reactions and interactions with you
> - Thoughts about what or whose voice might be missing from the setting
> - New questions and ideas that impact the research design

spective on a research topic specific to that setting, your relationships with participants, thoughts about a particular setting, ideas about how the data collection method is timely and appropriate for the research question(s), cautions you may have about possible methodological problems, and potential ethical and professional considerations. Reflective field notes often help "end" your descriptive field notes: You might reflect on how the new information supplements your knowledge of a particular phenomenon, what patterns or themes are emerging, and future points for clarification that relate to additional data collection sources, refined research questions, strategies for trustworthiness, and so forth. Case Example 8.1 (on page 232) includes descriptive and reflective field notes.

As you collect observational as well as other forms of data, you may have more extensive thoughts or reflections and want to jot these down without disrupting the "flow" of a field note. These longer pieces are often referred to as **memos** (Corbin & Strauss, 2008) and are an important data collection *as well as* data management and analysis tool. We recommend that you keep memos in a reflexive journal, a strategy described in Chapter 7.

We would like to highlight three influences on what gets included in a field note: stance, intended audience, and point of view. *Stance* refers to the researcher's orientation toward the topic itself and those being observed (Emerson et al., 1995). We believe that this stance originates from your conceptual framework. As fieldwork continues, your stance or perspective will likely change, affected by those you encounter. Another influence, the intended audience of your report, also impacts the content of what gets included in field notes. Try to write with an inconsistent voice and style, as your audience may change as your design evolves.

The final influence is point a view: that is, "through whose eyes events are seen as well as through whose voice they are described" (Emerson et al., 1995, p. 53). Whatever voice is used, the field note will be restricted in some way. For example, a first-person voice will likely include only the researcher's perspective, experience, and "take" on what participants are experiencing. Alternatively, a third-person voice will focus primarily on what others are thinking, saying, and doing, with occasional inclusion of researcher perspectives or a detached and "objective" stance. No matter the voice or point of view used, the researcher can attend to varying degrees and capture a broad or narrower written record.

ACTIVITY 8.2. Field Note Exercise

Taking field notes involves recording descriptions of both subjective and objective data from observing an individual, group, context, or all three. Considering the components listed in Table 8.1, practice writing field notes in dyads. Take turns whereby one person talks about his or her day for 5 minutes, and the other person records field notes. Switch roles. Discuss your field notes with each other and explore how you could expand them.

Strategies for Writing Field Notes

Imagine that you have spent several hours observing a special education classroom to examine students' behaviors toward a new student. Due to your role in the classroom as a teacher's assistant, you are only able to mentally note your observations. A couple of hours pass before you are alone with your thoughts about the data collection, and you begin to panic as your memory is failing you. All you can really remember is the conversations you had with the teacher about the observation! Actions and conversations among the students seem to be lost.

Time	Prompt or cue	Behavior	Comments

FIGURE 8.3. Field note template.

Date:
Time of Observation:
Location:
Observer:

Facts and Details in the Field Site	Observer Comments
[Insert verifiable sensory information in chronological order.]	*[Insert reflections/subjective responses to the facts and details of the setting.]*

Reflective Summary: *[Insert below the overall impressions of the observation as well as additional questions you have for future data collection.]*

FIGURE 8.4. Field note template.

This scenario is common with observations: Researchers tend to be overconfident during the observation that they will remember the details of a setting and events and be able to write an elaborate field note about the observation at a later time. To counter this pitfall we suggest the use of several important strategies for writing field notes.

First, write quickly and as much as possible. Constructing a detailed field note involves allowing ample time and giving ample attention to the data source. This activity will be particularly important if you are unable to write notes during the observational period itself. For instance, you probably don't want to take notes while observing a religious ceremony. Focus initial writing on remembering scenes and contexts rather than on the words to describe the scene; avoid being an "internal editor" too soon.

Field notes can be recorded in many forms that may include mental notes, jotted notes, or full notes, representing a continuum of less to more detailed note taking. Emerson and colleagues (1995) highlighted several strategies for expanding one's recall of what happened: (1) Start in chronological order; (2) begin with a salient moment or high point of an observational period, and then consider other significant events and interactions; or (3) focus more systematically on events that relate to topics of interest. We believe that constructing a record in chronological order is the most effective strategy.

As soon as you are able, construct (initially in a chronological manner) what happened when. Although you may want to organize your data source differently, such as by topic rather than by time, we find it is easier to recall detail if there is a systematic method for doing so. We believe that relying on topics to jog your memory is dangerous because there may be topics you leave out intentionally or unintentionally because you do not see them as salient.

Second, be committed to sufficiently documenting the data source. For every 30 minutes you spend observing a site, prepare to spend *at least* three times that amount of time reconstructing the period adequately. It is important to not leave anything out; you never know what might be important. Even when completing what you consider to be a thorough field note, we encourage you to go back and edit it. That is, read and reread your notes and continue to develop memos. We have found that after writing a field note, things get added as our memories continue to construct additional details. Furthermore, we have found that reflective field notes and memos become richer with a thorough review and revision. For example, if you were conducting the observation in the special education classroom, you would consider the perspectives of others in the room (e.g., new student, peers, teacher) and write a memo about these perspectives and how they might influence data collection and analysis. No matter your strategy for completing field notes, remember that "writing fieldnotes from jottings is not a straightforward remembering and filling in; rather, it is a much more active process of constructing relatively coherent sequences of action and evocations of scene and character" (Emerson et al., 1995, p. 51).

Be aware of your impact on the setting. Your influence on the setting and its participants is important to include in your reflective field notes and memos for your ongoing data collection and analysis. **Observer effect** refers to the unintentional effect you, as an observer, have on the research and the participants. In your notes ascertain normal behavior from behavior changed as a result of the researcher's presence. **Observer bias** refers to the subjective manner in which you, as an observer, selectively attend to particular individuals, events, and activities within an observation period. There are several ways to minimize observer effect and bias, including receiving adequate training, minimizing the time spent conducting each observation, video recording participants, maintaining audit trails, writing thorough field notes, using multiple observers, observing phenomena in multiple settings and at multiple times, altering your degree of involvement in one setting over time within one observational period as well as across data collections, and so on.

Finally, do not discuss with others the observation until you have a chance to construct a quality field note. As indicated in the scenario above, you may forget large chunks of details about an observation. Alternatively, others can bias your personal impressions of the data source, or worse, minimize its importance overall to your study.

CASE EXAMPLE 8.1. A Child with Autism in the Art Classroom

The following case was shared by graduate student Cheryl Shiflett (2008). Her reflective field notes are in italics.

"The art classroom is located in a local school built in 2007. Classroom size is approximately 40 feet by 35 feet, is well lit by natural and artificial light, and is decorated with art posters tacked onto the walls. The classroom has many amenities: two sinks, a kiln room, large areas for storage, and pottery wheels. Tables are adjustable for height. The chalkboard is covered with the directions for an ongoing assignment, and the American Sign Language (ASL) alphabet is posted. Many art materials are spread out on tables and spilling out of storage containers. The sink tops are covered with paintbrushes and clay projects.

"There is a general sense of disorganization and messiness. The art teacher is visibly upset and distracted by a personal matter that she disclosed to me upon my arrival.

"My observation took place on the final day of art class for this group of students. The teacher did not have the materials ready for the students upon their arrival, and much of the class time was spent sorting through accumulated artwork that students needed for the day's assignment or work that needed to be returned before the summer break. Throughout the class, R. V., the art teacher being observed, was distracted by this task.

"For observation purposes, I sat near the teacher's desk. There were a few times when I became a participant; a student asked me for help with finding materials, and I greeted the student with autism, as I have worked with him before in another setting."

Observation 1: Art Classroom

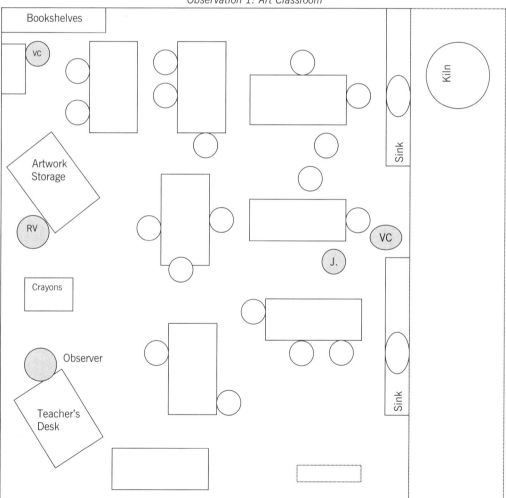

6/10/08 Observation One: Participants

R. V.—part-time, traditional art teacher in a local elementary school who has 30+ years of teaching experience. R. V. participated in an interview as well.

V. C.—a "floater" acting as J.'s assistant during art class. She is part of the self-contained special education classroom staff where J. is a student. A *floater* is a special education substitute who regularly fills in for special education staff who are absent.

J. is a 9-year-old male student with autism attending a self-contained classroom in a local elementary school where he has been mainstreamed into art for the 2007–2008 school year. He is in the fourth grade.

The class—traditional fourth graders.

6/10/08, 8:15 A.M., Descriptive Notes from Observation One: Art Class Instruction with Student with Autism Included

Regularly scheduled class arrives, with students chatting and jockeying for seats. Teacher reconfigures seating choices by limiting three students to each table.

J. enters the classroom wearing a baseball cap, unaccompanied, 3 minutes after the other students, and says, "Good morning!" brightly. *Where is his assistant? Why is he allowed to keep a baseball cap on when it is against school policy to wear one—is this an accommodation for his autism?*

R. V. asks if his assistant is coming.

J. does not respond and, without hesitance, sits down at a table with two boys.

At 8:24 A.M. J.'s assistant arrives and picks up a chair and moves to a corner of the classroom where she can see J. but is out of physical and hearing proximity. *How can she physically assist or give verbal/gestural cues if necessary?*

J. engages in self-talk while his table mates talk to each other.

R. V. calls student names to come pick up their artwork. R. V. specifically asks J. to retrieve his paper. Not responding to the first request, R. V. repeats the direction to come get his art and, fidgeting with his hat, J. walks to the teacher to get his paper and sits back down at his table.

The assistant (V. C.) picks up her chair and moves closer to J. *Apparently, she is realizing that she needs to be closer to J. in order to be effective.*

The boys at J.'s table continue to talk to each other. There are no verbal exchanges or interactions between the two boys and J.

J. stands up and approaches R. V., who is next to the art supply trays, and inquires, "What about crayons?" Distracted, the teacher does not respond to his question, and J. returns to the table. *I am impressed that J. does not take the crayons without the OK from his teacher.*

V. C. coaches J. to sit down.

R. V. says, "J., get your crayons." *Wow, doesn't this confuse J.? He requests something, is told to sit down, then is instructed to get up—a little "hokey pokey" . . .*

J. walks to the art supply trays at the front of the classroom, picks up his crayons and returns to the table to sit down.

The boys are sorting through their own crayons and make joke about the brown crayon looking like chocolate milk. The boys laugh, and J. laughs too. *It's difficult to determine whether J. gets the joke or is echolalic; however, to my perception, I don't believe he "got it."*

Laughing to himself, bouncing in his chair, and waving his arms intermittently, J. begins to color.

V. C. cues J. to put his arms down.

J. and one of his table mates have a brief verbal exchange. *This is the social interaction that is a primary goal for kids with autism.*

J. continues to talk to himself and color. *Other students do not seem distracted by his behavior.*

J. tosses his crayon up into the air, continues to rock in his chair and laughs. V. C. redirects J. to stop inappropriate behaviors. *Other students do not seem to notice this exchange.*

R. V. asks, "J., are you drawing some more stuff?" She reiterates the direction that J. should be using his crayons to create more images on his paper. *This is the first 1:1 interaction at the student's table.*

J. approaches the teacher's work area per her request. Two other students approach as well. R. V. irons J.'s paper image onto a piece of cloth.

R. V. asks J. to get a box of fabric markers.

J. appears unsure of what is being asked. Continuing to iron for other students, R. V. intermittently repeats the direction four times.

J. fiddles with the waistband of his pants and wanders around the classroom.

R. V. calls J. back to her and repeats the direction to use the fabric markers on the lightly faded image transfer to darken the cloth so that the image can be better seen.

J. states, "I don't want to draw." *J. seems resistant to using the markers on his drawing.*

V. C. redirects J. to go back to the table and encourages him to work on his "flag." *J.'s original drawing is a composition of neatly drawn animals. His transfer image is a faded copy of his original.*

J. diligently colors on the original drawing while his two table mates talk to each other. One student is not working on anything.

J., engaging in self-talk, is asked about his work by V. C.—J. does not respond.

J. continues to work on the original drawing rather than enhancing the cloth piece he was instructed to use. *J. is not following the teacher's direction. Is he expected to follow the direction? Does the teacher know he is not following her direction?*

V. C. walks around the class and chats with the other students about their artwork. *Does this normalize her attendance to the class with J.? How does the teacher feel about this? Is it appropriate?*

V. C. returns to J. and appears to recognize that he is not following the directions and encourages him to use the fabric markers on the material.

J. continues to color on the original drawing. *Stubborn.*

R. V., checking on what students have accomplished, stands in front of the classroom and asks J. to hold up his fabric flag.

J. says, "no," stomps his feet, groans, and continues to color on his paper.

V. C. encourages J. to hold up his fabric flag. *J. has done no work on the fabric.*

J. runs, stomping, to the front of the class, and shows R. V. his fabric. Without comment, J. runs and stomps back to the table. *R. V. makes no comment that he has not followed the direction. V. C. does not discuss this with R. V. either.*

R. V. says, "Line up."

J. cleans up, gets his book, and groans as he leaves. *J. has his planner with him to help with transitions, but he did not use it.*

V. C. redirects his agitated behaviors as they leave the classroom at 8:55 A.M.

7/19/2008, Field Reflections from Observation One

• *J. displayed behaviors typical of students with autism: self-talk, arm waving, and fidgeting in his seat and pulling at his clothes. Although these behaviors could potentially be distracting to his classmates, most students did not appear to notice.*

• *The student's assistant (V. C.) did not enter the art room at the same time as J. I am uncertain whether this was to allow J. a bit of independence and part of a strategy or if V. C. should have been with J. at all times. Because the art teacher asked J. the whereabouts of his assistant, I suspect that V. C. should have been with J. Initially, V. C. seemed unsure of her role by taking a chair and moving to a corner of the classroom away from J.'s table. However, once directions were given to J., V. C. seemed to recognize that she would need to return within a closer proximity to J. She appeared very responsive to his needs by redirecting inappropriate behaviors (arm waving, groans, running and stomping, etc.). She also encouraged him to follow the teacher's directions for completing the artwork.*

• *It did not appear that V. C. took any notes about J.'s time spent in art, nor did she communicate with the art teacher before, during, or after class. Student assistants are supposed to have a notebook for recording information. I'm uncertain whether the teacher or parents will be informed of J.'s participation successes and weaknesses.*

• *Although J. brought his communication planner, it did not appear that it was used to encourage his following directions (e.g., "Show me what you are working for?") or to transition out of the classroom. Perhaps if his book, typically used for communicating needs—which includes a visual schedule and incorporates a reinforcement tool for earning some privileges—had been utilized, some difficulties could have been ameliorated. For example, the planner could have been used to visually remind J. that in order for him to "earn" his privilege, he would need to follow the direction. Also, perhaps, if J. had been encouraged to check his book, then the transition out of the class would have been easier.*

• *Although J. sat at a table with two boys, there were minimal verbal exchanges and few attempts at sharing supplies. The table mates talked and joked with each other throughout the class time. J. spoke to one student briefly and laughed (most likely, echolaliacally). If one of the goals is to encourage social interactions with the student with autism, then any exchange, it seems, is expected to occur naturally. Neither the art teacher nor the student's assistant intervened to promote interaction (e.g., by limiting supplies for sharing).*

• *The art teacher did not seem to notice that J. did not follow the art directive. Rather than embellishing the cloth flag, J. continued to color on the original drawing. She made no attempt to redirect him. I'm not sure if she knows whether or not she is responsible for encouraging him to follow directions. J. became agitated when his assistant redirected him to work on the fabric.*

• *J. worked diligently throughout the class while many of his classmates talked and joked loudly. J. genuinely appeared to enjoy creating the art.*

   ACTIVITY 8.3. Observational Exercise

You and your co-researcher(s) are interested in communication patterns among university students, with a particular emphasis on the role of culture in communication patterns. Conduct a naturalistic inquiry in a setting of your choice in which you serve primarily in the observer or observer as participant role. Conduct fieldwork for no less than 20 minutes in your university and be sure to take field notes. Although there may be multiple researchers working with you, you are to work alone on your field notes.

Come back to the class, review your field notes, and add to them as needed for a few minutes. What things did you attend to during the observation? Why do you think you focused on certain things in the setting? To what degree were you involved with individuals in the setting? What challenges about the observation process do you note?

Discuss your findings with your research team. How did your teammates' field notes compare? Listen to other groups' field notes from other sites within the university. How did your observations compare? What initial themes about communication patterns and culture can you derive from multiple observations from multiple researchers?

Go back to your observation setting. Try to observe for 15 minutes without taking notes. What was this process like for you this time?

We would like to close this discussion on the process of observation by summarizing the steps typically involved in observational research:

1. Select setting or context in which to observe based on the case, unit of analysis, and research questions.

2. Determine degree of participation (see observation continuum in Figure 8.2).

3. Create a list of points you might expect based on your conceptual framework and other knowledge specific to the site or context. (As observations increase, develop a more refined observation rubric or protocol.)

4. Use the field notes template in Figure 8.4 on page 231 to develop preliminary thick description, outlining descriptive and reflective field notes as well as memos. (Consider researcher stance, intended audience, and point of view.)

5. Although what you observe will depend on your study, you may elect to observe setting characteristics, participant characteristics, and/or events (see Table 8.1).

6. Observe for brief periods, taking time to further develop initial thick description from field notes before returning to the field. It may be important to observe multiple settings, one setting at various times, or one setting from various angles.

INDIVIDUAL INTERVIEWS

Individual interviews are the most widely used qualitative data collection method (Nunkoosing, 2005; Sandelowski, 2002). Early ethnographers relied on informal interview structures with key informants to uncover characteristics about the "other" and their activities, while more in-depth interviews emerged from research traditions such as phenomenology (DiCicco-Bloom & Crabtree, 2006). Interviewing has guided much of early theory in education and mental health settings and continues to be a preferred option for unexplored and underexplored social phenomena.

Individual interviews generally consist of 5–10 questions, which may or may not include probing questions. Interviews typically last 30 minutes to 1 hour; however, this length varies depending on the purpose of the interview in the overall design. Expect to spend more than an hour interviewing in some cases. Developing an interview protocol or schedule usually begins with an outline of what is to be covered based on the research design. This outline consists of broad categories (Berg, 2004). For example, in a study I (Hays) conducted examining counselors' preparedness to work with clients who were in unhealthy relationships, some of the topics that made it to the outline were de-

TABLE 8.2. Advantages and Disadvantages of Individual Interviews

Advantages	Disadvantages
• Allows participant to describe what is meaningful or important using his or her own words. • Can gain participant's story. • Allows evaluator to probe for more details and ensure that participants are interpreting questions the way they are intended. • Depending on the skill level of the interviewer, there is great potential to uncover interesting and unexpected ideas and themes from participants. • May be less expensive than other data collection methods. • Can gain a lot of data in generally a simple format.	• Participants may not be able, or willing, to express their experiences accurately and thoroughly. That is, they may not be able to come up with answers to interviewer questions. Alternatively, the responses they do provide may not actually represent their realities, whether intentionally or unintentionally (Lambert & Loiselle, 2008). • Participants may wish to impress the interviewer, and/or they may be uncomfortable or unwilling to share all that an interviewer hopes to elicit. • Interviewers may not be skilled and thus fail to ask questions that facilitate detailed responses. • Interviews can change people even though not intentionally, creating potential ethical dilemmas. • May involve greater intrusiveness. • Interviewers need to be well trained.

mographics, training experience, training needs, definitions of healthy and unhealthy relationships, clinical experiences, and clinical interventions. These topics were then translated into nine questions. Table 8.2 provides advantages and disadvantages of the individual interview as a data collection method.

 ACTIVITY 8.4. Interview Practice

Select a classmate or friend to interview on a topic of interest to you both. Interview this person for 10 minutes on the topic. At the end of the interview, ask the interviewee to provide you with input on what types of questions and probes stimulated him or her to share the most.

Interactive Interviewing

Before we discuss types of interviews and specific interview question categories and considerations, we would like to highlight an emerging school of thought on the use of interactive interviewing. McMahan and Rogers (1994) described **interactive interviewing** as the interaction between interviewer and interviewee whereby the two engage in a conversational and open dialogue that involves the exchange of narratives. Special attention is given to both the content of the interview and the impact of the encounter itself on those involved. Interviews are seen as complex narratives that look at what happened and the interviewee's reflection and interpretation of those experiences. Thus, in addition to the content shared in the interview, the interpretation of that content by the interviewee and the complex interactions between the interviewee and interviewer— including the social and historical context of narratives—are addressed.

Kezar (2003) and Campbell, Adams, Wasco, Ahrens, and Sefl (2010) identified these elements of interactive interviewing:

- Diminishing the power differential that exists between the interviewer and interviewee by inviting the interviewee to question the dialogue that is taking place and by interviewer self-disclosure.

- Feelings of the interviewee and interviewer are processed as they arise.

- Two-way relationship rooted in mutual engagement by both.

- Mutual trust wherein the researcher has an inherent and sincere trust and belief in the interviewee (the interviewee is only challenged when the interviewer begins to not believe him or her).

- Reflexiveness of interviewer on his or her own biases.

- Commitment by the interviewer to be empathic and approach the interviewee with an ethic of care.

- Participation in this type of interviewing allows for greater action and advocacy.

Types of Individual Interviews

The first type of interview is the **structured interview**, which relies on a preestablished sequence and pace of questions that a researcher follows rigidly. Questions are asked exactly as written, and probes, if included, are also standardized. Qualitative researchers typically do not reveal anything personal about themselves and remain as neutral as possible. One advantage of this form of interview is that the same information (depth and breadth) is covered with all participants. Structured interviews are more likely to be used in survey research or telephone interviews (Esterberg, 2002). Some argue, however, that the more structured an interview becomes, the less "qualitative" the data are, since the interview is so controlled. That is, participants' voices are limited by the structure and increasingly defined by what the qualitative researcher wants to hear (Bogdan & Biklen, 2003).

The second type of interview, the **semistructured interview** (also referred to as an *in-depth interview*), typically uses an interview protocol that serves as a guide and starting point for the interview experience. Once the interview begins, the interviewee has more say in the structure and process. Even with those that do include a protocol, every interview question does not have to be asked, the sequence and pace of interview questions can change, and additional interview questions can be included to create a unique interview catered to fully describing the interviewee's experience. Often a sole data source in qualitative studies, the semistructured interview is typically scheduled in advance with a participant, perhaps outside the participant's typical setting (DiCicco-Bloom & Crabtree, 2006). Esterberg (2002) noted that this form of interview may be most culturally appropriate. We believe that although this type of interview does not ensure consistency of data collection experience across participants, it makes up for this disadvantage by including more participant voice, as appropriate, to provide a richer picture of a phenomenon under investigation.

The third type of interview, the **unstructured interview**, largely occurs as part of a participant observation (Esterberg, 2002) and often is associated with ethnography and perhaps other "in-the-field" research traditions. The label *unstructured* is mislead-ing, since no interview can truly be unstructured and is more likely a "guided conver-sation." Unstructured interviews focus on the surrounding context at the time of the interview. For example, ethnographers often observe and write a memo about the con-text, while approaching select participants (i.e., key informants, typically) to confirm their observations (DiCicco-Bloom & Crabtree, 2006). One disadvantage of this type of interview is that it may be difficult to synthesize the data.

⚠ WILD CARD 8.1. NO INTERVIEW IS THE SAME!

"Interviewers and interviewees are *not* interchangeable. No matter which form of inter-viewing you use, do not assume that you will gather the same types of data no matter who the interviewers or interviewees are. Both bring unique experiences, personality dynamics, cultural characteristics, and skills that make the interview process unique and thus the content variable. Interviewers have different ideas about the purpose of the interview: Are you trying to gain information or share information and create new meanings?

"I had a research team of 10 conducting individual interviews. Even though we used a semistructured interview format, transcripts varied greatly among the team members. Based on interviewer characteristics and abilities, as well as relationships with participants, some transcripts were more expansive than others. Some research team members asked the questions verbatim, others disclosed personal information to elicit responses, and others diverted from the protocol yet still provided relevant data."

—DGH

"I remember piloting a new structured interview protocol. We were asking questions about risky behavior—topics that typically included sex, drugs, and needle use. I found that certain people were less comfortable with the topics, and they would skip over these questions or not ask follow-up probes when participants gave answers that im-plicated risky behavior. Then there were interviewers who were *more* than comfortable with these topics, and at times asked questions that were too personal for participants. Because it was a pilot interview, I was able to regroup with the team and talk more about our comfort levels with the topic of risky behavior. This helped interviewers ask all the questions in the interview protocol, but we still had variance in some of the in-depth probes."

—AAS

The Interview Question

Researchers (Patton, 2002; Snow, Zurcher, & Sjoberg, 1982) have outlined several types of interview questions that serve as important templates when developing an interview protocol. These categories of questions, which we describe in the following sections, are likely suitable as primary questions or probes for most research traditions and set-tings. We believe it is important, no matter what your selected research tradition(s) or setting(s), to brainstorm examples of questions for each category (see Activity 8.5 on page 251). These questions can be asked using past, present, or future tense, as appropriate.

As we define and describe each category, we also illustrate it by providing examples of interview questions using a study involving mental health practitioners' experiences with the homeless population.

Background or Demographic Questions

Background or demographic questions are foundational questions that the interviewer should ask about the participant, setting, or phenomenon during the interview itself or in some written form, such as via a demographic questionnaire. If these questions are included in the interview itself, they should be kept to a minimum since responses to these types of questions are likely to be concrete and superficial. Examples include "What is your experience level as a mental health practitioner?" and "What gender do you identify as?"

Behavior or Experience Questions

This category of questions solicits information about participants' actions and their reflections on those actions. **Behavior or experience questions** are the "what versus why" questions; as an interviewer, you are concerned with gathering a thick description of what occurred by and for the participants rather than *why* things occurred. Examples include: "Tell me about what services, if any, you provide to the homeless population" and "How do your services for a client who is homeless compare to the services for someone who is not homeless?"

Opinion or Value Questions

These questions pertain to collective and individual beliefs about why things occur. **Opinion questions** seek participants' personal beliefs about a phenomenon. **Value questions** tap social norms in relation to individual beliefs. Examples include "How do you perceive that the homeless population is treated in this city?" and "What concerns, if any, do you have about a client who is homeless seeking mental health services?"

Knowledge Questions

Knowledge questions solicit responses from participants about the amount of information they possess regarding a phenomenon as well as where that knowledge originated. Examples include "Approximately what percentage of clients that come to your agency identifies as homeless?" and "What common concerns do clients who identify as homeless express?"

Feeling Questions

Departing from *what* and *why* interview questions, **feeling questions** are not directed toward eliciting the validity of how interviewees respond or what they know. Instead, these questions reflect interest in how participants feel about something. Examples include "What feelings arise for you when you are working with a client who identifies as homeless?" and "What emotional responses do you have when those clients are children?"

Sensory Questions

Using the five senses (i.e., sight, hearing, taste, smell, touch) in developing questions for this category, interviewers who use **sensory questions** are seeking information from participants about their bodily experiences. While this may seem strange at first, the use of sensory questions is useful for completing a picture of the interviewee's experience that is untapped in cognitive and affective responses. Examples include "Describe for me the sights and sounds of a recent group session that includes clients who identify as homeless" and "If I were to listen in on an intake session between you and your agency director about meeting the mental health needs of the homeless population in this community, what would I hear?"

Probing Questions

Seldom written out ahead of time, **probing questions** or probes are the "who, what, when, where, and how" questions that help to expand an interviewee's responses. Probing questions can be verbal, such as elaboration and clarification questions, or nonverbal, such as head nods. No matter what probes you use, the idea is to get interviewees to provide a richer interview because their voices are important (not because they are doing something wrong in the interview). Examples of probes are given in Table 8.3.

Use of Commentary

An interview question does not have to be a *question* at all. Snow and colleagues (1982) described obtaining information from a participant by using a statement rather than an interview question. Unlike an interview question, a comment does not pressure a participant to respond. That is, a participant can opt to respond or not, which is particularly important if he or she feels that the comment has little to no relevance to his or her experience. Types of comments include the following:

TABLE 8.3. Examples of Probes

- "Can you give me an example?"
- "Tell me a little more about that."
- "What happened next?"
- "How did that happen?"
- "What was that like for you?"
- "Where were you?"
- "Who else was there?"
- "How does *A* compare to *B*?"

- *Puzzlement*: Expression of ignorance (real or not) to demonstrate that the researcher is confused and in need of assistance. "I'm having a hard time making sense of what was done to you."

- *Humorous comments*: Use of sarcasm in a spontaneous manner to explore a sensitive issue. For example, in interviewing an instructor about his workload compensation, the interviewer commented, "I'm sure you don't have that much to do anyway, right?"

- *The replay*: A restatement or paraphrase immediately following a particular response or as a method of linking several responses to ensure clarification and elaboration. "I'm hearing you say that you are gaining a lot from the support group yet would like housing assistance." This is an important tool to ensure that the researcher has heard the participant correctly.

- *Descriptive comments*: Articulation of the concrete details of an experience that demonstrates the researcher's image of what the interviewee is stating; often the description is used to compare to other experiences. "I'm imagining several students talking out of turn and moving about frequently while you are trying to teach them. This seems similar to parents with whom I have spoken, who have experienced disruptive behaviors at home."

- *Outrageous comments*: An absurdity stated to induce a strong reaction from a participant when vague responses continue. For the workload compensation study mentioned above: "Maybe you should just work less since you will never make what you deserve."

- *Alter-casting comments*: Casting a participant in a role or identity congruent with an interview purpose to gauge rapport and appropriateness of including a particular participant in the study. "I bet you have had a lot of trouble getting what you need as a client from this agency."

- *Evaluative comments*: Solicitation of a participant's actual or suspected values, feelings, or opinions about a phenomenon. These comments can serve to compare how one should feel or think with how they do feel and think, illuminating social norms: "I wonder how social justice fits into your counseling philosophy."

Strategies for a "Good" Interview

It may difficult to determine what a "good" interview looks like, but there are a few general indicators. In general, as qualitative researchers conduct an interview, they listen carefully to participants, show personal interest and encourage them, and ask open-ended questions that allow them to speak freely and comfortably. In the following sections we describe a variety of more specific strategies.

Establish Rapport

Esterberg (2002) described interviewing as a relationship between a researcher and a participant. Because the qualitative interview is *not* a job interview, rapport building is absolutely necessary for a successful interview. Rapport building should occur before the interview process happens, as a result of prolonged engagement. However, we believe that there is also a necessary rapport-building process that takes place during the interview process itself.

Rapport building begins with entering the field, as discussed in Chapter 6. What is often missing from discussions of rapport building is the inherent role of the conflicts that arise at various stages of fieldwork: Establishing trust and building rapport isn't a linear and simplistic process, and roles constantly need to be evaluated and modified. Several issues arise in rapport building: the presence of multiple roles, the problem of "faking friendship," and differential understandings of the purpose of rapport among researchers and participants.

The first concern is that of the impact of multiple, often changing, roles in fieldwork. Throughout stages of fieldwork qualitative researchers negotiate and renegotiate a variety of social and power relationships as well as perform several activities within personal and professional contexts. As de Laine (2000) noted, researchers balance participation with observation, closeness with distance, and being an insider with being an outsider. Here are some other issues related to roles that arise as researchers enter the field and build rapport (Adler & Adler, 1987; de Laine, 2000; Reinharz, 1992):

- There are often dual and overlapping roles, such as those of friend and researcher, counselor or teacher and researcher, and so on.

- Roles can be defined as formal and/or informal—a multiplicity of roles creates ethical and professional dilemmas.

- Roles have been traditionally defined as the activities researchers "do" in fieldwork rather than who they "are."

- The way roles are conceptualized are largely based on choices in site selection and preferred methodology.

- Developing *real* closeness with participants may be impossible, and the best researchers can do is strive for roles that allow for "fake" friendship.

- Most friendships and efforts toward solidarity cultivated in the field are short-lived and unintentionally fraudulent.

- Based on the setting context and differences in characteristics among researchers and participants, researchers can have a peripheral, outsider role, and active, insider role, and/or a complete membership role with full commitment to group goals.

The second concern—the notion of "faking friendship" for rapport building—is an especially important one. Duncombe and Jessop (2002) noted that researchers "fake friendship" for scientific purposes: They learn to manage their appearance and purpose and pretend to not know what they will say, while at times pretending to know, to maintain rapport. It can often be a game of pretend to create the context for data collection:

> [Interviewers] should consciously dress and present themselves in a way that sends the correct message to the interviewee. That is, they must seat themselves not too far away but not too near; maintain a pleasant, encouraging half-smile and a lively (but not too lively) interest. They should keep eye contact, speak in a friendly tone, never chal-

lenge, and avoid inappropriate expressions of surprise or disapproval; and practice the art of the encouraging but "non-directive 'um.'" If this is "friendship," then it is a very detached form of it. (p. 110)

Although it is clearly impossible for participants to give their full informed consent, researchers rely on strengthening rapport to continue participant disclosure rather than engage in the complex nature of ongoing informed consent (see Chapter 3). "Ethical issues must inevitably arise where, increasingly, relatively unsuspecting interviewees are confronted by qualitative interviewers who are armed with a battery of skills in 'doing rapport' in interview relationships in order to achieve disclosure" (Duncombe & Jessop, 2002, p. 112). Even when researchers espouse a feminist or other postmodern paradigm that claims that the research relationship involves spontaneous and genuine rapport leading to mutual reciprocal disclosure, interview relationships likely fall somewhere on the continuum of genuine empathy and elements of "faking friendship" to obtain data. Qualitative researchers are to be reminded that interviewees are not totally powerless and have some opportunity to withhold their participation.

A final issue involves the different and often conflicting intentions of establishing rapport. Scholars (e.g., de Laine, 2000) have pointed out that researchers cannot assume that rapport has been established based on their being empathic toward participants, who seem to be agreeable to process. The problem with rapport building is that researchers often do it to meet research means: We often "trick" participants to get data, no matter how good our intentions are. Participants engage in the research process because they rely on the researcher's integrity, *not* the research's merit. No matter the intentional role the research takes, the participant is likely to engage and trust based on a perception of friendship or empathy and sympathy. Participants are not likely to engage in fieldwork for merits of research, even if the researcher assumes they are. Since there are role type, role conflict, role multiplicity, and power and cultural differences in fieldwork, researchers should be intentional about exercising control over the relationships established for research purposes (Burgess, 1991). As de Laine (2000) cautioned, "the fieldworker is sometimes required to perform a delicate balancing act to meet the obligations and responsibilities owed to various parties, and still promote their own research agenda" (p. 119). If not careful, qualitative researchers are just as likely to promote coercive relationships for the sake of research.

Make the Interview Not Feel Like an Interview

No matter how much rapport you build with a participant, sitting down to do an interview produces some rigidity to that relationship and may create anxiety for the participant to "say the right thing." Your job, then, is to take this pressure off as much as possible. Some strategies for making this happen include the following:

- Move from noncontroversial to more controversial questions.
- Ask for descriptions, then opinions, about a phenomenon.
- Watch your "nonverbal" interview questions.
- Use probes when possible to elicit expanded responses in personally meaningful ways.

- Ask both general and specific questions (drawing on participants' specific experiences whenever possible).
- Summarize what has been discussed in the interview as you proceed.
- Memorize questions when possible to minimize losing eye contact with the interviewee.

Finally, and most important, be sure to tell participants how helpful their responses are to the research topic. This can be done directly, like saying, "This has been very helpful," to more indirectly yet powerfully, such as, "That is really interesting—I have never thought of it that way." To ensure that your interview runs smoothly, we recommend that you pretest your interview questions (see Proposal Development 8.2 on p. 248).

Use Role-Playing or Simulation Questions as Appropriate

One successful method for engaging interviewees is by emphasizing their expertise on a phenomenon. **Role-playing questions** allow the participant to discuss a topic from a particular role of authority. The question stem, "What advice would you give," is an example of this type of question. **Simulation questions** request that participants verbally observe a phenomenon for the interviewer. That is, the interviewer asks the participant to place him- or herself in a situation. "Suppose I was present with you in that setting. What would I see?" is an example of a simulation question.

Make Assumptions When Relevant

While it is generally preferred that qualitative researchers ask questions in an open-ended manner to avoid influencing or limiting participant responses, sometimes it might be relevant to assume an experience of some phenomenon in a question to encourage participant elaboration. Using the scenario of an individual who has been abusing substances, and who has a high likelihood of comorbid disorders, **presupposition questions** might include: "Can you tell me about the depression or anxiety symptoms you have been experiencing?" and "How have your physical symptoms changed in severity since you began drinking?"

Use Illustrative Questions

At times, an initial interview question falls flat or the interviewee struggles with how to respond to a particular question. This can occur if a question is difficult to grasp or explain, or if the interviewee is resistant to respond. **Illustrative questions** are really comments that get across to the participant that you "have heard it all." That is, you present response extremes to illustrate a range of potential responses.

For example, when I (Hays) was interviewing supervisors in training about their perceptions of current practices in their training programs, I got very little information at first. So I illustrated potential responses, similar to the following, to expand the discussion: "Several students I have spoken with have discussed that there have been several challenges—like time constraints, problems establishing rapport with their supervisee, getting paperwork completed, and even wanting to leave the program for lack of support from faculty. Others have talked about how beneficial it has been to have several supervisees from various settings to practice supervision. I am wondering if any of you have experienced these things?"

Avoid Questions That Limit Participant Responses

Responses can be limited by various types of interview questions. For example, **dichotomous questions** (i.e., yes–no questions) or forced-choice responses require participants to select a response to a question without an opportunity to elaborate on why they responded in a particular way. Examples include: "Do you believe that college students are drinking more than during the last decade?" and "Have you noticed a change in the quality of students entering your graduate program?"

Second, **multiple questions** (or *double-barreled questions*) involve asking too many things at once. The problem you face with this is that participants may never answer all parts of the interview questions thoroughly or accurately. This makes it difficult to analyze interview responses. Consider this example: "What are the benefits and challenges of integrating special education students in the general classroom?" No matter how the participant responds, it will be difficult to determine which are descriptions of benefits and which are of challenges. Additionally, not having a singular focus or question regarding benefits, with an additional, separate focus on challenges, sends a message that independent attention to each is not warranted.

Do Not Attempt to Get the Participant "On Your Side"

Whether intentional or not, we as interviewers may let it be known to each participant what our thoughts and attitudes are regarding a phenomenon. To minimize this from happening nonverbally or through probes, avoid behaviors such as head nods and changes in facial expressions for particular responses (e.g., grimace, wider eyes), and verbal statements such as "right," "uh-huh," and "really." Essentially, you show interest in what participants are saying, but you do not give away your opinions and recommendations in a manner that disempowers their voice or that sways their attitudes or behaviors. **Leading questions** are more direct verbal questions that can be harmful to rigorous data collection as well as to the research relationship in general. These types of questions might begin with more overt stems such as "Don't you agree" and "Isn't it true"; however, leading questions can also be more subtle. For example, imagine that you are interviewing seventh-grade students about the effectiveness of a study skills program. Simply asking questions that assume only that the program was effective, rather than also including questions that uncover program challenges or other interventions altogether that have helped them improve their study skills, is considered leading.

Do Not Ask "Why" Questions

Similar to leading questions, we would like to caution against the use of "why" questions: Asking a participant why something occurred is likely to make him or her defensive. And, a "why" question might make an interviewee feel that he or she should know why something happened or why it is the way it is. Almost any why question can be reworded without the word *why*. For example, an interviewer puts the question, "Why is there more vandalism occurring in your high school?" to an administrator, who immediately bristles with defensiveness and wants to exit the interview as quickly as possible. Alternatively, the same question can be rephrased to "Tell me about the amount of vandalism that has occurred in your school over the past several years."

Prepare a One-Shot Question

A **one-shot question** is popular with opportunistic sampling (see Chapter 6). It refers to preparing one question to ask a key informant, should you get the opportunity to do so. Design decisions are often in response to researchers developing an understanding of and exposure to events or ideas. Because data collection can constantly change, we believe it is a good idea to prepare for possible interactions with participants you initially thought were inaccessible. For example, let's say you are studying the impact of budget cuts on faculty morale. A one-shot question might be the following, intended for the head of Human Resources, should you be able to interview her: "I am aware that your office collected data regarding faculty retention and university budget cuts. Could you tell me a little bit about your findings?"

PROPOSAL DEVELOPMENT 8.2. Developing an Interview Protocol

Develop 10 questions (or less, depending on your research questions and traditions). Review the question types as well as tips for conducting a successful interview presented in this chapter.
    Discuss your interview protocol with your research team or a peer.

1. Are the interview questions too limiting or leading? (Are they biased, so that certain "answers" will be generated that may falsely support what you expect to find?)

2. Are the questions too broad?

3. Are the questions clear, concise, and precise?

4. Is there evidence of cultural bias in your interview questions?

5. If you do find the "answer" to your interview question, what is the purpose (the "so what" factor)?

6. What are the strengths of your questions?

7. What are some suggestions for improving your protocol?

    Revise the interview protocol and document the process for your audit trail.
    As you collect and analyze data, be sure to continually evaluate your interview questions with your research team or peers, or perhaps with participants and other stakeholders.

Give Interviewees the Last Word

We suggest a couple of questions that should always end your interview: "Is there anything else important that you would like to add?" and "What else should I have asked you?" These questions allow participants to close the interview on their time and have the final say. We believe that this encourages their voice and provides closure to a strong interview.

Read the Results

Finally, the transcript can give a good indication of the quality of the interview. In reviewing the write-up, the participant's words should significantly outnumber the researcher's. Furthermore, qualitative researchers should encounter several details and examples given by participants, based on questions that elicited a deep exploration of a phenomenon or experience.

In reading a transcript, you are likely to find responses you want to follow up or phrases that need clarification. As a method of member checking (see Chapter 7), we encourage you to conduct multiple interviews with each participant. At the very least, in instances when you are unable to sit down with a participant again, we recommend that you have him or her review the transcript and insert comments to clarify any questions you have or to elaborate on points he or she made.

⚠ WILD CARD 8.2. LESSONS LEARNED FROM A "BAD INTERVIEW"

We asked our students and colleagues to talk about lessons learned from unsuccessful interviews. Here they are, in no particular order:

- Do not turn the tape off after the interview. Wait until you are completely done interacting with a participant. Some of the richest data come from conversations after the interview protocol is done.

- Avoid telephone interviews unless geographical location presents a problem. The face-to-face or video-streaming interactions are extremely important for their nonverbal cues during the interview.

- Practice your interview with someone. If not, your anxiety as an interviewer may cause you to rush through the interview and jump from topic to topic.

- Do not be afraid to steer away from an interview protocol. Expand on spontaneous conversations and note dynamics of the research relationship. Although it's hard to attend to both content and process during an interview, it is absolutely necessary.

- Conduct your interview in a natural setting, but without distractions when possible. This means no other people in the setting, no background noises, and no interruptions.

- Remind your participants of who you are and what the purpose of the interview is at the beginning of your interview. Sometimes participants are nervous and go off-topic, especially if they are members of a vulnerable group.

- Do not use "ten-dollar" words (e.g., *resilience*) in your interview, when you can use a simpler word or phrase that conveys the same meaning (e.g., *bounce back*). Definitely do not step away from the power you have as a researcher because your participants will see you as the "expert." But use this power to interact collaboratively with your participants as opposed to holding power over them as an interviewer.

- Avoid becoming the interviewee. If it feels too much like a conversation and you are the only one disclosing, it is likely no longer an interview. Disclose to build rapport, but step back to hear *their* voices.

- Relatedly, each question you ask takes time and space "away" from the interviewee. Be conscious about not firing away question after question. You do not want your participants to feel like they are being interrogated.

- Research questions are not interview questions. When you start translating your research questions directly to interview questions, you are likely to just get the responses you want. Be creative and seek help when developing your interview protocol.

- Watch your presentation. You should dress and conduct the interview in a way that does not make the interviewee guarded or resistant to being honest with you. More so than not, you will be leaving the suits at home.

Interviewing by Research Tradition

The type, content, and process of interviewing may depend on the research tradition. For example, a grounded theory approach might utilize a semistructured format (Fielding, 1994), whereas an ethnography might use a more informal or unstructured format (DiCicco-Bloom & Crabtree, 2006). One of the most predominant approaches in the literature is Siedman's phenomenological interviewing method.

Siedman's Phenomenological Interviewing

The purpose of Siedman's (2006) phenomenonological interviewing method is to elicit a description of the essence of an experience that several individuals have undergone. With a focus on the lived meanings of a phenomenon across individuals, this form of interview is conducted in three phases, with each phase having a central question with probes. Interviews should be spaced 3 days to 1 week apart.

    The first phase is the focused life history, which involves gathering a comprehensive picture of a participant's involvement, over time, with a phenomenon. For example, let's pretend that you want to conduct a case study of a high school recently affected by a school shooting. A focused life history would involve interviewing students about their overall experience in that setting, leading up to and during the school shooting: "Tell me about your experiences at this high school, including those surrounding the shooting."

    The second phase of this interview is focused on eliciting the details of an experience. Essentially, participants reconstruct the concrete details of the phenomenon. The use of critical incidents is very important in this phase. Using the school shooting example, here might be your central question: "What are the specific responses you had during the school shooting?"

The final phase of the interview is reflection on meaning (although participants reflect on meaning throughout the interview process). This third interview focuses heavily on meaning making and connecting thoughts and feelings from the first two interviews. Participants are asked to reflect on the meaning their experiences hold for them. With the school shooting study, an example of a third-phase central question might be the following: "Given your overall thoughts and feelings surrounding your experiences in this high school and those specific to the school shooting, how do you understand that school shooting today?"

ACTIVITY 8.5. Interviewing by Research Tradition

You are a part of a "research team" (dyad) that is interested in interviewing participants about public school education in comparison to private school education. You may choose which individual(s) to interview (e.g., students, community officials, school administrators, school counselors, parents, teachers). Select one (or two) of the research traditions below and develop an interview protocol.

Case study	Phenomenology	Grounded theory	CQR
Biography	Narratology	Ethnography	PAR
Heuristic inquiry	Hermeneutics	Ethnomethodology	Autoethnography
Life history	Semiotics	Symbolic interaction	

After you have developed the interview protocol, switch partners and reflect on the following:

- What type of interview (i.e., structured, semistructured, unstructured) does your protocol represent? What are the advantages and advantages of this?
- To what extent is the interview protocol appropriate for the research tradition?
- How might the sample affect the interview protocol? How might it influence the interview process?

- What personal characteristics do you possess that might affect your interviewing individuals about this topic? With this sample?
- To what degree do you feel that self-disclosure with participants during the interview itself might be appropriate?
- What changes should be made to the interview protocol?

FOCUS GROUP INTERVIEWS

Focus groups have been used in business and marketing disciplines (and briefly in sociology) since the 1940s. However, this format basically disappeared from the social sciences for a few decades due to some resistance toward qualitative research in general (Brotherson, 1994). Since the 1970s, the focus group format has been applied to other disciplines, including counseling, psychology, public health, and education (Wilkinson, 2003).

The focus group is a natural data collection method in clinical and educational settings. Kress and Shoffner (2007) stated that focus groups can be well suited to uncover information about the counseling process as well as the effectiveness of counseling programs and interventions. Focus groups offer unique opportunities for generating data from interactions among participants who share a common experience or are homogeneous in some manner. This format often serves as a catalyst for participant disclosure, connecting with others, and expanding on or challenging perspectives in a synergistic manner. We have found the focus group to be a great outlet for "brainstorming" about intervention and programmatic ideas as well as social phenomena underrepresented in the literature.

The focus group format can be used for needs assessment, program evaluation, and exploratory research. When conducting a needs assessment or program evaluation, qualitative researchers should ensure that the selected participants represent the demography of that setting. Furthermore, participants selected for exploratory research purposes should best represent the population of interest (Kress & Shoffner, 2007).

The primary purpose of a focus group is to discuss a particular topic of interest among a gathering of individuals who are homogeneous in some manner. Whenever possible, participants are selected for their similarities with regard to at least one particular characteristic related to a study topic, such as gender, education level, mental health disorder, occupation type, and so on. However, although focus groups may appear to be only a casual discussion among clients, students, administrators, special educators, college professors, and so forth, they are, "in fact, facilitated and purposeful data collection" (Kress & Shoffner, 2007, p. 191). Focus groups are valued because "group interactions may accentuate members' similarities and differences and give rich information about the range of perspectives and experiences" (Lambert & Loiselle, 2008, p. 229).

While focus group interview data can provide insight on the attitudes, beliefs, and experiences of individual participants, it is the *interactive* nature of this data collection format that produces data that cannot be obtained from individual interviews. That is, focus groups are intended to produce data from individuals that are based in their interpersonal interactions, not simply data from multiple individuals at once to save time. Focus group facilitators should ensure that a focus group interview session does not primarily become a counseling session or a venue for expressing complaints. Table 8.4 provides examples of focus group research in clinical and educational settings.

TABLE 8.4. The Focus Group Interview

Purpose	Reference	Description
Needs assessment	Ku, Lahman, Yeh, & Cheng (2008)	12 international doctoral students met twice per month for a year to discuss their needs in their programs.
Program evaluation	Quinlan (2009)	15 master's-level students enrolled in a multicultural counseling course participated in focus groups to assess the degree to which the course facilitated their multicultural counseling competency.
Exploratory research	Shoffner, Newsome, & Barrio (2005)	Students in grades 6–9 were asked about their opinions regarding careers in science, mathematics, and technology and what they might expect if they were to pursue more advanced coursework in these areas.

Advantages

There are several advantages of focus group data collection. First, it allows for direct contact between qualitative researchers and participants. This intimacy creates opportunities for researchers to ask follow-up or clarifying questions and to establish rapport. Provided that researchers are properly trained in conducting focus group interviews, they can manage interpersonal dynamics so that a topic is thoroughly addressed and each participant has an opportunity to contribute to the interview. Not only does this form of data collection involve a "focus" on a particular topic, it also creates a "focused" environment wherein participants are part of a captive audience that can speak about a topic in a safe setting without outside distractions.

Second, this format is also socially oriented, often creating a more relaxed feel than individual interviewing. Furthermore, Kress and Shoffner (2007) noted that focus groups may be a culturally sensitive and empowering data collection method. Since the purpose of focus groups is to bring together those with a common interest in a particular topic, the various points of view presented among participants may help to validate others' experiences as well as model respectful dialogue among diverse members of society.

Third, focus groups can facilitate self-exploration regarding the impact of the phenomenon under investigation. For example, imagine that you, as a counselor in a residential setting, are interested in improving programming for adolescents diagnosed with behavioral disorders. You conduct a focus group session with 10 clients and assess their mental health needs as well as helpful interventions for coping with symptoms. During this process several clients share personal information about their symptoms. As a result, other clients' experiences with those same symptoms are validated, and some clients become more familiar with symptoms of behavioral disorders to monitor in themselves. Furthermore, many clients might discuss helpful interventions that other clients have not yet experienced.

Fourth, focus groups allow for greater data collection in less time, particularly as compared to individual interviews. That is, qualitative researchers can obtain a larger number of participants to investigate a phenomenon with a minimum number of interview sessions. Focus groups are especially useful for gaining access to sites and other participants, site selection and sampling, and focused observations (Morgan, 1997). We would like to caution, however, that the focus group method should *never* be used solely to "save time": Selecting this data collection method is based on a need to investigate *interactive* data, not simply on a need to secure more data in a shorter amount of time. Since individual interviews differ from focus group interviews in purpose, process, and outcome, the decision to use the focus group method should be based on a sound rationale.

Finally, focus groups may be congruent with the counseling philosophy; counseling values such as respect for clients' views, encouragement, and promotion of insight are often mirrored in focus group interviews (Kress & Shoffner, 2007).

Disadvantages

Focus groups have many of the same disadvantages as those of groups in general. First, there is likely a pressure to fit into the group, such as producing socially desirable responses or other efforts at group conformity. This can manifest in several ways: Participants may be less likely to express opinions that are counter to the group majority; participants may want to please the qualitative researcher or avoid a contentious environment by withholding a nonpopular perspective; and participants may feel pressure to participate at a level that is uncomfortable to them. Thus, if not conducted carefully, the focus group interview can come to represent the voices of only a few participants.

Although facilitators should discuss the potential for bias in questions before conducting focus group interviews (Kress & Shoffner, 2007), it is often difficult for them to avoid biasing the interactions—particularly since they have the potential to be a large influence on the group. We recommend that focus group facilitators spend some time before and after the interview protocol establishing rapport and receiving feedback about the interview process, respectively.

Finally, focus group methods may not actually offer the same depth as individual interviews (e.g., recording methods often do not allow qualitative researchers to identify individual speakers), nor will they produce the rich contextual data of observations (Berg, 2004). Thus, they can be limiting if not used with other data collection methods.

Focus Group Structure

Generally, focus groups involve 6–12 individuals with one or two facilitators. While facilitators make the decision of how many to include based on the purpose of the qualitative inquiry, they must take into account the following: too few participants may cause some individuals to feel exposed in the group, whereas too many may risk side conversations (Brotherson, 1994).

A focus group interview typically includes three to eight interview questions. In addition to an interview protocol, there are likely specific probe and follow-up questions to facilitate interaction. Morgan (1988) reminds us that questions that directly assess experiences and views are helpful in the early stages of a focus group interview, but they do not facilitate a spontaneous, interactive quality among participants as the interview moves forward.

Facilitators (or *moderators,* as they are sometimes called) serve to promote extensive and meaningful interaction among focus group participants and to maintain the focus "on topic" (Kress & Shoffner, 2007). A facilitator should possess a strong skill set in conducting groups, whether it be those in a classroom, meeting or seminar room, mental health agency, and so forth. In the case of using two facilitators, one can serve as a process observer. That is, the process observer attends to the nonverbal communication and other subtle dynamics within the focus group, while the other facilitator more directly engages and directs the interactions. Alternatively, both facilitators may opt to trade off, and both solicit interviewee responses and take note of group process. Table 8.5 provides some strategies for facilitators; you may want to review other strategies presented under the Individual Interviewing section and apply those to focus group interviews.

Focus groups may contain significantly more than a dozen participants, such as in cases of a town hall meeting style or open forum method. Size does matter, however. Groups of a size much larger than 10 participants may garner less valuable results. People may be more hesitant to share feelings in larger groups, more participants require more time to adequately respond to questions, and researchers are less likely to maintain sufficient and even accurate field notes of larger focus groups.

TABLE 8.5. Strategies for Focus Group Facilitators

- Participate directly in focus group discussions with caution. The focus group discussion should flow naturally with few interjections overall from the facilitator(s). That is, participants should do most of the talking and interact with one another, not with the facilitator. To this end, a facilitator should be both skilled in "asking the right question" and then giving room for full individual participation and using silence and pauses, as appropriate.
- Adjust the number of questions based on the age and developmental level of focus group members.
- Use probing questions to encourage a deeper interaction among participants that facilitates the expression of potentially divergent attitudes, beliefs, and experiences.
- Avoid creating "rounds" wherein participants are pressured to respond to interview questions based on a sequencing of participants.
- Observe nonverbal behaviors.
- Interject themes derived from individual responses throughout the focus group interview. This collective "playback" often allows for a richer discussion of a topic of interest and increased participant disclosure.
- Be flexible and adapt to situations within the session whenever participants provide unexpected yet invaluable data regarding a topic. Given that a "good" facilitator will evoke more honest and richer individual responses, there will likely be times when these responses could conflict with one another. A facilitator should be prepared to deal with conflict or at least with changes in the conversation flow.
- Be present and genuinely interested in participant responses.
- Be aware of power differentials between the facilitators and the participants, as well as among participants.

Source: Kress and Shoffner (2007).

Establishing and Beginning the Focus Group

Participant selection is a vital component of a successful focus group interview. Hollander (2004) identified four contextual factors that influence the type and quality of interaction among participants: (1) degree of commonality among participants, (2) position or status among them, (3) nature and format of intended discussions, and (4) extent that facilitator(s) and participants are familiar with each other personally. These factors need to be weighed in relation to participant selection to maximize focus group interaction. We believe that focus groups should be composed of members who share similar characteristics and power in regard to the phenomenon of interest, and that facilitators should engage in an open and empowering dialogue with participants. The fourth factor, involving the relationships among members and facilitators, is less important when these preceding criteria are addressed. Otherwise, no matter how familiar participants are with each other and with facilitators, they may not be willing to disclose information. Finally, Morgan (1988) identified an additional contextual factor: participant diversity. That is, it is important to have diverse participants who share commonalities with respect to the phenomenon.

It is important to note that it is not always possible to select participants for a focus group interview. Groups form naturally in our everyday worlds, without prescreening and outside the researcher's control. Common groups for which participant preselection is likely impossible might include online chat rooms, students in a classroom, employees at a counseling agency, and so forth. Furthermore, they may include individuals whose characteristics aren't known to the qualitative researcher prior to, or during, the focus group interview. Qualitative researchers should consider the contextual factors discussed in the previous paragraph and note how a specific group's makeup creates both opportunities and challenges during data collection and analysis.

The initial stages of a focus group interview may seem parallel to securing informed consent in clinical settings, reviewing a syllabus or course outline in a classroom, or setting an agenda for a meeting among educators or administrators. At the beginning of a focus group session, a facilitator (1) explains the purpose of the qualitative study as well as the purpose of the focus group interview as a component of that research design; (2) sets the agenda for what the focus group interview will look like (e.g., approximate number of questions, duration of interview); (3) describes the roles of focus group members and facilitator(s); (4) discusses participant rights and responsibilities; and (5) develops ground rules for appropriate and inappropriate behaviors during the interview session (e.g., one person speaks at a time, there are no right or wrong answers, no side conversations).

Even with attention to these contextual factors prior to beginning the focus group, facilitators should still evaluate the quality of interactions after data are collected. The following questions can be used to guide that assessment:

- What were the salient issues discussed in the focus group, and how did members discuss those issues?
- In what instances did members demonstrate conflict?
- What unforeseen individual characteristics both helped and hindered focus group interactions?
- How did members, overall, respond to each other?
- Were there times that particular members were silenced by others or perhaps presented issues?
- How could what appeared as "group consensus" really be group conformity?

OTHER DATA COLLECTION CONSIDERATIONS

While we have provided some general information about the structure, advantages and disadvantages, and strategies for conducting observations and interviews, there are several other data collection considerations. Here are just a few of the more salient ones; others are introduced throughout the remainder of the text.

Recording Interview Data

Individual and focus group interviews can be recorded in many ways. The most common way to record individual and focus group data is to use a digital audio recorder, although video recording, typing, or handwriting verbatim or abbreviated interview responses can also be used. If you are using a recorder, be sure to bring extra batteries. We like to use two recorders during each data collection, just in case one does not operate correctly at the last minute.

Audio and video recorders tend to make participants nervous, so take this factor into account before beginning an interview. We suggest turning the recorder on about

5–10 minutes before beginning an interview. Eventually, most participants get used to having the recorder present and interact more naturally with the researcher.

Managing the Data, Initially

While we discuss many other data management tools in Chapter 10, it is important to note here that contact summary sheets are essential tools in data collection because they need to be filled out shortly after each data collection. A **contact summary sheet** is usually a cover sheet summarizing a single contact with a case. For each interview or observation that occurs in fieldwork, a contact sheet helps qualitative researchers capture their own reflections about the data, outline initial salient themes based on the interview process, and jot down additional questions to be asked of a participant or setting. Contact summary sheets serve as the first steps to qualitative data analysis, discussed in Chapters 10 and 11. Contact summary sheets should be completed within a couple of days following the data collection to best capture a researcher's impressions.

Miles and Huberman (1994) identified several areas that should be covered in a contact sheet:

- Identifying information about the contact (e.g., date, setting, method of contact, who or what was the subject of the contact, when the contact was made, when was contact summary sheet completed);
- Important issues and themes of the data collection;
- Individuals, events, settings, and processes involved in this contact;
- Brief responses to interview questions;
- Observation rubrics; and
- New or additional questions to be considered for the next contact.

While we provide one example of a contact summary sheet (see Figure 8.5 on the next page), we encourage you to review Miles and Huberman for additional formats.

Transcribing Interview Data

Transcripts, the typed responses of recorded interview data, are the main interview data sources. They are used not only as physical evidence of collected data but also as important data management and analysis tools. Transcribing is quite time-consuming; we have found that for every 15 minutes of recorded data, we spend about an hour transcribing the data.

We believe strongly that interview data should be transcribed verbatim as relevant. At times, it may be more convenient to save time by transcribing only interviewee responses to interview questions. However, a "good" interviewer is likely to have allowed participants to expand on the research questions, empowering them to speak freely and honestly. Thus, there may be invaluable nonverbal or extra data that become important in data analysis. Responses such as "okay," "yeah," "um," and "ah" may provide insightful information about the conversational content and flow. Whether you transcribe verbatim or not, it is important to reflect on how you transcribe. The amount of

---

Contact Summary Sheet

Interviewer: SC   Interviewee: T007

Contact Date: 1/15/09   Today's Date: 1/16/09

1. **What were the main issues or themes that stuck out for you in this contact?**
   - Good communication, respect, and valuing each other are components of healthy relationships. Control, power struggles, secrets, and dishonesty are components of an unhealthy relationship.
   - Seemed to have difficulty conceptualizing what types of clients would be easier to work with, but immediately knew types of clients that she would not have trouble working with.
   - Bases knowledge of unhealthy/healthy relationships and relationship violence on her own personal experiences with it (i.e., her relationships and her daughters').
   - A lot of anger against clients who are violent in relationships (i.e., abhors violence and those kinds of people).
   - Had difficulty expressing how to work with a client involved in a violent relationship.
   - What seemed to be most important in working with individuals in unhealthy relationships was the processing of her own baggage related to her own personal experiences in unhealthy relationships.
   - Took a course in couples counseling during master's program.
   - Felt that practical experience was the most valuable in learning how to work with clients who have relationship issues.

2. **What discrepancies, if any, did you note in the interviewee's responses?**
   - Knew how she would respond to those involved in violent relationships, but really unsure about her strengths for helping them. Seemed to indicate low self-efficacy rather than a lack of knowledge.

3. **Anything else that stuck out as salient, interesting, or important in this contact?**
   - Physical violence not mentioned in interview when discussing relationship violence and unhealthy relationships.
   - Focus on emotional/psychological pieces of violent relationships (i.e., anger, loss of control, lowered self-esteem), but not on the physical aspects of it.
   - Personal experiences, unresolved personal issues with relationship violence were seen as the main challenge to working with individuals in violent relationships.

4. **How does this compare to other data collections?**
   - Not applicable. This was my first data collection for this study.

FIGURE 8.5. Contact summary sheet example. The figure represents a contact summary sheet for an individual interview from a study examining counselors' and counselor trainees' understanding of healthy relationships.

detail of a transcription can be a result of your personal preferences, time and other constraints, or the research question(s).

Reviewing a transcript, you might take the written record at face value, as an accurate representation of the interactions of an audio or video recording. However, the qualitative researcher plays a large role in determining the rigor of the transcript and "makes choices about whether to transcribe, what to transcribe, and how to represent the record in text" (Lapadat & Lindsay, 1999, p. 66). Poland (1995) added that the quality of transcripts may be adversely affected by researcher alterations and other decisions, whether intentional or not. Thus, the final transcript is far from a neutral,

---

TABLE 8.6. Considerations in Data Transcription

- Should data be audio- or video-recorded, or both?
- What are the boundaries of the recording (e.g., start–stop time, duration)?
- How are data to be formatted on the page, and how might this format impact data analysis?
- How does the researcher negotiate the demands to present a succinct yet thick description of text?
- To what extent are verbal cues, pitch, volume, utterances, pacing of speech, length of silence, and intonation included in the record?
- To what extent are nonverbal cues, such as facial expressions, eye contact, and body movements, integrated into the transcript?
- Do language variations impact how data are recorded and interpreted?
- How does the audience type impact what gets included in the transcript?
- How might the conceptual framework and/or paradigm influence the final transcript?

Sources: Kvale and Brinkmann (2009) and Lapadat and Lindsay (1999).

---

comprehensive, and directly transferable indicator or what occurred in data collection. Unfortunately, the literature provides little direction on the transcription process. Lapadat and Lindsay (1999) and Kvale and Brinkmann (2009) noted many decisions that must be made during the transcription process (see Table 8.6).

Although there are a host of considerations related to transcribing data, we would like to focus on a few in Table 8.6 that we believe significantly impact data analysis. The first consideration relates to sentence content (e.g., problems with sentence structure, the use of quotation marks, omissions, and confusing phrases or words for others; Poland, 1995). Because people speak in run-on sentences or fragments, it is important that transcribers attend to where they place punctuation marks such as commas or periods because doing so can easily change the meaning of responses (DiCicco-Bloom & Crabtree, 2006). Additionally, information is sometimes altered intentionally or unintentionally: A certain amount is lost when transferring audio or video to written recordings (Poland, 1995). Poland provides examples of sentence content issues:

- *Sentence structure.* A period or comma is inserted in the wrong place and changes the sentence meaning: "I hate it, you know. I do" versus "I hate it. You know I do."

- *Use of quotation marks.* The transcriber fails to identify when an interviewee is quoting, mimicking, or paraphrasing someone else: "She was 'mortified' about the way teachers were 'fired'" versus "She was mortified about the way teachers were let go."

- *Omissions.* A transcriber wants to "tidy up" a transcript and leaves out several meaningful utterances and side conversations, or mistakenly leaves out a word ("I lost a very close friend of mine to cancer" instead of "I lost a very close friend of mine to lung cancer" in a transcript for a smoking cessation study).

- *Confusing words or phrases for others.* A digital recording is unclear: *Consultation* gets transcribed as *confrontation*.

Second, involuntary utterances—coughs, cries, laughs, and sneezes—can be meaningful or misleading, and your decision to include them needs to take into account how readers of the transcript will make sense of them in conjunction with the research question(s). When I (Hays) was interviewing individuals about university climate around multicultural issues, there were times where it was very relevant to note when participants laughed, as often the laugh indicated sarcasm or discomfort with an interview question.

Third, participant language is an important issue, particularly use of slang, accent considerations, and diction. How do you ensure that the meaning of slang words or euphemisms is properly conveyed to the reader? Should words (particularly when English is not the primary language) be transcribed as spoken, or should you "translate" them for the reader? What do you transcribe when words are mispronounced? How do you deal with grammatical errors for yourself and the participant? A related issue is how translation of text from non-native speakers impacts data management and interpretation. In some cases direct translation is not possible because words have different meanings in various contexts, or simply there are no direct translations. Qualitative researchers are encouraged to carefully consider how translation might impact their and audience data interpretation.

Even if you have the budget to hire a transcriptionist, we *adamantly* believe you should transcribe your own interviews. Since you conducted the interviews, you can include nonverbal aspects of the interview process that no transcriptionist can. Additionally, in cases where there is more than one interviewee (i.e., focus group interviews), you are likely able to identify "who said what," potentially enriching data analysis. If you have to hire a transcriptionist, we encourage you to work closely with him or her to ensure the accuracy and thoroughness of the transcript. It is important to review the transcript immediately to add pertinent information (e.g., nonverbal communication such as fidgeting, pointing, and hand gestures) or correct any misplaced punctuation or missed utterances (e.g., sighs, laughter, voice inflections). Table 8.7 provides some common transcription instructions (Poland, 1995) you may find useful as you transcribe data. Additionally, in Figure 8.6 on page 262 we present more pointers for formatting the transcript page.

Member Checking, Revisited

The concept of member checking was introduced in Chapter 7 as a strategy for maximizing trustworthiness. Regarding interview data, it can be done within the interview itself, after the recorded data have been transcribed, or after the transcripts have been analyzed. Use of probes, such as "Can you give me an example?", "Let me make sure I am clear on what you mean," and "Can you elaborate on that?" can be used for member checking within the interview. Furthermore, additional interviews with the same participant or participants can be scheduled to follow up on initial review of the first interviews after data have been analyzed.

If you would like to do member checking using transcripts, we have a few recommendations. First, have the participant review the transcript for accuracy. Encourage him or her to make corrections directly to the transcript. Second, request that the participant make notes to expand on any responses he or she would like to say more

TABLE 8.7. Transcriber Instructions

Pauses	Denote short phrases during talking by a series of dots (…). Denote pauses by the word *pause* in parentheses (pause) for 2- to 3-second breaks and "(long pause)" for pauses longer than 4 seconds.
Laughing	Indicate in parentheses: (laughing) or (laughter).
Coughing, etc.	Indicate in parentheses: (coughs), (sighs), or (sneezes), for example.
Interruptions	Use a hyphen (-) to show when someone's speech is broken midsentence (e.g., "What do you -").
Overlapping speech	Use a hyphen (-) to indicate when someone interrupts one speaker, include the speech of the other with "overlapping" in parentheses, then return to the original speaker: R: He said it was impos- I: (overlapping) Who, Bob? R: No, Larry.
Garbled speech	Flag unclear words with square brackets and a question mark. For example, "At that, Harry just [doubled? glossed?] over." Use *x* to denote undecipherable passages, with the number of *x*'s denoting the approximate unclear words. For example, "Gina went xxxxx xxxxx xxxxx xxxxx and then [came? went?] home."
Emphasis	Use caps to denote strong emphasis: "He did WHAT?"
Held sounds	Repeat the sounds that are held, separated by hyphens. If they are emphasized, then capitalize as well: "No-o-o-o, not exactly," or "I was VER-r-r-y-y-y happy."
Paraphrasing others	When it is assumed that an interviewee is parodying what someone else said or an inner voice in his or her head, use quotation marks and/or indicate mimicking voice. For example, R: Then you know what he came out with? He said (mimicking voice) "I'll be damned if I'm going to let YOU push ME around." And I thought to myself: "I'll show you."

Source: Poland (1995).

about in the existing transcript. For example, I (Hays) like to send the transcript to participants electronically and have them add comments directly onto the transcript in a different color. This makes for nice evidence during the auditing process. Finally, we engage in a conversation with participants about any problems they see with the interview or limitations to the interview process.

With respect to focus group interview transcripts specifically, Brotherson (1994) suggested selecting participants to review transcripts and respond to the following questions:

- Does the transcript represent accurately what transpired in the focus group?
- Are there any biases you note that the facilitators may have had in initial interpretation of data?
- Do you have any additional comments on the focus group process or content?

1   **Participant P001 Interview 1, Duration 34:20 minutes (1.18.09,**
2   **Transcribed by DGH)**
3
4   **DGH: Thank you for agreeing to participate in this study. As a**
5   **practitioner your responses will be helpful in training others**
6   **about working with those having relationship difficulties. So,**
7   **you know we are doing this relationship seminar. But before we talk**
8   **about relationship stuff, can you talk a little bit about your training?**
9
10 PA: Do you mean academically or could be professional training in
11 the community?
12
13 **DGH: Anything.**
14
15 PA: When I first started working with trauma and domestic violence,
16 and that's where I started right after graduation, I went through a
17 domestic violence training. They called it an institute but it was kind
18 of like a conference where we had 4–5 days of training with police
19 officers, it was with the Commonwealth's attorney...
20
21 **DGH: So it was all for these different disciplines?**
22
23 PA: Just different types of providers, right. It was open to anyone,
24 and I think it was at [university name]. It was really good. We got
25 a lot of different area's input. Dispatchers came and talked. I wouldn't
26 say it really taught us how to do things, but it made us more aware
27 of what was out there and systems we could use. I would say the
28 most training I got was I was on the Domestic Violence task force in
29 [Virginia city] and there was a lady there [female's name] just gave us
30 a lot of hands-on ... she was just like the domestic violence diva in
31 [Virginia city].
32
33 **DGH: So what was the task force for?**
34
35 PA: To change laws, to help the people. She was all about
36 education of police officers and working with the shelters.
37 She was really a real activist.
38
39 **DGH: And how long did you do that for?**
40
41 PA: I was on that team for about a year and a half, and
42 then I moved to juvenile detention and shifted my focus to juvenile
43 offenders.

On the first couple of lines, include information about who was interviewed (using codes), who interviewed and transcribed the data, and duration of the interview.

We like to use *PA* to represent the participant in individual interviews, with PA1, PA2, and so forth used in focus group interviews (when the transcriber can identify individuals).

Create ample margins for later data analysis. We usually leave at least 1.5-inch margins for memoing.

Include line numbers (continuous) on your document to make referencing easier during data analysis.

FIGURE 8.6. Excerpt from an interview transcript.

TRIANGULATING INDIVIDUAL AND FOCUS GROUP INTERVIEW DATA

Although we discuss triangulation of data collection methods more extensively in the next chapter, here we highlight integrating the findings of individual and focus group interviews because it is a common practice among practitioners of a variety of disciplines. There are several advantages to integrating individual and focus group interviews. First, individual interviews may offer an outlet for those who cannot or will not participate in focus group interviews (Lambert & Loiselle, 2008). However, qualitative researchers need to attend to whether there are systematic differences among those who select particular interviewing formats over others. Second, individual and focus group interviews may occur concurrently in qualitative inquiry to explore a phenomenon of interest using two varying sets of individuals. Third, one form of interviewing can occur after another form to compare and confirm findings.

However, some qualitative researchers may be making a large, easily contended, assumption: Interview data can translate across methods. When we combine interview methods, we should respect that they are very different and that the type of information obtained about a phenomenon is influenced by the method.

Can individual and focus group interviews *really* triangulate one another? We believe that the integration of individual and focus group interview data creates a more comprehensive picture of a phenomenon by searching for consistencies and inconsistencies in data across methods while actively analyzing how these methods present a quite different picture of a phenomenon. We agree, however, that "it may be challenging to determine if disparate views are expressed because different sources of data are used or because different methods are implemented" (Lambert & Loiselle, 2008, p. 230).

CHAPTER SUMMARY

In this chapter we provided information about primary data collection methods (which are often used together in qualitative inquiry): observations, individual interviews, and focus group interviews. We presented information about their format and characteristics and gave strategies to maximize success using each method. In deciding which methods are appropriate, qualitative researchers should consider which are most congruent with their research questions.

Observations are at the core of fieldwork in qualitative inquiry. Degree of researcher participation falls along a continuum: acting as an observer, observer as participant, participant as observer, and full participant. No matter your degree of participation as a researcher, creating a thick description of the setting (field notes) is important, as are the strategies we provided for doing so.

Individual interviews are the most common data collection method in qualitative research. There are three types of interviews—structured, semistructured, and unstructured—with unstructured interviews being the most commonly used. We also outlined various types of questions to include in your protocol, as well as strategies for conducting a "good interview." It is important to remember, however, that the questions in your interview protocol will be guided by your research tradition(s).

Focus group interviews are unique in that they highlight data from participants' interactions, something that cannot be captured by individual interviews. This chapter presents several advantages and disadvantages to focus group interviews, as well as discusses the unique considerations when integrating individual and focus group interview data.

Finally, additional considerations are discussed, including the recording of interviewing data, managing data using contact summary sheets, and conducting member checking.

RECOMMENDED READINGS

Berg, B. L. (2004). *Qualitative research methods for the social sciences* (5th ed.). Boston: Allyn & Bacon.

Emerson, R. M., Fretz, R. I., & Shaw, L. L. (1995). *Writing ethnographic fieldnotes.* Chicago: University of Chicago Press.

Kress, V. E., & Shoffner, M. F. (2007). Focus groups: A practical and applied research approach for counselors. *Journal of Counseling and Development, 85,* 189–195.

Siedman, I. (2006). *Interviewing as qualitative research: A guide for researchers in education and the social sciences* (3rd ed.). New York: Teachers College Press.

CHAPTER 9

Data Collection Using the Internet, Documents, or Arts-Based Methods

CHAPTER PREVIEW

In the last chapter we discussed observation, interviewing, and focus group data collection methods for qualitative research. However, often in clinical and educational research, your topic demands that you supplement traditional qualitative data collection methods (i.e., observations and interviews) with data from various media, including the Internet, photography, art, and written materials. In addition to discussing these methods, we review methods of using personal and public documents and archival data. Throughout the chapter we discuss the benefits and challenges of using each of these data collection methods.

GENERAL REMINDERS
ABOUT SELECTING DATA COLLECTION METHOD(S)

Before we dive into our discussion, we want to review a few guidelines we noted about selecting data collection method(s). We discuss many innovative, challenging, and creative ways to collect data in this chapter. You may feel tempted to incorporate some of these methods because they would seem "fun" or "cool" for you to do as a researcher. We urge you to be very cautious about heading down that road. Your main guideline in selecting data collection methods is to be able to understand your phenomenon of inquiry as fully as you can, guided by your research tradition and conceptual framework. Therefore, using photography, for instance, might seem like a great way to collect data from children. However, is it really the *best* way to understand your phenomenon? You can also create accountability for yourself in selecting data collection methods by asking, for example, "Would there be better data collection methods for me to use than photography in answering my research question?" As you read about the additional data collection methods in this chapter, keep in mind these types of questions as you make (or have made) decisions about the best data collection methods for your study.

MEDIA AS METHOD AND SOURCE OF DATA COLLECTION

When selecting a qualitative approach to study a particular phenomenon, the researcher is already working with an assumption that the data necessary to understand the study's focus cannot be necessarily quantified. In a similar way, there may be research topics in clinical and educational settings that do not lend themselves easily (or *only*) to one of the data collection methods discussed in Chapter 8. For instance, if you are seeking to understand how the trauma experiences of elementary school–age children affect their peer relationships, you might select participant observation as a method to collect data on peer interactions. However, because the literature on assessment of children's experiences of trauma often uses art as a way to understand these experiences, you may elect to supplement your participant observations with an art data collection method. In cases such as this, the researcher has the opportunity to examine how media can provide ways to more fully capture data about a phenomenon. Media are both a method and a source of data collection. We describe various types (or data sources) of media below: the Internet, photography and film, art and music, and written materials. We also discuss some of the ethical considerations that are inherent in using some forms of media (such as the Internet) as a method and data source.

USING THE INTERNET FOR DATA COLLECTION

The wide reach of the Internet has increased accessibility to information and knowledge to people around the world, and it has also provided immense opportunities and challenges for qualitative researchers. Cyberspace has "expanded the social researcher's toolkit" (Hookway, 2008, p. 91) and is increasingly used as a data collection source and method in qualitative research. From participant recruitment and e-mail interviews to using chat rooms as focus groups, there are many ways in which qualitative researchers can use the Internet to their studies' advantage. The opportunities include reaching individuals and groups who are historically marginalized and/or are difficult to access (Eagan, Chenoweth, & McAuliffe, 2006). For instance, see Perspectives 9.1 to read first-person accounts of reaching these types of groups.

• •

Perspectives 9.1. Researchers' Perspectives on Using the Internet for Data Collection

"I have used the Internet for qualitative research—specifically using it to conduct interviews online via Instant Messenger for a study examining online experiences of men who have sex with men. I used America Online because at the time I could create a profile. I would go into a chat room and people could look at my profile there. There was a link to my informed consent on the profile. I interviewed the participants using Instant Messenger technology. Basically, I cut and pasted the interview questions I had from a previously prepared word-processing document into the Instant Messenger 'window.' There were some technological problems because sometimes I would get disconnected from the Instant Messaging technology while I was interviewing a participant, and it could be really hard to find that person again to complete the interview. Some participants I interviewed were pretty

skeptical about whether I was for 'real' as a researcher conducting a qualitative study online. Some folks were skeptical and were afraid I was from an evangelical Christian perspective and would try to 'convert' them. One person called the IRB to complain that I was in a chat room invading his privacy—nothing came of that because I had previous IRB approval. Because I was online, there was no way for me as well to confirm that the participants were really who they said they were. I could have been interviewing someone underage or someone who wasn't the sex or gender he or she had said. On the other hand, because of the participants' anonymity, they were definitely more open with what they shared with me. A lot of people were excited about the topic I was studying. It was also pretty easy to recruit participants because I could just go online and find them. I didn't have to go into the community to find participants—they were readily available online. And I was able to get a diverse participant pool. I am proud of this study because I did it as a predissertation study as a graduate student in 2003. At that time, there were no studies out there talking about doing qualitative interviews online."

—MICHAEL CHANEY, PhD

"My field is applied linguistics and teacher education. I have become interested in practice-oriented research using the Internet due to some of my teaching experiences online. I am using WebCT Blackboard to put my entire course online. The students in my course are located all around the world. So, it is a live classroom where I can actually talk and type with students in a live session. I upload my presentation and ruminations, and students interact with one another in chat rooms to discuss class materials. The one assignment that I have them do is to read a nontheoretical book with three to four options. I set up literature circles where students meet together and talk about their book. In the past, I have only done that in WebCT Blackboard. I find this platform clumsy—and group work is somewhat clumsy for student–student interactions. There are some technical glitches, and students don't have as much group interaction. Now, I am experimenting with a Wiki classroom, and the student feedback I am getting is that it is superior to using Blackboard to facilitate group work. I am just now starting to collect data on this first group of 25 students. I am also interested in conducting qualitative interviews online on the topic of professional identity development—but doing this with people who live in France, China, and around the world. The Internet makes this type of interviewing more possible than ever before. The trick is that I am in linguistics, so I won't be able to 'see' their nonverbals as well—even if I am using a web camera. So, I as I design this study, I will need to account for how this might shape data collection and interpretation."

—KATHERINE KISS, PhD

"I have supervised student research using e-mail interviewing, but I think chat rooms can be better because you can have synchronous interactions. One study examined the experiences of classroom interactions of Chinese immigrant students in the United States—specifically, what types of contextual factors may be inhibiting their talking in class. A huge advantage of these chat rooms is that when you are working with participants for whom English is a second language, there is less pressure for the researcher and participants to reflect because you can pause the interaction in a chat room. It doesn't have to be rapid-fire questions and answers, which can help people feel less pressured. The other big advantage is that is there is no transcription—it's done when you are done with the interview! However, I also know that I get a lot out of doing the transcription. So, I am interested in what a researcher might lose in not doing a transcription. E-mail interviewing in that manner might be more analogous to having someone else do your transcript. You will have to reread it to get that sense of prolonged immersion in the data. The other disadvantage is you don't have body language

and intonation of participants, so you lose what you might have picked up with your other senses. One of the things I would encourage researchers to talk to participants about when collecting data online is to not worry about the spelling when they are communicating. A lot of participants will worry about that—so I tell them, don't let that impede what it is you are thinking—that's what spell check is for! One other thing is in using these types of technologies, it is important to find a technology that the participants feel comfortable with; it's best not to impose a technology on participants because it can create more anxiety for them. And don't just think about Internet technology as an age-related thing—big mistake! Using the Internet to collect data is a comfort thing for participants. For instance, there are probably some 19- to 20-year-olds who haven't used all the features of Skype because they are texting and Facebooking more; yet there may be lots of 40- to 60-year-old professionals who use Skype quite a bit. Use caution in the stereotypes you might have about using technology in your data collection—you might think that the younger your participants are, the more they will know how to use it—not true!"

—JANETTE HILL, PhD

• •

The immense opportunities the Internet provides for qualitative researchers in terms of participant recruitment and data collection should not be the only factors guiding your use of it in your study (Hamilton & Bowers, 2006). You must carefully consider the potential challenges of using the Internet as a method for, and source of, data collection—for there can be many. One challenge is the sheer numbers of people who use the Internet. Over 1.9 billion people, or 29% of the world's population, have access to the World Wide Web (Internet World Stats, 2010). As a researcher in cyberspace, you must continue to attend to the same critical issues of purposive and criterion sampling that you would use offline to describe your sampling method (James, 2007). How will you, as a researcher, ensure confidentiality of participants? What are the ethical considerations of engaging in your research topic online? How will you address the unique—and possibly unexpected—issues involved with research online?

If you are collecting data online, you should have a plan to address two major issues. First, you may encounter questions regarding the degree of honesty from online participants. Second, there will be issues of anonymity to address. Hookway (2008) uses Goffman's (1972) conceptualization of "face-work" to address these issues online. Goffman discussed face-work as a way to present a more socially desirable view of oneself; Hookway proposes a parallel "online mask." However, he also diverges from Goffman's notions of face-work when situated online, saying that the anonymity that online interactions provide actually assist people in "writing more honestly and candidly, mitigating potential impression management ... since they remain hidden from view" (p. 96). We believe it is important to acknowledge and address how face-work may influence your study's participants. For instance, you as a researcher may not be able to "control" the degree of honesty of your participants online. However, can we as researchers ever guarantee this in offline data collection? Additionally, if participants are potentially dishonest, how might this possibility contribute to the aim and understanding of your study? How might the Internet influence your participants' construction of self? Address these questions of face-work "head-on" (pun intended!) and you will strengthen the rationale for using the Internet for your study. Use the questions listed in Activity 9.1 to explore how using the Internet for data collection may be beneficial for your study.

ACTIVITY 9.1. Accessing the Internet for Your Study

Reflect on the following in your research teams:

- How could the Internet be used in your study?
- Would the Internet increase the availability of participants who have experienced the phenomenon you are studying?
- Are there challenges and/or benefits to participant confidentiality if you integrate the Internet into your study's design?
- Would the benefits of using the Internet for data collection outweigh the challenges?
- How will using the Internet to collect data influence researcher bias?

- If you use the Internet, how will you address "face-work" of participants?
- Are there any ethical issues that would encourage you to use the Internet or preclude you from using the Internet for data collection?
- If you have already used the Internet for data collection, how might your discussion within your research team guide you to revisit and refine your data collection methods?

Use the answers to these questions to identify how you will or will not use the Internet for collecting data.

Participant Recruitment Online

Imagine that you are considering conducting a PAR study on the effects of immigration policy on education access for Latin American students. As you think about participant selection and sampling concerns, you note one large barrier: You don't live in an area with a predominantly Latin American population, and you would like to obtain thick description from key informants in a more populated area. You locate various interest groups and chat rooms online, developed by policymakers, parents, students, and school personnel, to name a few. There are so many weblinks and so many questions as to where to start.

If going online for participants makes you nervous, we see this as a natural reaction. It is good to remember, however, that "qualitative researchers can apply long-standing principles of recruitment and interviewing to this new setting" (Hamilton & Bowers, 2006, p. 821). There are two criterion Hamilton and Bowers (2006) identify that should guide online participant recruitment. The first criterion, *appropriateness*, refers to how the researcher will select participants who have experience of the phenomenon to be studied. The appropriateness of a study's participant pool can be exponentially increased only when there is a large pool of potential participants online, which then increases the selection of the most appropriate participants for a study's focus. The second criterion, *adequacy*, is a common issue discussed in offline qualitative data collection. How will the online researcher determine that the number of participants is sufficient for the data the researcher hopes to collect?

Using the concepts of appropriateness and adequacy reminds the researcher using online data collection methods that the general guidelines of good qualitative scholarship still apply in cyberspace and should be guided by the researcher's selection of theoretical and methodological research traditions. For instance, an ethnographer using an online data collection component would determine the appropriateness and adequacy of participant recruitment much differently from a researcher using a grounded theory or phenomenological research tradition. The following sections explore the practical side of using data collection methods online.

E-mail Interviewing

E-mail has become a "given" for our everyday lives. It tends to be fast, reliable, and quick. These strengths of e-mail communication simultaneously become the challenges of conducting e-mail interviews with participants. Although the responses from participants can be quick, the researcher must have a structured, preplanned way to manage the incoming online data. What is the time frame for your data collection? How will you most effectively help participants understand the purpose of the e-mail interview and the topic of your research? What if using e-mail interviewing as a method of data collection "sounds" great, but the data you end up collecting from this source are not of sufficient quality, information, and/or detail?

If you are using e-mail interviews, think carefully about the type of questions you are asking. They should not be "yes–no" questions that will yield an abbreviated response from participants if you intend to collect rich, in-depth participant responses (Hamilton & Bowers, 2006). Rather, use open-ended questions that have primary and secondary probes. We advise doing a pilot of your e-mail interview to work out any potential kinks in your protocol that you may not be able to identify from your researcher perspective.

Other practical concerns with e-mail interviewing involve the time frame you give to participants to respond. What "makes sense" for your study, based on your research tradition? If you are conducting a phenomenology study, seeking to understand the lived experiences of Latina high school girls in after-school programs, the depth of a phenomenological design might guide you to use three e-mail interviews based on Siedman's (2006) phenomenological interviewing protocol discussed in Chapter 8. E-mail interviews within a case study research design that examines how a specific school addresses gay bullying with its students may have one e-mail interview protocol for students using their school e-mail address and have another e-mail interview protocol to determine school personnel responses to the gay bullying when it occurs.

One of the real advantages of e-mail interviewing is that it may be an inexpensive way to reach many people, rather than using the traditional audio-recorded interview. E-mail interviews can also be more convenient and comfortable for participants because they can respond in a time frame that works for them and in an environment that may be less anxiety-producing than a face-to-face interview (Eagan et al., 2006). Because e-mail interviews are essentially immediately available participant transcripts, they can be less cumbersome for researchers; they can also increase accuracy of participant sharing *and* increase the involvement of participants in the interpretation of data (Hamilton & Bowers, 2006). See Table 9.1 for an example of an e-mail interview protocol and instructions for participants used by an ethnographic study in examining how senior academics constructed their academic identities in various community settings (James, 2003). Pay particular attention to the level of detail within the researcher's writing in order to clearly communicate with his participants. This clear communication in writing is a key to successful e-mail interviewing.

TABLE 9.1. Sample E-mail Interview Questions and Instructions for Participants

Ethnography	Excerpts from James (2003)
E-mail interview questions	"How have your experiences shaped your professional identity? What images would you use to describe your professional identity? In what way has your professional identity been shaped by formative experiences? In what way is your professional identity shaped across communities of practice?" (p. 967)
E-mail interview instructions for participants	"A little while ago you completed a questionnaire, which considered professional identity and how it is managed across communities. You agreed to take part in an email interview, which will address the issues raised in that questionnaire. Please read the following guidelines and if you are still happy to take part in the interview, please reply to this email and I shall send you the first question. The email interviews will consider the issues that arose in the questionnaire in more depth. The data gathered through the email interviews will provide a narrative of your account. These accounts will be used to inform the research study. In undertaking the email interview please note the following guidelines:

1. If you are still willing to take part in this study, please reply to this email straightaway.
2. The interviews will be conducted in strictest confidence and your anonymity will be assured throughout the research project.
3. You will be asked eleven substantive questions.
4. These questions will be sent to you one at a time. Please respond to the question by email. Each question may be followed up by supplementary questions.
5. It is anticipated that an ongoing dialogue will occur. In order to achieve this, please ensure that you answer on top of the message question sent to you. PLEASE DO NOT ANSWER AT THE BOTTOM OF IT. This will be our record of the conversation.
6. Please reply to each email question within three working days if possible. I will also try to reply to your response within that timescale.
7. It is anticipated that the email dialogue will be completed within ten weeks.
8. Once the dialogue is complete you will be given an opportunity to take part in another email discussion." (p. 976)

Using Blogs and Vlogs

One of the most readily available sources of data collection on the Internet is in the exponentially increasing number of blogs and vlogs (VanDorn, Van Zoonen, & Wyatt, 2008). A **blog** (or weblog) is a type of journal that is either publicly or privately written online (Ellison & Wu, 2004). A **vlog** is the next generation of blogs (Runte, 2008) that uses video to integrate the diary-like component of blogs—and is also either in the public or private Internet domain. Of vlogs, Runte (2008) notes that vloggers "are constantly making the conscious choice to 'roll tape' as they move through the environments and events of their lives, they are essentially engaged in interpreting their lives through the lens of their camcorders" (p. 315). Because there are few studies using vlogs currently, we focus our discussion on blogs and encourage the reader to apply the principles discussed to vlog data collection.

Like e-mail interviewing, blogs leverage the inexpensive, publicly available, and unobtrusive aspects of data collection. Without the boundaries—and potential barriers—of digital or tape recorders and face-to-face interviews, blogs truly are "naturalistic data in textual form" (Hookway, 2008, p. 92). In this manner, blogs provide a "peek" into the very private lives of participants, which happens to be communicated in a very public way. Because blogs are increasingly popular for individuals and groups as a way to communicate with others, there is a huge variety of them.

A first step for a researcher who is considering using blogs for data collection is to consider whether he or she wants to sample existing participant blogs and/or ask participants to blog about a certain topic. Ellison and Wu (2008) integrated blogging into educational learning in the classroom and qualitatively examined students' perceptions of blogs as useful for learning. They drew on existing literature on educational learning—such as Gill's (2006) considerations when determining effectiveness of online communications technology in the classroom. These considerations included the degree of voluntary participation and satisfaction of students, in addition to the assessment of the educational outcomes and objectives met. Using these criteria to guide their examination of students blogging in the classroom, Ellison and Wu's findings were many. Among these findings were that students viewed working on blogs "less seriously" than writing traditional papers. Ethical questions were also raised—such as the degree to which students would have anonymity on their blogs in the future. A sample of how the authors encouraged the use of pseudonyms is included in Table 9.2.

Hookway (2008) suggests that it is best to establish a "road map" when using blogs to collect qualitative data. This road map has four quadrants. The first quadrant is to identify how to find blogs. He lists many different blog content management systems (BCMSs), such as Blogster, LiveJournal, Xanga, and Blogger. The second quadrant involves actually sampling the identified blogs. For instance, researchers may be interested in bloggers with certain demographic characteristics—say, African American men living with depression or college students living away from home for the first time. The type of search engine on the blog may lead a researcher to select or avoid a certain BCMS because that particular search engine may or may not allow the researcher to locate the participant samples needed for their study.

The third quadrant of the road map is to establish a researcher presence online. This may entail initiating a blog account, which then facilitates researcher entry and allows for participant sampling and data collection. The fourth and final quadrant in the road map of blog data collection involves the actual data collection, which Hookway (2008) divided into two phases for his qualitative study on morality. In the first phase, he

---

TABLE 9.2. Ethical Considerations: Encouraging the Use of Pseudonyms in Blogging

"For this class, you will be asked to create a blog and to post some of your written work online. If you wish, you may create a blog that uses a pseudonym (a made-up name), or you may use your real name if you wish. This decision is yours and will have absolutely no bearing on your grade. . . . Keep in mind that blogs are a 'public space.' This means that anyone in the world—including future employers, future close friends, family, etc.—can and may have access to your individual writings. You should monitor your own writings with this in mind."

Source: Ellison and Wu (2008, pp. 117–118).

passively reviewed various blogs for a sample purposively selected for his study. The second phase—which he experienced as much more useful than the first phase—included active solicitation of blogs from participants. In this phase he (1) posted a research request on a potential participant's blog, (2) responded to a participant's agreement to be in the study, and (3) was invited by the blogger to view the blog or was sent certain links to various sections of the participant's blog that were pertinent to the study's focus.

In another example of qualitative data collection using blogs, VanDorn and colleagues (2007) examined gender identity presentations on blogs. The authors found that the bloggers they sampled narrated their everyday experiences in blogs within the traditional gender binary of woman and man. However, they also discovered that the expression of femininity and masculinity was less aligned with the gender binary. In their final manuscript, the authors excerpted samples from the blogs that illustrated their findings.

Online Focus Groups, Discussion Boards, Chat Rooms, and Social Networking Sites

Just as blogs and vlogs are a naturally occurring source for online data collection, there are other groupings of individuals on the Internet that you may want to tap for your study. The groupings we discuss in this section are online focus groups, discussion boards, chat rooms, and social networking sites—all of which overlap with one another. Take a look at Figure 9.1 of a posting from the social networking site Facebook. What are your reactions to the contents of the questionnaire? How might this form of Internet media (social networking) be beneficial in a qualitative study? What might be some challenges of it to you as the researcher?

In Chapter 8 we discussed the benefits of integrating focus groups as a data collection method. Conducting focus groups online can address some of the challenges that exist in holding focus groups offline. The anonymity of online focus groups can increase trust and sharing of participants. Using the Internet to hold focus groups can also reach individuals who share a common experience of a phenomenon that might be rare and/or a difficult subject to discuss in a group of people. The use of an online focus group really has burgeoned over the last few years as a data collection method for social sciences research, but this format was actually a popular tool of marketing analysis long before academia utilized it (Stewart & Williams, 2005).

Researchers can artificially create **online focus groups**—similar to offline focus groups—wherein they recruit and organize an online meeting of several participants who share an experience of a phenomenon. An example would be a study investigating the coping resources of parents who have children with autism. In this example, a researcher might recruit participants through web postings and/or e-mail announcements to offline and online support groups that focus on this area. An advantage of online focus groups is that larger numbers of participants may be accommodated than their offline counterparts (LeBosco, 2004). Additionally, they may provide "more considered narratives, providing a depth that might be absent in uttered data" (Stewart & Williams, 2005, p. 413).

Once participants are contacted for the online focus group, the researcher can organize an Internet space such as a chat room in which to conduct the session. Chat

Here is an example of an "application" that was downloaded from Facebook by a teenager:

[x] Gotten detention. (Lunch detention . . . that's all)
[ ] Gotten suspended.
[x] Gotten caught chewing gum.
[x] Gotten caught cheating on a test.
[ ] Gotten phone taken away in class.

[ ] Arrived late to class more than 5 times.
[x] Didn't do homework over 5 times.
[ ] Turned in at least 3 projects late.
[x] Missed school 'cause you felt like it.
[ ] Laughed so loud you got kicked out of class.

[ ] Got your mom/dad, etc., to get you out of school.
[ ] Texted people during class.
[x] Passed notes.
[ ] Threw stuff across the room.
[x] Laughed at the teacher.

[ ] Pulled down the fire alarm.
[ ] Went on MySpace, Facebook, Xanga, etc., on the computer at school. (How do you do that?)
[x] Took pictures during school hours. (Photography class doesn't count.)
[x] Called someone during school hours.
[x] Listened to an IPod, CD, etc., during class.

[ ] Threw something at the teacher.
[ ] Went outside the classroom with permission.
[ ] Broke the dress code.
[ ] Failed a class.
[x] Ate food during class.

[x] Gotten a call from school.
[ ] Couldn't go on a field trip 'cause you behaved badly.
[x] Didn't take your stuff to school.
[ ] Gotten a detention and didn't go.
[ ] Stuck up your middle finger at a teacher when they weren't looking.
[x] Cursed in class loud enough so the teacher could hear.

[x] Faked your parent's signature.
[x] Slept in class.
[ ] Cursed at a teacher to their face.
[x] Copied homework.

TOTAL: 17

MULTIPLY THE TOTAL BY THREE: **17** $\times$ **3 = 51**

Tag 10 of your friends.

Then repost this and put the title as "I screwed up ____% of my teenage life."

FIGURE 9.1. Facebook questionnaire.

rooms are bound online spaces that are either preestablished by online users and Internet providers (Moloney, Dietrich, Strickland, & Myerburg, 2003) or that users spontaneously create as they interact with one another around a common topic. Online focus groups are most effective when the social group is naturally occurring on the Internet. In these cases, the researcher does not plan the online focus group in advance. An example is a discussion board, which is "an ongoing site participants are free to log on at any time, read others' postings, and post their own thoughts" (Moloney et al., p. 275). Discussion boards and chat rooms both provide the advantage of having ready-made transcripts, so there is an ease to data collection. Often, as you read in Perspectives 9.1, researchers just have to copy, cut, and paste participants' sharing into a word-processing document—rather than transcribing data—so it is ready for data interpretation.

A critical role to consider for the researcher is how to manage or "moderate" online discussions in focus group or chat room formats. The role of the moderator may range from being more active in an online setting where participant-to-participant interaction is slow moving to a more passive role where these interactions are happening spontaneously and quickly (Moloney et al., 2003). Another moderator role may be to actively respond to those who may be distrustful of the researcher's intention and/or of the purpose of the study. Because online spaces are often unmoderated, especially when a researcher is joining a ready-made online focus group, discussion board, or chat room, it is important to be prepared for those who feel that the presence of a researcher is an invasion of their "privacy" online. Another moderator role is being prepared to manage the technical challenges of conducting research online; Internet technology can fail or disconnect during important researcher–participant exchanges (Moloney et al., 2003). It can also be challenging to track the participants who are sharing in an online format due to large numbers of participants or use of participant pseudonyms that may be similar to one another or unfamiliar to the researcher. These challenges contribute to the overall disorientation researchers may feel when conducting online research (Hookway, 2008). However, as with the primary data collection methods reviewed in Chapter 8, researchers must weigh the pros and cons of using each approach. See Table 9.3 for a summary of the opportunities and challenge of online data collection methods discussed thus far. Also see Perspectives 9.2 for student researcher experiences in using instant messaging and social networking sites—both of which are the cutting edge of Internet data collection practices.

Ethical Considerations When Using Online Data Collection

In Table 9.3 we touch on the ethical considerations you want to consider when using online data collection. Additional ethical considerations can also be found in Chapter 3. The issue of informed consent is a serious one when collecting data online. As Mike Chaney shared in Perspectives 9.1, there was no way for him to verify his participants' identity online. However, it was still critical for him to seek informed consent and follow the rules of the IRB at his university. The way he addressed this issue was to have a link to his IRB approval, description of his study, and informed consent forms within the description of who he was on his instant messaging technology.

Mike's study examined the experiences of adults, but he also acknowledged that because he was not able to verify his participants' identities, he might have had some participants who were not over the age of 18 years old. The best way to address this

TABLE 9.3. Opportunities and Challenges of Online Data Collection Methods		
Data collection method	Opportunities	Challenges
E-mail interviewing (Hamilton & Bowers, 2006)	• Inexpensive • No transcription—cut and paste • Increased accuracy • Ability to follow up with participants • Increased ability to integrate participants in data analysis, member checking, etc. • Potentially fast data collection	• Participants' understanding of study may be limited • Developing questions that are open-ended • Ensuring participants give rich responses to questions • May feel cumbersome for participants • Being prepared to manage incoming data • Excludes those without access to Internet • Asynchronous data collection
Blogs and vlogs (Hookway, 2008)	• Available in public domain • No transcription—cut and paste • Naturalistic • Anonymous • Inexpensive • Global reach • Active or passive data collection	• Ethical considerations—use of pseudonyms, future access of public to blogs, etc. • Overwhelming to select blogs to sample • Establishing researcher presence online • Demographics of participants sometimes difficult to identify (e.g., geographical region)
Online focus groups, discussion boards, chat rooms, and social networking sites (Stewart & Williams, 2005)	• Potential anonymity • Inexpensive • Defined online spaces for data collection • Wide reach of participants experiencing a rare phenomenon • Increased depth of participant sharing • Ease of scheduling • Ready-made transcripts • Potentially synchronous data collection	• Defining group characteristics may not be useful for a study's focus • Fewer social cues among participant–participant and researcher–participant interactions • Ethical challenges • Participants may feel privacy is "invaded" • Technical glitches

uncertainty, in our experience, is to have a clearly worded statement about the age requirement in your informed consent forms and in your description of who you are. Boldface and highlight the font you use so that this information stands out. Also, before you conduct data collection with a particular participant, you should *ask again* about his or her age, explain the parameters of your informed consent forms, and specifically *ask again* if he or she understands the informed consent procedures. And, of course, if you are in the middle of data collection and your participant discloses that he or she is outside your age parameters, discontinue the interview in a way that is respectful and explain the age restrictions for your study to the participant. Always remember that even in online data collection, *you must obtain parental consent* (and we suggest, and most IRBs require, child/adolescent assent) for participating in your study.

Sometimes the issue of informed consent becomes even stickier, according to van Eeden-Moorefield, Proulx, and Pasley (2008). These authors acknowledge that the traditional, signed informed consent documents cannot be obtained by the online researcher. However, they summarize two common ways online researchers have secured

Perspectives 9.2. *Student Researchers and Online Data Collection*

"My dissertation study is about anime fans who role-play people from anime in online games—using Instant Messenger and LiveJournal as their platform for their role plays. Therefore, the data that I collected pertained to these platforms. I collected instant messaging logs of gameplay, as well as Live-Journal posts and unofficial LiveJournal interviews. I liked that this data collection was naturalistic, more or less—I was collecting data in the environment that I was studying, using their means for interaction in a natural way. It wasn't artificial, or imposing online methodology onto an offline study. I used a theoretical frame of pop culture studies out of the media field, and my methodology was case study with ethnographic data collection techniques. The only challenge was with my ability to keep up with it all! It was actually tremendously easy to collect data because it's all generated and stored electronically, so there's no need for in-person interviews, transcription, scheduling—just some asynchronous collection, and some synchronous data collection. It all flowed really well. For others doing an online ethnographic study, my main advice is 'know thy participants.' If they are night people, do not attempt to collect synchronous data in the morning! If they use certain kinds of messengers and bulletin boards/blogs—go to them. Do not make them step out of their comfort zones."

—ACHARIYA REZAK

"I used Myspace and Facebook to send messages to participants and ask follow-up questions from face-to-face interviews. I conducted a series of interviews on the perceptions of reading by struggling eighth-grade readers. During transcription, my research partner and I had some additional follow-up questions to ask some of the students. However, school was out and the students were very busy in their summer schedules. So I used Myspace and Facebook to connect with the students. I messaged the student with the questions and they responded, much like I am answering your questions through e-mail. Also, we were able to see how these students represented themselves on the social networking sites. The challenge was short answers. The students typed a short answer to most questions. When I asked for more, they wrote a little more. I know that they would have verbalized more if they had been sitting with me in an interview session, but didn't want to take the time to type it all out. The benefits were easy access. These students didn't drive and were scattered across the country due to summer break and traveling vacations, but they stay connected to their friends through social networking sites. I was able to connect with them wherever they were and ask our questions. It depends on the research questions and the participants. My participants were students who were labeled as struggling readers and writers by the school. This label may have played into their reluctance to write long answers. So my advice is, know your participants. I knew mine were on Facebook and Myspace, which allowed me to finish up a study, but I would rather have talked to them in person."

—EMILY PENDERGRASS

this consent. They first describe the method Mike Chaney shared in Perspectives 9.1, where potential participants are referred to a weblink with a description of the study where they can decide either to not participate or to engage in the chat room or other online forum where the data will be collected. Eeden-Moorefield and colleagues note that a disclaimer statement is included, which states that informed consent is given when the participant enters the chat room or other online data collection forum. Second, the authors discuss the approach of using e-mail to send potential participants a description of the study and a copy of the informed consent document. Informed consent is given via the participants' reply to the e-mail. We would just add to both of these common approaches that you can ask participants to cut and paste the informed consent in the window of the chat room to indicate their informed consent (with the first approach to obtaining informed consent) or ask them to e-mail you a copy of the informed consent with their electronic signature (with the second approach). Of course, with our latter approach, anonymity is lost, which might be a critical aspect of your study. Work closely with your IRB to establish the best informed consent procedures for your own online data collection, and definitely keep an eye on the literature regarding the ethics of online data collection. This is a rapidly growing body of literature with many helpful guidelines and thorny ethical issues addressed.

USING VISUAL METHODS FOR DATA COLLECTION

Whereas one of the disadvantages of using the Internet to collect data is that your study is limited to those with convenient and consistent Internet access through home or school computers, one of the advantages of using visual (i.e., arts-based) methods for data collection is that you, as a researcher, can literally put a tool of research in participants' hands. Visual methods, in general, provide participants with an opportunity to express themselves in a nonverbal manner that may access deeper aspects of their understanding and/or experience of a phenomenon. A main advantage of using visual methods as a data collection strategy is that they include a wide variety of data collection sources: photography, drawing and painting, film and video, sculpture, collage, murals, print making, craft making, mixed media, and multimedia. In this chapter we focus on visual arts-based media such as photography and drawing or painting.

Finley (2008) stated that visually based qualitative research can be transformative, can aim toward social justice goals, and can provide the flexibility necessary to work with diverse communities. She emphasized that these data collection methods can be complex and challenging to describe because of the many varied forms art can take: "Arts-based inquiry can explore multiple, new, and diverse ways of understanding and living in the world" (p. 71). Cole and Knowles (2008) assert that arts-based data collection methods can assist participants in translating the meaning and value of their experiences of a phenomenon into a visual format. In one of their studies that examined the life histories of teacher educators, the authors noticed that their participants tended to use metaphorical and pictorial language in describing their histories. This type of participant sharing inspired the use of art as a result of their research. Other times, arts-based methods are used to more powerfully communicate the narratives of participants. In a study of university graduates living with disabilities, Gillies (2007) used drawing and poetic strategies to portray her participants' transition to living in communities after university life. Because arts-based forms do disrupt traditional ways of communication (Cole & Knowles, 2008), it is important for researchers to find ways to "trust" the process when they use it as a data collection strategy to help them "understand [participants] and see them in a unique light" (Estrella & Forinash, 2007, p. 379). See Table 9.4 for tips on how to think about incorporating visual-based data collection methods in your study.

TABLE 9.4. Tips for Including Visual Data Collection Methods in Your Study

1. Select an art form that can be easily used by your participants. Making art does not always appeal to every age group and/or participant. Some may even have negative experiences associated with art. Consider the comfort level of your participants with the arts-based data collection method you select.

2. Plan for anticipated and unanticipated challenges in using art to collect data. For instance, what if a participant's camera does not work? How many supplies will you need for each of the participants?

3. Question yourself. Are you using arts-based data collection strategies because they fit your research tradition and theoretical framework?

4. Anticipate questions your participants may have about the art medium you are using. Consider having a prepared list of instructions for participants, especially if they will be engaged in the art outside the researcher's presence.

5. Consult with an expert in the area of the arts-based medium you will use. This expertise can save you time, money, and frustration and help you focus your study.

6. Ensure that you have sufficient funds for the art medium you would like participants to use. You don't want to run out of necessary supplies for your participants.

7. Revisit your data collection arts-based methods often. How might they need to be refined?

Photography

Qualitative researchers select photography for data collection typically to supplement the primary collection methods discussed in Chapter 8. Photographs can be "found" or may be taken, as instructed, by a researcher. This data collection strategy is often used with children or other groups where words alone may not capture the depth of participants' experiences of a phenomenon. There are many ways you might consider incorporating photography into data collection in your project. You can send participants into their communities with a camera to document a phenomenon—such as stressors or sources of resilience in their lives. You could also hold a focus group with participants around a certain topic—for example, inviting middle school students to photograph school factors that increase their sense of belonging in school.

We "photograph" things in our settings as practitioners all the times, and taking photographs allows for permanence, and thus potentially for more intense data analysis, whether for formal research processes or not. For example, a doctoral supervisor in training of mine (Hays) began a master's-level clinical supervision group one semester by asking his supervisees to take pictures of their office environments. The supervisees were instructed to take pictures only of the physical setting, not of clients or students. They brought the photographs to group supervision the following week when my student discussed how the environment might affect those deciding to seek counseling services, and how the trainees could make the environment more inviting to them.

Photovoice (Wang & Burris, 1997) is a well-known qualitative data collection strategy using photography as a way to document visual information. As with other data collection strategies, your theoretical and research traditions should guide your selection of this strategy. For instance, in a study of children's obesity, Darbyshire, MacDougall, and Shiller (2005) used Photovoice only because children are "unable to articulate their experiences and thus capable only of visual expression" (p. 423). The authors' theoretical and research design led them to "believe that if a respectful and sensitive inquiry approach was taken, children could and would describe their perceptions, experiences, and understandings related to the central questions of physical activity, places and spaces in their lives" (p. 423). Figure 9.2 is a photograph taken as part of a homelessness study (McBride, 2008), wherein the researcher asked participants (individuals who were homeless) to take photos of their daily lives. The study was aimed at illuminating needs and resources of these individuals; this photograph, taken in a city park, is of one individual's primary lodging.

Photography "in and of itself carries meaning prior to even considering the content of the image" (Mitchell & Allnutt, 2008, p. 258). The use of photography as a supplemental data collection method can be especially useful with ethnographic, case study, and phenomenological designs that seek an in-depth understanding of a phenomenon. We discuss how existing photographs can be used as archival data collection sources later in this chapter. Regardless of how photography is used as a medium, there is an empowerment approach embedded in this data collection strategy because the participants are valued for the images they themselves create.

Other advantages of this medium include the potential for participatory action and social change during and after the research process—such as Flint's (2009) Youth Violence Prevention Center's Photovoice Project, which emerged out of a research project and continued as a community intervention. Disadvantages of using photography can be the cost involved if researchers provide cameras for participants. Other challenges include ensuring that participants understand the purpose of using the photographs. One way to address this challenge is to print an instruction sheet with guiding questions about the study's focus that participants may take with them as they take photographs.

Other studies have specifically used visual ethnography to document a phenomenon. **Visual ethnography** involves the use of images, such as photographs or paintings,

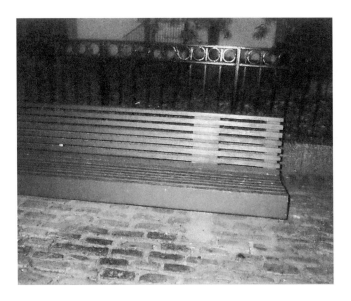

FIGURE 9.2. A day in the life of homelessness.

to understand a culture-sharing group. Previous to conducting any data collection in visual ethnography, however, it remains important to consider the role of research reflexivity and the context in which the visual data are collected and then interpreted. For instance, Banks (2001) discusses context in terms of the external and internal narrative an image possesses: The external narrative serves as the context for the image, whereas the internal narrative is the interpretation of the image by those who view it.

Visual images may stand on their own as a data collection method. After they are collected, these images are then interpreted for themes. Visual images may also be used in tandem with other data collection methods in seeking to understand a phenomenon. For instance, in a study of transformative education, Guajardo, Guajardo, and Del Carmen Casaperalta (2008) used an activist methodology to use visual media for data collection and to encourage Mexican American students to become "authors" and storytellers of their own lives. The authors first equipped the high school students with cameras, tripods, and audiotape machines to collect oral narratives of the elders in their community. As the students transcribed the elders' immigration stories, they reflected on their own immigrant backgrounds and used photography as a way to document these narratives. One student shared: "When I was encouraged to reflect on my immigrant experience, I slowly began to understand that my story was not something to be ashamed of … to the contrary, I began to feel proud of my story and didn't mind sharing very emotional things that I went through" (p. 11). (See Figure 9.3.)

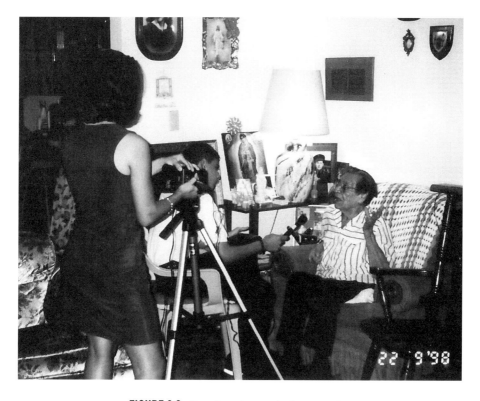

FIGURE 9.3. Immigration and photography.

Participant Artwork

Participant artwork is another data source that allows visual documentation of behaviors and contexts that are often unconscious, giving researchers access to participants' subjective worlds. Artwork not only expresses a particular moment but also can suggest why and how it was obtained, what it represents about the participant, and socially constructed meanings participants and researchers may communicate at various times. Finally, it often generates interview data, and this is typically triangulated with interviews or other data methods (Rhodes & Fitzgerald, 2006). Collectively, being able to present findings in both visual and verbal formats allows a thicker description of participants' experience.

Figure 9.4 depicts a section of a collage created by a 13-year-old female, asked to depict what a healthy dating relationship looks like (see Hays, Forman, & Sikes, 2009). This collage contains artwork, writings, and photographs. Figure 9.5 portrays a drawing by a 14-year-old who was asked to draw what first came to mind for her when thinking about unhealthy dating relationships. With both examples, you can get a sense of the richness that comes with arts-based data collection. These examples are from younger participants, where arts-based media may be even more in line with seeking to understand their experiences of a phenomenon when they might not have the cognitive skills to describe them.

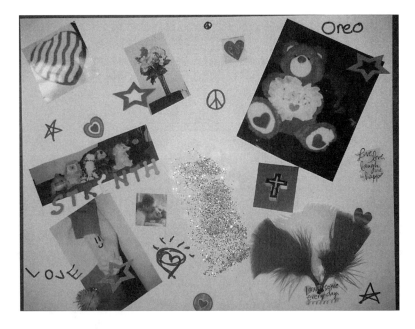

FIGURE 9.4. Healthy relationships collage artwork.

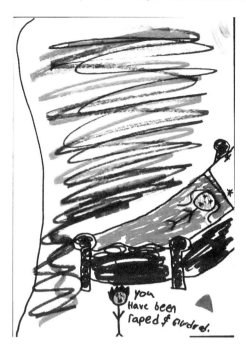

FIGURE 9.5. Adolescent's perspectives on an unhealthy relationship.

Additional Visual Methods

In addition to these arts-based data collection methods, there are other forms of art you may select to incorporate in your study to collect data. The focus of your study should drive the type of art you use. Whether you select music, film, expressive writing, sculpture, poetic writing, or other forms of art, it is best to identify which arts-based data collection strategies you will use in advance of your study. It is also important to keep a keen eye on the needs of your participants in "telling their story." See Perspectives 9.3 to read how a researcher integrated music into a qualitative study.

● ●

Perspectives 9.3. Using Music in a Qualitative Inquiry

"I initially became interested in using music in research when writing about Tupac Shakur for an undergraduate project. I had been thinking about Tupac's lyrics as important to analyze because the lyrics discussed racism and sexism explicitly. I had the students analyze his music in terms of masculinity, hypermasculinity, racism, and sexism. That's when I decided to start using music in qualitative research. The biggest challenge in using music in qualitative research is that it is a lot harder to analyze because there is so much context to music, and in many ways a lot more subjectivity. Also, I definitely had to be aware from the beginning of my own personal bias as a researcher with regard to his lyrics. I think the most beneficial part of using music in qualitative research is that as a researcher you can dive more deeply into significant themes; you can even build theory through identifying the aspects of your participants' experience of music. For instance, what exactly are the mechanisms and

thoughts that go on in terms of how people use and experience music? These dimensions are exceptionally hard to capture if you are using quantitative measures.

"The advice I would give to others is that you must have a solid qualitative paradigm—you need a good methodology. Creswell was my mentor. I used phenomenology as a paradigm—it describes the essence of the meaning of the phenomenon I wanted to study in rap music. So, phenomenology guided my research question. I would say, just because you are using music does not mean that you should throw out your theory and research tradition! Be open to all the types of creative aspects you can use in music as well—such as how music can be an outlet for clients. I would love to study that too. I have used music as a way to establish a common ground on which to bond with my participants around a topic as well. Music helps participants express their feelings more because they are talking about themselves through the music. Especially when you are exploring sensitive topics, such as racism and sexism, music can be an easier medium than a more upfront question like 'What have been your experiences of racism?' I have used this type of approach with music and research in a youth development center, and it has been a powerful way to collect data."

—DEREK IWAMOTO, *PhD*

USING WRITTEN MATERIALS FOR DATA COLLECTION

Written materials can be an important source of data collection. Similar to interviews and focus groups, written materials can provide insight into your participants' experiences of a phenomenon. However, written materials are distinct from interviews and focus groups because they offer a less invasive manner to collect data. This lack of invasiveness may be important if you are researching a sensitive topic; writing can give participants the opportunity to express themselves in a more private manner and/or have more time to reflect on a phenomenon. Your research focus can also benefit from your collecting written materials when they provide source information critical to understanding a phenomenon. For instance, if you are studying the intergenerational experiences of educational attainment of white rural students in Georgia, participants' grade reports, diplomas, and other educational materials have the potential to elucidate understanding about this phenomenon. There is a vast array of written materials you can select for data collection, some of which may include participant journals or diaries, notes, lists, records, reports, and many more.

For some studies, you may elect to have participants write or journal as a way to collect data. Often, this can be an unobtrusive way to supplement your data collection. Especially for phenomenological, life history, and case study examinations, participants' written material can help you more fully understand the phenomenon you are studying. You may be specifically studying writing—such as Stanford's (2009) examination of the self-efficacy perceptions of postsecondary learners. In this study, the author solicited narrative compositions from participants as data. Then the author used focus groups to explore these written narratives and supplemented this data collection with participant observations in class.

More often, written materials are used as supplemental data collection. DiSalvo (2009) examined how school principals use strategic communication skills in different contexts with different audiences. The primary data collection strategy was the semistructured interview, which was then supplemented with samples of participant writings. Using participants' written material can invite a participatory component into your study. Cullen (2009) integrated participants' writings into a PAR project with student affairs professionals regarding the development of an antiracist professional identity. The project included group meetings wherein participants discussed becoming an antiracist as a white person in student affairs. In addition to semistructured interviews pre- and postgroup experience, the participants kept written journals after each group session. These written reflections helped the researcher document the various schemas in white identity development, which might not have been captured as fully in the group sessions alone.

In counseling, Mackrill (2008) encouraged the use of participant **diaries** in qualitative research. He points to the use of client diaries in the work of many famous psychotherapists such as Carl Rogers and Irwin Yalom. He discusses the advantages of using this data collection strategy, including the ability to show change over a period of time and to showcase the context of participants' lived experiences. Mackrill points out that diaries can be solicited as a form of qualitative data collection or unsolicited (a personal document that may be used as a source of data collection; we discuss this further in the next section).

Additional strengths of using diaries for qualitative data collection include what they reveal that participants might not feel comfortable sharing openly, fearing that the subject is "taboo," and that they can help researchers understand the differences between participants' experiences of a phenomenon. Mackrill also identifies some of the challenges in using participant diaries—namely, the presumption that participants have the skills to write and feel comfortable writing and the participants' motivation to write within the structure (e.g., time, duration, frequency) prescribed by the researcher. See Table 9.5 on the next page for an excerpt from a qualitative study of mentoring with Bangladeshi girls, using solicited participant diary entries in qualitative data collection.

In Table 9.5 we can see how the use of diaries provides rich, in-depth information about participants' experiences that might not be identified using other data collection methods. Especially with regard to the interpersonal aspects and emotions documented in the diaries, there is an enriched, firsthand description of these experiences.

Now that we have discussed many different forms of media that you can use for data collection, see Activities 9.2 and 9.3 to explore how you might use media to more fully explore your research topic.

 ACTIVITY 9.2. Assessing Use of Media for Data Collection

Select two to three forms of media—Internet, photography, drawing, music, written materials, etc. Answer the following questions for each of the media you selected:

- How would you use this type of media in data collection for your research topic?
- What information will this medium allow you to collect?
- What information will be more challenging to collect using this media method?

- If you have already used media data collection methods, how might your answers to the previous questions guide you to revisit and refine your methods?

TABLE 9.5. Using Diaries as Data Collection Methods

Excerpts from Sperandio (2008)

Diary and focus-group themes

"Participants' diaries, notes from focus-group discussions, and informal interviews were analyzed for common themes. Four themes were identified that appeared to be of particular interest to the hostel girls. These were the decisions made by their mentors regarding balancing work/family, their mentors' interactions with others in the workplace, the personal advice and encouragement they received from their mentors, and reflections of their own abilities and skills in the context of their observations. . . .

"The level of control mentors appeared to exert over their life events, as well as their decision making and life planning, received frequent comment. One participant recorded in her diary, 'has utilized her education very well.' Another stated, 'She said she feels that to become successful you will need support from other people, but the most important thing is having your own willpower and determination.' Other diary entries included, 'Most of the women in our country cannot finish their studies, but she finished her studies, though she gave credit to her parents for this but she also deserves credit for it. Besides, she finished her studies and then got married'; 'Most of the people cannot plan for their lives, but she has planned her life very well'; and 'Though she is a woman, she is working in a good position.' " (pp. 214–215)

"The most striking aspect of the diaries was the strong emotional response the girls showed toward the personal interest, sympathy, and understanding they received from their mentors. A typical diary entry in this category was:

> The fact that D frankly spoke to me about her personal family life was very heartwarming. She spoke to me as though I was her daughter. Despite being such a well-reputed member of IS, she spoke to me patiently and pleasantly. She gave me unconditional support throughout. She dealt with me with such care and respect that it was overwhelming. When I told her about my life and my background, she consoled me a lot. She also comforted me, saying that I would reach heights in life someday. That really cheered me up. I am grateful for her constant support. Her behavior and sense of responsibility was lovely!

"Other hostel girls echoed these sentiments: 'When I told her about my life, she [teacher] consoled me. This soothing moment will be embedded in my heart for life.' Another girl described how a teacher had shared her life history and how they had formed a close emotional bond: 'She told me not to feel shy to ask her any kind of questions. At first I was a bit scared, but after she told me to feel comfortable, I gained strength and started to ask her questions.' Other comments endorsed the perceptions the girls had of the relationship building that took place: 'I appreciated the fact that a Bengali teacher came up to me in one of the classes and asked about myself. She was genuinely very pleased to see me there. It filled my heart with joy'; and 'I liked it when the ayahs were talking to me openly. The ayahs smiled when they saw me—I liked that.'" (p. 216)

ACTIVITY 9.3. Exploring Use of Media for Data Collection

Can media serve alone as a data collection tool? If so, brainstorm possible research topics or professional issues that could be addressed through the use of media as method. If not, discuss why you believe that media offer only a supplemental method to the primary data collection methods discussed in Chapter 8. If you have already used media data collection methods, what did you learn from the process? What might you need to revisit and/or refine as a result of using media as a data collection method in your study?

USING OTHER DOCUMENTS FOR DATA COLLECTION

A researcher may elect to use a variety of other documents in data collection. Qualitative researchers may use documents as secondary data collection when there would be an important aspect of a study left unexamined or not understood without the documents. Also, when traditional qualitative interviews, focus groups, and participant observations are not available with the participants and/or focus of your study, documents may become a primary source of your data collection (Rapley, 2007). In these documents researchers may examine not only their contents but also the style of what is written and the themes (Rapley). Often, it is the text of documents in which researchers are most interested for data collection; however, there may also be other items in the documents (e.g., graphic images, tables) that may supplement researchers' understanding of their topic (Mason, 2002). We separate our discussion of using documents in data collection into personal and public documents and archival data.

Personal and Public Documents

Personal and public documents can be rich sources of secondary data collection. **Personal documents** are typically solicited to help understand the culture and context of participants' experiences of a phenomenon. Personal documents have a naturalistic value, for they emerge from participants' own environments (Mason, 2002). Examples of personal documents include letters, books, health care records, diaries or journals, financial records, report cards or grading sheets, homework assignments, legal documents, and any other artifacts that may elucidate the phenomenon you are studying. For instance, artifacts such as family documents handed down through generations may provide insight into your participants' lived experiences. In another example, say, you are conducting a study on the intergenerational transmission of trauma. You might elect to explore personal artifacts within a participant's family that he or she states is important to review in order to understand the history of trauma in that family. This might entail family records surrounding a family's experience of trauma—which could include photographs, medical records, and other documents involving major stressors within or outside the family. Often in school counseling research, evaluations of group interventions involve use of secondary personal documents such as school attendance and tardiness, grade reports, and teacher assessments of classroom performance.

Similar to personal documents, **public documents** also have a wide variety of sources. Official records, newspapers, newsletters, magazines, reports, tax records, legal reports, and other public data may serve as public documents. Mason (2002) expands this list to include "insurance policies; bank statements; accounts and balance sheets; company reports; wills; minutes of meetings … menus; advertisements, websites and other materials on the Internet" (p. 103). This should give you perspective on the numerous available public documents you may elect to use in your study. Rapley (2007) provides excellent examples of public data collection that are microscopic in focus—analyzing a small sample of text in a document—to a macroscopic focus such as collecting documents that cover a lengthy period of time.

Archival Data

Archival data are ready-to-use data that are typically collected by government and other institutional research organizations. These data have been described as "raw" data waiting to be used by a researcher. LeCompte and Schensul (1999) describe these raw data "as data sets or sources [that] are available in their unanalyzed and uninterpreted formats (case records, questionnaires, applications, forms, or numerical or text data coded and formatted into computer-readable data sets). They are organized and stored in their original sampling frames and units (e.g., cases of individuals, households, classrooms, communities, and countries)" (p. 202). Archival data can be a helpful supplement to primary data collection because they can provide an enhanced understanding of your study's focus. For instance, you may be studying the mental health of recent immigrants from Ethiopia to the southeastern United States. Incorporating data from the U.S. Census Bureau and other government agencies tracking the migration of Ethiopian residents to the United States can help you understand the larger contextual factors influencing the individuals you are studying.

Archival data can be in any format—written materials, statistics, etc.—and are maintained by a variety of organizations. Recently, there has been an increase in maintaining qualitative archival data. For instance, the Inter-University Consortium for Political and Social Research (ICPSR) in Michigan and the United Kingdom Data Archive (UKDA) store qualitative data digitally for research. These data collection storehouses are excellent resources for researchers and facilitate both national and international collaborations in qualitative work.

Although managing archival data analysis can be overwhelming, it may make sense to include this type of data in your study. Gladstone and Volpe (2008) discussed five types of possible archival data analysis. First is *supra analysis*, which is a form of secondary qualitative analysis that goes beyond the initial focus and explores new research questions. The second type is *supplementary analysis*, involving a more microscopic examination of the initial data that was outside of the first study's focus. With the third type, *reanalysis*, the researcher revisits the original data collection and examines the congruence of the initial analysis. In the fourth type, *amplified analysis*, qualitative data from several studies are analyzed to increase the sample size with a research topic. Finally, the fifth type is *assorted analysis*, where the researcher uses a combination of data that is naturalistic or from an initial data collection with analysis of an archival data set.

Gladstone, Volpe, and Boydell (2007) conducted a supra analysis of an original qualitative study they had conducted with 60 persons living with schizophrenia. They revisited the data set and asked a new question of the portion of the parents' data. The authors outline several challenges in using archival data in this manner, namely, how to ensure the quality, context, and ethics of reexamining these data. In terms addressing issues of quality, the authors note that researchers should consider if the rigor and trustworthiness of examining previously collected qualitative data remain similar in the second examination. Also important for establishing quality is the degree of availability of the initial qualitative data products—are items available or not available, and how this degree of availability will influence the way the data "speak" after the initial analysis. With regard to the context of secondary data analysis, the authors urge

TABLE 9.6. Considerations in Using Documents as Data

You should be able to answer the following questions when incorporating documents into your study for data collection:

1. What are the benefits or challenges of using documents in your study?
2. What is your rationale for using documents for data collection in your study?
3. What is the context of when the documents were created? You may even want to know the sociopolitical and cultural environment of the documents.
4. Who were the authors of the documents? What is their expertise?
5. What are the credibility and trustworthiness of the documents?
6. If you do not use the documents as data, will an integral aspect of your study be left undiscovered?

researchers to examine the important influences on the data—from the history and biography of those collecting the original data and the theoretical frame that guided the data collection. Finally, in terms of ethics, the authors cite IRB challenges, including whether reexamining the data is covered within the informed consent participants signed. Researchers should also consider the ease with which they may contact previous participants, and if this is feasible, the appropriateness of contacting these participants if necessary for a secondary analysis. See Table 9.6 for considerations when using documents as secondary data collection.

We have reviewed many types of secondary data collection in this chapter. However, there are instances where there may not be secondary data collection methods available to you as you conduct your research. See Activity 9.4 to brainstorm ways to address this situation in your study. Then, see Wild Card 9.1 for some general tips to help you think about data collection in your study.

 ACTIVITY 9.4. When There Are No Secondary Data

Brainstorm professional issues in which there are no secondary data collection methods available. Discuss the following in your research groups:

• Think of two to three examples of research topics in your field that would preclude secondary data collection methods.
• When there are no available records, documents, archival data, or media tools that verify the existence of a phenomenon, what would you do?

⚠ WILD CARD 9.1. TIPS TO KEEP IN MIND AS YOU USE MEDIA

It is challenging just to think about traditional data collection methods in your study, much less be open to using media and other secondary data collection tools as well. Use the following tips to keep your mind open to various data collection strategies:

- Let your research focus, research tradition, and theoretical framework guide your use of secondary data collection strategies. It may sound "cool" to use social networking sites to gather data for a case study on families with autism—but it might not be the best fit for your study's design.

- Embrace the ambiguity that media data collection can provide. You may not have as much researcher "control" as in traditional data collection, but you may open the door to more fully understanding your participants.

- This may seem contradictory to the preceding point, but have a plan for data collection. Using media and embracing ambiguity should *not* translate into "anything goes" in your data collection. You should have a plan to manage the solicitation of data and the potential rapid responses (especially if you are working online) of participants.

- Wear your ethical hat at all times. Remember that entering the world of data collection via the Internet and other arts-based data collection strategies can be disorienting. This disorientation does not mean that you should abandon your use of similar ethical guidelines in interacting with participants. Is it smart to accept a Facebook request from a participant, for example? What if your blog research suggests negative findings related to your participants that could be damaging to them? There are no quick and easy answers to these questions. However, you can use your good sense of personal and professional ethics and your good knowledge of your research area and of research methods to guide you.

- Use long-standing principles of qualitative data collection and apply them to innovative data collection methods. For instance, if you are asking participants to vlog about their experiences of living with social anxiety, be sure to have discussions about how, when, where, and why this data collection will take place.

- Expand your ideas of data collection—but not too much! Have conversations with your peers and research mentors about which data collection methods might be "too much" or "too little" for your project. You don't want to overcollect data and drain or burden your participants. You also don't want to miss out on a creative way to collect data that might be less obtrusive for participants and/or help you understand their experiences more fully. It's like that overused mantra we all hear often about life: "It's all about balance!"

- Consistently revisit your data collection methods, assess how they are going, and refine the components that need to be adjusted accordingly so that they reflect the highest integrity and quality.

CHAPTER SUMMARY

In this chapter we have discussed the many ways in which secondary data collection can be conducted in qualitative research. Similar to the primary data collection strategies discussed in Chapter 8, the researcher should be guided by the research tradition and theoretical framework for the study. Secondary data collection methods include a wide variety of media. From the expansive reach of the Internet to the hands-on visual methods of photography and artwork, these secondary data collection strategies can enhance the researcher's understanding of a particular phenomenon. Additionally, personal and public documents as well as archival data may be useful as secondary data sources. No matter which secondary data collection strategy you select, you should have a thorough understanding of its possible impact on participants. A more sensitive research topic, for instance, may require secondary data collection methods that are less intrusive to best meet the needs of participants; a topic that requires access to participants who are difficult to reach may require the use of the Internet to cast a wider "net." Regardless, consider your use of secondary data collection as carefully as you would select primary data collection methods in order to gain the best understanding of your phenomenon.

RECOMMENDED READINGS

Cole, A. L., & Knowles, J. G. (2008). Arts-informed research. In J. G. Knowles & A. L. Cole (Eds.), *Handbook of the arts in qualitative research* (pp. 55–70). Thousand Oaks, CA: Sage.

Hamilton, R. J., & Bowers, B. J. (2006). Internet recruitment and e-mail interviews in qualitative studies. *Qualitative Health Research, 16*(6), 821–835.

Hookway, N. (2008). "Entering the blogosphere": Some strategies for using blogs in social research. *Qualitative Research, 8*(1), 91–113.

VanDorn, N., Van Zoonen, L., & Wyatt, S. (2007). Writing from experience: Presentations of gender identity on weblogs. *European Journal of Women's Studies, 14*(2), 143–159.

Wang, C., & Burris, M. A. (1997). Photovoice: Concept, methodology, and use for participatory needs assessment. *Health Education and Behavior, 24*(3), 369–387.

CHAPTER 10

The Basics of Qualitative Data Management and Analysis

CHAPTER PREVIEW

Greater attention to the components and processes associated with qualitative data management and analysis is needed in qualitative research studies today. In this and the next chapter, you will hopefully find some helpful information to guide your qualitative data management and analysis. In this chapter we provide some basics for qualitative data management and analysis—what we consider to be more generic steps and components, regardless of your selected research traditions. In Chapter 11 we discuss qualitative data analysis more specifically in relation to the different research traditions. First we present some foundational information as you embark on your present qualitative research proposal and beyond. Qualitative data management, a process of both data collection and analysis, is discussed later in the chapter. Figure 10.1 depicts the key components and sequencing of qualitative data management and analysis.

QUALITATIVE DATA ANALYSIS

What is qualitative data analysis, and why is there so little written about it? Part of the reason is that *it is not quantitative data analysis*: There are no statistical formulas or standardized rules for analyzing data; there are no specific, straightforward statistical tests for significance, reliability, validity, and so forth (there are no "click here" options with an "answer" appearing); generalizability is questionable in the sense that qualitative researchers' actions cannot be precisely replicated in another context; and the boundaries around data collection and analysis are less clear with qualitative inquiry.

Second, qualitative data analysis has been noted as challenging, time-consuming, and requiring creativity. Making sense of massive amounts of data that cannot simply be accommodated by computer programs can be a daunting task, with few doing it *really well* and even fewer writing about the process itself. In essence, trustworthy qualitative data analysis relies on the researcher as an individual as well as a skilled professional. Patton (2002) described the complexities of qualitative data analysis:

> [It] involves us not just making sense of the world but also in making sense of our relationship to the world and therefore in discovering things about ourselves even as we discover things about some phenomenon of interest. ... Because qualitative inquiry depends, at every stage, on the skills, training, insights, and capabilities of the inquirer, qualitative analysis ultimately depends on the analytical intellect and style of the analyst. The human factor is a great strength and the fundamental weakness of qualitative inquiry and analysis—a scientific two-edged sword. (pp. 432–433)

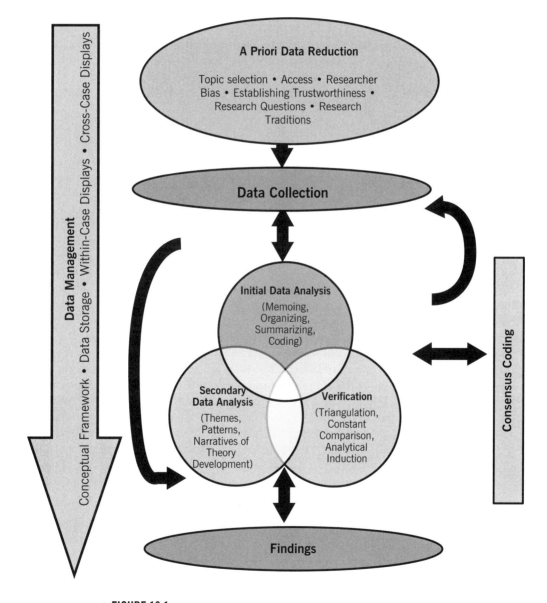

FIGURE 10.1. Qualitative data management and analysis process.

Finally, there may be little written, and we can assume less understood, about the qualitative data analysis process since it *should* occur concurrently with qualitative data collection. Refer back to Chapter 1 when we discussed one of our top 10 pieces of advice for qualitative inquiry: *Qualitative data collection and analysis must occur concurrently.* Unfortunately, many qualitative researchers fail to interweave these processes due to lack of time, interest, or knowledge of the power of simultaneous data collection and analysis (see Wild Card 10.1). We believe that it is not possible to have a rigorous research design without beginning qualitative data analysis with the first data source—if not before—and continuing throughout data collection because lacking the analysis, there is no way to speak to the trustworthiness of the study, and, furthermore, there are ethical considerations. If you wait until all data are collected, how do you investigate emerging research questions? How do you follow up with participants? If a distinguishing and important characteristic of qualitative inquiry is providing dialogical opportunities for often-silenced participants, how do we do that in a responsible way if we wait to listen to them at the end of a study? The major fallacy of postponing data analysis can be summed up with a trite expression: "If only I had known then what I know now!" Since there are few opportunities to gather a thick description of participant perspectives as well as contextual information, it is a professional and ethical imperative that we think of qualitative data analysis as something that continually influences research design from the very beginning of the study.

⚠ WILD CARD 10.1. THE "QUICK" QUALITATIVE STUDY

One of the common misconceptions of qualitative inquiry is that it is quicker and easier to do than quantitative research. This is certainly not true! And if a researcher is operating with this mindset, the potential for conducting an unethical study is immense. Unfortunately, researchers may attempt to get through a qualitative investigation as quickly as possible. A common way to conduct a quick study is to collect all data and then analyze them all at once, without going back to participants to check findings or allowing room to modify the research design.

We have seen several *published* studies, as you probably have, that have simply tapped several data sources (often, via interviews) and then presented themes extracted from these sources. In essence, the design was so rigid that there were no built-in opportunities to revise data collection as data analysis occurred. Participants were not offered a chance to verify the findings. New data sources to better address the research questions were not made available, nor were revisions in data collection methods allowed.

Remember, ethically and socially responsible data analysis is more likely to occur throughout data collection the "looser" your design is initially. The tighter your design, the more rigid your questions, the less open you are to making changes as you start collecting data. *Never, ever* sacrifice your research design to simply save time. Leave enough room in your plan to change your data collection plan. Otherwise, you may complete a study quickly, but practitioners in counseling and education will likely not trust the findings.

STEPS OF QUALITATIVE DATA ANALYSIS

Miles and Huberman (1994) viewed qualitative data analysis as a cyclical process of the following components: reduce data, display data, draw conclusions, and verify. Data reduction—the process of organizing, segmenting, and analyzing text—or visual material really begins even before data collection begins. What we attend to and ask about is based largely on our researcher biases, our conceptual framework, and other components discussed in Part II of this volume. Qualitative data analysis involves categorizing text or keywords that are similar to one another (i.e., **coding**), as well as connecting text or keywords that influence one another (i.e., relationships among codes). Connections among codes are often displayed in narratives or case presentations (Maxwell & Miller, 2008). We discuss later the processes of coding and identifying themes and patterns from these codes. Coding has also been referred to by many names, including *template analysis* and *thematic coding* (King, 1998). However, coding is only a small part of qualitative data analysis.

As we interact in a setting and collect more data, we further reduce data and then chunk it into summaries, memos, codes, themes, clusters of themes, patterns, and so forth. Jorgensen (1989) noted: "Analysis is a breaking up, separating or disassembling of research materials into pieces, parts, elements, or units. ... The researcher sorts and sifts them, searching for types, classes, sequences, processes, patterns or wholes" (p. 107). This assembling and disassembling (and reassembling) process refers to coding. Additionally, Miles and Huberman (1994) recommended displaying data as they are reduced (data displays are discussed later in this chapter as data management tools) to assist in organizing the data to draw "final" conclusions.

What steps are involved in analyzing qualitative data? McLeod (2001) has been one of the few to propose a generic qualitative data analysis process that we believe fits nicely with Miles and Huberman's (1994) vision of qualitative data analysis. We integrate McLeod's steps in our presentation. These steps are *most directly applicable to analyzing text* derived from certain data collection methods, such as in the case of interview transcripts, documents, observation and field notes, contact summary sheets, document summary forms, and so forth. However, the steps can also be applied to non-textual items such as visual materials (see Chapter 9). Special analysis considerations for nontextual data collection methods are discussed later in this section.

This chapter highlights generic, more universal steps, as noted, and the next chapter presents analytic procedures across research traditions. What you will likely surmise after reviewing these two chapters on qualitative data analysis is that there is an underlying basic process to analysis; however, various research traditions label it differently. Although we present these steps linearly, it is important to note that they are cyclical and recursive as you collect and manage data.

We use data from one qualitative study to illustrate these steps. This grounded theory study explored aspects of diagnostic variance in the clinical decision-making process of 41 counselors and counselor trainees (Hays, McLeod, & Prosek, 2009). As you will see as we move through the steps, analysis moved from a priori data reduction, to several iterations of analysis, to data management as a tool in collection and analysis, to presentation of findings of how counselors vary in their clinical decision making.

Step 1: Reduce Data

Referring to Figure 10.1, notice that data analysis begins before data collection. How is this possible? What you decide to investigate, why, and with whom are all data reduction strategies. That is, you narrow your focus of analysis because it is necessary to do so. You cannot study everything, so you limit data analysis (and collection) options. Your selected topic, research questions, research bias, conceptual framework, access to participants and settings, and plans for establishing trustworthiness initially guide what you are likely to find as important concepts. Once initial "data" are reduced, you can make decisions about data collection. Proposal Development 10.1 may assist you with the initial step.

PROPOSAL DEVELOPMENT 10.1. Data Reduction

Revisit your evolving audit trail and responses from early proposal development activities. Create an initial list of keywords related to each of the following areas. That is, what information or terms do you associate with each of these data reduction techniques?

Topic: _____

Research question(s): _____

_____

_____

Your role and assumptions about the study:

_____

_____

_____

Previous literature and pilot data:

_____

_____

_____

Access to participants and setting:

_____

_____

_____

Trustworthiness strategies:

_____

_____

_____

Step 2: Collect Data

Data collection methods were discussed in Chapters 8 and 9, so here we just briefly mention them. Data collection methods include individual and focus group interviews, observations, documents, and visual data, to name a few. Decisions on these methods are largely based on your research questions and access to a population. For the diagnosis study (Hays, McLeod, & Prosek, 2009), the data collection method consisted of individual interviews.

Step 3: Memo and Summarize

Recall from Chapter 8 that "memoing," or jotting field notes immediately following data collection, is an important part of data collection. Memoing is also an important component of data analysis because this is often the initial analysis that occurs with new data. For the diagnosis study, the authors and research assistants noted their impressions of potential findings directly following an interview and then again after the interview text had been organized (i.e., transcribed). After interviewing a 28-year-old white female school counselor about the process she used to diagnose a 32-year-old Latina female, a research assistant created the following memo:

> I was struck with how this school counselor assumed that the client was in denial about her symptoms, and how quick she was to assume that this person had a personality disorder! She seemed to note a lot of symptoms for this client, yet focused in on such a pathologizing diagnosis, even though she became even more uncertain with her decision as we talked. She did mention that ethnicity and gender played a role in symptoms, but I do not think she talked about it when she presented the diagnosis. ... I wonder if this participant's clinical decision making is partly a result of the notion that she is a school counselor and does not work with 32-year-old clients.

Memos can be used in conjunction with other data analysis steps to summarize preliminary findings, what McLeod (2001) referred to as a **preliminary descriptive summary**. This summary is likely to go beyond a memo to more broadly describe the data source. For the above participant example, a descriptive summary might include more detailed information about the interviewee and the participant, the clinical decision-making process, cultural factors, treatment recommendations noted, perceived prognosis, and so forth. In essence, this is an initial narrative that will be expanded upon throughout data analysis.

Step 4: Organize Text

Organizing the text usually refers to transcribing textual data, converting and expanding upon field notes, and creating data management tools such as contact summary sheets and document summary forms. You may refer to Chapters 8 and 9 for examples of data management tools. Figure 10.2 presents an excerpt of an interview from the diagnosis study (Hays, McLeod, & Prosek, 2009), with some initial codes (Step 5).

Interview transcribed by CRB: Interviewee ID # 016D 05/14/07, Duration: 36:58   *Include information about the data and length of the interview when you organize text.*

CRB: What diagnosis or diagnoses would you give this client?

PA: With this individual I think I would diagnose her with major depressive disorder and a personality disorder, probably borderline personality disorder.   *Major depressive disorder and borderline personality disorder*

CRB: How would you summarize the symptoms used to arrive at your diagnosis?

PA: Well, this individual has multiple symptoms prior, she has a couple of episodes of rage, she mentions crying almost daily within the last month, the attempted suicide, she is eating more lately, she has gained weight, poor concentration, difficulty getting out of bed, she is doing impulsive things, she spent like $10,000 in a short period of time.   *Availability—broad*

CRB: Are there other diagnoses that could explain the client's symptoms?

PA: Yeah, I think there might be some as well. Um, possibly, I don't think she has schizophrenia, but she has schizophrenia-like symptoms, but not full-blown schizophrenia, possibly bipolar, but I don't know if she's that extreme to be bipolar. There are some things here and there, but I don't know if I would diagnose her with, but I think it is a good possibility because she has such a variation of symptoms.   *Uncertainty*

Diagnosis rule-out (bipolar and schizophrenia)

CRB: What aspects of the case did you use to arrive at your diagnosis?

PA: OK, the multiple symptoms that she has—the weight gain, the eating, her lack of interest in doing things, her problems at work, she thinks the people that she works with are watching her, she has trouble getting out of bed, she worries, and a lot of these things have happened within the last 2–3 months. Very rapidly. She spent over $10,000, she has used her credit card a lot lately, and she is hearing voices. I learned at [University] that these symptoms tend to relate to a mood disorder.   *Availability—academic*

CRB: Were there any particular salient criteria for you?

PA: Definitely. The extreme shifts in mood stand out to me.   *Vividness criterion*

CRB: What cultural characteristics, if any, are important to this client's presenting problem? How so?

PA: Um, well (long pause), I guess the fact that she is female, and as far as her changing her mood, I think that would be, well as far as her weight gain, that's really not that uncommon, but the fact that she is female, and she is Latin American, but I think there is a huge variation that she is having that is alarming.   *Gender*

Race/ethnicity

CRB: What cultural characteristics, if any, are important to your diagnostic decision? How so?

PA: (long pause) Well, I think the fact that she is Latin; we can look at her culture because it talks about in her summary that she is isolated and doesn't want to interact with others. I think it would be important to look at her culture and see if that is something Latin Americans like to do; they may not like to be very social. That may be very common for her culture. It also talks about her stress, and it could be that there are some things here and there that are appropriate for her culture and, you know, she may not be doing anything out of the ordinary for her culture.   *Race/ethnicity*

Uncertainty about cultural "norms"

Race/ethnicity

[Transcript break]

(cont.)

FIGURE 10.2. Interview excerpt for diagnosis study. *Source*: Hays, McLeod, and Prosek (2009).

CRB: How would you describe this client's level of functioning? How, if at all, do you see this changing with treatment?

PA: She definitely needs some sort of treatment, and I think I mentioned before that she does have a variation in her symptoms, and they are pretty extreme as far as she has had a lot of the symptoms within the last 2–3 months and that is pretty alarming. Right now I think her level of functioning—I think she is able to function on one level, but she certainly needs some sort of continuous treatment. I wouldn't with this patient. She has had outpatient treatment for, um, painkillers, so I would be wary to prescribe medication. It may be something that she needs, but I would be wary of doing that.

Needing treatment

"Alarming" symptoms [emic code]

Cautious about future medication

[Transcript break]

CRB: And what might make it difficult to get the information for diagnosing the client?

PA: Well, I think on this is, I want to point out assuming that she is having, some of these things say that she denies that. But I think of the things that may be accurate so I think that to focus on the things that she is having instead of what she denies. I guess maybe a lack of information. I don't, I wouldn't want to know what she does not or what she denies. I would want to know what she is and I would want it to state what she has or what is going on instead of what she denies.

Client "resistance"

FIGURE 10.2. *(cont.)*

Step 5: Code

A **code** is a label or tag that "chunks" various amounts of data based on the defined case or unit of analysis. It may be referred to by many other terms, including *domain, factor, theme, subtheme,* and *item,* to name a few. Codes can be descriptive or interpretive, and they can be specifically labeled by participants themselves (**emic codes**) and/or by the researcher (**etic codes**). Codes can originate from predetermined categories or from the data. Complete Activity 10.1 to become more familiar with the coding process.

    ACTIVITY 10.1. Coding Exercise

In small groups, review annual top 100 music lists for the past 5 years. (The *Billboard* annual top 100 lists are good ones; visit *www.billboard.com.*) The purpose of this "research study" is to investigate popular music according to a ranking system. Your group decides what categories are important to attend to as you develop a codebook or coding system. First, create individual coding lists for your five documents (one for each of the 5 years covered by this study). How might you categorize list entries? Then come to consensus with group members about your classification system. Develop a list of codes based on your coding system, working for approximately 15 minutes.

Discuss your coding system with the entire class. What were the similarities and differences in the coding systems of your groups? How might the way the data were reduced influence this coding system? What other forms of data could be used to investigate popular music? How might these other forms affect your current coding system?

As you code, focus primarily on thickly describing the code before trying to shorten it. A code should be described thoroughly, using examples to illustrate it, so that another researcher could readily identify the code for a data source, based on your detailed, operational definition of it. Miles and Huberman (1994) conceptualized codes as the abbreviations rather than the words; however, we believe that phrases should be abbreviated later, rather than earlier, in the coding process to avoid confusion.

So, what do you code? How do you begin? Earlier steps have mentioned data organization strategies so that you can more easily see what information you have in front of you. First, code before you collect data, as appropriate (see Step 1): Examine your conceptual framework and jot down several key phrases from previous literature, researcher assumptions, pilot findings, and so forth. This framework provides insights into possible codes and will likely be revised as data are collected. Place these "codes" aside. Table 10.1 presents some codes for Step 1 in the diagnosis study (Hays, McLeod, & Prosek, 2009).

Second, take the organized text and visual data and consider them in the context of your research purpose. Some researchers argue that coding should be guided strictly by the research question(s) since there are so many data sources, whereas others assert that it is better to remain more "open" and code using various methods. Table 10.2 presents possible coding sources. Finally, with written text, you have to decide if you will code by word, phrase, sentence, or paragraph. We find that, although it may be related to your research purpose, the unit of analysis you code is a matter of personal preference.

A few other coding considerations are important to note. First, qualitative researchers should code specific data sources as soon as possible after data are collected. Second, if a code is used a lot, then create subcodes, even early in data analysis. (For example, in Figure 10.2, you will notice that the code "Availability" has two subcodes: *Broad* indicates a broad range of symptoms, and *Academic* refers to the notion that a diagnosis is made on the basis of academic training. *Availability* refers to the notion that certain material is more available to us.) Third, continue to memo. You will find that additional impressions about your overall research design, including future data collection and analysis, will emerge as you code. Be sure to write memos about codes and add to your codebook. Finally, you can code manually (e.g., writing directly on organized text, creating index cards of codes) or electronically (use of computer software). We actually prefer to code manually after organizing text with word-processing or PDF documents; however, this method can become cumbersome quickly as data accumulate. Remember, software does not analyze data; it facilitates data storage, coding, retrieval, comparing, and linking. (Computer software is discussed later in this chapter.)

Step 6: Identify Themes and Patterns

Themes or patterns are higher-order codes (*pattern codes*), or codes that have been chunked together to more fully describe a phenomenon (McLeod, 2001). Miles and Huberman (1994) asserted that themes and patterns are "meta-codes" or codes of codes in the previous step. They appear as themes, causes, or explanations; relationships among people; more theoretical constructs; and so forth. Maxwell and Miller (2008) described this step as implementing connecting strategies to identify relationships among codes. *Patterns* are also known as *structures* (LeCompte & Schensul, 1999).

Similar to factor analysis in quantitative research, identifying patterns involves examining codes and brainstorming ways in which the codes "chunk together." LeCompte

TABLE 10.1. Codes Noted in Literature on Diagnostic Variance

	Description	Example(s)
Representativeness	Likelihood that a criterion belongs to a specific diagnosis; we expect to see (and subsequently confirm) certain disorders for certain populations.	Depression expected for females; crying spells a salient criterion for depression.
Availability	Certain events or criteria are more available to us because they are salient and relate closely to a disorder; we are more familiar with criteria, or they are easier to retrieve.	Someone with a lot of experience with particular disorders will have those cues more available and will naturally lean toward certain diagnostic decisions. Certain symptoms may be personal for us.
Vividness criterion	Some criteria are more intense in their presentation and heavily influence our decisions.	Withdrawal symptoms as evidence of dependence
Anchoring	Earlier clinical data hold more weight in final decisions; propensity to focus on later data that support earlier clinical data (or later data not viewed as salient).	Initial Mental Status Exam shows thought disorder symptoms and thus more likely to identify psychotic symptoms in intake to support diagnosis
Locus of attribution (dispositional vs. situational)	What caused the problem—is it biological or external?	Irritability seen as a result of chemical imbalance or as a maladaptive way of coping with an overwhelming situation.
Confirmation bias	This tool overlaps with some of the others; we look for clinical evidence to support our diagnosis, versus looking for symptoms that would lead us to select another diagnosis.	
Gender	Gender stereotypes (overdiagnosis)	More severe diagnoses for females; women overrepresented with personality disorder diagnoses.
Race/ethnicity	Racial and ethnic stereotypes (overdiagnosis)	More severe diagnoses for racial/ethnic minorities; more negative symptoms noted for racial/ethnic minorities, even when they receive the same diagnoses as majority group members.
Underdiagnosis	When symptoms (1) do not fit an existing category, (2) are congruent with gender roles, (3) are more prominent for an oppressed group (the dominant group avoids the diagnosis), and (4) are viewed as happening *to* them versus *because* of them (locus of attribution issue). Also, the more resources we perceive the client to have (this can be connected to awareness of oppression issues), the more we will underdiagnose or avoid more severe diagnoses.	

TABLE 10.2. Coding Sources

- Research questions
- Interview questions
- Observation rubrics
- Other researchers
- Conceptual framework
- Who, what, when, where, how, why questions
- Participant actions
- Participant activities

- Participant meanings
- Discrepancies (use of terms such as *never*, *always*, and *should*)
- Silences and other nonverbal communication
- Relationships among participants
- Setting information
- Absence of codes
- What participants label as codes (emic codes)
- What theory and practice determine are codes (etic codes)

and Schensul (1999) noted that patterns emerge from several factors, including (1) declaration (informant identifies the pattern); (2) frequency of omissions (something notable missing); (3) similarity; (4) co-occurrence of codes; (5) triangulation and corroboration; and (6) sequences of items or events. Two of the themes (with sample codes or subthemes following in parentheses) from the diagnosis study include Forms of Diagnostic Variance (information variance, observation variance, criterion variance); and Use of Cognitive Tools (representativeness, availability bias, vividness criterion, anchoring, and locus of attribution).

Comparative Pattern Analysis

Identifying themes and patterns should not stop there. Patton (2002) discussed a more elaborate process known as **comparative pattern analysis**. This involves researchers moving back and forth through chunked data to understand how the categories are alike and how they are different. Considering participant and contextual (e.g., time, setting, culture) factors, how might similarly coded text be coded (i.e., what are the meta-codes)? More specifically, Patton described this process as one of making sense of convergence (internal homogeneity) and divergence (external homogeneity) within a data source as well as across data sources. In his text he used an apple versus orange metaphor to illustrate comparative pattern analysis: Although apples and oranges are both types of fruit with other similar characteristics, there are ways in which they diverge or vary (e.g., texture of external layer, color, shelf-life). It is important to note that comparative pattern analysis creates the meta-codes that are not likely visible from directly reviewing data. This type of analysis requires studying the processing and sequencing of data and attending to where, how, why, and by whom that the data occurred. In addition, researchers seek and examine sequences and changes across time while triangulating data sources. Activity 10.2 may be a useful tool for understanding comparative pattern analysis.

An example from the diagnosis research might clarify what comparative pattern analysis involves. After carefully coding, chunking data, and developing themes for the 41 interviews, my research team and I (Hays) noted that participants became more uncertain (and less confident) about their diagnostic decisions as we interviewed them. Furthermore, my research team and I found that many would defer to a professional whom they perceived was more competent (e.g., psychiatrist, psychologist) for a final decision. This led us to an important training implication: Educators in mental health professions need to discuss attitudes associated with diagnosing and the importance of counselors believing in their competency and their right to diagnose. Comparative pattern analysis led to two of many important meta-codes that we included in our codebook: "regressive uncertainty" and "perceived incompetence."

 ACTIVITY 10.2. Coding Exercise, Revisited

Return to your small groups and review your coding system for the top 100 music lists from Activity 10.1. What patterns might be visible as you apply a more revised coding system to your five data categories? How do these patterns relate to "participants" (e.g., music artists, audience) and context (e.g., time, sequence)? What are the meta-codes?

Noting patterns, particularly through comparative pattern analysis, can be a fun and creative endeavor. However, we caution that you should not create pattern codes too soon. And, not every code will be chunked into a larger pattern or theme: Sometimes we code something initially, and it "goes nowhere" as far as explaining a more complex aspect of a phenomenon. Finally, when you have developed patterns, check these codes in future data collections.

Step 7: Create a Codebook

A codebook is a document that lists codes, subcodes, and patterns. A codebook also can contain a definition or description of each code, examples from data, and direct quotes or references to aspects of visual data. Although we list the codebook as Step 7, this step really starts once you begin coding, and revisions occur as you code more data and reach consensus. Figure 10.3 presents an abbreviated version of the codebook from the diagnosis study (Hays, McLeod, & Prosek, 2009).

Constant comparison is an important component of developing a strong codebook. It refers to the continuous process of using earlier coding systems to code future data sources (Lincoln & Guba, 1985). Constant comparison works like this: Use codes from your evolving codebook to label new data sources; add new codes to your codebook when existing codes do not readily fit data; reach consensus about all codebook edits; make decisions about collapsing codes in codebook after all data are analyzed (but not before!); and go back and recode data sources with the more final codebook.

Now, let us turn to your data. Activity 10.3 will assist you in beginning the coding process. All you need is a single data source to get started.

 ACTIVITY 10.3. Beginning the Coding Process

Using a data source, such as an interview transcript or some other form of textual data, review for codes and labels. Code by phrase, sentence, line, or paragraph. You can code using various sources (see Table 10.2). Note whether each code is etic or emic, descriptive or interpretive. Feel free to write a memo on the data source itself. Then revisit the codes and develop themes, if possible. Create a codebook for this data source, perhaps a listing of codes with some basic definitions. Present your codes in dyads and discuss the features and challenges of the coding process. How was this coding experience for you? What might you do differently next time?

Create Multiple Codebooks

One major issue that we have seen (and encountered) is the creation of only one codebook for all data sources and methods. This means there would be one reference guide to code all sources with similar labels. Initially, this might seem to make intuitive sense: such a codebook streamlines the process of developing a main narrative or theory (Step 8). However, it really defeats the purpose of triangulating data collection methods. That is, if we, as researchers, are triangulating data to confirm (and to disconfirm) findings, we need to assess them independently and note what codes are similar and dissimilar across data methods, and why. We recommend strongly that you create a codebook for *each* data collection method you use in a study. Then, examine each "final" codebook

REPRESENTATIVENESS_CRITERIA	Likelihood that a criterion belongs to a certain diagnosis (alludes to rigid adherence to DSM criteria), understanding of differential diagnosis (e.g., knowing that a criterion does not solely belong to a certain diagnosis)
REPRESENTATIVENESS_CULTURE	Likelihood that certain disorders belong to certain cultural groups (e.g., depression in females)
ANCHORING	Earlier clinical data hold more weight in final decisions, propensity to focus on later data that support it (or later data not viewed as important) (e.g., MSE shows thought disorder symptoms, and thus likely to find psychotic symptoms in intake to support diagnosis)
AVAILABILITY_EXPERIENCE	Diagnosis made based on clinical/personal experience; certain symptoms/disorders as available/familiar due to experience
AVAILABILITY_ACADEMIC	Diagnosis made based on general cluster of symptoms learned in academic training; certain symptoms/disorders as available/familiar due to classroom learning
AVAILABILITY_CONTEXT	Diagnosis made based on general cluster of symptoms from environmental factors (usually indicative of giving a less severe diagnosis); symptoms familiar or common for certain environmental stressors
AVAILABILITY_BROAD	Integrates a broad range of symptoms as identified symptoms
VIVIDNESS	Some criteria are more intense in their presentation and heavily influence diagnostic decisions (e.g., withdrawal symptoms as evidence of dependence)
NO_VIVIDNESS	No criteria were salient in the diagnostic decision
DXCHANGE_SEVERE	Transitioned from a less severe to more severe diagnosis for the final diagnosis (e.g., MDD to bipolar; bipolar to schizophrenia)
DXCHANGE_LESS_SEVERE	Transitioned from a more severe to a less severe diagnosis for the final diagnosis (e.g., schizophrenia to MDD)
DX_RULEOUT	Discussed a rule-out diagnosis
DX_CONSIDERATION	Listed possible diagnoses considered but not additional processes to rule out
DX_DEFER	Deferring a more severe diagnosis to avoid unnecessary labeling
SITUATIONAL	Locus of attribution that focuses on external factors as causing the problem or presenting symptoms
DISPOSITIONAL	Locus of attribution that focuses on internal/biological factors as causing the problem or presenting symptoms
INFORMATION_VARIANCE	Limitations of self-report in diagnosis; clients may not present all information about what is really going on (unintentionally); amount or type of data collected is limited by how much clients report as well as how much counselors seek
OBSERVATION_VARIANCE	There is variability in how the same data are interpreted among different counselors

(cont.)

FIGURE 10.3. Diagnostic variance codebook. *Source*: Hays, McLeod, and Prosek (2009). Reprinted with permission from Taylor & Francis. MSE, Mental Status Exam; MDD, major depressive disorder.

OBV_PERCEIVED_INCOMPETENCE	Subcode of OBSERVATION_VARIANCE; information is interpreted differently based on experience level; participant reports incompetence as compared to other professionals (e.g., perceives not able to give more severe diagnosis because not an MD, psychologist)
CRITERION_VARIANCE	Use of different criteria to diagnose; similar criteria can fit multiple diagnoses—alludes to the ambiguity/subjective nature of diagnosing; has insight into cognitive error/tools, i.e., confirmation bias
UNCERTAIN_INFO	Participant reports uncertainty for the diagnosis given due to information presented in the case
UNCERTAIN_EXPERIENCE	Participant reports uncertainty for the diagnosis given due to his/her clinical or personal experience
CERTAIN_INFO	Participant reports certainty for the diagnosis given due to information presented in the case
CERTAIN_EXPERIENCE	Participant reports certainty for the diagnosis given due to his/her clinical or personal experience
REGRESSIVE_UNCERTAINTY	Participant initially comfortable or certain about diagnosis yet regresses in decision making throughout interview to a lesser degree of certainty with the diagnosis given
PROGRESSIVE_CERTAINTY	Participant becomes more comfortable with the diagnosis given throughout the interview
DXATTITUDE_POSITIVE	Likes to diagnose; sees diagnosing as helpful

FIGURE 10.3. *(cont.)*

for parallel findings. We have often found that more advanced pattern codes are evident through comparative pattern analysis when we examine the codebooks by method.

Step 8: Develop a Main Narrative or Theory

The final step of qualitative data analysis is bringing together the patterns identified in multiple data sources and methods, and examining how categories or concepts relate back to research questions and also how they relate to each other. This step is often analogous to report writing, discussed in the last section of the text. However, Step 8 may lead back to Steps 2–7 as you review the larger findings and discover that more data collection and analysis need to occur.

The main narrative or theory will be presented differently for each qualitative report, depending on your research tradition, audience, and personal preference. Table 10.3 provides some ideas to consider for developing a main narrative.

Visual Data and the Coding Process

Although a majority of the eight "universal" steps of qualitative data analysis can easily apply to visual data, we would like to highlight a few additional considerations. Visual data include media such as film, newspapers and newsletters, artwork, advertisement

> ### TABLE 10.3. Developing a Main Narrative.
>
> - Use research questions to structure.
> - Create vignettes (e.g., normative depiction of phenomenon, typical day for participants, dramatic account to get reader's attention, use of critical events/stories).
> - Provide a historical account of phenomenon.
> - Describe a social process.
> - Create summaries of interview results or individual profiles.
> - Create a conceptual framework or other display (e.g., contrast table, event lists, matrices, scatterplots, conceptual diagrams, tree diagrams, pie charts, Venn diagrams, flowcharts, sociograms).
> - Develop metaphor (for central meaning).
> - Describe functions or organizational structure of group (i.e., basic components, operations, interconnections/relationships).
> - Write up critical events in chronological order.
>
> *Source:* LeCompte and Schensul (1999).

posters, DVDs, movies, photographs, artifacts such as graffiti and clothing, and so forth. Organizing visual data can be challenging, but whenever possible, create an electronic, storable representation of the data. This can include a DVD with observation notes, a PDF or JPEG file of a newsletter article or photo with an accompanying document summary form, a photo of a building or landscape converted into an electronic format, and so on. With respect to coding, Grbich (2007) provided three key strategies: (1) Evaluate for content and context (i.e., What is the image? Why, when, how, and by whom was it produced? What meanings are conveyed?); (2) look for links (i.e., how does the image relate to other aspects of the phenomenon of interest?); and (3) interpret (i.e., what are the dominant reviews of the data? What are alternate reviews of the data?).

CASE EXAMPLE 10.1. Coding Visual Data

Use the steps of the coding process and Grbich's (2007) coding strategies to code the following political cartoon.

- At first glance, what would you say are the content and context of the image?
- This is a cartoon featured in an article on classroom discipline. How does knowing this affect your coding of the cartoon?
- What additional information might be useful to interpret the image?
- How does the cartoon relate to other experiences you may have had with the phenomenon of classroom discipline?
- Create a preliminary descriptive summary and a list of preliminary codes for the cartoon.
- Compare your findings in small groups. Discuss how the coding process differs for each group member.

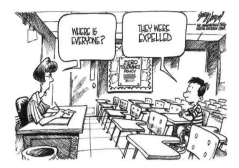

Source: New Hampshire Union Leader. (n.d.). Retrieved April 2, 2009, from *www.unionleader.com/up-loads/media-items/cartoons/2006/411cartoon.jpg*. Reprinted with permission from Creators Syndicate.

CODING CONSIDERATIONS

With some basic coding methods presented, let's now move on to additional coding considerations that impact some of the steps. These include analytic induction, consensus coding, frequency counting, use of multiple classifications, taking a vacation from data, and member checking.

Analytic Induction

Qualitative data analysis is rarely purely inductive. We alluded to this point from the beginning of this volume: Our choices about research paradigms and traditions, research questions, topic, participant and site selection, researcher role considerations, and conceptual framework development (among many others) are affected by the data we expect to find. Although these expectations may unfortunately be guided at times by what we need or want to find, often they are guided by preexisting "codes" in our everyday lives. Thus, no matter how open and inductive we strive to be, we often have predetermined ideas about a phenomenon that guide which codes we select. Because qualitative research is not purely inductive, Hammersley (2008) emphasized that researchers should consider their research questions as working assumptions that are allowed to change as data are collected and analyzed.

Additionally, at some point in collecting and analyzing data, we have to verify what we are finding. Verification involves seeking out cases to disconfirm present codes and themes in order to strengthen emerging models; this component is a presented in Figure 10.1 as a part of analysis. (Recall in Chapter 7 the discussion on verification strategies of negative case analysis and referential adequacy.) In essence, initial data collection may be somewhat inductive, but later data collection, as a result of ongoing data analysis, focuses on more deductive methods, and researchers challenge their working assumptions along the way. The process by which qualitative data analysis moves from exploratory to confirmatory methods is known as **analytic induction**.

Johnson (1998) identified the primary purpose of analytic induction as theory development, although we feel that this process can be applied to other research purposes. Johnson noted four key phases: (1) gain access to phenomenon; (2) define the phenomenon and identify case variations (or case categories); (3) create an initial list of features for each case category, identify deviant cases and either modify categories or list of case features, then compare across categories; and (4) present theoretical explanations of variance for a phenomenon. Hammersley (2008) noted:

> What analytic induction proposes is that inquiry must start from some sort of puzzle about why a particular event occurs, followed by the abduction of hypothetical causal principles—in other words, theoretical ideas—from study of a few cases. There is an iterative process by which, through examination of further cases and careful reflection, the theoretical hypothesis and/or the initial formulation of the type of event to be explained may be refined or transformed. The aim is to produce a theory that conceptualises a process of systematic causation that will operate when particular conditions are met. (p. 85)

Analytic induction, then, allows for the way a phenomenon is explained to change, as well as permits the phenomenon to change altogether as part of theory development.

Consensus Coding and Reliability

Recall from Chapter 7 that the triangulation of multiple researchers is a strategy for establishing trustworthiness. Use of multiple researchers is particularly important for **consensus coding.** We recommend that you independently code a data source, and then reach agreement on a code with your research team, discussing and agreeing on an operational definition of a code.

Consensus coding is one of the most important aspects of qualitative data analysis: By discussing and arriving at a shared operational definition of each code, researchers are co-creating new knowledge about the phenomenon at hand. Consensus coding is best accomplished through somewhat structured consensus meetings. Adapted from Miles and Huberman (1994), Figure 10.4 provides a template of a consensus meeting form that can be used to discuss each independently coded case. This form is analogous to the contact summary sheet presented in Chapter 8: It is a cover sheet for a consensus meeting. Prior to beginning the consensus meeting, the research team should pick a recorder to take notes on the form.

Computing interrater or intercoder reliability (also referred to as **reproducibility reliability**; see Weber, 1990) is another method for determining consistency or agreement among research team members. **Interrater reliability** is a ratio between research team members about the appropriateness for use of each code or pattern in textual or visual data. Miles and Huberman (1994) determine reliability with the following formula:

$$\text{Reliability} = \frac{\text{No. of agreements}}{\text{Total no. of agreements} + \text{disagreements}}$$

Saris-Gallhofer, Saris, and Morton (1978) noted that reliabilities are likely to vary by unit of analysis, with words and phrases typically having higher reliabilities than coding at the sentence, paragraph, or document level. Regardless of selected unit of analysis, Miles and Huberman (1994) established .70 as an acceptable cutoff for intercoder reliability, which we believe is adequate.

Project ID: _____

Consensus Meeting Form

Date: _____   **Case or Cases Discussed:** _____

Research Team Members Present:

_____

_____

New Codes and Definitions:

Main Themes:

Salient Quotes/Key Phrases:

Primary Reflections: *Reflections* refer to member impressions of the case, and can be impressions held by the majority (primary) or those held by a minority (rival).

Rival Reflections:

Case Narrative:

Next Steps: Future directions for qualitative data collection are written here.

Codebook Revisions:

FIGURE 10.4. Consensus meeting form.

If you decide to compute interrater agreement, be sure that you and your research team members are in agreement about the definitions and labels of codes. There are several benefits and challenges to using consensus coding or interrater reliability (or both), and you have to determine what is most useful for your qualitative study as well as what your personal preference is (see Reflexive Activity 10.1).

One last form of reliability we encourage you to use is **stability reliability**, which is analogous to test–retest reliability in quantitative research and refers to the extent that the same researcher codes text the same way more than once (Weber, 1990). To compute stability reliability, a researcher may want to identify codes in a transcript and then later recode that transcript similarly. Another way to compute this rating is to examine how data of similar characteristics within the same data source are coded: If a keyword is used repeatedly to indicate similar data, then the data source may have stability reliability. It is important to note, however, that the longer duration between recoding, the more likely codes or keywords might change simply given the fact that codebooks get revised. When interpreting stability reliability, the qualitative researcher needs to consider the tension for time that elapses between recoding a data source and potential changes in research design and data analysis.

REFLEXIVE ACTIVITY 10.1.
Consensus Coding versus Interrater Reliability

Journal about the benefits and challenges for using both consensus coding and interrater reliability. Should you use both in establishing triangulation of investigators? Why or why not?

We have presented two methods that can be used when triangulating investigators. Complete Proposal Development 10.2 using one or both of these triangulation strategies.

PROPOSAL DEVELOPMENT 10.2. Reaching Agreement in the Coding Process

Using a data source that you and a research team member have independently coded, meet to reach agreement on codes and any patterns for that data source. You may decide to code for consensus, compute interrater reliability, or both. What was this process like for you? How might you reach agreement differently in the future?

Frequency Counting

The issue of frequency counts is a tough one, and quite a debated topic! **Frequency counting** refers to tallying the number of times a code occurs for a data source. After a data source has been developed into a written record and the text has been analyzed, qualitative researchers review documents and count the frequency of each code related to the research purpose and then rank-order codes by frequency. Some argue that counting the number of times codes occur (or fail to occur) can denote an important theme or pattern that can be used to address a research question. So, the more a code appears, the more salient it is assumed to be. We see frequency counting as potentially valuable in observations of human behavior and needs assessments of new or existing clinical and educational programs. In seeking grants for various programs, for example, having numbers tied to qualitative data can "legitimize" a need.

However, we believe more times than not frequency counting is neither necessary nor helpful. The key assumption of frequency counting—that more is better—easily goes against the spirit of qualitative inquiry. How so? Well, let's say you are conducting several focus groups with parents of children with special needs, and you are interested in their experiences in a local school system. After interviewing 20 parents, you decide to rank-order their experiences for each identified group with which they interacted:

Contact group	Theme	Frequency
Teachers	Provide extra attention	45
	Ignore child	15
	Meet regularly with parents	15
	Show concern for special need	13
Teacher assistants	Show concern for special need	36
	Provide extra attention	30
	Collaborate with school personnel	5
	Meet regularly with parents	1
School counselors	Meet regularly with parents	5
	Meet regularly with child	5
	Ignore child	2
Principals	Ignore parents	55
	Ignore child	50
	Collaborate with school personnel	3
Other parents	Ignore parents	2
	Meet regularly with parents	1
Child's peers	Ignore child	1
	Show concern for special need	1

You might draw certain conclusions from these data. The most salient themes were that parents perceived principals as ignoring them and their children, and that they perceived teachers as providing the most extra attention for their children. You might also conclude that other parents and peers were not involved in parents' experiences with the school system. Examining further, you might guess that parents perceive that teachers are more willing to meet with them than teacher assistants, school counselors, or others in a particular school. From this interpretation you might want to examine training opportunities with school personnel of all levels on more effective interactions with parents of children with special needs. But wait: What if we told you that most of the interview questions involved teachers' roles in working with their children? Also, what if in one of the focus group interview sessions parents spent most of the time discussing their principals, whereas in another focus group there was no mention of principals?

This example illustrates two cautionary points we make about frequency counting. First, frequency counts must be considered *in context*. By the very nature of talking about one topic for a significant period of time, more codes about that topic are likely to appear. So, if an interviewer is probing an interview question regarding experiences with principals, it is likely that parents will talk more about principals. If an interviewer runs out of time in most of the focus groups and cannot discuss the role of other parents and peers, it is likely that parents will not discuss these two groups. One can easily see that whatever information is solicited, the degree to which researchers and participants attend to a topic, and the notion that certain topics may not be covered well, create a complicated picture for interpreting frequency counts. Based on these issues, we caution strongly to not "count too soon" and to ensure maximum opportunities to cover topics adequately as possible.

Furthermore, themes with low frequency counts (e.g., 1 or 2) may be just as meaningful as those with high frequency counts (e.g., 50 or 55). One of the key characteristics of qualitative inquiry that we mention throughout this volume is that this research approach is designed to give voice to various perspectives and groups. So, with the parent focus group example, let's assume that there were plenty of opportunities in each group to explore parents' experiences within the school system. And, parents report only 2 counts of other parents ignoring them. Should researchers ignore this theme because it has a low count? We believe, absolutely not! Perhaps the parent that raised this issue felt silenced in the focus group. Perhaps that participant "represents" many others with that opinion who were not able to participate in the focus groups. Thus, there are so many challenges with frequency counting that we caution against solely relying on them. We highlight some of our views on frequency counting in Perspectives 10.1.

Single versus Multiple Classifications

No matter what you decide for your unit of analysis in coding, you will collapse or chunk codes into larger categories, typically themes or patterns. Insch, Moore, and Murphy (1997) noted that qualitative researchers have the options of single classification (i.e., codes assigned to one category, the category of "best fit") and multiple classification (i.e., placing codes in more than one category). Weber (1990) asserted that although single classification maximizes validity (because only codes directly applicable to one category get included), there is the potential that important codes describing dynamics across categories may be missed. Insch and colleagues remind us that codes in multiple categories may not be considered independent concepts. To minimize challenges during interpretation of these categories, we recommend that you consider creating a category that describes the overlap itself.

Perspectives 10.1. The Pros and Cons of Frequency Counting

"I can share two experiences from qualitative studies I completed recently, one where I used frequency counts and another where I decided that they were a bad idea. The first study involved examining counselors' attitudes toward, and actions related to, social justice advocacy in their work with clients, wherein I assessed responses from 206 counselors (see Hays, Chang, & Chaney, 2011). In this study, I computed frequency counts for each of the responses. Since there were so many participants in this study (and thus so many data) who were fairly representative of various demographic variables, work settings, and disciplines, I felt it would be me more helpful to the reader to present the findings in counts to illustrate the frequency of various social advocacy attitudes and actions. In essence, the findings served as a needs assessment for working with practitioners and training students to remove barriers to social advocacy in their communities.

"For the second study (Hays, Cole, et al., 2011), I could not imagine conducting frequency counts. I worked with a group of adolescents ages 12–14 and discussed their conceptualizations of healthy dating relationships and experiences with dating violence. Given that there was a small group of participants (n = 7) with very diverse experiences and feelings toward unhealthy relationships (dating and otherwise), I felt it was important to portray their stories rather than count the most frequent responses. Thus, I felt that no one's experiences (no matter how common they were) were more valuable to presenting the findings."

—DGH

"I also have two stories that readily come to mind regarding frequency counting. In a mixed methods study of social justice advocacy by counseling psychology trainees on internship (Singh, Hofhess, et al., 2010), we solicited quantitative and qualitative data through an online survey. Our research team went back and forth about the pros and cons of using frequency counting with the qualitative responses. After an initial look at the data, we identified large domains and subcategories that were consistent throughout the qualitative responses. In the end, we decided not to use frequency counting because of our small sample size (n = 40) and in order to stay true to our participants' voices.

"In other phenomenological examinations I have conducted of resilience in historically marginalized groups (Singh, Hays, Chung, & Watson, 2010; Singh, Hays, & Watson, 2011) I would not say that I used the traditional definition of frequency counting. However, I did count the number of participant responses that may not have been shared by all participants, but were shared by a majority of participants. Because both of these studies examined new areas of inquiry—South Asian American survivors of sexual abuse and transgender people—I wanted to make sure that we communicated as much information as we could to our 'audience members' about their experiences in the hopes that future research will examine these topics in more depth."

—AAS

Take a Vacation

Take time off from your data. That's right! You have probably realized by this point that qualitative data collection and analysis (and we haven't even gotten to data management yet) are time-consuming and require a lot of reflection. With any complex research project, you can start to lose your focus and thus may not be able to thoughtfully arrive at patterns and themes, brainstorm about future data collection methods, or revise your conceptual framework and/or theory. Taking time off from data does not necessarily have to mean not focusing on some aspect of the project: For example, you may want to take some time off and read some new literature on the topic or develop stronger relationships with participants and settings. We all have unique work styles, so the amount of time needed will vary by individual.

Member Checking, Revisited

We come back to member checking, as we have in our discussion of data collection methods, to remind you of the importance of including participant voices in qualitative analysis. Participants can be helpful during several qualitative analysis steps, including having them review initial codes and patterns individually or in focus groups, as well as the Results section of the final report. As qualitative researchers, it is a professional and ethical responsibility to be transparent with participants as to how we arrived at a particular coding system, and to have them provide judgments on that system to the extent relevant. In sum, we encourage continued dialogue with participants, from initial data collection to the final qualitative report.

ADDITIONAL "GENERIC" STRATEGIES OF QUALITATIVE DATA ANALYSIS

In the final section of qualitative data analysis we discuss three other labels for the coding process we have encountered in the clinical and education literature. Specific data analysis processes and strategies for various research traditions are presented in Chapter 11. We do not claim that the two "generic" strategies we cover are exhaustive; however, we have seen them applied to a variety of research traditions. These include content analysis and attributional coding.

Content Analysis

Content analysis, a process of examining content and themes in written documents, is a popular term we have seen in several qualitative studies (and some quantitative studies) used interchangeably (likely erroneously) with the coding process described above. However, there are some unique features of content analysis. It generally involves unobtrusive data sources (see Chapter 9), often using data that were previously collected *not* for research purposes. Additionally, frequency counting is an integral part of content analysis, and thus findings are amenable to statistical procedures.

Insch and colleagues (1997) identified 11 cyclical steps for conducting a content analysis, which we highlight in Table 10.4. You will likely note that many of these steps parallel those of our general data analysis steps. However, there are some minor differences. First, the developers emphasize the importance of creating a strong coding scheme with pilot data before more extensive data collection. Second, there is greater attention to reliability and validity.

Insch and colleagues (1997) noted several benefits of content analysis. These include potential for high reliability; use of qualitative and quantitative approaches; typically unobtrusive, which minimizes participant reactivity bias; and use of a priori codes. Some challenges, however, have also been noted. First, researcher bias, as in other data analysis strategies, occurs in the type and form of data selected for analysis, and coding schemes (codebooks) are biased in that there is no way to confirm the universality of codes or themes. The second major cluster of challenges relates to what to code once data are selected. Specifically, these involve assigning weight to codes (i.e., do codes carry equal values in a codebook?), assessing the value of missing data, and inattention to nonverbal cues and insufficient attention to other contextual information.

TABLE 10.4. Content Analysis Steps

Steps	Characteristics
1. Identify research questions and constructs.	Review the literature to articulate research questions and important concepts or words to be counted.
2. Identify texts to be examined.	Determine which texts or data sources are appropriate for the phenomenon of interest (i.e., **source validity**).
3. Specify the unit of analysis.	Unit of analysis can be a word, phrase, sentence, paragraph, or entire document. Selection should be based on consideration of the study purpose.
4. Specify the categories.	Chunk codes into categories and consider the categories in three ways: single vs. multiple classifications, assumed (a priori) vs. inferred ("emerging") categories, and use of existing content analysis dictionaries.
5. Generate sample coding scheme.	Consider the **face validity** of the category definitions (i.e., researchers' definitions of concepts and the definitions of categories used to evaluate them).
6. Collect data (pretest).	Pretest the coding scheme.
7. Purify the coding scheme.	Examine pilot/pretest results and ensure that those familiar with the words in each category (themes) agree that they have similar meanings or relate to a category similarly (i.e., **semantic validity**).
8. Collect data.	Refer back to Step 2 and collect additional data. Be sure to make adjustments to coding protocol based on text type (e.g., a local newsletter article may be coded differently from a major newspaper article).
9. Assess reliability.	Inadequate reliability may be indicative of an inappropriate coding scheme or codebook.
10. Assess construct validity.	Examine how well themes represent underlying constructs.
11. Analyze data.	Begin data analysis and consider both qualitative and quantitative analysis techniques.

Sources: Insch, Moore, and Murphy (1997) and Weber (1990).

Attributional Coding

Attributional coding involves analyzing public attributions individuals make during spoken or written discourse, indicating their understanding of the causes of various events of interest (Silvester, 1998). There are five major stages of attributional coding. Stage 1 identifies the source of attributions. Typically derived from transcripts of dialogues or written documents, public exchanges are identified based on the relevance to a research question. Stage 2 refers to extracting the attributions; that is, identifying a speaker's statements about causes and their consequences. The speaker is defined as the participant of interest. Stage 3 involves identifying agents and targets. Agent–target coding, which is initial coding in attributional coding, means that a researcher analyzes what the speaker states is causing something to happen (agent) and what the impact is (target). Agent–target pairings generally refer to individuals, groups, or entities. Stage 4 is coding attributions on causal dimensions. These dimensions or continua include stable–unstable (permanence of cause of an attribution); global–specific (degree of importance of cause); internal–external (whether a cause of an attribution originates within or outside the speaker); personal–universal (extent that a cause is individual or culturally specific); and controllable–uncontrollable (degree of control a speaker perceives over the cause). Stage 5 involves analyzing data. Readers are encouraged to review Silvester (1998) for additional information on attributional coding.

QUALITATIVE DATA MANAGEMENT

Recall in Chapters 8 and 9 that we began discussing qualitative data management with data collection. Some forms of qualitative data management, such as contact summary sheets, memos, and document summary forms, are applied immediately, as data are collected. As we move forward, you will quickly see that data management is a job in itself, as data will pile up rather quickly! We advise strongly that you develop a data management system early and revise it, as necessary, as you proceed.

Storing Data

While you are likely to develop a data management system that works for you, we would like to provide a few tips. First, we recommend that you format data similarly. Particularly for textual data, structure transcripts, contact sheets, memos, etc., use a template for each. This is especially important if you are working with multiple research team members. In addition, templates make it easier for an external auditor to review your audit trail. In sum, each data source should look as similar as possible, as if only one researcher formatted them.

Second, convert all data (to the extent possible) to electronic format using word processors and scanners and retain the hard copies (or originals) of data. Use binders and tabs for physical copies and an organized computer system for electronic formats. In essence, divide and label your audit trail carefully. (We discussed the contents of an audit trail in Chapter 7.)

Third, you will need a well-organized and secure physical space for storage. Keep physical data, removed from participant identifying information to the extent possible, in a locked file cabinet. Ensure that electronic data are password protected. We recommend that you keep data at least 5–7 years upon completion of a project.

Our final tip relates to managing data during the coding process. As you create codebooks, you may find that you need to cross-reference data sources, even as you keep them separate initially for data analysis. Cross-referencing will be extremely helpful as you make sense of multiple codebooks to develop a main narrative or theory (Step 8). We like to keep a journal or log with memos about the data sources themselves, particularly to jot notes about potential codes that seem to overlap for data sources. Additionally, cross-reference the data sources themselves. For example, it may be important to cross-reference a meeting agenda that a participant mentions during an individual interview.

CASE DISPLAYS

A **case display**, a graphic depiction of reduced (and chunked) data, is one of the most valuable data management tools available. We cannot imagine conducting a qualitative inquiry without displays as part of our initial thinking about research design and throughout data collection and analysis. Case displays are initially created for each individual case (**within-case display**) and then are later consolidated to examine concepts and variables across cases (**cross-case display**) for increased understanding of themes and patterns and to enhance generalizability.

Let's provide an example of how case displays are useful. Say you want to complete a study on the impact of student activities organizations on first-year student retention in a particular university. You interview 15 first-year students, five student organization leaders, and three university administrators. Since the amount of data for these 23 participants will likely become overwhelming, you want to create "snapshots" of each (i.e., within-group displays), identifying variables such as the role and actions associated with participating in student organizations and activities; personal characteristics of participants, including demographics, academic needs, and experience with the university; and the reported satisfaction with student organizations and activities as well as other academic and extracurricular components, to name a few. Upon completion of individual profiles, you may want to group participants with common characteristics (e.g., role, time and duration of participation, gender, major) and look at data collectively (i.e., cross-case display) to address the research question. By individualizing data management, analyzing each data source, and then collapsing this process to examine themes and codes across data sources, you are more likely to develop an organized, easily accessible, and more comprehensive picture of your findings.

Case displays serve four basic yet interconnected purposes: They help qualitative researchers explore, describe, explain, and predict phenomena. By reducing data sources into one display per unit of analysis (let's say, integrating and graphically presenting findings from an individual interview and multiple observations for one participant), qualitative researchers have data and analysis in one place and can likely draw more valid conclusions. Other benefits of data displays are that researchers can absorb large amounts of information quickly, compare different data sets, and make direct use of results in qualitative reports (Miles & Huberman, 1994).

Case displays are formatted using matrices or networks. A matrix format involves using rows and columns to portray major concepts or variables. A network uses points or nodes with links between them. Often, the purpose of a network display is to show causal links or chronology among variables. Your choice of display format will be driven by your research question as well as emerging codes.

You will likely address your research question(s) one case at a time, moving to a more complex answer to your question(s) as you integrate your findings across cases in a cross-case display or displays. With cross-case displays, data usually are oriented by case or variable, although we recommend that you combine these strategies. These orientations can be presented using matrices or networks. Case-oriented displays focus on (1) structuring individual cases similarly to see if they match previous ones (Yin, 1984), (2) analyzing each case for essential components and presenting these components in a particular order in a larger display (Denzin, 1989), or (3) clustering cases that are similar and can be considered to be a "family" of cases (Lofland & Lofland, 1995). Variable-oriented cross-case displays involve looking for themes that cut across cases (Miles & Huberman, 1994). Similar to Yin's strategy with case-oriented displays, the goal is to synthesize similar components.

Miles and Huberman (1994) wrote extensively about the use of case displays as an analysis tool. We highlight some basic information about various types and purposes of case displays, and we encourage you to review their text for a more thorough coverage of the displays. Table 10.5 includes some general strategies for developing and interpreting case displays, and Table 10.6 shows common approaches to case displays.

Exploring and Describing Data Using Case Displays

Whether you are interested in developing a within-case or cross-case display, there are some basic types of displays used for *exploring and describing* data. These include partially ordered, time-ordered, role-ordered, and conceptually ordered displays. For each of these displays, it is important to construct a narrative to "tell the story" for a case or across cases. This narrative will help in future data analysis as well as in report writing.

Partially Ordered Displays

Partially ordered displays are quite useful in the initial stages of data analysis, as qualitative researchers can attend to a variable of interest and its subcomponents, as well as look at the various roles of those involved in a particular setting. There are two types of within-case and one type of cross-case partially ordered displays we mention briefly here. The within-case partially ordered displays are the context chart and the checklist matrix. A **context chart** is a network that depicts the interrelationships among those in a particular setting, related to a behavior of interest. Context charts help to identify an underlying meaning of a behavior as the individual associations are mapped out for a particular context (the case). A **checklist matrix** can outline a major variable of interest and compare data from all key respondents. For this display, the case can be considered the variable of interest. A cross-case partially ordered display is the **partially ordered meta-matrix**. This display can be thought of as a "master chart" of descriptive data across all cases. To create this display, cluster all relevant data into major categories.

TABLE 10.5. Case Display Tips

Designing displays

- Be clear about the purpose of your case display: Are you trying to describe a phenomenon or explain one?
- Choose whether you want to display data for an individual case or for multiple cases.
- Decide if order or placement of variables in a display matters. For example, you may find that strength or intensity of themes is important to show.
- Does time have a significant role in your research question(s)? If the ordering of variables is related to time, investigate time-ordered displays to allow for analysis of sequence, flow, causes, and effects.
- Determine how many dimensions your display needs. We have found that most projects are two-dimensional, yet your study may be better suited to a three-dimensional (or more) display.
- Limit to four or five rows for matrices.
- Use both variable- and case-oriented cross-case displays.
- Write down decision rules or criteria for selecting and removing data from displays.

Entering data

- Be clear about the amount and level of data you want to enter in any display. (When in doubt, enter more!)
- Include any of the following in cells or nodes: codes, quotes, summaries, researcher reflections, ratings, or any of these combined.
- Note in the matrix or network when data are missing or unclear.
- Use a coding system to locate important material in original data sources.
- Include a detailed reference to salient quotes, as appropriate.
- Understand each case individually before lumping cases.
- Write a narrative for individual case displays if possible.
- Look for typologies, case "families," or those that cluster easily together due to similar characteristics.

Interpreting data

- Be aware that your display will likely change design as you interpret data.
- Cluster themes.
- Note patterns among themes.
- Investigate further into "deviant" cases (i.e., individual cases that vary from those that are easily synthesized and replicated).

Sources: Mishler (1986) and Miles and Huberman (1994).

Then sort for each cluster and, finally, examine the display for cross-category clustering.

To illustrate these forms of partially ordered displays, consider a study investigating degree of preparedness among counselors and counselor trainees for working with clients involved in unhealthy relationships. Figures 10.5, 10.6, and 10.7 are useful for describing the phenomenon of preparedness. Figure 10.5 on page 320 shows a context chart of the coding process for data from 10 trainees (represented by T followed by an identification number) by 10 researchers (represented by R followed by an identification number), all graduate students at university X, with relationships to the responsible project investigator. Figure 10.6 on page 321 depicts various training components that six key participants have received regarding intervening in unhealthy relationships. (The case or unit of analysis is training experience.) Finally, Figure 10.7 on page 322 uses a matrix format to display participants' conceptualizations of unhealthy relationships.

TABLE 10.6. Case Displays

	Within-case displays	Cross-case displays
Explore and describe		
Partially ordered	Context chart Checklist matrix	Partially ordered meta-matrix
Time ordered	Event listing Critical incident chart Activity record Decision modeling	Scatterplot over time
Role ordered	Role × time matrix	Contrast table Scatterplot
Conceptually ordered	Thematic conceptual matrix Cognitive map Folk taxonomy	Content-analytic summary table Decision tree modeling
Explain and predict		
Effects matrices	Explanatory effects matrix Case dynamics matrix	Case-ordered effects matrix Case-ordered predictor–outcome matrix Variable-by-variable network
Causal networks	Causal network	Cross-case causal network

Source: Miles and Huberman (1994).

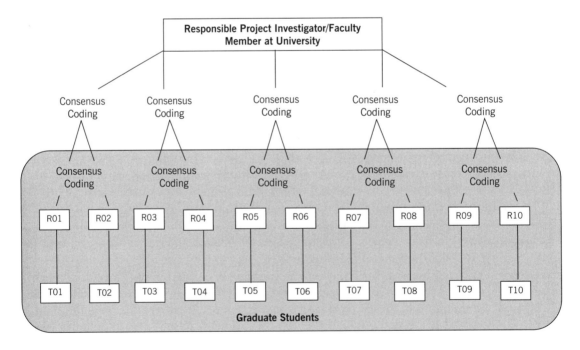

FIGURE 10.5. Context chart of researchers and participants at university *X*. R, researcher; T, trainee.

Training Experiences for Intervening in Unhealthy Relationships						
	T01	T02	T03	T04	T05	T06
Workshop	Yes	No	No	No	No	Yes
Couple Counseling Course	Yes	Yes	Yes	No	No	No
Families Course	Yes	Yes	Yes	Yes	No	Yes
Child/Adolescent Course	No	No	Yes	No	No	No
Internship	No	No	No	Yes	Yes	No
Journals	Yes	Yes	Yes	Yes	Yes	Yes
Books	No	No	Yes	Yes	Yes	Yes

FIGURE 10.6. Checklist matrix of training experiences of six counselor trainees.

Time-Ordered Displays

A **time-ordered display** depicts a sequence or flow of events or processes of a phenomenon of interest. Essentially, it orders data by time and sequence. We highlight four within-case and one cross-case time-ordered displays. The first type of within-case time-ordered display we find helpful is the **event listing**, which organizes a series of events or actions by time periods, and then sorted into categories. This display shows how events are connected to each other. The second type, a **critical incident chart**, is similar to an event listing but limits the display to those events that are particularly salient for each period. Thus, the event listing can be considered more comprehensive overall, whereas the critical incident chart might hit the key points for a particular period of time. The third type, an **activity record**, displays a specific activity from the beginning to final phases or steps, making explicit each detailed step of each phase. The final type of within-case time-ordered display that we highlight is a **decision model**, which can be considered a "decision tree" of yes–no responses regarding the thoughts and actions associated with an activity record. Figure 10.8 on page 323 is an event listing that outlines one school psychologist's participation at three schools in a study of school psychologists' involvement in evaluations in a school system.

We have found one cross-case time-ordered display as helpful in data management and analysis: the **scatterplot over time**. This display provides a picture of a similar variable or concept over two or more time periods. In Figure 10.9 on page 323, the school psychologist was interested in the relationship between number of psychological and educational evaluations for schools in school district *A* and the degree of support for 2 academic years.

Role-Ordered Case Displays

A **role-ordered case display** depicts social interactions for a setting or variable of interest; it provides a "role occupant" view for each key participant (Miles & Huberman, 1994). Thus, the organizing principle for this is participant *role*. We highlight one within-case and two cross-case role-ordered displays that we particularly like, using a

Trainee	Knowledge	Abuse Survivor	Forms of Abuse	Consequences	Client Influences	Participant Influences
T01	Defines as making someone feel unworthy, having limited communication, being at an impasse in a relationship	Female or Male	Physical and emotional	Physical: isolation Psychological: delayed awareness of situation, depression/suicidality, decreased self-esteem, self-blame	Media (television, movies)	States has never been in a violent relationship but sees them "all around" her
T02	Defines as having feelings of not being loved, being unhappy, having negative affect	Female or Male	Physical	Physical: bruises, high blood pressure, chest pains Psychological: loss of focus, stress	None noted	Witnessed domestic violence at age 7 or 8; parents' model of healthy relationship
T03	Refers to as being taken advantage of, not supported, manipulated or controlled, having a loss of identity and being someone "not strong enough" to leave a bad relationship	Female or Male	Physical and emotional	Physical: isolation Psychological: decreased self-esteem (may have already been low), denial, dependency	How they were raised, media, something in their lives making them more vulnerable/ more accepting of relationship problems	Parents as model—it as "never an option"; trying to emulate healthy relationship in own marriage, media (television)
T04	Defines as degradation, putting someone down, having a selfish partner, limiting communication, not valuing, lacking trust and safety, both partners likely have a history of abuse	Female	Physical, emotional, and sexual	Physical: lowered self-esteem	Previous history of trauma, their parents' relationship, culture	Own parents' relationship (they divorced and then entered healthy relationships) "shaped what I wanted"; marriage and family development course taught her about gender differences in communication; watched sister in an unhealthy relationship
T05	Refers to as abusing one another, being obsessive, and lacking trust	Female or Male	Physical, emotional, and sexual	Psychological: emotional harm, low self-esteem, feelings of worthlessness, suicidality, depression, feeling inadequate or incapable	Media (television, movies), friends who have been in a bad relationship	Coursework, own abusive relationship
T06	Involves not being valued, having a power struggle, limiting communication	Female	Physical and emotional	Psychological: dependency, lowered self-esteem, less personal value, degradation of person, personality changes	Family/peer socialization, upbringing, media, cultural acceptance of violence, coping/ resilience, personal factors	Personal and family experiences with violence most salient—"I know in my own life I had a hard time dealing with those types of people"; coursework

FIGURE 10.7. Partially ordered meta-matrix of conceptualization of unhealthy relationships.

School	Aug–Dec 2009	Jan–Apr 2010
Craigen Elementary	• 3 evaluations • 2 students referred to special education classes (7-year-old white female; 9-year-old Latin American male)	• 8 evaluations • No referrals made
Parks Elementary	• 12 evaluations • Consulted with parents for 2 students (8-year-old white male; 8-year-old African American female) regarding remediation • Recommended further psychological testing for 4 students (5-year-old white male; 5-year-old Asian female; 10-year-old African American male; 10-year-old multiracial male)	• 1 evaluation • Continued work with IEP (pending disposition)
Wood Middle School	• 2 evaluations • 1 student pulled into a general classroom (13-year-old multiracial female)	• No evaluations conducted

FIGURE 10.8. Event listing for a school psychologist in school district *A*.

study exploring university administrators' perceptions of the financial aid profession. First, a **role × time matrix** is a within-case role-ordered display that is useful in cases in which *when* something is done is just as important as *who* is doing it. Typically, roles are listed in columns and time periods are listed in rows, or vice versa. Figure 10.10 depicts the administrators' views of the degree to which financial aid officers at university *Z* met job expectations.

The two cross-case displays are the contrast table and the scatterplot. A **contrast table** shows two variables of interest. Figure 10.11 depicts a contrast table examining financial aid officers' job responsibilities and the perceptions from administrators of several colleges and universities. A **scatterplot** displays data from all cases on two or

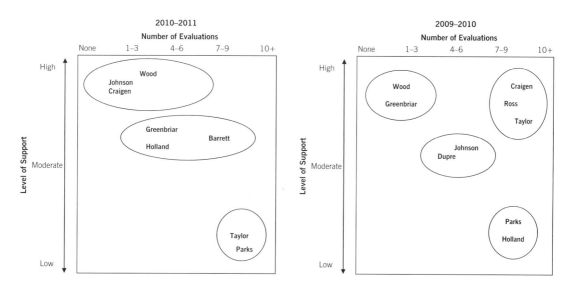

FIGURE 10.9. Scatterplot over time: School evaluations.

Provost	Moderate	High	High	Moderate	High
President	Low	Low	Moderate	Moderate	High
Faculty	Low	Moderate	Moderate	Moderate	Not reported
Graduate Students	Moderate	Moderate	Low	Moderate	High
Undergraduate Students	Low	Low	Low	Moderate	Moderate
	2007–08	2008–09	2009–10	2010–11	2011–12

FIGURE 10.10. Role × time matrix of financial aid officers' job expectations.

	Berry University President	Lane College Dept. Chair	Belle College Provost	Hardy University Dean
Analyze financial information from applicants	Exceeds expectations	Satisfactory	Satisfactory	Unsatisfactory
Develop financial aid policies	Exceeds expectations	Satisfactory	Satisfactory	Unsatisfactory
Coordinate a work–study program	Satisfactory	Unsatisfactory	Satisfactory	Unsatisfactory
Manage financial loan programs	Satisfactory	Unsatisfactory	Exceeds expectations	Unsatisfactory
Prepare detailed financial reports	Unsatisfactory	Unsatisfactory	Exceeds expectations	Unsatisfactory

FIGURE 10.11. Contrast table example of financial aid officers' job ratings.

more dimensions conceptualized as related to each other. Figure 10.12 portrays data for job satisfaction and job ratings regarding 10 financial aid officers.

Conceptually Ordered Case Displays

A **conceptually ordered case display** is helpful when the concept itself is the organizing principle, rather than time periods or roles (Miles & Huberman, 1994). Although any display can "look like" a conceptually ordered one, it must be organized by a concept or variable to be considered one. We have already presented a conceptually ordered display in Chapter 4: the conceptual framework. As you recall, this network portrayed the major nodes of a conceptual framework, including previous literature, personal experience, thought experiments, and pilot or exploratory data.

We highlight three within-case and two cross-case conceptually ordered displays. The within-case displays include a thematic conceptual matrix, a cognitive map, and a folk taxonomy. A **thematic conceptual matrix** portrays data by themes, rather than by individuals or roles. You have already created an example of the second type, the **cognitive map**. Chapter 4 discussed developing components of the conceptual framework, and a conceptual framework (open to revisions as your study progresses) is essentially

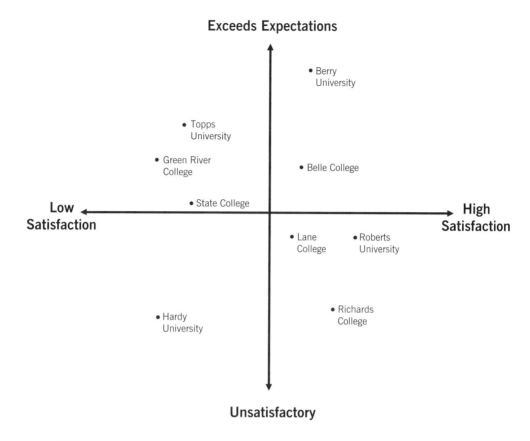

FIGURE 10.12. Scatterplot of job ratings and financial aid officers' job satisfaction.

your thoughts of the important elements that organize your study. Thus, the conceptual framework is an example of a cognitive map. Finally, a **folk taxonomy** is analogous to a hierarchical tree diagram. Miles and Huberman (1994) suggested that a folk taxonomy can be created initially by using a batch of cards; each card has a key code or theme on it. Then the cards are sorted. Figures 10.13 and 10.14 display a thematic conceptual framework and a folk taxonomy for a study examining an agency sexual assault counselor's experience with vicarious traumatization and self-care (Forman, 2009).

The two cross-case displays are the content-analytic summary table and the decision tree model. A **content-analytic summary table** portrays the common elements or factors underlying a phenomenon of interest more so than each case. (In fact, you might not even mention from which cases the content originated.) First, you must determine how many cases share similar characteristics. Then sort each major characteristic and identify how prevalent that characteristic (or subcharacteristic) is in a case. **Decision tree modeling** is used to depict a model or theory of "how something works" by piecing together individual decision trees to show the basic process across several cases. This can be conceptualized as a cross-case decision modeling described earlier in this section. Figure 10.15 pn page 327 depicts a content-analytic summary table of 15 sexual assault counselors' coping strategies. You will note that this is the same type of

Theoretical Aspects	Vicarious Traumatization	Burnout	Self-Care	Work Environment
Components	Intimacy, trust, control	None noted	None noted	None noted
Agency	Frequency of agency discussion—twice per month	Frequency of agency discussion—rarely	Addressed twice per week	Funding concerns, client load high, low salary, supervision inadequate, underlying politics
Others	Frequency of school's acknowledgment—once per year	Frequency of state's acknowledgment—trainings at state and school level	Acknowledgment by others; not addressed at all—had to learn for herself	Involvement of family
Experiences	Dreams, memory, safety changes at work, home, world, travel	Supervisee boundary issues, staff support, too many clients and paperwork	See Coping Strategies	Mention of protection measures—safety concerns
Coping Strategies	None noted	None noted	Education (learning Spanish), reading, and media; use of humor; leisure activities and volunteer work; processing with colleagues; receiving support	Informal and formal training; therapy for counselor

FIGURE 10.13. Thematic conceptual matrix for a sexual assault counselor's experiences.

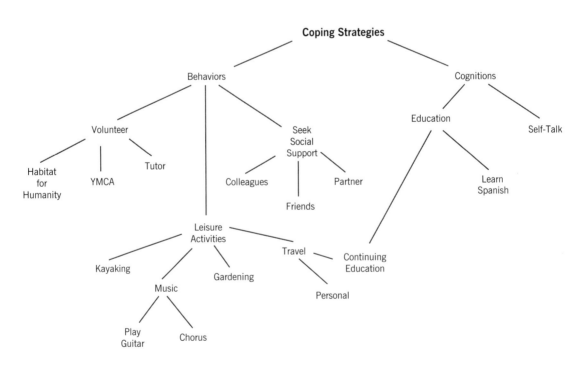

FIGURE 10.14. Folk taxonomy of a sexual assault counselor's self-care strategies.

Volunteer	Leisure	Social Support	Cognitive Strategies
Habitat for Humanity (3) Food Bank (1) YMCA (7) Local schools (6) Tutoring (1)	Kayaking (1) Gardening (2) Traveling to conferences (1) Traveling to other trainings (7) Personal travel (9) Reading (9) Playing guitar (1) Singing (2) Listening to music (12) Exercise (1) None (2)	Colleagues (11) Partner (10) Friends (2) None (3)	Learn Spanish (1) Workshops and seminars (8) Self-talk (13)

FIGURE 10.15. Content-analytic summary table of sexual assault counselors' coping strategies.

content presented by the folk taxonomy in Figure 10.14. (The number in parentheses indicates how many participants reported a particular strategy.)

PROPOSAL DEVELOPMENT 10.3. Creating Case Displays

Based on your research purpose and available data, select two of the case displays used for exploration and description presented here (preferably within-case displays).

- Use your evolving codebook to develop a case display. Memo about your displays.
- Work with your research team members and review each "final" display. What are some recommendations made to alter the display? How, if at all, has the display solidified future data collection? How is this useful for data analysis?
- Now compare the two displays. What are some advantages and disadvantages of each? Are there other displays that might be helpful for your study? Why or why not?
- Continue to develop with pilot data within-case and cross-case displays to describe and explore your findings. Add these displays to your audit trail.

Explaining and Predicting Using Case Displays

Case displays can also play a significant role in theory or model building, a goal of many research traditions and research questions. Displays that are suitable for explanation and prediction often move beyond those that are used for exploring and describing, to make "causal" statements and predictions about descriptive components. The phrase *explaining data* refers to supporting a claim and making causal statements; *predicting data* involves using explanatory statements to estimate what is likely to happen in the future involving which factors for a phenomenon of interest (Miles & Huberman, 1994). Case displays that are used for explanation and prediction are likely to include reference to antecedents, short-term and long-term consequences, and/or predictor and outcome variables. This second form of case display may be categorized as effects matrices and causal networks.

Effects Matrices

We highlight two within-case displays and three cross-case displays that are considered effects matrices. The two within-case displays are explanatory effects matrix and case dynamics matrix. An **explanatory effects matrix** depicts short- and long-term outcomes for a particular variable of interest with a primary purpose of explaining those outcomes. In fact, there is often a column used to note researcher explanations of outcomes. A **case dynamics matrix** traces consequences of outcomes for particularly salient or dynamic issues. In essence, the display depicts the process used to arrive at a particular outcome or outcomes for a particular "dynamic" issue.

To illustrate these effects matrices, consider a program evaluation of a social work program that addressed several initiatives to recruit and retain racial- and ethnic-minority students. This program has run for 3 years. As you can see from Figure 10.16, future programming can be easily inferred from the effects and outcomes of important issues.

The three cross-case effects matrices are case-ordered effects matrix, case-ordered predictor–outcome matrix, and variable-by-variable matrix. A **case-ordered effects matrix** is used when an important "cause" has a variety of results. (This is different from a causal model, discussed in the next section, which highlights a variety of causes for an important outcome.) This matrix focuses on the outcomes that may present themselves as a function of the cases. Cases are sorted for a major cause by intensity, with more intense or strong cases typically presented toward the top of the matrix. Figure 10.17 on page 330 provides an example of the case-ordered effects matrix.

A **case-ordered predictor–outcome matrix** orders cases on a main outcome or criterion variable and provides data for each case on the antecedents for that outcome. Cases are sorted and ordered in the matrix by variable. A **variable-by-variable matrix** has two main variables in its rows and columns, and cell entries are case names. Figure 10.18 depicts a variable-by-variable matrix using the social work program evaluation, highlighting responses from 12 students of color.

Causal Networks

A **causal network** is a display of the most important variables, showing directions and sequences rather than relationships (e.g., the case with displays used to explore and describe). In essence, it is a network of variables or factors with causal connections between them for theory building. A workable concept network usually has three variations: concept A, then concept B; when concept A, always concept B; and another concept links concepts A and B (Miles & Huberman, 1994)

To create a causal network, Miles and Huberman (1994) recommend the following steps: (1) start with whichever factors influence each other, typically those that appear together; (2) determine which variables happen first, later, etc.; (3) rate the importance of each variable in explaining and predicting (e.g., high, moderate, low); (4) determine antecedent variables, mediating variables, and outcomes; (5) construct a narrative; (6)

Initiative	Details	Short-Term Effects	Long-Term Consequences	Researcher's Explanation
Increase professional development mentorship.	Create a diversity interest network. Provide targeted research funding. Recruit racial and ethnic minorities for student leadership positions.	The number of racial- and ethnic-minority students involved in program activities increase. Approximately half of students participate in independent research projects.	Students of color report increased stress and state that they are having difficulty academically. White students perceive they are not as professionally supported.	Faculty not ensuring self-care for students? Students may feel pressure to participate, or afraid to ask for help?
Create a supportive environment.	Address diversity issues in social work curriculum. Invite students to contribute their perspectives in written program materials.	Several white students become more resistant to curriculum. Teacher evaluations decrease.	Cultural tensions develop in the program during the first year. Students of color report increased program satisfaction and a sense of belonging.	Need to address cultural resistance throughout the coursework? Targeted prejudice prevention?
Increase communication.	Present faculty and student expectations regarding diversity issues at monthly meetings. Develop a monthly column in program newsletter that communicates diversity-related issues.	Diversity issues are discussed orally and in writing.	Students of color collaborate with faculty and work with student organizations at a high rate.	Greater communication, greater safety?
Conduct ongoing assessment of students' needs.	Conduct interviews with students at the end of their first semester and again at clinical internship. Assess faculty and administrators' views annually on recruitment and retention issues.	Students of color report feelings of limited mentorship and feeling invisible. They report being grateful for the space to present their voices.	Assessment data reveal that feelings of belonging continue to increase.	The more voice given to participants, the greater sense of belonging.
Build relationships with other social work-related programs.	Develop database on undergraduate and graduate programs for marketing purposes.	Over 100 programs are contacted and presented with marketing materials.	Students of color from national undergraduate programs select the social work graduate program.	Continued networking and creative communication increases the program's reputation as being inclusive.

FIGURE 10.16. An explanatory effects matrix of a social work program evaluation.

Effects	Intense ← Causes Moderate →		Low
Academic difficulty	Students' fear of soliciting assistance	Lack of self-care education	Psychological concerns
Funding disparities	Perceived threats by whites	Limited funding	Fewer white students are seeking funding
Increased prejudice	Lack of prejudice prevention education	Recent racialized event in program	Limited communication among students and faculty

FIGURE 10.17. A case-ordered effects matrix of recruitment and retention initiatives.

Initiatives	Strategies	Enrollment	Curriculum	Climate	Professional Development Activities
Professional Development Opportunities	Diversity interest network Funding	Elle	Mary Chris Rebecca	Claudine Thomas	Rebecca Maya
Support	Curriculum changes Student voice in materials	Cynthia James	Maya	Martin	Todd Elle
Assessment	Interviews Faculty surveys	Thomas	Amos		Amos

FIGURE 10.18. A variable-by-variable matrix of changes resulting from program.

refer back to existing theory and research about connections among variables; and (7) solicit feedback from participants, research team members, and auditors.

Figure 10.19 presents a causal network for a cross-case display. This display explores privilege and oppression awareness of counselor trainees (see Hays et al., 2004) and depicts which variables create changes in levels of individuals' awareness.

A variation of the causal network for cross-case displays is the **cross-case causal network**. This display allows for a comparative analysis of individual cases, using the most influential variables accounting for a particular outcome as the organizing principle. This display rates antecedents found across cases and links variables and processes.

 ACTIVITY 10.4. Reviewing Case Displays

There are a lot of case displays from which to select when managing and analyzing qualitative data, many more than we had space to cover in this chapter. In small groups, review the various types of case displays and compare them. What are their respective purposes? What are advantages and disadvantages of each?

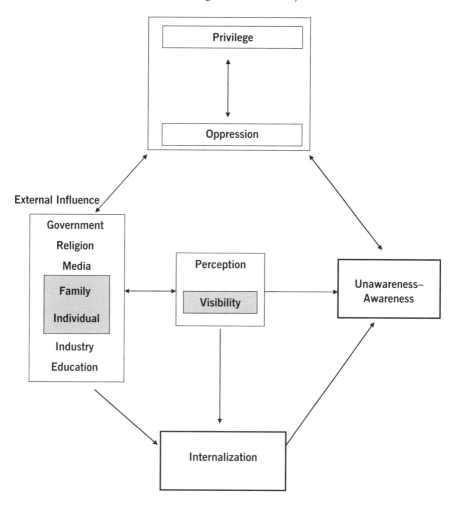

FIGURE 10.19. A causal network of developing privilege and oppression awareness. *Source*: Hays, Chang, and Dean (2004). Reprinted with permission from the American Counseling Association.

Postscript: Developing a "Theory"

How do you know when you have constructed an ideal display, useful for explaining and predicting a phenomenon of interest? That is, how do you judge if you have a good theory or model in front of you? When do you stop analyzing and presenting data within a source and across sources? When have you addressed your research question(s) sufficiently? Is a "final" framework, model, or theory acceptable?

   First, a good "theory" in qualitative inquiry can be defined as one that can be applied to several cases (Glaser, 1978). As you construct within-case displays and integrate them to create cross-case displays, you may notice that the core explanation of what is going on is almost universal across individuals. Although there may be variations in how codes and themes are expressed, all cases typically possess common categories. Second, a sound theory will seem to connect "disorderly data," whereby carefully labeled codes, and the placement and sequencing of those codes, seem to glue the data together to explain and predict data for a research question. In essence, a theory references two requisite causality components: time and sequence. Finally, a sound theory is open to change and is modifiable (Glaser, 1978). Since qualitative findings are contextual and involve a particular set of data, a theory should be developed to represent the fluid nature of a phenomenon of interest.

So, create a theory but understand the limitations of that theory. Your model or theory may be strengthened by conducting similar investigations across different contexts, as you work to disconfirm a present theory. Recall from Chapter 7 that important strategies of trustworthiness involve negative case analysis and triangulation of multiple researchers, data sources, data methods, and theories to investigate a phenomenon. These strategies are quite useful when presenting your model or theory. We caution, however, that even with methodological rigor and good intentions, a theory is undoubtedly open to scrutiny (see Wild Card 10.2).

⚠ WILD CARD 10.2. POTENTIAL CHALLENGES IN THEORY DEVELOPMENT

In our own as well as our students' and colleagues' qualitative investigations over the past several years, we have noted some common challenges that seriously impact a study's rigor. We present some of them here and hope that you will solicit outside feedback (e.g., peer debriefer, research team, auditor, existing theories and scholarship) before preparing and developing a theory for a particular research question.

- Theory development when our research tradition(s) and research question(s) do not support it as a goal

- Use of data that are not adequate or sufficient to explain or predict

- Failure to return to the literature to confirm that there are no existing theories or models that already explain the "emerging" theory

- Too much attention to ambiguous data

- Construction of a scenario or narrative to force a sequence or order to emerging data

- Assignment of causal explanations to random events

- Failure to consult others who do not have a vested interest in the study being published

---

QUALITATIVE SOFTWARE

Since the 1970s qualitative software has continued to evolve from single-text file coding and retrieval programs to more elaborate multiple texts and media files for theory building and "quasi-coding" programs (Grbich, 2007). Furthermore, software to assist in the transcription of data is available. Finally, we cannot forget about the software right at our desks, the word-processing program. Word-processing software accommodates everything from data management and storage (e.g., creating displays, developing transcripts) to initial coding (e.g., inserting comments in margins, using "Find" option to search for word frequencies).

Below we present software related to various phases of the qualitative research process. Miles and Huberman (1994) highlighted some key questions that may be useful in selecting qualitative software (see pp. 313–315 in their text). These questions include: (1) What kind of computer user are you? (Are you new to computers or able to manage complex software?), (2) what kind of database and project are involved? (How many data sources and cases are you working with?), and (3) what kind of analysis is anticipated? (Are you exploring or confirming phenomena, using single or multiple classification, intending to display findings, and wanting to blend quantitative data into findings?) Upon reflecting on these questions, you may find that qualitative software is not for you, and that's okay! We just ask that you educate yourself about the functions and types of qualitative software before making that decision. Table 10.7 presents some of the common functions of qualitative software. We highlight the types of software in the remainder of this section.

Transcription Software

Transcription software can be an invaluable resource for you, particularly if you have several interviews to transcribe or memos and field notes to develop. *Dragon Naturally-Speaking* (*www.nuance.com*) is probably the most well-known speech recognition software. It allows you to talk to your computer (at a normal pace) or use handheld recorders and watch what is said appear on your computer monitor! The software is available in three versions that allow you to do computer tasks (e.g., surf the Internet, write e-mails) with your voice commands.

TABLE 10.7. Functions of Qualitative Software

- Composing field notes and memos
- Transcribing interviews or other data sources
- Developing contact summary sheets, document summary forms, or other data collection templates
- Storing text
- Coding key words, phrases, or sentences
- Searching and retrieving codes and key phrases
- Linking data across files
- Displaying data in matrices, charts, graphs, or networks
- Counting frequencies of codes
- Building theory
- Preparing proposals and writing reports

Express Scribe is audio playback software to assist with audio recordings (*www.nch. com.au*). It is designed to be used with the Dragon NaturallySpeaking software, although it may be used without it. Express Scribe is free to download, and there is an optional foot pedal for purchase. Express Scribe works with word-processing applications to give you control of transcription tasks. Additional information can be found at *www.nch.com. au/scribe/index.html*.

Coding Software

There are many coding software options available. If you want to simply tag codes and categories in a text document and do more of the coding process online, you can do so with coding and retrieval programs. If you want to compare several different documents and files at the same time and use the programs to generate theory and/or conceptual networks as well as address some issues of validity and reliability, you can select theory generation programs. Finally, if you are interested strictly in computing word and category frequencies for textual documents, a content analysis program might be right for you.

Ethnograph v6 (*www.qualisresearch.com*) is a common coding and retrieval program that allows you to perform several functions with written text. It allows you to code imported data files, segment text, create a codebook, do a single-code or linked-code search within documents, and write memos. Two tutorials are available online that make this user-friendly software.

Atlas.ti 5.0 (*www.atlasti.com*) is a theory generation program that also has the capabilities of coding and retrieval programs. With this software you can input word processing, spreadsheets, PowerPoints, sound files, video files, and many graphics files. It allows you to code, create patterns, build models, and work with multiple files at once for both text and visual data. It comes with two manuals and provides online demonstrations and several examples of the program's capabilities at the website.

NVIVO 8 (*www.qsr.com*) serves similar functions as Atlas.ti 5.0, allowing for coding, retrieving, indexing, and theory building. It also supports various data sources, including audio, video, word-processing documents, PDFs, and photos. The software allows you to create "mini-transcripts" or memos as you review visual data; use coding tools to tab "nodes"; create "Sets" to link sources or codes; display findings in text, charts, or models; and export files to web pages. As with other software, there are plenty of tutorials available online.

QDA Miner 2.0 (*www.provalisresearch.com*) is a content analysis software that allows files to include up to 2,030 variables. It works with two other software programs from the Provalis Research Company, *WordStat* (text-mining capabilities) and *SimStat* (statistical analysis capabilities). QDA Miner 2.0 also allows for computing interrater reliabilities. The website provides tutorials of the software and allows for a 30-day free trial period. Lewis and Maas (2007) provide an excellent review of this software.

HyperRESEARCH (*www.researchware.com*) was introduced in 1991 and functions primarily as a coding and retrieval service. Some of the software capabilities include autocoding, memoing, theory building, and code mapping. Additionally, the software works with multiple media. The website provides a free version to download without a time limit.

Challenges of Qualitative Software

If you investigate qualitative computer software options, try them, and do not fall in love with them, you are not alone. In fact, several challenges have been documented related to the use of software (see Fielding & Lee, 1991; Grbich, 2007). First, the notion of software for qualitative research implies increased control and manipulation. This increased structure may create a scenario wherein a computer program influences our understanding of the phenomenon of interest as we decontextualize data for software compliance purposes. As Grbich (2007) noted:

> In creating computer tools for the management of data, we cannot avoid shaping both the outcomes of our data interpretation and our perceptions of the outcomes. Each tool creates artifacts and metaphors (frames) which are not neutral in effect and which change our ways of thinking and seeking. "Reality" has to be segmented, truncated and textured to prepare data to "fit" a particular form of programming. (p. 230)

Relatedly, a second challenge is that as we rely on software to assist with qualitative inquiry, we decrease the interactive nature of research design proposed by Maxwell (2005; see Part II of this text). Using various framing processes mandates segmenting text at very early stages of data analysis, creating a very linear coding process for the steps described earlier in this chapter. It is harder to go back and recode and examine pattern codes if the data are stripped so early from their context.

A third challenge is that qualitative software, particularly programs that assist in theory generation and concept networking, minimize the gap between quantitative and qualitative research. In essence, recent software programs (e.g., NVIVO 8, Atlas. ti) interface with quantitative software programs (e.g., Statistical Package for the Social Sciences [SPSS]) to allow for statistical analyses. On the surface, this may seem to help legitimize the value of qualitative research. However, there are significant conceptual differences between these two research approaches that impact sampling techniques, sample size, and degree of variable control that do not create parallel data. So, using qualitative data for quantitative interpretation can create a scenario wherein qualitative findings appear statistically insignificant and thus to some critics not as important as quantitative findings.

Grbich (2007) notes another challenge: Qualitative software programs that allow computer-to-computer or person-to-computer communication are *not* analogous to face-to-face consensus coding. Reviewing data in person is a spontaneous and interactive process that develops findings in a very different way from the structured and (often time-delayed) consensus process involved in computer use.

A final challenge is the reputation and increased visibility of qualitative computer software. Software companies highlight features of new and/or updated software that can handle massive amounts of data, compute frequencies across multiple data files, interface with quantitative methods, and so forth. The message is clear to us: Qualitative research can be quick and easy to do, and more and more data can be considered. However, we believe that more technology is not necessarily good news. It may encourage what Fielding and Lee (1991) label as "quick and dirty research," with overinterpretation and abuse of software capabilities. And, those of us who may not be comfortable with computer software may find that it takes more time to use these programs than not.

CHAPTER SUMMARY

Qualitative data analysis is an integral component of qualitative inquiry in clinical and educational settings; it is constantly linked to qualitative data collection. We introduced qualitative data management strategies beginning in Chapter 8 and continue the discussion here to show the value of case displays in qualitative data analysis.

While various research traditions present their own analysis methods, we present eight steps of qualitative data analysis that seem to be found across research traditions (even though they may be labeled differently for the research traditions). The steps include (1) reducing data, (2) collecting data, (3) memoing and summarizing, (4) organizing text, (5) coding, (6) identifying themes and patterns, (7) creating a codebook, and (8) developing a main narrative or theory. These steps are appropriate for textual and visual data sources.

Several coding considerations were also presented, including a description of analytic induction procedures, consensus coding, and establishing reliability; debates about whether to use frequency counts; single versus multiple codes or classifications; the importance of taking a break from data; and the importance of using member checking during data analysis steps. Finally, related to data analysis, content analysis and attributional coding were discussed as two "generic" forms of qualitative data analysis.

Case displays are data management tools that allow for exploring, describing, explaining, and predicting phenomena. This chapter presented multiple examples of case displays as well as tips for developing them.

The chapter ended with a brief presentation of qualitative software. There are several functions of software, and various software programs perform various operations on your data. We presented some common examples of transcription and coding software, as well as general challenges to qualitative software to help you make an informed decision regarding what (if any) software is appropriate to use for your study.

RECOMMENDED READINGS

Grbich, C. (2007). *Qualitative data analysis: An introduction.* Thousand Oaks, CA: Sage.

Insch, G. S., Moore, J. E., & Murphy, L. D. (1997). Content analysis in leadership research: Examples, procedures, and suggestions for future use. *Leadership Quarterly, 8*(1), 1–25.

Miles, M. B., & Huberman, A. M. (1994). *Qualitative data analysis: An expanded sourcebook.* Thousand Oaks, CA: Sage.

Poland, B. D. (1995). Transcription quality as an aspect of rigor in qualitative research. *Qualitative Inquiry, 1*(3), 290–310.

CHAPTER 11

Qualitative Data Analysis by Research Tradition

CHAPTER PREVIEW

In this chapter we review the approach of each qualitative research tradition to data analysis. We begin the chapter with some general thoughts about data analysis across the research traditions. Then we examine qualitative data analysis across the five research tradition clusters discussed in Chapter 2 (see Figure 11.1). We begin our review with the "universal" tradition in qualitative designs: the case study. The four remaining clusters involve traditions that address experience and theory formulation, those that investigate the meaning of symbol and text, approaches that explore cultural expressions of process and experience, and the tradition that views research as a change agent. With each tradition, we highlight the similarities and differences among data analysis approaches. We also include several case examples to bring to life what data analysis "looks like" for each research tradition. We refer to researcher reflexivity in data analysis across the clusters; you may want to return to our in-depth discussion of researcher reflexivity in Chapter 5. At the end of the chapter, Table 11.10 summarizes data analytic approaches across the research traditions.

GENERAL THINKING ON QUALITATIVE DATA ANALYSIS ACROSS TRADITIONS

So, you have collected your data—hooray! We also know that this is the moment when the panic can really start to set in. We have already discussed the importance of inviting recursivity into the ways you collect and analyze your data. However, before we get started on our review of data analysis in each of the research traditions, let's revisit this "panic" for a moment. There are so many things embedded within this feeling. You want to "stay true" to your participants. You are quite possibly (and hopefully) immersed in your study's data. You may even have come to care about your participants and/or feel a sense of injustice or a desire for justice based on your participants' stories. Or you might

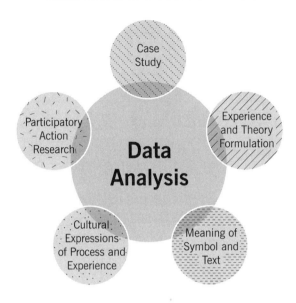

FIGURE 11.1. Qualitative data analysis by research tradition.

just be feeling the need to make your dissertation a "done" dissertation. Regardless of why the panic is there, just know that it is a pretty natural part of analyzing data. By now, you know we like top 10 lists, so see Table 11.1 for suggestions to remember before we dive into the specifics of qualitative data analysis for various research traditions.

Another general thought on data analysis is that *you should have a data analysis plan.* You can call it a strategy—it might even feel like a "plan of battle" at times (although we think it is always best to not position yourself as a researcher "opposite" of your data but find ways to work *with* your data). Establish your data analysis plan ahead of time and closely align your data analysis activities with this plan. Often this plan includes developing a codebook of some kind (introduced in Chapter 10), where you track the large domains and categories of data, in addition to the subcategories and subdomains of your data.

Also, remember to not lose sight of how your theoretical framework is a lens through which to view your data as you engage in analysis. For example, in our phenomenological study of the resilience of child sexual abuse survivors, we had a feminist and critical theory framework (Singh, Hays, et al., 2010). So, we had a solid data analysis plan. However, as we conducted data analysis, we continually invited our research paradigms into this analysis. The question we asked ourselves was "How true are we being to our theoretical framework?" In this study, this question translated into the extent to which our data analysis focused on themes of empowerment and acknowledgment of contextual factors and experiences of privilege and/or oppression—exactly what our theories demanded we do in our data analysis.

Before we delve into the distinct methods of data analysis within each tradition, we emphasize the "generic" steps of qualitative data analysis presented in Chapter 10. Additionally, Miles and Huberman (1994) provide a list of common features of qualitative data analysis among the research traditions:

TABLE 11.1. Top 10 List for Qualitative Data Analysis

When you feel the panic start to take over, remember that you dog-eared this page so you can reread this list (and engage in some deep breathing) to get back on track. Many of these tips are reminders from previous chapters.

1. Data do not "emerge." We are researchers who "identify" findings. Acknowledge your researcher role and how your biases and assumptions influence how you analyze data.

2. The point above is actually a good thing. We are researchers for a reason—we bring expertise to the data analysis. We are experts on our participants' data. We can (and should) own this if we are to be able to communicate our findings to an audience postanalysis in the most effective way.

3. It's not always possible to form one, but remember that a research team increases the quality of your data analysis. Try not to go solo on data analysis.

4. Multiple sources of data require multiple ways to analyze them. Many of these methods we discuss in this chapter. However, the qualitative field evolves and grows constantly. Read this book—*and* consider any new ways of analyzing data based on your field.

5. Think about how you "think" best, and talk about how this style or process is in common, or not, with your research team members. You don't want differences in style to be a barrier to your data analysis process.

6. Remember that it's best to try to disprove and "argue" with your data along the way to ensure that you are doing the best possible data analysis.

7. Be creative. Sometimes you will be challenged in how to proceed with data analysis. This can actually be useful as long as you are not just making things up to make the process easy or to take a shortcut, and are straying incredibly far from your theory and research tradition (which both guide you in your data analysis).

8. Take a vacation from your data analysis and you will often come back "fresh" to see your data in a new light.

9. When you get stuck, revisit your data again and again ... and again. Your participants' voices will often point to your path out of the quicksand.

10. Be familiar and have some facility with the range of data analysis techniques across research traditions. You may borrow from a few different traditions. Again, this shouldn't happen just because you don't know what else to do, but rather because you have a solid rationale for doing so, and the techniques help you understand, interpret, and communicate your findings most effectively.

1. Affixing codes to a set of field notes drawn from observations or interviews

2. Noting reflections or other remarks in the margins

3. Sorting and sifting through these materials to identify similar phrases, relationships between variables, patterns, themes, distinct differences between subgroups, and common sequences

4. Isolating these patterns and processes, commonalities and differences, and taking them out to the field in the next wave of data collection

5. Gradually elaborating a small set of generalizations that cover the consistencies discerned in the database

6. Confronting those generalizations with a formalized body of knowledge in the form of constructs or theories. (p. 91)

You will notice that similar processes are described with different terms in the different research traditions. Honestly, this used to frustrate us! Now, we see it actually as a comfort. Each research tradition is undergirded with a particular philosophical bent—and this does and *should* emerge in how data analysis is described within each one. We think that the best way to learn the most about the research tradition that is best for your research project is to get to know all of the various differences and similarities across the research traditions. A helpful way to learn them is to take your research topic and situate them in each of the research traditions. We have several activities in which you can apply data analysis in research traditions and get a true "feel" for the ways each distinctly approaches analyzing data. Let's get started!

QUALITATIVE DATA ANALYSIS
WITH THE UNIVERSAL TRADITION: THE CASE STUDY

We have discussed previously the unique position the case study has in qualitative research as the "universal" tradition. Case studies are most often used when a researcher seeks to understand a phenomenon for which there is no in-depth understanding at that point in time (Creswell, 2006). Case studies are "bounded systems"—that is, they have boundaries of time, place, and other delineations (Yin, 2008). Therefore, the researcher tends to have multiple sources of data about the processes within the case study, and thus multiple decisions to make about how to approach data analysis (Schwandt, 2001). These multiple decisions, however, should be guided by the *case* itself and not by the many factors surrounding and/or involved in the case. This is one of the largest challenges in qualitative data analysis with the case study research tradition. It can be tempting to veer off in many interesting directions, which, although interesting, may not illuminate the case itself.

A good way to stay on track with data analysis is to remember what led you to study the case in the first place. The case study strategy is "preferred when the inquirer seeks answers to how or why questions, when the inquirer has little control over events being studied, when the object of study is a contemporary phenomenon in a real-life context, when boundaries between the phenomenon and the context are not clear, and when it is desirable to use multiple sources of evidence" (Schwandt, 2001, p. 23).

So, if you are examining a single case of an immigrant Latina woman living with bulimia and her treatment outcomes in a residential treatment center, there will be numerous "pulls" on you as a researcher to examine the variables influencing the case—such as the family or the media—rather than the case itself. This does not mean you should limit your analysis of numerous data sources. For instance, you may conduct interviews with the participant herself, the family, and her treatment team of counselors and physicians, among others. However, when you begin analyzing data in these interviews that take you away from the case itself, be sure to come back to the research question guiding your case study.

Stake (1995) discussed four major forms of data analysis with case study designs. First, there is **categorical aggregation**, where you examine several occurrences for critical incidents, concerns, and issues within the data you have collected. For our sample study above, the researcher may create broad categories of influences on the Latina woman that have meaning for the case itself. For instance, in interviews with treatment team members, the Latina woman, and her family, you may identify broad categories of media influence, peer relationships, religious influences, family dynamics, cultural factors, and negative self-concept.

Distinct from the first is the second form of case study data analysis—**direct interpretation**—the researcher directly interprets the meaning of a singular critical incident, concern, or issue within the data. This process is similar to taking a single puzzle piece and carefully analyzing this data for meaning before interpreting it within the whole case for its meaning. For our sample study, this could mean taking an influence on the case or a chronological event—the family's decision to participate in family counseling within her treatment plan, for instance—and separating that critical incident from the case itself to examine its meaning, then placing this meaning within the context of the meaning it lends to the case as a whole.

The third form of data analysis Stake (1995) discussed is **pattern identification**, wherein the researcher examines broad categories within the case for their relationships or interactions. Returning to our sample study, say the researcher has used direct interpretation of the family's participation in their daughter's family counseling treatment plan, and the researcher has also identified the participation of the Latina participant's partner in couple counseling. From the data collected, the researcher might elect to examine the data from the family counseling and the couple counseling (e.g., critical incidents, broad categories) in terms of their impact on the case. In the fourth form of case study data analysis, **naturalistic generalization**, the researcher actively interprets the data with an eye toward the ways an audience would be able to transfer or apply the broad categories or findings from the case study to another case(s). With our example of a Latina woman living with disordered eating, naturalistic generalization may include identifying influences on healing and recovery from disordered eating that are rooted in cultural factors.

Creswell (2006) supplemented Stake's (1995) suggestions for case study data analysis with two additions. First, he recommended that if the researcher notes a chronological sequence of events in a case to use this sequence to guide data analysis. A good example of this type of data analysis was used in Murphy-Berman, Berman, and Melton's (2008) examination of child abuse and neglect in South Carolina. The researchers used a multiple case study design to explore a sequence of three critical incidents or events in a large child abuse and neglect prevention program in three different communities in South Carolina.

Creswell (2006) also encouraged case study researchers to analyze the **case description** itself—the details and facts of the case. The tendency in case study data analysis can be to identify the major findings that help an audience understand the phenomenon, its boundaries, and its context more fully—but leave out some of the important details. If you take that approach, it is challenging to "paint a full picture" of the case. So, describe the case—how would you "tell the story" of your data based on your analysis. Remember, this shouldn't be a magazine article about your case, but it should include the most salient facts and details of the case. Returning to our sample case study of a Latina woman in treatment for bulimia, the details and facts would probably include her diagnosis, her presenting issues, the duration of her treatment, the major "players" in her treatment, in addition to demographic details such as her age, socioeconomic status, and so forth.

Yin (2008) outlined four principles to guide researchers in case study data analysis. First, the researcher should ensure that all data relevant to the case(s) have been the subject of analysis. A good gut check with this principle is to ask yourself "What data have I ignored and/or neglected to analyze that might contribute to the understanding of this case(s)?" Second, Yin asserted that rigorous case study data analysis should maintain not just the findings that are congruent with one another, but also search out what we discussed before as negative case analysis. The gut check question here is "What in my analysis of this case(s) is indicating a finding that appears to go against major identified findings?"

Third, Yin (2008) gave the researcher permission to highlight the most significant, meaningful findings of the case study in the process of analysis. This point aligns with our previous caution to "stay on course" with understanding your case—as opposed to veering down interesting (but perhaps not as important) roads in data analysis that take you further away from understanding the boundaries of your case rather than bringing you closer to this understanding. Another cautionary note here: Try not to lose the rich complexity and trustworthiness of your data analysis in this process (Drisko, 1997). The gut check question for the researcher here is "Does my analysis reflect the most important findings I have identified in the case?" Finally, Yin advised that the researcher *must* rely on and use his or her previous knowledge (which could be considered expertise) about the case to drive the analysis forward. This might be the most complex of his principles for case study data analysis. It is not enough to "just observe" the various data of a case study. The researcher brings him- or herself to the data analysis—and should embrace, own, and consider how to use this perspective to produce the highest possible quality of analysis. The gut check question here is "Where am I leaving my expertise as a researcher out of the data analysis?"

Data analysis methods in case study research are inductive because the researcher does not know what the important research challenges of theoretical issues will be before the research commences (Paulus, Horvitz, & Shi, 2006). Therefore, it can be challenging to predict the time necessary to complete case study data collection and analysis. Reis and Diaz (1999) used a case study method to examine academically successful urban female students for a time span of 2½ years. Not every case study, of course, will take this long. What is important about this study is that the research tradition, question, and data collection and analysis process required this amount of time to achieve the researchers' ultimate goal of describing a case. This particular study also used a blend of analytic techniques across grounded theory (e.g., using axial and selective coding and saturation of the data, which we discuss in the next section).

A first step of case study data analysis often involves a "bounding of the data" (Paulus et al., 2006, p. 366). Based on the suggestions by Stake (1995), Creswell (2006), and Yin (2008), we believe that case study data analysis should strive for a balance of presenting the major facts of a case with a complexity of findings and interpretation that will illuminate prior misunderstandings and/or lack of information about a case and delineate the case from the context in which it resides. We also believe that there is a balance between drowning in the multiple sources of data you have collected and conducting a general analysis of all these sources, and coming up for air and relying on your qualitative data analysis skills. It's okay to trust in yourself and your own expertise to guide qualitative data analysis. Just make sure that you are answering our "gut check" questions along the way! See Activity 11.1 to put some of these questions into action with case study data analysis.

ACTIVITY 11.1. "Gut Check" Questions for Case Study Data Analysis

In your research team, take your research topic (whether it is a case study design or not) and consider it within a case study design. You are looking at the data you have collected and analyzed. Answer the following questions with regard to your data analysis:

1. What data have I ignored and/or neglected to analyze that might contribute to the understanding of this case(s)?
2. What, in my analysis of this case(s), indicates a finding that appears to go against major identified findings?
3. Does my analysis reflect the most important findings I have identified in the case?
4. Where am I leaving my expertise as a researcher out of the data analysis?
5. How might my research tradition guide me to return to my data collection and analysis and shift the lens with which I analyze my data?

In addition to the "gut check" questions in Activity 11.1, we offer the following tips for qualitative data analysis for a case study tradition:

- Your data analysis should be guided by the case(s) itself, not the factors that influence the case. For instance, in a case study of an urban college counseling center partnership with a local school, you may analyze data from staff members. However, the analysis should focus on how these data elucidate the case itself. Aim to stay "on course" with your analysis. Write your research question on an index card and keep it near you during data analysis, or post your research question on your codebook to help you stay on track.

- Construct a strategy for your data analysis. Is it based on the chronological sequence of events or other boundaries of the case? Use this strategy consistently throughout your analysis.

- Consider the benefits and drawbacks of using each of Stake's (1995) four recommendations for case study data analysis. You may not use each recommendation, but have a good rationale for which approach you do or don't use.

- Flyvbjerg (2004) advises that good data analysis and interpretation of case studies should be able to ward off the "so what" question—meaning that the reader of a study should not have this question come to mind at all if the data analysis has been well thought out and guided by the case study itself. (We like this guy's thinking!)

Case Example 11.1 offers an example of qualitative data analysis for the case study tradition.

CASE EXAMPLE 11.1. Teacher Community in an Early Childhood Education Center

Blank, J. (2009). Life in the village: Teacher community and autonomy in an early childhood education center. *Early Childhood Education Journal, 36,* 373–380.

In this case study, Blank (2009) investigated the extent to which an early childhood education center included a focus on teacher community. She defined teacher community as entailing connections between teachers and students, an emphasis on professional development, sources of innovation in teaching, reflective practice, and a culture of its own, among other factors. Blank's data included participant observations of classrooms and participant development opportunities, in addition to interviews with key school personnel (e.g., principal, teachers).

Blank's initial analysis involved immersing herself in the data through multiple readings of the participant observations and interview transcripts. This first analysis was general, and she began to identify large codes and to begin to set the stage for comparing her data. She used Stake's (1995) categorical aggregation and pattern identification to guide this process. The following quote illustrates some of the ins and outs of her data analysis:

> I utilized memo-ing (Stake, 2006), "contact summary reports, and periodic interim reports as tools for grouping codes, to show that they are instances of a general concept or themes pertaining to teachers' views on community that were constructed through analysis: (a) shifting priorities, and (b) preference for privacy. Teachers' values, school knowledge, external interests, and changes in leadership are examples of codes used to construct understandings of the teachers' shifting priorities. Interaction contexts, teacher feedback, and recognition of good teaching are examples of codes that were categorized as teachers' preference for privacy." (2009, p. 376)

Here is a visual portrayal of Blank's case study data analysis plan:

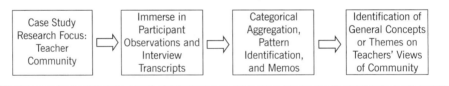

QUALITATIVE DATA ANALYSIS IN EXPERIENCE AND THEORY FORMULATION: GROUNDED THEORY, CONSENSUAL QUALITATIVE RESEARCH, PHENOMENOLOGY, AND HEURISTIC INQUIRY

In this section, we discuss data analysis for the research traditions of Cluster 2 (see Chapter 2): grounded theory, consensual qualitative research, phenomenology, and heuristic inquiry. We discuss each individually, and you will notice some overlap in concepts because data analysis in all four traditions seeks to understand an experience and/or generate a theory. We distinguish where some of these overlapping data analysis strategies use similar analytic techniques, yet have different names in the four traditions. We also interweave case examples to bring data analysis "to life" for each tradition. After reviewing the four traditions, see Activity 11.2 on page 357.

Grounded Theory

Grounded theory, as we have discussed previously, seeks to generate a theory of a phenomenon (Glaser & Strauss, 1967). Grounded theory data analysis "simultaneously employs techniques of induction, deduction, and verification to develop theory" (Schwandt, 2001, p. 110). It can be overwhelming to consider how your data analysis will identify a theory of a phenomenon without understanding that there are specific steps to take in this process. Out of all the traditions we discuss, grounded theory is one of the traditions used most often across disciplines (e.g., constructivist grounded theory by Charmaz, 2005) in numerous ways, so there are several ways to methodically approach its data analysis. We summarize eight steps for grounded theory data analysis (Figure 11.2 on page 350), whether you are working as a researcher alone or on a research team.

First, the researcher (or research team) reads through the participants' transcripts. Ideally, grounded theory data collection and analysis are recursive, so the first data analysis may entail one researcher or several research team members initially looking at one participant transcript that has been collected. Identifying large codes to comprise a codebook, the researcher or research team then comes to consensus on the codes "seen" in the data. Then, the researcher or research team collects and analyzes subsequent data based on this initial codebook. The codebook is then refined between each step of data collection and analysis. Within this refining of data collection and analysis is a process called constant comparison. Schwandt (2001) describes **constant comparison** as follows:

> Empirical indicators from the data (actions and events observed, recorded, or described in documents in the words of interviewees and respondents) are compared, searching for similarities and differences. From this process, the analysis identifies underlying uniformities in the indicators and produces a coded category or concept. Concepts are compared with more empirical indicators and with each other to sharpen the definition of the concept and to define its properties. (p. 110)

In other words, the researcher or research team is constantly comparing previous data collection and analysis to subsequent data collection and analysis.

As the larger domains are identified and constant comparison is used, the researcher or research team uses a coding process entailing open, axial, and selective coding (Corbin & Strauss, 2008). **Open coding** is a type of wide review of the data answering the question "What large general domains am I seeing in the data?" This might involve key words or phrases provided by the participants or the researchers. Then, **axial coding** is a process that begins to refine the open coding and examine relationships among the large open codes to understand more in-depth what the data are revealing with regard to theory building. Axial coding is a second-tier process by which open codes are collapsed into broader categories or codes. Next, **selective coding** is used to further refine axial codes. Selective coding is truly the step that begins to "look like" a grounded theory of your phenomenon. Selective coding is the most complex coding process in grounded theory, whereby patterns, processes, and sequences are identified among axial codes to generate a theory about a phenomenon.

Corbin and Strauss (2008) urged grounded theory analysts to develop their own unique style of, and techniques for, coding in these three categories. Are you a visual person? You might want to color-code everything. Do you like sticky notes? They might be lifesavers to help you stay organized and track your coding. Whatever helps you keep sight of your goal and purpose—theory building—those are the techniques and style you want to maintain throughout the process.

Let's take a look at what open coding in a transcript looked like in Singh, Urbano, Haston, and McMahon's (2010) study of school counselor advocates' strategies for social justice change. Here is a "raw" transcript excerpt from one participant. (The underlined portions became an exemplar of an open code we defined as "relationship building.")

> You really have to, especially in the position that I am speaking from now, the administrators at local schools are really, is really the key, that you really need to be able to work with. Number one, I think that they will be immediately available to listen to the data that you gather as a school counselor, and any social justice issues that you will have to raise. <u>Forming good relationships with them and making sure they know your job is to be an advocate for students</u>—having them understand that you're there for students, you care, you do a good job—that is key if you want to make change.

As my colleagues and I (Singh) delved into the axial coding process and revisited transcripts in our research meetings, we identified in the data that the broad open code of "relationship building" involved an action about their role as participants. We had identified a selective code that became "educating others about school counselors' roles as advocates." Toward the end of the data analysis, selective coding involved identifying relationships among the selective codes, which we decided to portray in a visual model that signified the close relationships among them. Case Example 11.2 presents additional information about grounded theory analysis for this study, and Perspectives 11.1 (on page 348) highlights research team reflections on grounded theory data analysis.

CASE EXAMPLE 11.2. School Counselor Advocates' Strategies for Social Justice Change

Singh, A. A., Urbano, A., Haston, M., & McMahon, E. (2010). School counselors' social justice change: A grounded theory of what works in the real world. *Professional School Counseling, 13,* 135–145.

"Researchers built recursivity into each stage of the research process so that simultaneous data collection and analysis continuously informed each other and, in turn, the emerging grounded theory After the first two interviews were transcribed, four research team members individually reviewed and coded the transcripts using an open coding process. Open coding involved analyzing each line or paragraph of the transcripts for codes reflecting each participant's experiences. More specifically, each discrete idea, event, or experience was given a name (e.g., 'courage,' 'dialoguing,' 'student empowerment'). To create a codebook for the remaining interviews, researchers used constant comparison with their discrete codes to identify categories that related to a common overarching concept and to discern any discrepancies between their discrete codes.

"After each interview was conducted, transcribed, and coded using this codebook, axial coding was utilized to examine the relationship between each of the pre-established categories. During this stage, the research team created higher-level categories based on the data (e.g., 'methods of consciousness raising'), thereby contributing to the initial development of a grounded theory of the phenomenon under study. Finally, selective coding was used to refine the theoretical model based on the identification of an overarching core category that accounted for most of the variation in the previously identified categories (e.g., 'school counselors' strategies for systemic change'). Researchers reviewed each participant's transcript using the codebook until saturation of findings was attained at participant sixteen, where no new data were identified.

"Verification standards and procedures were built into each stage of the research process. Member checking of transcripts, researcher reflexive journals, routine team meetings, the use of multiple data analysts, and peer debriefing were utilized to maximize trustworthiness of findings. Researchers identified thick descriptions of the phenomena to demonstrate credibility of findings. The researchers' immersion in the data for a year, during which time the team continually reviewed and coded data as data were collected and analyzed, further strengthened the credibility of findings. Throughout the research process, a school counselor served as an internal auditor by attending research meetings regularly and reviewing the data for accuracy of the coding and theory-building process. An external auditor reviewed the products of the study (i.e., transcripts, research team notes, emergent model) for accuracy. Finally, the research team searched for evidence to disconfirm the emerging theory and modified the theory when necessary to ensure accurate representation of the data" (p. 13).

Here is the visual portrayal of this grounded theory study:

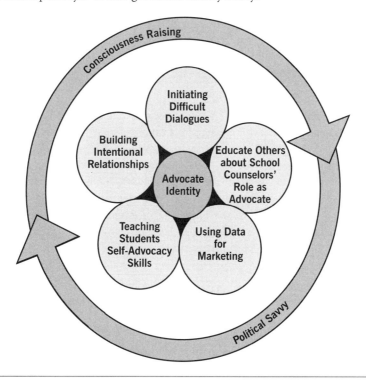

As you proceed with these three types of coding, as a researcher or a team, you begin to look for causal conditions, intervening conditions, and consequences (Creswell, 2006). **Causal conditions** are factors influencing the phenomenon you are studying. In the Singh, Urbano, and colleagues (2010) study above, the causal conditions included the school context and the need for advocacy on social justice issues (i.e., achievement gap, overrepresentation of students of color in special education classes). **Intervening conditions** are ways in which participants address these influencing factors. For the Singh and colleagues study, the intervening conditions included the political savvy and consciousness raising that the school counselors reported were infused throughout their advocacy strategies in school. Finally, the **consequences** are the results of intervening conditions for participants. In the Singh and colleagues study, the consequences included the five general strategies the school counselors reported using for social justice change: initiating difficult dialogues, educating others about school counselors' roles as advocates, using data for marketing, teaching students self-advocacy skills, and building intentional relationships.

• •

Perspectives 11.1. Grounded Theory Research Team Members Look Back on Data Analysis

The perspectives below are from three research team members working on the Singh, Urbano, and colleagues (2010) grounded theory study. Read their perspectives to get a sense of how working on a grounded theory research team "feels" in the data analysis stage.

"The grounded theory data analysis process allowed me to get very close to the experiences and voices of our participants through our data. We became heavily immersed in their collective perspectives, and where these perspectives overlapped in concrete, meaningful ways. The challenges were that the process is messy. It often seemed that we had a swirling, nebulous mass of data that somehow we needed to bring order and structure to. This can be overwhelming, and it takes a lot of conceptual work to develop this structure. I think you have to get comfortable with the constant shifting of structures and rearranging of your model as the theory emerges from your data. I enjoyed the collaborative and intellectually engaged nature of the process. The constant conceptualization and reconceptualization of what you are seeing develop from your data is challenging, exciting, and fun. This is a very active process, and hashing out with your team what your data mean and how they fit in the larger context of your emergent theory is a wonderful experience. I learned tremendously from the perspectives of my colleagues as we wrestled with our data. Because grounded theory data analysis is such a collaborative and interactive process, I think it is important to have a great research team. It's also important to set the tenor of the analysis process as an open, collegial, communicative process, where all voices and perspectives are valued—those of the participants and also those of the researchers in analyzing the data."

—ELEANOR MCMAHON, MS

"Prior to becoming part of this research team, most of my research experience had involved quantitative data. Hearing our participants speak to their experiences, and then working to develop a model that honored these voices, was thus new territory for me. Connecting with the participants during the interviews made the data analysis process feel all the more significant to me—having heard the participants' stories in person, having been granted the privilege of documenting their experiences—made it seem all the more crucial that we develop a model that was truly reflective of their collective message. One of the elements of the data analysis process that seemed most challenging was that the sheer amount of data—the ideas, themes, and concepts that emerged—made it difficult to select those themes that were most significant and that were threaded throughout each of the participants' stories. In addition, it was also striking to me how I, as a researcher, approached the data that I

collected personally, and the data that I didn't collect personally. More specifically, there are themes that emerge clearly on the page as you read the transcripts, and then there are feelings, ideas, 'senses' that you get when you speak to someone in person. I, and we as a team, had to challenge ourselves always to come back to the data, to the words on the page, to be sure that the themes that were emerging were truly grounded in the written word, and not just in our own interpretations or the feelings we got when we spoke to the participants. To anyone interested in working with qualitative data, I would advise that patience is key. The process of working in the grounded theory paradigm is a long one and can feel unclear at times. It is so important for all members of the team to trust the process—to know that if the team is committed to the data, and to the voices of the participants, the themes and the model that emerge will indeed be a grounded theory."

—MEG HASTON, MS

"The data analysis process for our grounded theory study was a complicated and rewarding one. We collected about 400 pages of rich data, which were initially overwhelming to sort through. We relied on each other—our research team members—to keep us grounded as we initially sorted through the volume of data during the open coding stage. Our team was passionate about the topic of social justice and became progressively more excited about the emerging theory as we moved from the open coding stage to the axial and selective coding stages. We used our analytic, creative, visual, and comedic selves throughout the analysis process and experienced a shared sense of excitement when our theory eventually reached its final form. One of the greatest opportunities of completing a grounded theory study is the chance to work collaboratively with a group of individuals who share a common interest. Another unique opportunity is the inevitable intimacy of the data analysis process, both among the researchers and with the participants (through their transcribed voices). By the end of the data analysis process, I felt empowered by and connected to 16 social justice advocates (our participants) and three inspirational colleagues (the research team)—quite an incredible experience!

"For me, the greatest challenge of the data analysis process involved sorting through the huge volume of data, which was a circuitous process rather than a linear one. The real challenge here was accepting that the process was not going to be tidy, organized, and straight. I think I would give two pieces of advice for anyone embarking on the data analysis process of a qualitative study. First, select a supportive team that shares a passion or interest for the topic at hand. Second, accept before you even begin analyzing the data that it will be a circuitous process rather than a linear one."

—ALESSANDRA URBANO, PhD

In selective coding, Corbin and Strauss (2008) emphasized two tasks: identifying a central category and integrating variation into data analysis. The authors discuss the central category as having "analytic power" (p. 146) that is like a black hole: It is a central category that brings all the other codes together. When identifying a central category, they cite Strauss's (1987) criteria, including that it is an idea that (1) appears frequently, (2) is not forced, (3) is named or phrased in a way that could be further researched in other studies, and (4) evolves in its depth and power to explain the phenomenon. The central idea should also be capable of accounting for variation, or varying explanations, of the phenomenon. Speaking of variation, Corbin and Strauss assert that the variation represented in a final grounded theory data analysis is ultimately important because no phenomenon is static. Ideas ebb and flow within our data—"there is variability with dif-

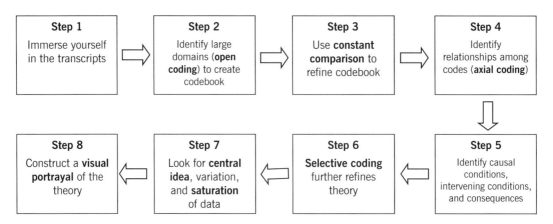

FIGURE 11.2. Grounded theory data analysis steps.

ferent people, organizations, and groups falling at different dimensional points along some properties. … We want to bring out the variations both within and between categories" (pp. 160–161). Using the Singh, Urbano, and colleagues (2010) study, for instance, the central idea was the advocate's identity. Each participant's advocate identity contained within it variations—contradictions, divergences, and other ways in which the selective codes indicated variability. We identified and discussed this variability.

So, if this all sounds like a good deal of coding—it is! How do you know when you are "finished" with your data collection and analysis? That is where **saturation** of the data comes into play in grounded theory analysis. Saturation of the data occurs in the axial coding step, where you as a researcher or research team identify no "new" data in subsequent participants' transcripts. See Figure 11.2 for a summary of eight steps to organize your grounded theory data analysis.

Consensual Qualitative Research

As we discuss data analysis in consensual qualitative research (CQR), you will see the many similarities it has with grounded theory data analysis. Some of the key features that distinguish CQR analysis are its emphases on consensus, shared power, and frequency counting. There are five main data analysis components in CQR (Hill et al., 1997, 2005). First, a primary research team conducts a **domain development and coding** process. In this step, each research team member immerses him- or herself in all of the data, reading each participant transcript. As team members read these data, their analysis begins by identifying a list of large domains, categories, or themes. Then the research team meets as a collective group, and each member presents his or her identified domains to one another. The team members argue, debate, and come to consensus on one group of large domains. Then the individual members revisit the data through a second analysis using these large domains to code.

Second, the research team abstracts core ideas within domains (**domain abstraction**). As the team members reimmerse themselves in the data, they keep an eye out for core ideas that illuminate aspects of domains they have previously selected to examine. Third, members of the research team meet and attempt to reach consensus on these core ideas through a process of **cross-analysis**, wherein categories are developed by team members through a consensus-building process. In this process team members examine each category for evidence across all, some, and/or none of the participants. Once the list of categories is finalized, the team members then return to the data and code all participant interviews within these categories. This cross-analysis should result in a separate document that includes a list of domains and within-domain categories common to all participants and any participant data that were not common across participants and/or were not included in another domain or subdomain.

The fourth key component of CQR is the use of an **external audit**. In this process, a secondary research team comes in to assess the accuracy of the cross-analysis and the creation of domains and subdomains common to all participants. The auditors also examine the data and categories listed as *not* common to all participants and/or placed in an "other" category. The auditors then communicate their audit to the primary research team, suggesting alterations, revisions, and/or data that were not addressed by the original abstraction of core ideas and cross-analysis. You can see how this process of using what might be termed a primary research team and a secondary research team can be complex, and perhaps even burdensome. However, this is the heart of the rigor of CQR, so it is a critical interaction between these two research teams.

Finally, the fifth data analysis step with CQR involves **frequency analysis**. Now, we have already discussed in Chapter 10 how we feel about frequency—the benefits and the challenges of frequency counts. Regardless of the epistemological challenges we believe are inherent in "counting" responses in qualitative research, this is a critical aspect of the way Hill and colleagues (1997, 2005) constructed CQR's data analysis. In this final step, research team members categorize domains into one of four categories: **general** (all or all but one case), **typical** (more than half of the cases up to the cutoff for general), **variant** (at least two cases up to the cutoff of typical), and **rare** (used for sample sizes greater than 15, two or three cases). See Table 11.2 to see what CQR findings "look like" at the end of the five steps of data analysis.

Okubo, Yeh, Lin, Fujita, and Shea (2007) used CQR to examine the career decision-making processes of eight Chinese immigrant youth. The authors developed and coded the data from transcripts into large domains and subdomains for an initial list, or codebook. Then, the research team members reread each transcript, using the codebook to indicate the domains and subdomains in the data. They invited recursivity into their data analysis by revising the codebook at several stages, based on what they were "seeing" in the data. When abstracting core ideas within domains, the research team members "constructed core ideas individually and then came to consensus" (p. 442). Next, the cross-analysis of data included "bringing all the transcripts together" (p. 442) and utilizing an auditor to assess the accuracy of the data analysis thus far. Finally, the research team addressed frequency issues and categorized their domains as *general*, *typical*, or *variant*, and then portrayed them in a table because CQR asserts that "representativeness can be plotted on [a] table to clearly show the results" (p. 443). The researchers did not note any rare domains.

At the end of Okubo and colleagues' (2007) CQR data analysis, the research team had identified 10 domains in participants' transcripts and between three and eight subdomains per domain. Interestingly, all the subdomains were either typical or variant in their frequency. See Figure 11.3 on page 353 for a visual portrayal of the CQR data analysis steps Okubo and colleagues used in their study.

TABLE 11.2. An Example of Data Analysis in Consensual Qualitative Research Data

Domain/category	Illustrative core idea	Frequency
1. The homeless experience		
a. Negative feelings about being homeless	Depression, shame, frustration, injustice, helplessness	Typical
b. Greater empathy for the homeless	Changed attitudes, greater sympathy	Typical
c. Homeless persons struggle with substance use, mental illness, and physical illness	Alcohol, drugs, mental and physical illness are problems	Typical
d. Dichotomy of homelessness	There are two different types of homeless individuals—those who choose to be homeless and individuals who are not homeless by choice	Typical
2. Perceptions of men and masculinity		
a. Man as the "breadwinner"	Breadwinner, provider, worker	General
b. No changes in masculinity since becoming homeless	A succinct "no" when asked if they viewed their masculinity differently since becoming homeless	Typical
c. Others perceive homeless men negatively	Viewed as drunk, looked down upon, outcast	Typical
3. Changing social status		
a. Aspirations for upward mobility	Desires to change to a higher social class, including not being homeless anymore and discussion of home, family, and job	Typical
b. Barriers to change identified	"Myself," financial situation, substance abuse, and/or health	Typical

Source: Liu, Stinson, Hernandez, Shepard, and Haang (2009, p. 137).

Phenomenology

Phenomenological data analysis differs from grounded theory and CQR in that although all three traditions examine participants' experiences, phenomenology's sole focus is to understand the depth and meaning of these experiences (Moustakas, 1994) rather than to generate a theory. One of the reasons we chose to discuss the data analysis of these three traditions in the same section is that the unique similarities and differences in the data analysis among the three can be more easily understood when grouped together. When one engages in phenomenological data analysis, it can be tempting to begin down a road of theory building. However, the integrity and quality of phenomenological data analysis are retained more when the researcher refrains from this temptation. Phenomenology—and its focus on understanding the meaning of participants' lived experiences—is a powerful perspective in its own right!

Moustakas (1994) is probably most influential in revisiting phenomenological data analysis techniques, summarizing, and expanding the steps for analysis. We include two reviews: Moustakas's modification of van Kaam's (1959, 1966) phenomenological data analysis, which includes seven steps, in Table 11.3 on page 354; and his modification of the Stevick–Colaizzi–Keen phenomenological data analysis in Table 11.4 on page 355. Creswell (2006) asserts that he sees the Stevick–Colaizzi–Keen approach used more

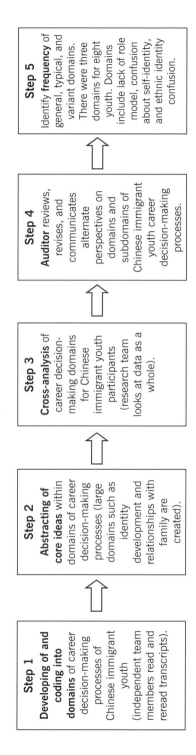

Step 1
Developing of and coding into domains of career decision-making processes of Chinese immigrant youth (independent team members read and reread transcripts).

Step 2
Abstracting of core ideas within domains of career decision-making processes (large domains such as identity development and relationships with family are created).

Step 3
Cross-analysis of career decision-making domains for Chinese immigrant youth participants (research team looks at data as a whole).

Step 4
Auditor reviews, revises, and communicates alternate perspectives on domains and subdomains of Chinese immigrant youth career decision-making processes.

Step 5
Identify **frequency** of general, typical, and variant domains. There were three domains for eight youth. Domains include lack of role model, confusion about self-identity, and ethnic identity confusion.

FIGURE 11.3. Steps in Okubo and colleagues' (2007) CQR data analysis.

353

often recently. We believe both modifications provide helpful ways to analyze phenomenological data. See Tables 11.3 and 11.4 for helpful guides through the intricacies of phenomenological data analysis. Specifically, in Table 11.3, we have reproduced Moustakas's guidelines for phenomenological analysis. For now, we discuss the following components of phenomenological data analysis in greater depth: bracketing, horizontalization, textural description, and structural description.

Padgett (2004) used the phrase of "burrowing inward" to describe phenomenological data analysis—appropriate words to remind us of its purpose: to understand the depth and essence of participants' lived experiences. At the outset of phenomenological data analysis, the researcher immerses him- or herself in the data. A critical pre–data analysis step is the **bracketing** of researcher bias and assumptions about the study's focus.

Just as grounded theory and CQR begin a coding process (open, axial, and selective coding, and development of codes, abstracting core ideas, and cross-analysis, respectively), phenomenological data analysis begins with large domains or categories of text. The term used to describe this process is **horizontalization**. As discussed in Table 11.4, the research team begins to identify nonrepetitive, nonoverlapping statements in participants' transcripts. This is an important first step not only in analyzing the data,

---

TABLE 11.3. Moustakas's (1994) Modification of van Kaam's (1959, 1966) Phenomenological Data Analysis

Using the complete transcription of each research participant:

1. *Listing and Preliminary Grouping*: List every expression relevant to the experience. (Horizontalization)

2. *Reduction and Elimination:* To determine the invariant constituents:
   Test each expression for two requirements:
   a. Does it contain a moment of the experience that is a necessary and sufficient constituent for understanding it?
   b. Is it possible to abstract and label it? If so, it is a horizon of the experience. Expressions not meeting the above requirements are eliminated. Overlapping, repetitive, and vague expressions are also eliminated or presented in more exact descriptive terms. The horizons that remain are the invariant constituents of the experience.

3. *Clustering and Thematizing the Invariant Constituents*: Cluster the invariant constituents of the experience that are related into a thematic label. The clustered and labeled constituents are the core themes of the experience.

4. *Final Identification of the Invariant Constituents and Themes by Application*: Validation

   Check the invariant constituents and their accompanying theme against the complete record of the research participant. (a) Are they expressed explicitly in the complete transcription? (b) Are they compatible if not explicitly expressed? (c) If they are not explicit or compatible, they are not relevant to the co-researcher's experience and should be deleted.

5. Using the relevant, validated invariant constituents and themes, construct for each co-researcher an *Individual Textural Description* of the experience. Include verbatim examples from the transcribed interview.

6. Construct for each co-researcher an *individual structural description* of the experience based on the *Individual Textural Description* and *Imaginative Variation*.

7. Construct *for each research participant* a *textural–structural description* of the meanings and essences of the experience, incorporating the invariant constituents and themes.

From the individual textural–structural descriptions, develop a composite description of the meanings and essences of the experience, representing the group as a whole.

Source: Moustakas (1994, pp. 120–121).

TABLE 11.4. Moustakas's (1994) Modification of Stevick–Colaizzi–Keen Phenomenological Data Analysis

1. Using a phenomenological approach, obtain a full description of your own experience of the phenomenon.
2. From the verbatim transcript of your experience complete the following steps:
   a. Consider each statement with respect to significance for description of the experience.
   b. Record all relevant statements.
   c. List each nonrepetitive, nonoverlapping statement. These are the invariant horizons or meaning units of the experience.
   d. Relate and cluster the invariant meaning units into themes.
   e. Synthesize the invariant meaning units and themes into *a description of the textures of the experience.* Include verbatim examples.
   f. Reflect on your own textural description. Through imaginative variation, construct *a description of the structures of your experience.*
   g. Construct a *textural–structural description* of the meanings and essences of your experience.
3. From the verbatim transcript of the experience of *each* of the other *co-researchers*, complete the above steps, *a* through *g*.
4. From the individual textural–structural descriptions of all co-researchers' experiences, construct *a composite textural–structural description of the meanings and essences of the experience* integrating all individual textural–structural description into a universal description of the experience representing the group as a whole. (p. 122)

Source: Moustakas (1994, p. 122).

but also in managing the data in a way that is efficient. The **textural description** is similar to the process of how grounded theory and CQR begin to refine the data into new categories. However, the real distinction here is that the textural description always strives to understand the *meaning* and *depth* of the essence of the experience.

Depending on how the researcher chooses to manage the phenomenological data analysis, he or she may have a list or visual model that represents not a theory, but the experiences of participants. The list is a result of refining the horizontalization of data into a textural description of the phenomenon's essence. Then a **structural description** is identified by the researcher and/or team, identifying multiple potential meanings within the textural description, in addition to variations among these meanings (i.e., what is identified as "opposites" or as "tensions" in the data). You can think of structural description as similar to grounded theory's axial coding, wherein relationships are identified and understanding of their complexity is sought; or as somewhat similar to CQR's identification of the general, typical, and variant themes *if* the tensions between these were fully examined for the essence of their meaning.

Because the goal of phenomenological data analysis is to deeply understand a phenomenon's essence, we advise that you be familiar with Moustakas's modifications in Tables 11.3 and 11.4. However, we also encourage you to utilize any techniques with your data analysis that you think are necessary to best understand the essence of your study. Often, this entails creating a case display or writing the "essence" of the phenomenon for each participant, and then combining these individual essences into one composite essence. Think of your phenomenological data analysis via horizontalization and textural and structural description as a metaphorical "sieve" through which to filter all the participant descriptions. What is left in your sieve is the essence of participants' lived experiences—and your data analysis is continually aiming to get closer and closer

• •

Perspectives 11.2. The "Essence" of Phenomenological Data Analysis

"In our phenomenological study (Singh, Hays, et al., 2010) of the resilience strategies of South Asian American child sexual abuse survivors, I remember that Danica Hays and I often found ourselves musing about when we would arrive at the "essence" of the phenomenon we sought. We had case displays. We had long debates, discussions, and meetings about each participant's experience of resilience and child sexual abuse. We bracketed our own assumptions and biases consistently. We talked about horizontalization and structural and textural description, and we kept sifting through an immense amount of data. And then one research meeting, it hit us. The essence of participants' experience was speaking to us through the data. It felt like a moment out of that movie The Matrix, *when the 'grid' comes to light! It felt like a magical moment. But the truth was that we spent many long weeks laboring over the data, digging deep into participants' descriptions of the phenomenon. I probably could have recited Moustakas's modifications of phenomenological data analysis in my sleep! In the end, we had a rich, complex visual model of participants' experiences that captured their essence indeed."*

—AAS

"One of the many challenges of phenomenological studies for me has been to honor and illuminate their great contribution—providing the essence of a lived experience of a phenomenon, stripped of my experiences of that phenomenon. Being able to bracket and refrain from theory generation is a valuable skill to hone. Bracketing is difficult at times because it takes practice to 'set aside' our own experiences and judgments of those experiences. Saying to myself, 'This, what I know and have experienced, has to be placed outside the study so that I can provide space for what my participants contribute. There is no need to try to take their experience and apply it to others. This only limits others' descriptions of their essence of the same phenomenon.' No matter the degree to which I have experienced a phenomenon, it is not as 'valuable' to the study as the experiences of those participants with whom I am interacting. Furthermore, their essence does not necessarily apply to others outside the study. (There is a reason you wanted to tell their story in the first place!) Saturation, common in other traditions, is irrelevant. The greatest joy of phenomenology and phenomenological analysis is to be present for your participants and give justice descriptively to their story."

—DGH

• •

to that essence. See Perspectives 11.2 for our descriptions of the frustrations and joys of phenomenological data analysis.

Heuristic Inquiry

There are many overlaps between heuristic inquiry and phenomenological data analysis because they both "seek to understand the wholeness and the unique patterns of human experiences in a scientifically organized and disciplined way ... requiring the researcher to dwell intensely with subjective descriptions and to search for underlying themes or essences that illuminate the meaning of the phenomenon" (Casterline, 2009, p. 2). Moustakas (1990) noted that heuristic inquiry is different from phenomenology in terms of the role of the researcher. In heuristic inquiry the role of the researcher is to not separate his- or herself from the phenomenon being studied. Often, the researcher has an experience of the phenomenon and thus brings not only his or her expertise to the data analysis, but also experience that must be analyzed.

Moustakas (1990) outlined important steps of data analysis for heuristic inquiry. He used the term **illumination** to describe the quest of the researcher to identify categories, themes, and patterns of the phenomenon within the data. In this quest, the researcher begins to recognize the depth and meaning of the phenomenon. He also discusses a stage of data analysis called **explication**, wherein the researcher uses self-reflection to further analyze the structural and textural descriptions that were described in the previous section on phenomenological data analysis. Moustakas then describes the final task of data analysis in heuristic inquiry as **creative synthesis**. Similar to the final stage of phenomenological data analysis, the researcher seeks the best way to portray the findings as a composite whole. The key difference between this final stage is, again, the experience the researcher has of the phenomenon. Case Example 11.3 illustrates the data analysis steps of a heuristic inquiry.

CASE EXAMPLE 11.3. A Teacher's Heuristic Inquiry of Gifted Education

Eger, K. S. (2008). Powerless to affect positive change for the gifted students in an urban school district as revealed through one teacher's heuristic inquiry. *Dissertation Abstracts International Section A: Humanities and Social Sciences, 69*(3-A), 827.

In this study, Eger (2008) used heuristic inquiry to examine feelings of disempowerment as a teacher advocating for change within a gifted program in an urban school district. During the illumination phase, she identified large domains of common themes across interview data she had collected from key informants within the school and from the research literature in gifted education. In the explication stage, Eger self-reflected on her personal experiences as a researcher and on her shared experiences with the phenomenon. The final data analysis in her study involved creative synthesis, wherein she visually portrayed her findings to depict the essence of the feelings she experienced and the context in which she experienced them.

 ACTIVITY 11.2. Experience and Theory Formulation

Within your research groups, answer the following questions:

1. What are the unique differences and similarities between grounded theory and CQR data analysis?
2. With your research topic, what would be your data analysis steps if you used a grounded theory approach versus a phenomenological one?
3. What are the unique differences and similarities between data analysis with phenomenology and heuristic inquiry?
4. Take the four data analysis approaches with experience and theory formulation we have discussed in this section. Toward which approach do you naturally gravitate? Which approach do you find challenging?
5. If you have already collected and analyzed your data from an experience and theory formulation research tradition, how might you return to your analysis and refine it based on your discussion within your group?

QUALITATIVE DATA ANALYSIS WITH SYMBOL AND TEXT: NARRATOLOGY, BIOGRAPHY, AND HERMENEUTICS

In this section we review the analytic strategies that employ narratology, biography, and hermeneutics. Especially regarding the analysis of symbol and text in these traditions, we encourage you to immerse yourself in the literature of the field because there are many creative and innovative analytic strategies continually being developed. We focus our review of symbol and text analysis on various aspects of narrative analysis. As a researcher, you should consider tailoring these aspects of analysis to the various other research paradigms within the cluster of symbol and text we have discussed previously (i.e., symbolic interaction, semiotics, life history) and/or applying the more generic data analysis techniques we discussed in Chapter 10.

Narratology

Narrative data analysis is used in the narratology tradition. We highlight Avdi and Georgaca's (2007) review of narrative data analysis techniques used in examining psychotherapy because of the specificity of their types. The authors note five types of analytic approaches that have been used in examining details of client narratives. These five types are distinct in terms of the focus of their data analysis (see Table 11.5).

First is an approach involving general analysis of themes in the client narrative, or **thematic analysis**. This is a method wherein the researcher identifies central themes and subthemes and their development across counseling sessions. The authors discuss studies that use this analytic technique to note a larger storyline in which these themes and subthemes are subsumed. Other approaches might include analyzing critical incidents within therapy sessions or examining the data for intrapersonal and interpersonal processes within various modalities of psychotherapy.

Second are investigations into the typology of clients' narratives, or **typological analysis**. *Typology* refers to a type of presenting issue clients bring into psychotherapy. They cited Dimaggio and Semerari's (2001) distinction between "effective" and "ineffective" narratives that are categorized based on the level of organization, integration, and assessment of meaning, coherence, and continuity of clients' stories. In this type of analysis, Avdi and Georgaca (2007) noted that the focus is on the individual client narrative more than the interaction within psychotherapy or the content.

TABLE 11.5. Types of Narrative Data Analysis

1. Thematic analysis
2. Typological analysis
3. Dialogical analysis
4. Narrative process coding system
5. Whole client narrative analysis

Source: Avdi and Georgaca (2007).

The third type the authors discussed is less common: data analysis that takes a dialogical approach to a client narrative, or **dialogical analysis**. They cite Lysaker, Lancaster, and Lysaker's (2003) study of the narratives of clients living with schizophrenia. These researchers focused on where the dialogue failed in psychotherapy and suggested that the failure was evidence of a lack of organization in the narrative or a lack of interaction. Avid and Georgaca (2007) see this type of narrative data analysis as promising for noticing positive change in psychotherapy, and they suggest a focus on the psychotherapist's role in the discourse as well.

Fourth, Avdi and Georgaca (2007) reviewed studies that emphasize the processes within the client narratives, termed **narrative process coding system** (NPCS; Angus, Levitt, & Hardtke, 1999). There are three analytic techniques within NPCS. The first, external narrative sequences, describes events. The second, internal narrative sequences, builds on a description of clients' subjective experiences (e.g., thoughts and emotions) and expands these descriptions. The third, reflexive narrative sequences, analyzes the meaning of client narratives. These three analytic techniques enable "the researcher to track shifts both in the topics discussed and in the types of narrative processes involved in a client narrative, within and across sessions" (p. 413).

Fifth, Avdi and Georgaca (2007) reviewed a diverse group of studies that focuses on the whole client narrative, or **whole client narrative analysis**. The authors explain that this type of narrative analysis is similar to case study data analysis, which emphasizes analysis that illuminates the entire "case" of the narrative rather than its diverse parts. They cite McLeod and Lynch's (2000) study of a female client's narrative of the satisfaction she experiences with her life as she copes with depression. The analysis focuses not only on the client's narratives and perspective, but also on those of the psychotherapist—and how both intersect with one another to build a "whole" client narrative.

Kelly and Howie (2007) also outline steps for narrative data analysis in a study they conducted with psychiatric nurses in Gestalt therapy training. Their data analysis entailed eight steps:

1. Connecting with the participant's story.
2. Attention to Dollard's (1946) life history method.
3. Chronological ordering of events and experiences.
4. Core story creation.
5. Verification of core stories.
6. Examination of plots and subplots to identify a theme that discloses their significance.
7. Examination of plot structure.
8. Emplotted whole narratives. (pp. 139–141)

Some of the above steps will sound familiar to you from other analytic techniques we have reviewed. In Step 1 Kelly and Howie (2007) immersed themselves in the data by reading and rereading the transcripts and listening to original audiotapes. Step 2 involved examining the data through the lens of Dollard's (1946) life history analytic techniques to identify the narrative development of cultural context, character values, key players, actions and decisions of character, plot lines, history, and the start–middle–ending of the narrative. Step 3 used the chronology of the narrative to analyze it. The authors color-coded sections of the transcripts according to events during, before, and after the Gestalt therapy training. Step 4 involved the core story creation, which included identifying thematic fragments and subplots of four stories. In Step 5 the authors shared the four identified core stories with their participants to determine the accuracy of their data analysis. Step 6 investigated the plots and subplots to determine the meaning and significance of the narratives. Step 7 focused on the plot structure, returning to the core stories in a microsopic manner. The authors used diagrams to break down each core story and identify major influences on the plot. Finally, Step 8 involved restructuring the four core stories in order to create an entire whole narrative that subsumed them all. In the final version of their manuscript, the authors provided an example of a core story—the story of Mary—as a whole narrative example.

We have presented two strategies for narrative data analysis. Let's turn to Activity 11.3 to practice analyzing narrative data.

 ACTIVITY 11.3. Narrative Data Analysis

Select a favorite children's book and analyze the narrative using one or both of the narrative data analysis strategies discussed in this chapter. (As a class decide on a possible research question to guide the analysis.) Work in small groups to discuss some of the benefits and challenges of narrative data analysis. Discuss your analysis as a class. How might it be useful for a research topic in counseling or education?

Biography

Data analysis with biography focuses on the life events and experiences of participants. Creswell (2006) outlined six steps for analysis of the data within the biography tradition. We use an example of a biography of an expert in trauma in order to bring these steps "alive." In the first step, Creswell encourages the researcher to **organize data files** into a framework that will facilitate coding. For our example, we may have a series of interviews with the expert herself, in addition to interviews with her peers, clients, and trainees. A natural strategy might to organize the interview transcripts according to the role of the person interviewed. In the second step of data analysis, the researcher combs through the transcripts to identify **broad codes** or **domains**. For the biography of a trauma expert, we might identify broad codes in the interviews with her clients as including empowerment interventions, attention to interpersonal skills, and cultivation of hope.

For the third step of data analysis in biography, Creswell (2006) discussed the importance of **description** that focuses on the chronology of the participant's experiences in life. With our example, this might entail describing the critical incidents the participant identified as pivotal in the development of her interest in trauma, such as witnessing a traumatic event within her family and/or surviving a traumatic event herself. The fourth step involves pinpointing the stories, **epiphanies**, and any contextual materials of the participant's life. For our trauma expert, this could mean identifying stories she tells about her own trauma practice with clients. We might also describe epiphanies she has had in the development of her trauma experience—such as a particular mentoring or training experience. Then we could explore the contextual materials of these stories and epiphanies that have shaped her—possibly influential texts she read or cultural artifacts in her life.

In the fifth step Creswell (2006) encouraged the researcher to **work toward a theory**, or a framework, that serves as an organizing structure containing the patterns and meanings identified in the data analysis. In our example, we might identify patterns and meanings of "rebirth" after tragic circumstances or resilience in the face of adversity. Thus, an organizing structure of resilience might be the framework or theory we propose in which we are able to describe the many subthemes within the biography. Finally, in the sixth step, the researcher expands the theory or framework in the fifth step to highlight both the distinct and more ordinary aspects of the participant's life. Back to our example, the biography of our trauma expert might describe both the everyday and extraordinary experiences of resilience within her life.

Hermeneutics

Hermeneutic data analysis involves interpreting "sacred" textual data. Recall from Chapter 2 that hermeneutics can be closely aligned with, or even intentionally paired with, phenomenology due to its emphasis on understanding the *meaning* of text or narratives (Grant & Boersma, 2005).

Diekelmann and Ironside (2005) described the process of hermeneutical data analysis that we categorize in six steps. First, interview transcripts are read in their entirety by members of the research team (which the authors describe as the foundation of hermeneutical analysis of data), and broad domains are identified. In the second step, the research team members initiate dialogue with one another regarding their interpretations of the interview transcripts; this dialogue entails checking analysis of specific text with one another. A third step involves refinement of the broad domains into more distinct categories or abandoning themes that do not hold up across the team members' analysis. Also, team members may identify new broad themes—a step that may require looking to future participant interviews to confirm. The fourth step requires research team members to explore any contradictions or data analysis unaccounted for in the previous identification of codes. This step may entail interviewing previous participants again.

In the fifth step team members should "read across all texts and write critiques of the interpretations ... to extend, support, or overcome the themes and patterns identified by hermeneutics" (Diekelmann & Ironside, 2005, pp. 260–261). In the sixth step, the research team identifies patterns that explain the relationship between the domains. This final step does not entail a conclusion. Rather, the authors assert that hermeneutic data analysis does not have an ending, and they cite Benner's (1994, p. 116) quote that "cycles of understanding, interpretation, and critique" continue. In this manner, researchers are reminded of the importance of acknowledging their own role in deciding when data analysis ends—in addition to analyzing how, why, and when this end point was selected.

Hummelvoll and Severinsson (2001) used a hermeneutic data analysis in a study of health professionals working in an acute psychiatric ward and the care provided in that setting. First, they read their field notes and other textual data several times to become immersed in the data before proceeding with analysis. Second, the authors identified text in the transcripts that revealed the health professionals' views about the care they provided in the setting. Third, the authors distinguished central themes that were related to their research question. Fourth, they revisited the data to illuminate the central themes by providing examples from the text. Throughout the hermeneutic analysis, others analyzed their researcher reflections and analysis as the process unfolded. See Table 11.6 for an excerpt of their central themes identified in this study's data analysis. Also see Activity 11.4 to delve further into data analysis with symbol and text.

TABLE 11.6. Table of Central Themes, Content, and Statements from Hummelvoll and Severinsson's (2001) Study of Health Care Professionals' Provision of Care in an Acute Psychiatric Ward

Themes	Content	Statements
Thriving	Professional development	"Clinical supervision means a lot to me. I experience both personal and professional development."
	Significant work	"It is rewarding to establish good relations, observing the patient improve and being a part of his/her progress."
	Good collegiate relations	"We function as a team and consult each other. We have a tone which allows both joking and being serious."
	Being valued	"My opinions are considered, and I can influence decisions concerning treatment and care."
Strain	Unpredictable climate and work-related stress	"Efficiency is measured in terms of admissions, and not what we really achieve with our patients." "You never know what you have to deal with when starting your shift—especially during late evenings and weekends."
	Feeling inadequate	"It happens that I have a guilty conscience when I come home after my shift because I have partly left my primary patients unattended due to having too many tasks."
	Diffuse directions in the work situation	"Long-lasting seclusion without clarified attitudes and guidelines causes strain."
	The patients' suffering and inadequate quality of care	"It's hard to experience patients' suffering. We do not have time to talk with each patient. It leaves me with a guilty conscience."
	Sole responsibility	"Sick leaves, constantly shifting of assistants, and new colleagues make me busy trying to get acquainted with them and to know what I can expect from them if urgent problems arise."
	Detrimental physical milieu	"The furniture is worn out, the cleaning is inadequate, and the seclusion unit is not suitable for its purpose."

ACTIVITY 11.4. Data Analysis with Symbol and Text

In your research teams, answer the following questions:

1. What are the strengths and challenges of narrative data analysis and hermeneutic analysis for your research topic?
2. What type of research team would you want to build for each of these two traditions? Would your research team differ or be the same in each tradition?
3. What similarities and differences do you see across narrative data analysis and hermeneutic analysis?
4. If you have already collected and analyzed your data from a symbol and text research tradition, how might you return to your analysis and refine it based on your discussion within your group?

QUALITATIVE DATA ANALYSIS OF CULTURAL EXPRESSIONS OF PROCESS AND EXPERIENCE: ETHNOGRAPHY, ETHNOMETHODOLOGY, AND AUTOETHNOGRAPHY

As we discussed previously, ethnography is distinct because it is "the process and the product of describing and interpreting cultural behavior" (Schwandt, 2001, p. 80). In this section, we explore data analysis with ethnography, ethnomethodology, and autoethnography. There are several similarities in the philosophies of the three traditions because they each seek to understand cultural aspects. Let's review the distinctions in their process of data analysis.

Ethnography

Similar to other research traditions, ethnographic data analysis, at its best, should have recursivity built into the data collection and analysis processes, such that the ethnographer begins data analysis immediately. Immersing him- or herself in the data, the ethnographer then **identifies broad patterns**, categories that exemplify the culture-sharing group. As these categories and patterns are identified, the ethnographer refines them by **seeking exemplar data** that "tell the story" of a culture-sharing group. Ethnographic data collection—much like case study data collection—may entail a variety of data sources from interviews, participant observations, and focus groups to reviewing public and personal documents and other artifacts relevant to understanding the culture.

Creswell (2006) cited three of Wolcott's (1994) data analysis techniques as important for ethnographic design: description, analysis, and interpretation of a culture-sharing group. First, the ethnographer uses **description** by using a chronological, sequential, or some other type of order to describe a culture-sharing group. This might remind you of some of the techniques used in case study data analysis. It should, because the approaches share a similarity: to describe the main events, occurrences, interactions, perspectives, key players, storylines, and so on, of a culture-sharing group. Say, you are conducting an ethnography of graduate students in a qualitative course (you might have already wondered about conducting a similar study of your own class experience—we sure did!). The order could be framed by the syllabus, progression of topics introduced, themes in class discussions, group dynamics (e.g., who speaks when, how class participation occurs), and/or by other frameworks that would help you the most, as an ethnographer, to understand the culture of that graduate qualitative class.

Once you have decided on the order most appropriate to describe the data, **analysis** is a "sorting procedure … [that] involves highlighting specific material introduced in the descriptive phase or displaying findings through tables, charts, diagrams, and figures" (Creswell, 2006, p. 182). This is a stage of data analysis wherein you might find yourself using more general qualitative data analysis tools, such as identifying patterns in the data (Wolcott, 1994, as cited in Creswell, 2006). It can be important to identify these patterns not just within the culture-sharing group, such as within our qualitative research class example, but also in terms of "comparing the cultural group to others, evaluating the group in terms of standards, and drawing connections between the culture-sharing group and larger theoretical frameworks … critiquing the research process and proposing a redesign for the study" (Creswell, 2006, pp. 152–153).

Applying this analysis to the example of an ethnography of a graduate qualitative course, you might build on the description of the phenomenon and examine what patterns the ethnographer notes across data sources. You might use some of the data management techniques discussed in Chapter 9, such as case displays or concept mapping, to track these patterns. Examining the patterns in your reflexive journal, comparing the course to another very similar or opposite course, and identifying connections within the patterns might be important to elucidate the culture-sharing group. As the analysis continues to build the description of the culture-sharing group, there may also be patterns and/or themes that you notice as an ethnographer that demand future study or suggest a restructuring of an ethnography for this group. For instance, maybe you notice that the culture of this qualitative class is influenced by fatigue due to a shortened semester, and you note that a longer semester might allow more of the culture-sharing group to be studied. Really, when you are conducting ethnography, it's the content and process of the culture-sharing group you are analyzing, in addition to your role as a researcher.

How will you analyze your role and influence in the ethnographic research process? This brings us to the idea of the "insider" versus "outsider" discussion with regard to ethnography. Dwyer and Buckle (2009) contend that the issue of whether or not researchers should share "insider" status with their participants is not a dichotomous question. We agree. So if you are conducting ethnographic analysis, be sure to analyze your perspective and the space you occupy as a researcher along the insider–outsider continuum. It is typically not an "either–or" situation. Dwyer and Buckle note:

> There are complexities inherent in occupying the space between. Perhaps, as researchers we can only ever occupy the space between. We may be closer to the insider position or closer to the outsider position, but because our perspective is shaped by our position or closer to our position as a researcher (which includes having read much literature on the research topic), we cannot fully occupy one or the other of those positions. (p. 67)

Hammersley and Atkinson (2007) assert that ethnographic analysis should also seek to examine the situated meaning of a culture-sharing group. *Situated meaning* refers to the ways that a local culture experiences and makes meaning of the events within their group. The authors also note that **triangulation** of data sources is important, comparing data from different chronological stages of data collection and various settings within the culture-sharing group.

    Content analysis and **domain analysis** are also terms used commonly in ethnographic research to describe the process of identifying codes in the data. Content analysis seeks to identify relationships and patterns among words, phrases, and ideas within the data (Altheide, 1987; Graneheim & Lundman, 2004). Domain analysis is a similar process (Spradley, 1979); here is an excerpt from an ethnographic data analysis using domain analysis to examine the use of a reflecting team in couple therapy:

> In this study the general research question was "What are couple and therapist perceptions of reflecting team practice?" … [In] transcripts, each sentence is analyzed through what is called a domain analysis to identify emergent themes and categories across interviews from different people in the same setting or culture (Spradley, 1979). In a domain analysis, long, complex sentences are broken down into shorter semantic relationships of meaning. A domain can be represented whenever someone makes a statement about something. That statement can be broken down into three parts: (a) the main concept being talked about—the cover term, (b) the other terms we use to describe that main concept—included terms, and (c) the relationship between the included terms and a cover term—semantic relationship. (Sells, Smith, Coe, Yoshioka, & Robbins, 1994, p. 250)

Floersch (2004) defined **practice ethnography** as ethnography that "examines the process of practice and investigates how practitioners use theory in practice" (p. 79). He acknowledges that in the study of mental health care or educational settings, an ethnographer must become familiar with the culture of a setting through its specific language and by becoming a witness to the daily lived experiences within the culture. We believe that this type of ethnography is well suited to designs in counseling and education. Floersch includes five steps in practice ethnography:

1. Identification of the disciplinary knowledge/power, or strengths language.
2. Recording the oral narratives of management events.
3. Reading the written text (i.e., case record) corresponding to the event.
4. Comparing the oral and written strengths of narratives with the invented or situated language.
5. Interviewing managers to confirm whether or not the language I identified as situated was a language acknowledged by the practitioner. (p. 81)

Floersch uses an example of his study of medication management in a mental health care setting to demonstrate data analysis with practice ethnography. He used the above techniques to analyze case records, interview transcripts, and his own role as the researcher in this study.

    We also encourage you to consider Agar's (2006) discussion of the five parameters of an ethnography that we think can help guide your data analysis. First, he discusses *control*: whether you as a researcher have more of a tendency to "take charge" or to "go with the flow" (p. 7) in your approach to data analysis. Second, he discusses the *focus* of your ethnographic study. Staying on course with that focus during your data analysis is critical. Third, he discusses the *scale* of your ethnography. Are you interested in an in-depth examination of a particular phenomenon (e.g., individual experiences) or are you seeking a more global or broader understanding of your topic? Fourth, the *events* of your ethnography can guide your data analysis. Are you examining one event in one setting or multiple settings and multiple people interacting in those settings? Finally, Agar discusses *event links*, the recognition that events are particularly situated in time and can be influenced both backward and forward in time and space. How might this be important for analyzing your data?

Ethnomethodology

Remember that it is easy to begin to think that ethnography and ethnomethodology are more similar than they actually are. Ethnomethodology is both a method and a theory of a culture-sharing group (Pollner & Emerson, 2001), and this is a difference whose uniqueness translates in terms of how one approaches data analysis with ethnography versus with ethnomethodology. *Discourse analysis* (Edwards & Potter, 1992) or *conversation analysis* (Sacks, 1992) are terms you may see used in relationship to ethnomethodology. See Table 11.7 for a comparison of ethnographic, ethnomethodological, and autoethnographic (discussed in the next section) analytic strategies.

A first step in ethnomethodological data analysis is to select if and how you will address the cultural context of the text. De Kok (2008) outlined three issues that complicate this decision. First, ethnomethodology tends to analyze natural speech patterns rather than using, for instance, interview data for analysis. The conversation itself is valued as important—the text and interactions—rather than the interpretation of the

---

TABLE 11.7. Comparison of Data Analysis in Ethnography, Ethnomethodology, and Autoethnography

Ethnography

- Prioritizes analysis of contextual and cultural factors.
- Focuses on recursivity of data collection and analysis.
- Identifies situated meanings within culture-sharing group.

Ethnomethodology

- Prioritizes conversational text in analysis, rather than interpretation of context surrounding text, and stays close to details of text.
- Identifies critical sequential events and meaningful interactions.
- Asks questions of the text to fine-tune data analysis.

Autoethnography

- Uses analytic strategies from ethnography.
- Produces a descriptive narrative about the relationship of the ethnographer to the phenomenon.
- Ranges in researcher focus from "objective" stance of details and facts to a more "subjective" description of the relationships between researcher and phenomenon and attention to feelings.

context surrounding it. Second, the numerous contexts at play surrounding any conversation, text, and interactions are viewed as an important reason to stay closer to the details of the occurrence rather than to the contextual factors. Third, acknowledgment of the context is viewed as removing the agency of participants' text and interactions by placing them into "boxes" of assumptions about their culture (e.g., race/ethnicity, gender). Next, the ethnomethodologist reads transcripts, identifies critical incidents that are sequential, and interactions that are meaningful. Coding is often used to track this identification process. Questions may be asked of the data during analysis to fine-tune ways in which the data can "answer" these questions to illuminate the phenomenon studied. Here is an excerpt from de Kok's study in Malawi with women and men on the issue of infertility:

> Recordings of interviews were transcribed verbatim, according to a simplified version of the standard [conversation analysis] transcription notation (see e.g., Atkinson & Heritage, 1984). In order to be able to examine the sequential organization of talk and the co-construction of meaning, I obtained translations of the interactions between interpreters and respondents (displayed in the extracts in italics). After reading and re-reading the transcripts, I coded the interviews provisionally, based on content, utterance design (i.e., kinds of words, phrases or examples used), or actions performed (e.g., "discarding responsibility").
>
> Preliminary analysis of the data drew my attention to recurrent reference to the cultural content. I therefore selected extracts in which explicit reference was made to "culture," "tradition," "society" or "community" for more detailed analysis, leaving out extracts in which the interviewer explicitly asked about cultural or traditional issues.
>
> I used several "tools" in the analysis. First, I asked certain questions of the data, such as "what is the participant doing in this turn?" (Pomerantz & Fehr, 1997) and "why this (utterance/phrase/action) now?" (Hutchby & Wooffitt, 1998). Second, I made use of findings regarding discursive devices and their functions as reported in the discourse analysis and conversation analysis literature. Third, I paid attention to deviant cases; if a particular extract did not fit in with an analytic claim, I adjusted the claim in order to account for the anomaly, unless certain features in the extracts made them recognizably different from the "average" extract (Potter & Wetherell, 1987; Schegloff, 1968). Throughout the analysis I adhered to the principle that claims should be based on the participants' orientations and interpretations as displayed in their utterances. (p. 891)

Autoethnography

Autoethnography may typically be thought of as solely the autobiography of the ethnographer. However, it has recently become a tradition that attempts to hold both the culture-sharing group *and* the ethnographer in the ultimate data collection and analysis (Schwandt, 2001). The data analysis techniques used in ethnography apply to autoethnography. The difference is that the aim of autoethnographic data analysis is to produce a descriptive narrative about the relationship of the ethnographer to the phenomenon. Because autoethnography can range in its focus from a more "objective" (entailing attention to the details and facts) stance of the researcher to a more "subjective" description of the relationships between researcher and phenomenon (entailing attention to feelings), the focus of data analysis will necessarily be distinct depending on the researcher focus (Anderson, 2006). However, Duncan (2004) urges autoethnog-

---

TABLE 11.8. Tips for Data Analysis with Culture-Sharing Groups

1. Address the context of the culture-sharing group. If you elect not to do so, have a strong rationale.
2. Keep your purpose of the study at the forefront of your mind. What are you seeking to describe and why?
3. Select an order or framework for describing the culture-sharing group and/or your relationship to it. Note how chronology, sequence of events, critical incidents, etc., will structure your description.
4. Triangulate data sources (e.g., transcripts, records, artifacts) in your analysis.
5. Look for variation within your description. Where are the "tensions" or inconsistencies within the culture-sharing group?
6. Use general coding techniques throughout your analysis to stay organized.
7. Don't forget to analyze and code your own researcher reflexivity.

---

raphers to not give over to feelings in autoethnography, but rather to have authenticity about their motivations to conduct an autoethnography, and to locate their research experience within a theoretical framework to increase the quality of data analysis. Wall (2008) notes the challenges in data analysis of autoethnography, including the degree of honesty and authenticity, or what she terms as "acceptability," both within academia and with her own self with regard to her autoethnography.

Pennington's (2007) investigation of autoethnography as a technique used with white preservice teachers in elementary schools working with students of color is a wonderful example of addressing some of the challenges mentioned above. She used critical race theory as a theoretical framework to analyze her own racism in the classroom and her experiences as both an educator and a researcher. She used her theoretical framework, critical race theory, to situate explorations of counternarratives to racism. Pennington also uses her own researcher reflexivity to describe her relationship to the topic of racism and preservice elementary school teachers. Guided by her theory and research tradition, she stays on course with her topic through self-analysis and description of the interaction between her own culture and the culture-sharing group of students and teachers. She writes: "I used myself to understand my participants. I used the similarities we shared, our skin color, our background as white women, and our placement in a school and community of color to provoke and process the discussions about race" (Pennington, 2007, p. 107). See Table 11.8 for tips on data analysis with culture-sharing groups in ethnography, ethnomethodology, and autoethnography.

QUALITATIVE DATA ANALYSIS WHEN RESEARCH IS A CHANGE AGENT: PARTICIPATORY ACTION RESEARCH

Participatory action research (PAR) should, of course, incorporate participatory data analysis methods. Stoecker (2005) asserted that PAR approaches have three common elements: an emphasis on utility, a use of diverse methods, and a focus on collaboration. Similar to case study analysis, the management and analysis of data are often immense tasks because the data come from a variety of sources. Just as a case study must endeavor to stay true to the case and not veer off course to data analysis that might be interesting, PAR data analysis must not lose its focus on its action, community and/or stakeholder involvement, and change (McTaggart, 1997). For instance, in a PAR study seeking to increase advocacy for persons with intellectual disabilities, participants were invited to (1) play important roles in each step of the data analysis, (2) identify sites of change in the systems in which they were involved during data analysis, and (3) take action steps during the process of data analysis. In this manner, developing your data analysis strategy in a PAR study must include some flexibility so that you can build in numerous places for you to analyze data collaboratively with your participants.

Another critical aspect of PAR data analysis is reflection. PAR researchers are often guided by a think–act–look focus in their community partnerships; however, self-reflection is an integral process in each of these stages (Koch, Mann, Kralik, & van Loon, 2005). This reflection is important because it helps identify both within, and as a result of, the data analysis opportunities for the next most effective action steps. There-fore, a guiding force of PAR includes ensuring that periods of reflection are recursively built into the data collection, action, and analysis process. See Figure 11.4 of Riel's (2007) visual portrayal of progressive problem solving with action research.

Similar to many other qualitative research traditions, the data collection and analy-sis should be recursive. We believe it is best to have key informants from the community you are working with on your research team. However, this is not always possible. If it is not, an important initial decision in your data analysis will be to identify how you will integrate participant voices into the data analysis process (Kidd & Kral, 2005). Often, the dialogue or reflection session is used to create a space wherein participants speak

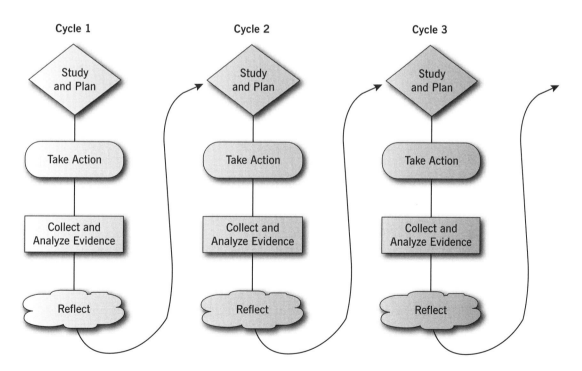

FIGURE 11.4. Riel's (2007) visual portrayal of progressive problem solving with action research. Re-printed with permission from Margaret Riel.

with one another and the researcher about the actions they are planning and/or implementing and the experiences they are having in the process (McTaggart, 1997).

These sessions can also serve as spaces in which data analysis is simultaneously conducted. For instance, if your PAR study is a peer-led intervention in middle schools on decreasing bullying and violence, your reflection and dialogue sessions may entail planning, identifying sites of change, and reporting on activities from participants and researchers. Within this meeting, the researcher can also present data—whether they are broad domains the researcher and/or research team is identifying about the change process within the school or analysis of the participation levels of each individual in the PAR sessions—and invite analysis in that moment.

Because of the level of **involvement of the researcher** *and* participants in PAR designs, the researcher *must* be well organized and track how the collaborative partnership is analyzing data because the participants may be already overtaxed by the systems in which they are working. Whereas in other research traditions, the researcher decides when the data analysis ends—such as reaching saturation in grounded theory approaches or illuminating the boundaries of a case study—best practices in PAR should really follow the will and experiences of the participants and/or community in deciding when data analysis should end. Kidd and Kral (2005) remind those engaging in PAR that "the interaction of PAR with local culture can itself be a source of study along with the more specific course and outcome of groups' efforts" (p. 188). See Table 11.9 for a list of tips for data analysis steps in PAR designs.

Nastasi and colleagues (2000) noted that the **cultural/contextual variables** specific to this local culture should drive the data collection and analysis. Therefore, collaboratively identifying these variables can be an important way to frame PAR data analysis. We would like to add that data analysis with PAR may borrow analytic strategies from other traditions when it "makes sense" for PAR's aim toward social change. See Case Example 11.4 for an excerpt from a PAR manuscript describing this approach to data analysis.

CASE EXAMPLE 11.4. Family–School Participatory Action Research

Ho, B. S. (2002). Application of participatory action research to family–school intervention. *School Psychology Review, 31*(1), 106–121.

"As a first step toward organizing the data, three members of the research team analyzed the responses independently. Each survey that had a written response was counted as one response. This step of the process involved each member reading over the comments several times while keeping a separate running list of major ideas. A primitive coding system of classifications in which data were initially sorted was developed based on the notes. As a second step, the three independent coders compared their lists, and the numerous codes generated were systematically examined to discern emerging patterns. They transformed these patterns into categories or themes based on inductive content analysis guidelines (Coffey & Atkinson, 1996). This process involved the coders first sharing and discussing their generated codes and the frequency, extensiveness, intensity, or uniqueness of certain ones, and then obtaining consensus on the most important themes that emerged from this discussion. For the third step, these themes were used for the final sorting of the comments; each coder independently sorted the comments based on the four mutually exclusive identified themes. (p. 113)

TABLE 11.9. Tips for Data Analysis in PAR Designs

- Your participants should be guiding your data analysis—optimally, in person as integral members of the research team. If this is not possible, collaboratively identify with your participants and/or community how you will integrate their voices into the data analysis.

- Strongly consider a dialogue or reflection meeting wherein an exchange of knowledge is conducted. Bring your expertise and ideas for the PAR and present various potential ways to collect and analyze data. Then be quiet and listen to your participants and/or community partners as they discuss their ideas and needs for social change. Let this discussion guide your data analysis plan.

- Be flexible. Once you collaboratively identify the best data analysis plan for your PAR study, the subsequent actions and research involved may demand changes. Flexibility does not mean throwing all your plans out the window. Being flexible means you should collaboratively identify ways you and your participants will address challenges—both expected and unexpected—along the way.

- Analyze the process, not just the outcome, of your PAR study. If you focus only on an end "result," you may not only be disappointed, but you will also likely miss out on opportunities to use data analysis of the process to inform the subsequent actions needed to produce social change.

- Collaboratively identify local cultural/contextual variables of the setting in which the change will be located, for these variables may provide a more structured framework for data analysis.

- Use the following questions to guide your data analysis: How is this PAR producing change? What are the opportunities for change based on community needs, and how is this occurring in the PAR? What are the barriers and facilitators for change in the PAR?

- Determine early in the process how will you collaboratively decide when the data analysis will end. Have a specific discussion about this point with your stakeholders. You don't have to have a magic ball to do this—just brainstorm with them possible indicators that the data analysis is complete.

- Are there analytic strategies that make "more sense" for the social change the PAR is seeking to affect?

- Be sure to bring all your organizing skills to a PAR study. You may be the person with the best ability to ensure that the products and processes of the data collection and analysis are brought to research meetings, dialogue and reflection sessions, and other aspects of the action research.

"The four themes identified in this PAR data analysis were:

1. Requests for more communication.
2. Requests for information on ways to help their children.
3. Expressed satisfaction with school.
4. Requests for special parental consideration. (p. 111)

These themes were organized with other data by the school psychologist in the study and shared with the community. The research team met with stakeholders to identify action steps for family–school partnerships, which included:

1. Develop mechanisms for decreasing language, cultural, and overall communication barriers to improve parents' involvement with the school.
2. Increase efforts to help parents become involved in reading and learning activities at home.
3. Increase opportunities for communication with parents about their individual child's educational progress and needs, and to provide families with resources." (pp. 114–115)

ACTIVITY 11.5. Building Action Components into Your Research Design

In your research groups, answer the following questions:

1. How would your research topic change (or not) with a PAR design?
2. Are there action components you could add to your study based on what you have learned about the purpose, focus, and outcome of PAR?
3. What do you think are the challenges to PAR in terms of managing your influence and power as a researcher using PAR techniques?
4. *Empowerment* is a word that is often misunderstood. We don't believe that we empower people, but rather that we create spaces wherein participants empower themselves. How might your research, whether a PAR design or not, create spaces with the potential for empowerment and change?
5. If you have already collected and analyzed your data from a research and action tradition, how might you return to your analysis and refine it based on your discussion within your group?

⚠ WILD CARD 11.1. CAUTIONS FOR THE DATA ANALYSIS "ROAD"

Here are a few general tips for you across the research traditions for data analysis:

1. Stay on course with your research tradition. How is it guiding your data analysis?

2. Balance your expertise and your power of interpretation with listening to the voices of your participants and the data.

3. Ask different questions of your data. It's not a bad thing if your data offer different, and even diverging, types of evidence. Variation is a good thing in data analysis; it helps you more fully represent your data.

4. Don't be haphazard in selecting data analysis approaches. Know why an approach is the best fit for your topic. This may mean a blend across traditions—but have a strong rationale for doing this!

5. Don't rely on one qualitative text (even ours!) to teach you about data analysis. Use this book to get your repertoire of data analysis techniques down. Then, read, read, and read some more about how data analysis is conducted within your field and across disciplines—not just with your topic, but also with your research tradition.

6. Don't throw in the towel during data analysis! This is a time to persevere, endeavor to do your best quality work, and challenge yourself. If your study were a marathon, the data analysis might feel like the point when you "hit the wall" and your roll might begin to slow. Get reenergized and pour that energy into your analysis.

7. Be creative. Even all the data analysis techniques we have discussed might not provide a specific answer or guide about how to analyze a particular piece of data. Consider the general analytic techniques such as coding, identifying themes, triangulation, and so on, and then acknowledge that you may have to supplement these with a creative approach that makes sense for your data.

8. Be open to pausing your active data analysis to return to data collection if your data are requiring this. Repeat after us: Recursivity, recursivity, recursivity!

9. Don't get overwhelmed by all the different terms used for data analysis techniques across the research traditions. Turn that anxiety into energy and get to know the similarities and differences in each form of data analysis. You not only will learn the tradition you are using better, you also will become a better qualitative researcher!

10. Don't forget to analyze your own researcher reflexivity. Yes, we know you have already acknowledged your biases and assumptions at the beginning of your study. But good analysis demands that we analyze how and why we are examining certain aspects of data and not others—it matters in terms of where our analysis ends up!

POSTSCRIPT:
A FINAL NOTE ON QUALITATIVE DATA ANALYSIS

We have spent a good deal of time reviewing the tools each research tradition uses for analysis. Corbin and Strauss (2008) discussed the importance of embracing the researcher's role in the interpretation of one's data analysis. They note that beginning qualitative researchers tend to shy away from the power of interpretation, feeling nervous about being "off" in their analysis of the data. Corbin and Strauss agree that data analysis will vary in quality of standards. However, they encourage researchers to "push forward with analysis. With [analysis], we have more to gain than we have to lose" (p. 49). We wholeheartedly agree. Make sure that you are an ethical researcher staying close and true to the data you have collected as you interpret.

There will also come a time when you must "abandon" your interpretation by deciding that your analysis is at a stopping point. Notice that we did not say "*done*" with your analysis. The process of data analysis and interpretation is one that actually has no end point, so it will feel as if you are abandoning your data. And you are. However, you as the researcher should abandon your data with full disclosure of when, how, and why your decisions are the right ones for your study and are guided by your research tradition, theoretical framework, knowledge of your data, and analytical skills. That is when your interpretation ends ... *for now.*

CHAPTER SUMMARY

In this chapter we have traveled the long road of data analysis, identifying the unique similarities and differences in approaches to handing data across the research traditions (see Table 11.10). Each of the research traditions has some version of categorizing data and "cooking" them down into a description or portrayal that illuminates a phenomenon. However, it is the philosophy of each of the traditions that becomes evident in *how* that categorization occurs. We have provided numerous examples from studies using the analytic techniques so that you can get a picture of what the data analysis may look like for your study.

TABLE 11.10. Qualitative Data Analysis by Research Tradition

Research tradition	Central principle	Step 1: Reduce data	Step 2: Collect data	Step 3: Memo and summarize	Step 4: Organize text	Step 5: Code	Step 6: Identify themes and patterns	Step 7: Create a codebook	Step 8: Develop a main narrative or theory
Case study	Case description					Categorical aggregation and direct interpretation (Stake, 1995)	Pattern identification and naturalistic generalization (Stake, 1995) Noting sequences (Creswell, 2006)		Case description (Creswell, 2006)
Grounded theory	Theory development					Open coding (Corbin & Strauss, 2008)	Axial coding and selective coding; noting causal conditions, intervening conditions, and consequences (Corbin & Strauss, 2008)	Constant comparison and saturation (Corbin & Strauss, 2008; Creswell, 2006)	Central idea, variations, and visual portrayal of theory (Corbin & Strauss, 2008)
Consensual qualitative research	Consensus on experience					Development and coding of domains, researcher consensus (Hill et al., 2005; Okubo et al., 2007)	Abstracts core ideas of domains, cross-analysis, external audit (Hill et al., 2005; Okubo et al., 2007)	Noting frequencies of categories (general, typical, variant, rare; Hill et al., 2005; Okubo et al., 2007)	Presentation of phenomenon
Phenomenology	Essence of phenomenon					Horizontalization, reduction, and elimination (Moustakas, 1994)	Structural and textural descriptions (Moustakas, 1994)	Individualized structural–textural descriptions (Moustakas, 1994)	Provide composite description of the essence of experience (Moustakas, 1994)
Heuristic inquiry	Integration of researcher in participant experience						Illumination and explication (Moustakas, 1990)		Creative synthesis (Moustakas, 1990)
Narratology	Narrative plots					Thematic analysis, typological analysis, dialogical analysis, narrative process	Chronologically ordering events and experiences (Kelly & Howie, 2007)	Core story creation, verification of core stories, examination of plots and subplots,	Emplotted whole narratives (Kelly & Howie, 2007)

Tradition	Data				
Biography	Participant story	coding system, and whole client narrative analysis (Advi & Georgaca, 2007; connect with story and attend to Dollard's (1946) life history (Kelly & Howie, 2007)		examination of plot structure (Kelly & Howie, 2007)	Expand theory or participant story (Creswell, 2006)
Hermeneutics	Sacred texts	Identify broad codes and domains (Creswell, 2006); Dialogues in research teams and reach consensus (Diekelmann & Ironside, 2005)	Identify broad themes, explore contradictions, and identify patterns (Diekelmann & Ironside, 2005); Description of chronology epiphanies (Creswell, 2006)	Create organizational structure (Creswell, 2006)	Describe symbols embedded in sacred text
Ethnography	Culture-sharing group	Content analysis (Altheide, 1987; Graneheim & Lundman, 2004) and domain analysis (Spradley, 1979)	Description and analysis through fieldwork (Wolcott, 1994)	Situated meanings of a culture-sharing group (Hammersley & Atkinson, 2007)	Describe culture-sharing group
Ethnomethodology	Natural speech patterns	Discourse analysis (Edwards & Potter, 1992) and conversation analysis (Sacks, 1992)			Identify discourse within social interactions
Autoethnography	Autobiography of ethnographer	Same as ethnography	Same as ethnography	Same as ethnography	Describe researcher's role in culture-sharing group
Participatory action research	Change agent	Study field and reflect on previous action (Riel, 2007)			Take action, present data to create change for participants

Note. This table includes selected research traditions in which qualitative data analysis steps have been discussed in the literature.

We began this chapter discussing data analysis strategies for the universal tradition, the case study. Here we emphasized the importance of having the case itself lead the data analysis and the caution about veering into analytic directions that might be interesting influences on the case but that do not elucidate the case itself. Then we reviewed analytic strategies used in experience and theory formulation. Data analytic strategies for grounded theory, phenomenology, and heuristic inquiry use a variety of coding methods designed to identify a theory or the essence and meaning of a phenomenon for participants. Next, we reviewed data analysis with symbol and text. These analytic approaches also use coding strategies, but typically they have a focus on narrative analysis, building a structure for analysis (whether by chronology of events, time, etc.), and/or using the generic coding methods discussed in Chapter 10. We explored cultural expressions of process and experience with ethnography, ethnomethodology, and autoethnography and identified the unique analytic approaches among the three involving the role and perspective of the researcher and the analysis of contextual or cultural influences. Finally, we discussed data analysis used as a change agent in PAR designs, where the process of analysis is guided by social action and, ideally, analytic collaboration with key stakeholders.

RECOMMENDED READINGS

Brydon-Miller, M. (1997). Participatory action research: Psychology and social change. *Journal of Social Issues, 53,* 657–666.

Hill, C. E., Thompson, B. J., & Williams, E. (1997). A guide to conducting consensual qualitative research. *The Counseling Psychologist, 25,* 517–572.

Kelly, T., & Howie, L. (2007). Working with stories in nursing research: Procedures used in narrative analysis. *International Journal of Mental Health Nursing, 16,* 136–144.

McTaggart, R. (1997). Guiding principles for participatory action research. In R. McTaggart (Ed.), *Participatory action research: International contexts and consequences* (pp. 1–24). Albany: State University of New York Press.

Moustakas, C. E. (1990). *Heuristic research: Design, methodology, and applications.* Newbury Park, CA: Sage.

Moustakas, C. E. (1994). *Phenomenological research methods.* Thousand Oaks, CA: Sage.

Yin, R. (2008). *Case study research: Design and methods* (4th ed.). Newbury Park, CA: Sage.

PART IV

PRESENTING YOUR QUALITATIVE RESEARCH

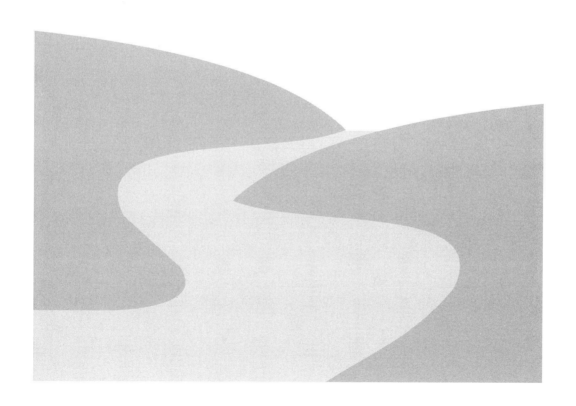

CHAPTER 12

Writing and Presenting Qualitative Research

CHAPTER PREVIEW

In this chapter we discuss the fundamentals of writing and presenting qualitative research. Conducting a rigorous qualitative study demands an equally as thorough writing process. First, we describe foundational writing techniques you will need to convey your study from beginning to end. These include the basics of developing a research proposal and writing a qualitative report across research traditions. Next, we explore guidelines for submitting, publishing, and presenting qualitative studies. Throughout the chapter, exercises guide you to assess the quality and basic components in writing and presenting your research study. Figure 12.1 presents an overview of the main topics covered in this chapter. Additionally, see Appendix B for sample qualitative proposals.

DEVELOPING A RESEARCH PROPOSAL

Now that you know the basics of conducting qualitative research that is meticulous and rigorous in its methods, it is time to learn how to convey all of your hard work to an audience. It may seem overwhelming to compile all of the steps of your research process into an integrative document. However, remembering that in writing and presenting your qualitative study, your main goal is to be true to your participants will pull you out of any overwhelmed state. This goal can be achieved by understanding your philosophy about academic writing. This philosophy will guide your entire approach to composing your qualitative report.

By now, you have probably read several qualitative study articles in journals both within and outside your discipline in order to understand your phenomenon of inquiry. You may have noticed that, as we discussed in Chapter 7, the way that authors select writing techniques depends on which of the positions they hold about "truth" in qualitative research. Do you hold Position 1, the *holy trinity* position, which asserts that qualitative research is a valid approach only to the extent that it looks like quantitative approaches? From this position, you should select a writing philosophy that seeks to be more similar to typical quantitative proposal writing. For instance, you should use

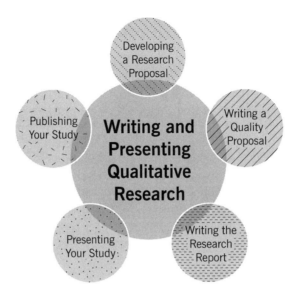

FIGURE 12.1. Writing and presenting qualitative research.

language that is "unadorned and disembodied" (Golden-Biddle & Locke, 2007) and asserts a more objective stance of representing truth in your writing. Rather than exploring the many varying ways to represent truth, Position 1 guides you to help your reader see that qualitative studies can be written similarly to quantitative approaches. A good example of this type of writing is positivist language, as opposed to more tentative language that would acknowledge varying perspectives on representing truth. You might title your findings section *Results*, as quantitative writing would use, rather than using a word such as *Findings*. The latter is a more tentative word implying a discovery-oriented approach as opposed to *Results*, which implies a finality of the research process.

If you are more aligned with Position 2, the *translation approach*, your proposal writing will seek to establish the "gold standard" of qualitative research (i.e., credibility, transferability, dependability, and confirmability; Lincoln & Guba, 1985). This gold standard is translated from the quantitative standards of validity and reliability. From this perspective, you will use language in your writing that conveys the components of the gold standard. You might conceptualize this writing approach as helping the reader understand that there are rigorous criteria for evaluating qualitative research, and your proposal will reflect these criteria. For instance, you would provide a definition of confirmability and the other gold standard components. Then, you would seek to convey how you accounted for the subjective nature of qualitative research throughout your proposal writing using these components. Position 2 guides you to use more tentative language than used in Position 1. However, you are still asserting the expertise of the researcher in describing the details of the research process.

Position 3, the *emergence of qualitative criteria* position, asserts that qualitative research should have its own emergent definitions of what truth is according to one's individual study. Therefore, proposal writing from this perspective should use language exploring the topic of inquiry from an approach recognizing that there are many ways to understand—and therefore write about—the phenomenon. For example, this position guides your writing to define and explore these multiple ways to represent truth. However, a simple exploration does not suffice. Rather, Position 3 encourages you to identify why the selected approach to representing data is the most appropriate one, out of the multiple approaches that exist.

Those who identify more with Position 4, which defines qualitative truth as *relative and changing*, do not look to established criteria for their writing approach. Position 4 asserts that there should be no consensus of criteria for qualitative "truth," but rather increased acceptance that these criteria are constantly emerging. From this perspective, your language in writing should identify and "bring to life" the process by which you arrived at your topic. For instance, the words you use to describe the researcher and research process might be rich and vibrant in detail—perhaps, the very opposite of the "disembodied and unadorned" words you would use in Position 1. Position 4 guides you to write in the way that best represents the relative and changing criteria that exist even within your own study. Was there a point where you collected data and realized your research question needed to recursively change in its focus? This would be an opportunity to convey this recursive process in detail, using descriptive language to help your audience understand its relevance for your phenomenon of inquiry. In Table 12.1 we summarize the writing philosophies guided by each of the positions. We encourage you to carefully consider the four positions and how they might guide your overall approach to your writing. This encouragement is not to select one approach over another; in actuality you might blend positions in your writing. Ultimately, being aware of your philosophical approach to representing the "truth" in your writing will be a helpful

TABLE 12.1. Qualitative Proposal Writing Guided by the Four Positions on "Truth"

The four philosophical positions on "truth" in qualitative designs	Proposal-writing philosophies
Position 1: *Holy Trinity*	Follow quantitative guidelines for writing (e.g., *Results* as opposed to *Findings*).
	Use words that convey an objective stance of the researcher and research process.
Position 2: *Translation of Qualitative Criteria*	Follow gold standard guidelines (i.e., credibility, transferability, dependability, and confirmability) for writing.
	Use language that explains how the gold standard guidelines translate to quantitative approaches to truth.
	Use words that convey the subjective nature of the researcher and research process.
Position 3: *Emergence of Qualitative Criteria*	Since qualitative research should have its own universal set of criteria, acknowledge the many different criteria for establishing truth.
	Use language that is tentative in nature and explores the most effective way to represent the researcher and the research process in writing according to your study.
Position 4: *Criteria as Relative and Emerging*	Acknowledge the identified criteria you have selected for establishing truth in your writing according to your study.
	Use language that identifies the most effective way to represent the researcher and research process that is relevant to your study.

place to come back to any time you feel "stuck" in what language to use to convey your study to your audience. Proposal Development 12.1 assists you in brainstorming writing strategies based on the position you select.

PROPOSAL DEVELOPMENT 12.1. Brainstorming Strategies on Writing the "Truth" in Your Research Proposal

Select one of the four positions on representing "truth" in qualitative research that you think is most aligned with the way you want to approach your research proposal writing. Draw a table with two columns and write "Strengths" and "Challenges" at the top of each of the columns. List everything that you see as a strength of this position in terms of how it would influence your writing. Next, list the challenges of this position and how they would shape your writing. Which of the strengths will be most helpful for your research proposal writing? How will you address the challenges you have identified as you write?

Writing about Your Conceptual Framework

When writing your research proposal, an initial consideration across traditions is your conceptual framework. We discussed the development of your conceptual framework in detail in Chapter 4. As a reminder, the conceptual framework develops from experience, pilot and exploratory findings, available literature, and thought experiments (Maxwell, 2005). In essence, your conceptual framework is comprised of your literature review, research tradition, and any selected personal and professional theories that act as a lens to understand your research approach (Bell, 2005). As you write about your conceptual framework, the components should be fully defined within the research proposal. However, these components should additionally be defined in regard to the interrelationships among them. For example, if you are using a feminist theory and a phenomenological research tradition (in addition to your literature review), you can begin with defining the feminist theory. Because feminist theory has numerous branches (e.g., liberal, radical, social) and subbranches (e.g., womanist, intersectionality), defining the particular feminist theory in appropriate detail is important. We like to think of providing appropriate detail as akin to whether your uncle, who works in computer technology (about as far away as you can get from qualitative inquiry!), could understand the theoretical perspective for your study. We will call this the "uncle" test of accountability, which you can use as you write any aspect of your research proposal. Then do the same for your research tradition. Tell the reader why it is a critical method with which to understand your phenomenon. We encourage you to revisit the original sources for both your theory and research tradition, so that you are clearly articulating their aims.

Once you have described your theory and research tradition in detail, next you should clearly explain to your audience the interrelationships among them and how they are appropriate for your study. In our previous example, a phenomenological tradition (Moustakas, 1994) and feminist theory (hooks, 2000) might share three major interrelationships that are critical in writing up a qualitative study of the educational experiences of children who live in poverty. First, both emphasize the importance of honoring participant voices in understanding their truth. Second, there is attention to the role of researcher bias within feminist theory and phenomenological designs. Third, both value the role of contextual factors in the lives of participants—with feminism, through recognizing the impact of oppression, and with phenomenology, through the valuing of daily lived experiences.

To give you a clear understanding of how you might describe your conceptual framework in your qualitative report, we highlight an exemplar from education of how to articulate a conceptual framework. Dr. Michelle Espino's study of Latina professionals and their journeys in obtaining their doctoral degrees used critical race theory (CRT) from a Latino perspective (LatCrit; Solórzano & Delgado Bernal, 2001) and social constructionism (Berger & Luckmann, 1966) to ground her qualitative study, a "conceptual model ... to explain the complex relationship between marginalized communities and the dominant culture in reproducing and resisting master narratives" (p. 3). We highlight Espino's discussion of theory related to her conceptual framework. In discussing how Espino has undergirded her study of 33 Latina doctoral-level professionals in higher education, she initially defines and contextualizes CRT:

> Although the critical race theory (CRT) movement began with legal scholars, educational researchers noted its applicability to analyzing the experiences of students of color, discussing critical pedagogy, uncovering racial microaggressions, and developing best practices (Parker & Stovall, 2004; Solórzano, 1998; Solórzano, Ceja, & Yosso, 2000). CRT offered an opportunity to design studies that would "identify, analyze, and transform those structural, cultural, and interpersonal aspects of education that maintain the subordination of [students] of color" (Solórzano, 1998, p. 123).

After she has defined and contextualized the use of CRT in her conceptual framework, Espino's writing shares her research positionality as it relates to her topic. Recalling Kline's standards of presentational rigor, her writing about her own positionality, as it relates to her theory, builds trustworthiness with her audience:

> Believing that research should lead to transformation and that CRT, as a framework, could illuminate new stories not yet shared in the literature, I devised a study of the life narratives of 33 Mexican American Ph.D.s (Espino, 2008). I was intrigued by the way participants told stories about their families and educational experiences because embedded within the stories were responses to societal messages about their communities. Consistent with challenging the dominant ideology, one of five main tenets in CRT, my goal was to deconstruct ideologies that blame Mexican American communities for low levels of educational attainment (for a discussion of the five tenets, see Solórzano & Yosso, 2000).

It becomes clear to her audience the centrality of her role as a researcher and her related assumptions. Rather than defining all of the tenets of CRT, Espino defines the specific component of the theory she is using to frame her qualitative inquiry. Then she cites an article the reader can reference for further details on additional CRT tenets. In addition to building trustworthiness, Espino has additionally set the writing stage to highlight forthcoming methodological and analytic rigor and to showcase the complexity of her findings. Her researcher positionality continues to invite complexity as she narratively describes the "surprises" entailed in her research process:

However, I found that calling attention to these ideologies or master narratives led to more complicated, perhaps controversial considerations about power and oppression within U.S. society. (Re)presenting the findings from my study not only meant uncovering master narratives and counternarratives, but also addressing the reproduction of master narratives within Mexican American communities themselves.

Our only critique of Espino's description of the position of her theory in her research is that we bet it could be revised slightly to pass the "uncle" test. For instance, the uncle test might guide her to define terms such as *master* and *counternarratives* and *power* and *oppression*. Overall, however, we believe that Espino hits the mark in her writing as she clearly communicates to the reader exactly *how* theory is a critical component in understanding her study. See Figure 12.2 for a pictorial description of all the components within her conceptual framework.

Additionally, you can think about writing your conceptual framework in terms of answering the questions of *what, who, how,* and *why*. See Table 12.2 for a listing of these questions and considerations related to our earlier example of studying the educational attainment of children who live in poverty.

Writing about Your Research Tradition

Your research tradition is a key component of your conceptual framework; we have discussed this point throughout this text. So, you want to make certain that you convey the importance of your research tradition through your writing. We discuss the politics of

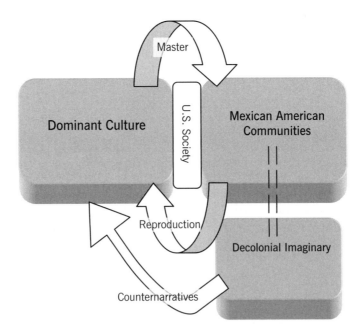

FIGURE 12.2. Conceptual framework of the relationship between the dominant culture and Mexican American communities, master narratives and counternarratives, and the location of the decolonial imaginary. *Source*: Espino (2008). Reprinted with permission from Michelle Espino.

TABLE 12.2. Sample Questions and Considerations for Writing about Your Conceptual Framework

Let's say you are studying the educational attainment of children who live in poverty, and you are using phenomenology as your research tradition and feminism as your theory. In the left column are the questions you want to ask yourself about your conceptual framework. In the right column are considerations you want to keep in mind as you seek to answer these questions; the considerations in italics apply directly to our example of children's education attainment:

Question	Considerations
What	What are the relevant tenets of your theory and research tradition?
	Phenomenology assisted the researcher to understand the essence and meaning of the educational attainment of children who live in poverty.
	Feminist theory guided the researcher to explore the contextual influences of poverty (e.g., classism) on children's educational attainment and to value their responses as the truth of their experiences.
	What are the critical constructs within your theory and research tradition?
	Phenomenological designs allowed the researcher to seek an in-depth understanding of participants' daily lived experiences.
	Important constructs within feminist theory, as used in qualitative traditions, are the development of a collaborative relationship between the researcher and participants, in addition to seeking to understand participants' experiences of empowerment despite oppressive systems in society.
Who	Who are the major players within your theory and research tradition?
	The researcher will use the tenets of phenomenology described by Moustakas (1994).
	There are many strands of feminist theory. The researcher used the Chicana feminist theory articulated by Gloria Anzaldua (1987), specifically her approach to exploring the "borderlands" where divergent cultures meet and intersect.
How	How will the combination of your research tradition and theory(s) influence your study?
	The combination of phenomenology and Anzaldua's Chicana feminism guided the researcher to specifically seek to understand the essence and meaning of how Latina children who live in poverty engage educational systems at the "borderlands" where their race/ethnicity and social class meet.
Why	Why not pick another research tradition and/or theory(s)?
	Although quantitative inquiries of Latina children's educational attainment have been conducted, there is not an in-depth exploration from the children's perspective about their daily lived experiences. The researcher considered a grounded theory design. However, the goal of the research was not to build a theory of Latina children's experiences, but rather to understand the essence and meaning of their educational attainment.

publishing qualitative research later in the chapter (see Publishing Your Findings section) where you might be asked to shorten your description of your research tradition. However, we believe that the best qualitative proposal writing aims to clearly articulate the research tradition as a way to contextualize the study. We lead you through what we consider to be an example of strong writing on the rationale for a research tradition from Okech and Kline's (2004) article, a grounded theory of group coleader relationships. Their writing begins with their reason for selecting grounded theory:

> This research used the grounded theory approach because of its ability to describe patterns and complex relationships between data and its sensitivity to process. Grounded theory uses systematic analysis (e.g., open, axial, and selective coding) and analytic tools (e.g., constant comparison, asking questions, etc.) to build theory. During the data collection and analytic processes, researchers continuously compare data provided by participants with their emerging theoretical concepts, thus developing a theory consistent with participants' perceptions of the phenomenon under study. (p. 175)

You can see that the authors defined the research tradition themselves in three sentences. You may possibly need more, but we advise not much more, because you have much more to write! Plus, rather than simply defining your research tradition in your own words, you might want your writing to also showcase that you know something about the original texts upon which the tradition is based. Okech and Kline (2004) then cite Strauss and Corbin's (1998) description of grounded theory. They select an excerpt from Strauss and Corbin that further illuminated the key points of the research tradition:

> "They mean theory that is derived from data, systematically gathered and analyzed through the research process. In this method, data collection, analysis, and eventual theory stand in close relationship to one another. A researcher does not begin a project with a preconceived theory in mind (unless his or her purpose is to elaborate and extend existing theory). Rather, the researcher begins with an area of study and allows the theory to emerge from the data" (p. 12). (Okech & Kline, 2004, p. 175)

Next, Okech and Kline (2004) directly link their tradition to their phenomenon of inquiry: group coleader relationships. Again, their writing is simple to understand, but not simplified beyond holding meaning for the reader:

> Grounded theory, therefore, offered a structure for the conceptualization of the social and psychological processes of participants based on their experiences and perceptions. It did this not only by incorporating the perspectives and voices of the participants (Denzin & Lincoln, 1998) but also by involving the "verification" of the collected data with the participants. (p. 175)

As you can see, in two sentences Okech and Kline foreground their coming discussion of their data collection and analysis process. However, this foregrounding involved just a hint at this point, not a full discussion, to help the reader move from the definition of the research tradition and building a rationale for why it is an appropriate research tradition for their topic, to a brief statement on what grounded theory techniques "looked like" within their study. As the authors wrap up this portion on their research tradition, they explicitly restate its relevance. You might notice that although their language is not repetitive, it does have some aspects of the initial definition. Okech and Kline are helping their audience—who might be reading about grounded theory designs for the first time—understand the tradition's utility with their topic. They are also garnering respect from their readers who know a good deal about grounded theory, as they are further defining the theory and identifying the rationale for its use:

> Grounded theory methodology is a scientific method that features the systematic analysis of data gathered through interviews with the participants under study to build a theory of their experiences (Strauss & Corbin, 1998). The emerging theory, because it grounds its concepts in data provided by the participants, is consistent with the phenomenon under study (Strauss & Corbin). Therefore, the used of grounded theory methodology was essential to the goals of the study. (p. 175)

WRITING A QUALITY PROPOSAL

What constitutes "quality" in qualitative proposal writing has been much discussed in qualitative inquiry across disciplines and research traditions. Although there are no easy answers to this question, we explore the important components that we believe constitute quality writing.

Presentational Rigor

Kline (2008) described the importance of *presentational rigor*—"the combination of trustworthiness, methodological and analytic rigor, and coherence" (p. 212)—in evaluating quality writing. We have described trustworthiness in detail in Chapter 7. Writing that conveys *trustworthiness* in the research proposal should include *methodological and analytic rigor*. For instance, trustworthiness in research proposal writing involves providing sufficient information about the participants, settings, and data collection and analysis techniques as you write the research proposal. The degree of rigor your research proposal conveys is also important. Kline asserts that *rigor* in qualitative writing is reflected in sentences that detail the researchers' beginning conceptualization and use of methods. For instance, he suggests that *rigor* includes

> researchers' prior experiences with and assumptions about the topic being researched, the rationale for the specific qualitative approach used as it relates to the research questions, and the presentation of sampling and data collection methods. In addition, researchers have the responsibility of describing how their biases influenced data analysis and how their relationships with participants affected their interpretation of data and findings. Finally, a rigorously presented manuscript includes implications that findings have for professional practice. (p. 211)

Coherence is an additional component of quality proposal writing. Coherence, discussed in Chapter 7, is the degree to which the proposal is epistemologically consistent from its purpose statement and use of tradition to its data collection and analytic techniques. There are certainly instances where the phenomenon of inquiry may not allow the researcher to maintain a high degree of coherence throughout a manuscript, for a variety of reasons. For instance, in a recent study colleagues and I (Singh) conducted of transgender (female-to-male, or FTM) experiences of sexual orientation and gender identity (Dickey, Burnes, & Singh, 2011), our opportunity for sampling rested on a one-time data collection of semistructured interviews at a conference geared toward transgender people. Therefore, our ultimate research study was not able to maintain a rigorous degree of coherence throughout our writing because we extracted data analytic techniques (axial coding from grounded theory) that were inconsistent with grounded theory demands for recursivity in the process of data collection and analysis. The study was important, and the one-time-only data collection reflected a reality of working with a historically marginalized group. However, this reality also positioned our writing as less coherent than we would have liked. We share this example to illustrate that you may not always be able to achieve all of the standards of quality involved in rigorous and coherent qualitative writing. But don't throw the baby out with the bathwater at this point. Consider the components of quality research proposal writing, and if you do not meet all the criteria—write about *why* this is so. Below is an excerpt from our research proposal as an example of how we addressed limited coherence in the Discussion section (Dickey et al., 2011):

> There are also several research implications from this study. Unlike traditional grounded theory designs where the researchers can revisit initial participant interviews and invite recursivity into the qualitative design, the participants in this study were interviewed only once. There were several times during the data analysis where the authors would have liked to follow up with questions about the participant interviews. The decision to interview participants once was based on the fact that it remains challenging to access a readily available FTM sample (Namaste, 2000). Future research should integrate online components to supplement semi-structured interviews. For instance, use of Instant Communication Technology (e.g., instant messenger, Skype) may be a less intrusive way to follow-up with participants. Indeed, future studies may consider conducting email interviews or video interviews that would increase access to potential participants. The drawback of this approach would be that the sample would be limited to participants who had online access, which may limit understanding of FTMs who have lower socioeconomic and/or educational status. (p. 27)

Tell a Good "Story" of Your Study

Many qualitative writing experts have highlighted the importance of telling the *story* of your study (Golden-Biddle & Locke, 2007; Richardson, 2003; Wolcott, 2008). If you think of the great storytellers in your life, you can sense that this ability is both a skill and a gift. The gift of telling the story of your study through your writing is either there or it is not. However, fortunately it is also a skill, especially when it comes to crafting a story through your writing.

This skill may well be among the most important criteria of qualitative writing because it has many implications. A good story should have a beginning, middle, and end. *Boring, disinterested, disconnected*—these are words that you would not associate with a good story. Golden-Biddle and Locke (2007) describe the importance of deciding about the "authorial character" of the researcher. In other words, you as a researcher are a character in your story, so what authorial decisions will you make as you write to convey yourself as a character/storyteller? The authors discuss the tension that exists and the choices you will have to make along the way as you write. Will you be the "character of the institutional scientist, carrying the marks of the Academy" (one end of the continuum) or will you recognize that "personal human depictions are equally crafted as the human scientist" (pp. 78–79)? Or will you write somewhere in the middle of that continuum?

Wolcott (2008) added that telling the story of your study includes addressing the *problem of focus*. He shares that there is indeed a challenge if you are struggling with writing, for instance, a purpose statement. He does encourage people to seek outside support in talking through the focus of the story you will tell of your study. However, we really appreciate that he refers the researcher *back to the written word*. Rather than seeking to come up with solutions prior to writing, Wolcott sends us back to the paper to use our storytelling as a way to *resolve* the problem of focus, so writing, then, is not framed as the source of the problem in telling the story of your study.

In her discussion of writing about the focus of qualitative research, Sandelowski (1998) takes a different approach; she emphasizes that one must *determine the point of the story*. She asserts that quality writing about the story of your research will not happen until you are able to state the story of your study in one sentence. Her rationale is that if you cannot tell the story of your research in one sentence, then you are still unclear as to the point of your study. *Hmm.* We do not think this means that you are back at the drawing board if you cannot achieve the story-in-one-sentence task or elevator speech, discussed earlier in the text. However, we do think it is a useful organizing tool to ensure that the "point" of your study is always in your mind to support the continued (and what Golden-Biddle & Locke, 2007, call "theorized") story of your research.

Refer Back to Your Favorite Qualitative Authors

A significant aspect of telling a good story about your study is having some reference point for your writing. Let's take this a step further and say that this reference point is an author (or authors) who inspires you. Pratt (2009) explicitly describes this as *modeling someone whose style you like or who consistently publishes qualitative work*. He asserts that as the number of strong qualitative studies increases, there are more opportunities to find a diverse array of authors with whom you may resonate in terms of writing style. We would add that this number has increased across disciplines as well, so the typical advantages of reading deeply in the literature across disciplines (e.g., finding similarities and/or differences in how different fields discuss a topic of inquiry) are maximized further when you find a model to inspire you. Pratt advocates an additional goal of looking for your exemplar writers across disciplines because journals themselves, due to their individual review processes and related editorial criteria for evaluating strong qualitative studies, differ considerably. Later in the chapter, we share an example of one journal's criteria for qualitative writing. See Perspectives 12.1 for our discussion of some of the writers who have influenced our approach to qualitative writing.

Avoid the Danger Zone: Cautions to Take When Writing

In addition to the key components you need to include in your proposal, a large component of writing a quality research proposal is making sure that you know what *not* to include in your writing. Pratt (2009) called stepping into this terrain "wan-

Perspectives 12.1. Writers Who Have Influenced Our Qualitative Work

"I remember clearly when I found that 'one' article that inspired me. It actually wasn't a qualitative article. It was a conceptual article on traumatology by Burstow (2003). Because my research agenda was looking at trauma in South Asian communities from a feminist perspective, I had difficulty finding relevant articles that had a resilience perspective. Burstow inspired me with every word she wrote. She was basically calling the entire trauma field to take an empowerment perspective, which was perfect for my literature review and for a good dose of inspiration. For qualitative writers, the two members of my writing group—Stephanie Jones and Corey Johnson—consistently push me to think differently, creatively, and with imagination about the use of words in writing. Reading their work on a regular basis has naturally influenced my writing. Stephanie is in early childhood education and Corey is in recreation and leisure studies—so the added bonus is getting to read across disciplines. I have learned new theories and different writing techniques along the way."

—AAS

"There are so many scholars that contribute to how I write up qualitative research! First, the works of Creswell, Miles, Huberman, Patton, Lincoln, Guba, Denzin, Lather, and others sprinkled throughout the text indicate that these are some of the major contributors that influence how I conceptualize and participate in qualitative inquiry. Second, one of the scholars to whom we dedicate this volume, Dr. Joel Meyers, serves as a foundational model for me. He is an ethnographer and advocate for educational issues, whose writing not only captures rigorous aspects of a qualitative report, but has findings that directly translate to educational practice. Finally, I cannot forget the importance of promising and budding scholars with whom I have the privilege to interact on a daily basis: my students in counseling, higher education, curriculum and instruction, special education, early literacy education, K–12 education, and other disciplines. No matter if I am instructing them in coursework and witnessing their development of qualitative projects, or if I am working alongside them on research projects, they remind me of the importance of collaboration, interdisciplinary research, and thinking outside the box in qualitative inquiry. I truly am inspired by them every day."

—DGH

dering down dangerous paths" (p. 857). In general, it is important in any academic writing to avoid using casual or dramatic language or even using "ten-dollar" words. Examples of casual writing are, "The researcher *wishes* to convey … " and "The researcher *hopes* to convey. … " You could easily revise these two sentence stems to better reflect academic writing: "The researcher *aims* to convey … " and "The researcher *seeks* to convey. … " As you can see, you really do not have to use ten-dollar words to replace casual writing with academic writing. It's a simple but important shift in your use of language.

You want to be cautious in using dramatic language because it detracts from your content. This might be tough to enforce, as it is likely that you are passionate about your topic—which might draw you to use more dramatic language. Also, as you build your rationale for studying a phenomenon, you do want to convey to your audience how necessary understanding the phenomenon is for your field. It is fine to write so that you build the reader's understanding of the need to study a phenomenon. However, as you build your case, you do not want your writing to be so dramatic that when the audience reads the details of your actual study, they are so distracted they miss the important components. Using words such as *alarming, frightening, distressing,* or *shocking* are good examples of dramatic language *not* to use. Instead, more academic language, if you were describing the prevalence of a problem, might include *increasing, concerning,* or *rising.* Even the word *escalating* would be a good compromise here because it has a hint of the dramatic, but would not overshadow the words that come next. Take a look at the difference below—and notice what part of the sentence you are drawn to the most. You want your reader's eye to be drawn to the focus of your topic primarily:

> *There is a frightening increase in the rates of children who are living in poverty.*
> versus
> *There is an escalating increase in the rates of children who are living in poverty.*

As you have read various types of qualitative writing, you might have also noticed that there is an abundance of folks who are fond of using ten-dollar words or phrases that require second, third, and fourth readings in order to understand them. Avoid this kind of language for the same reason you want to avoid the casual or dramatic in your writing: It minimizes the importance of your topic because the reader is distracted. We have a personal belief that those folks using the ten-dollar words have a wee bit of insecurity issues they might need to work out. Our belief is that if you want your audience to care about your topic (why would you spend all that time on your study anyway, right?), you want your writing to be invitational. Let's take another look at some examples. Again, pay attention to where your eye goes as a reader. Ideally, you want to aim for your reader's eye to go to the focus of your topic:

Using ten-dollar words in a sentence:

> *The representational nature of grounded theory designs mimics epistemological complications where the interface between researcher and subject is maximized.*

Hopefully you can see that writing in this manner creates a significant barrier between the author and the audience in terms of understanding—*and* the meaning of the sentence is somewhat lost amidst the verbiage. Next, we revise the above sentence to use academic language that is also invitational and allows the reader to easily understand the author's focus:

> *The goal of grounded theory designs is to seek the "truth" of what participants describe as their daily experiences of living in poverty. The role of the researcher and the participants is clearly defined in grounded theory studies and requires a collaborative relationship.*

If you continue to struggle with using casual writing, dramatic language, or too many ten-dollar words, don't get too down on yourself. We don't want to see you on another slippery slope—the dreaded writer's block! Keep writing as you would for your first draft so that you can get something down on paper. Then go back and use the nifty thesaurus in your word-processing program or ask for your instructor and/or peers to take a look at your writing.

In addition to giving thorough attention to your choice of words in your writing, keep in mind Pratt's (2009) five writing paths, which you do *not* want to wander down. He discusses two main "perilous paths" that can lead you, as a writer, down the wrong road (p. 857). First, Pratt described what he often sees in weak qualitative writing as *lacking a balance between theory and data*. We have already touched on achieving high-quality writing about theory within your conceptual framework, and we talk about quality writing in describing your findings in the next major section in this chapter. However, Pratt's reference to finding a balance between theory and data refers to keeping an eye on this balance within the entire qualitative research report. He encourages writers to maintain a balance between writing about the findings of a study and including all the data for the reader. Additionally, Pratt urged writers to not overfocus on showcasing the data for the reader without using the theory (part of the conceptual framework in this volume) to interpret the data. From this perspective it might seem that Pratt is focusing on the Method section of your report (which we talk about in detail in the next section). However, we interpret his encouragement of seeking balance to apply to the entire report. Richardson (2003) similarly discussed writing a "layered text" as a way to achieve this balance in your writing and integrate the researcher's voice, your findings, and your conceptual framework throughout your qualitative report. A good way to double-check that you have achieved a balance in your writing between theory and data is to do an actual word count of how often you are talking about both; there should be a rough equivalence (although not exact) between the two. If you are not the type to like this approach, you can also read through your paper (or ask a peer or mentor to do so) while actively holding the questions of, "How am I maintaining this balance between theory and data?" and "Where are the instances in my report where I am not maintaining this balance between theory and data?" And, of course, you do not want to merely hold these two questions. You want to identify the answers and make revisions accordingly.

Form a Writing Group

We have discussed a mixture of the "dos" and "don'ts" of writing up your qualitative report. A definite "to do" that we have found helpful is the formation of a writing group. We know, we know. It feels like you don't have time to conduct your study—yet alone call together a circle of writers who also do not have the time. Maybe you have heard or hold a stereotype that writing groups are for "serious" writers or geared more toward creative writing. You also might not be the type of person who likes to do anything in a group (even some of the group exercises we have asked you to do in this volume).

Whatever your initial reaction is to thinking about developing a writing group, we encourage you to be open to it! A writing group can give you structure when you are struggling to give yourself that structure. There is nothing like the accountability that comes when you have a deadline for writing that is set by a group rather than by yourself. Writing groups can, in this manner, increase your productivity *and* the quality of your work. If writer's block is something you experience, as if you can hardly put pen to paper (or, rather, fingers to the keyboard), a writing group can make the block feel less gigantic and less impossible to penetrate. In addition, you might have discovered this in the route to pursuing the PhD; the journey is an individual one ultimately, and research and the act of writing can be isolating for some. Being a member of a writing group not only combats that isolation but also can give you specific steps to take and inspiration to feel when it is tough to generate those for yourself. We list some helpful considerations to guide you in forming a writing group in Table 12.3.

In Figure 12.3, we visually summarize the important components of quality writing in your qualitative research report.

TABLE 12.3. How to Start a Writing Group

- *Consider the focus of the group you would like to form.* Is it to complete your qualitative report? Is it to give and exchange writing feedback? Is it a place to simply check in on the status of your report and brainstorm with your writing group members?

- *Keep it small.* In our experience, a writing group of three people is the ideal size. With only two people, the meetings and feedback more easily become routinized and stale. Yet it is still comfortably small so that the meetings are not stressful—especially if you are committing to reading each others' writing before the writing group meets.

- *Create some clear structure.* How long will each meeting last? Where will you meet? Over what period of time will you meet? Any structure you agree upon in advance will help you through the inevitable challenges (e.g., busy schedules, emergencies) that will arise.

- *Set individual and group goals.* On member might want to improve his or her writing in the Discussion section. Another might struggle with the Introduction section and literature review. The third might have trouble knowing where to begin writing or how to approach academic writing at all. Knowing each other's goals can help you check in on one another. Having a shared group goal (which might be general or specific) can help as well.

- *Commit to attending and supporting one another.* If one of you misses the group or cannot make a previously scheduled meeting, talk in advance about whether you will reschedule so that everyone can be present.

- *Protect your writing group time!* This goes back to the point about structure. A critical aspect of your writing group is to support you in writing *better*. So, if the time is not protected … well, you can probably figure that one out.

- *Celebrate your accomplishments along the way.* Each member has (ideally) set individual goals, which are not achieved overnight but rather step by step. Celebrate these individual steps and soon all of you will have behaviorally reinforced for yourselves the fact that the act of writing is good and an important part of qualitative research.

FIGURE 12.3. Components of "quality" in your qualitative report.

WRITING THE RESEARCH REPORT

We always kid one another about our personality types and how they influence our interactions with the world—and, naturally, how our personality shapes the process of our writing. My colleague (Hays) is quite fond of telling her classes that my (Singh) personality tends toward less structured and more "anything goes" approaches to life. I actually experience my life very differently. Structure—especially in my writing—keeps me sane and focused. However, I believe that my colleague (Hays) is *so* structured that I "look" free-flowing in comparison. I am sure we will continue to enjoy this back-and-forth debate for many years to come. However, for now, my true "structured" colors come out in Table 12.4, where I share a sample structure for a qualitative research report.

Your Introductory Sentence(s)

You want your introductory sentence(s) to serve three functions. First, your introductory sentence should immediately contain the topic of your qualitative inquiry. We have both reviewed several qualitative manuscripts for publications that waited too long to tell the reader exactly what was being studied. The writing may be good, but it is also a waste of time for your audience and, worse, can confuse your reader as to the topic of your manuscript. So, immediately dive into your topic in that first sentence. If you have conducted a case study of school reform, discuss school reform in the first sentence. Second, you want to give some type of pressing rationale as to *why* the topic is important. Using school reform as an example, you might note that school reform is traditionally understood in terms of policies, but that there is little known, from the policymakers' point of view, about *how* they engage in the school reform process. You might even decide to define the constructs early in your introductory sentences if the topic is poorly understood in general, drawing on previous literature. Finally, you want your introductory sentences to "pop." Although we are avoiding dramatic language, we also do not want to bore the reader to death. We provide an example here from student Kim Molee (2009) from her study on school reform entitled *School Reform from a Legislator's Point of View*:

> The nature of a republic requires the general population to elect our representatives, who then create policies that affect all our lives. An example of such a policy is the public school reform movement, and its impact on students, teachers and the public school system. There are many professionals, within different disciplines, such as social science scholars, policy makers and education practitioners making efforts to improve and reform our education system. Yet often these people work for similar goals and do not collaborate. Given this assumption, there is a need for more information about school reform to improve collaboration among scholars, policy makers and education practitioners. Finally, this information can be of value to the general public as well, if we are to be informed, participatory citizens. (p. 10)

You can see that Kim does something a little different with her introductory sentence. Its "pop" factor is present in that she "paints" with a broad stroke the implications of policymaking for all people's lives. Then, she drills down to the specific topic of her study: educational reform. Kim's study specifically focuses on how collaboration occurs

TABLE 12.4. A Structured Approach to Qualitative Report Writing

Components of a qualitative report	Sample page length
Introduction/Rationale • Introductory sentence stating the topic • Inclusion of relevant background information (e.g., statistics, important gaps in the research literature)	3–4 pages
Literature Review • Review of the most relevant and recent (within 5–10 years) literature related to topic • Include older research (more than 10 years) only when seminal theory and research related to topic • Include purpose statement • Introduce research tradition if used in a novel or innovative manner • See Chapter 4 for more information on writing a literature review.	5–6 pages
Method • Describe research tradition (if not introduced in previous section) • Describe participants • Provide demographic information • Outline the procedure for study • Describe research bias and research team • Describe instruments (e.g., semistructured interviews, researcher as instrument) • Describe data collection • Describe data analysis • Describe standards for and strategies of trustworthiness	5–6 pages
Findings • Provide introductory sentences describing overall findings • Provide thick description in describing findings	7–8 pages
Discussion • Provide summary sentences of findings • Describe relationship of findings to previous literature review • Identify implications of study • Discuss limitations of the study	5–6 pages
Conclusion	1–2 paragraphs

Note. This table outlines suggested parameters in terms of page length and organization for a 25- to 30-page qualitative report (a page length often requested by journals due to space limitations). It is incredibly challenging to condense a rigorous qualitative report that includes rich, thick descriptions of participants' voices. This outline is provided to give those of you who love structure an overall visual of your report. Of course, we encourage you to *not* use this suggested outline as a one-size-fits-all approach, but rather to stimulate your own reflections on a comprehensive picture of your report.

within educational reform policymaking, which she states within her first few introductory sentences. Our only suggestion to strengthen her introductory sentences might be to add statistical information or other specific information to help the reader define the construct of policy reform. However, since that information can also come in the second paragraph, we think Kim actually did a nice job of using her writing to invite her readers to care about her topic. That's what we call success in answering the "so what" question about your study. Case Example 12.1 provides another excellent model of introductory sentences.

CASE EXAMPLE 12.1. The Introductory Sentence(s)

Anne M. P. Michalek, *The Experience of Success for Adolescents Diagnosed with Attention-Deficit/Hyperactivity Disorder.*

The following is the introduction of her study on the experiences of adolescents diagnosed with ADHD. The reader begins the proposal with a description of ADHD.

> Attention-deficit/hyperactivity disorder (ADHD) is one of the most frequently cited medical/behavioral conditions and the most common childhood disorder (Barkley, 1997). Barkley (1997) describes ADHD as a developmental disorder affecting a child's ability to regulate behavior, control behavior, or keep future goals and consequences in mind. These deficits are manifested and demonstrated through a variety of behaviors, including an inability to sustain attention, effectively regulate levels of activity according to the situation, and effectively plan and complete tasks.

(Please see Appendix B for full proposal.)

The Purpose Statement across Traditions

Numerous qualitative scholars have discussed the importance of writing a strong purpose statement in the qualitative report (e.g., Creswell, 2006; Merriam, 2002; Wolcott, 2008). A strong purpose statement forms the transition from the rationale for and introduction of your study and related literature to a specific statement of the study's purpose (sometimes called the "problem statement"). In other words, your writing guides the reader from your curiosity about and exploration of your topic to a "problem that can be addressed through research" (Merriam, 2002, p. 11). Wolcott (2008) urges writers to dive right into the purpose statement and be explicit, using a sentence stem of "*The purpose of this research is . . .*" (p. 70). Your purpose statement should have several important components within it. Take a look at doctoral student Sesha Joi Moon's purpose statement for her study on *The Subsistence and Impact of Tokenism on the Doctoral Experiences of African American Females* (2009):

> The purpose of this study is to investigate the subsistence of tokenism in higher education and its perceived impact on the doctoral experience by African American females at traditionally White institutions. (p. 2)

You can see that Sesha clearly states her study's problem in her purpose statement. Her writing avoids extraneous words and language that are uninviting, obtrusive, or

> The purpose of this _____ (narrative, phenomenological, grounded theory, ethnographic, case) study is (was? will be?) to _____ (understand? describe? develop? discover?) the _____ (central phenomenon of the study) for _____ (the participant) at _____ (the site). At this stage in this research, the _____ (central phenomenon) will be generally defined as _____ (a general definition of the central concept).

FIGURE 12.4. Creswell's (2006, pp. 103–104) formula for a purpose statement.

unclear to her audience. Writing a purpose statement can vary across traditions in that these different research traditions, as we discussed in Chapter 2, require different research problems to be answered. See Figure 12.4 for Creswell's "formula" for a strong purpose statement across the research approaches. We especially like his formulaic approach for beginning writers of qualitative studies because learning his structure initially can help you later become more creative in crafting your purpose statement.

Another advantage of using Creswell's formula for the purpose statement is that it clearly showcases the function of the purpose statement to transition your report to the Method section. However, before you move on to writing the Method section, we suggest that you briefly write two to four additional sentences to "unpack" your purpose statement and link it back to the focus of your study. To illustrate, let's return to Sesha's purpose statement and how she links it to her research tradition and important constructs in her study's examination:

> The purpose of this study is to investigate the subsistence of tokenism in higher education and its perceived impact on the doctoral experience by African American females at traditionally White institutions. A qualitative methodological approach was used to report the findings from a series of interviews with one (1) participant that intends to reveal the respondent's life history experience. Tokenism is operationalized as a person that is assigned to a group as a result of their auxiliary differentiations from the dominant group (Blalock, 1967; Kanter, 1977). Race and gender classifications are defined according to the participant's self-identification as African American and female. (p. 5)

Sesha did a beautiful job in her writing of moving from a clearly articulated purpose statement to introduction of the use of life history as her research tradition. Next, she described tokenism and race and gender classifications in a manner that is accessible to the reader. She intentionally used words such as *defined* and *operationalized* to guide the reader to more fully understand the context of her purpose statement.

The Researcher's and Participants' Voices in the Report

We discussed the issue of *voice* in qualitative research in Chapter 5. Now, let's revisit that issue so you understand how to *write* about voice—your voice, as the researcher, and the voices of your participants. Prior to writing, you need to make a decision about the degree to which your voice or your participants' will be present. As Sandelowski (1998) notes, "this decision involves thorny issues concerning authorial presence and power" (p. xx). It is a serious issue in your writing, however, so own that in making the decision, you are holding power. How does holding this power influence the way you write, what you write about, and the basics of whether you will write in the first or third person?

Sandelowski (1998) asserted that qualitative researchers often *write* that their participants' voices will hold prevalence in the report—yet the researchers' voice still predominates and/or participants' voices are boiled down to one voice. She cites Richardson's (1994) encouragement to write a *polyvocal text*, wherein the writer integrates several points of voice in the report. A polyvocal approach echoes the idea of the "layered text" we discussed previously. Essentially, you want your writing to incorporate your voice as the researcher and your participants' voices in a format that contrasts the multiple perspectives, rather than writing in a singular (e.g., participant voices showcased while neglecting your own voice as a researcher) or dichotomous (e.g., delineating sections where you write about your voice from sections where you write about participants' voices) manner. We touch briefly on the politics of publishing in the last section of this chapter, but we do want to acknowledge Sandelowski's implication that writing from a polyvocal stance may be challenging to more traditional journals that still view qualitative research from Position 1 (the *holy trinity*) or Position 2 (*translation of methods*). We encourage you to make your decisions in writing about voice in your report guided by what your conceptual framework and research questions demand of you. For now, engage in Proposal Development 12.2 to explore how the issue of voice will influence your writing in the report.

PROPOSAL DEVELOPMENT 12.2. Exploring the Issue of Voice in Your Report

Develop an outline for a research report or proposal that is specific to your selected research tradition(s) and paradigm(s). What type of voice will you use in your writing? To what degree do you feel that you could thickly describe your findings?

The Participant Section of Your Report

In writing the participant section of your report, think about your participants. This might seem like a pretty obvious statement! However, we often read participant sections of manuscripts that do not fully describe the demographics of participants. Any data that you collected about participants' demographics should be shared in this section. Hopefully, you have collected a good deal of demographic information. We suggest that you consider including the major identity categories of demographics listed below that are relevant to your phenomenon of inquiry:

- Gender identity and/or sex
- Race/ethnicity

- Socioeconomic status or social class
- Sexual orientation
- Ability identity
- Religious/spiritual affiliation
- National origin
- Geographic region

Of course, you may not include all of these demographics (or decide to add other categories), but try to interrogate yourself when you decide not to include a certain demographic component of your participants. What might the reader miss in understanding your study as a result of not having access to this demographic information? For instance, when Michelle Espino makes presentations on her study of the pursuit of higher education by Latinas, she often discusses how, at the time of the study, she was so focused on the race/ethnicity and gender of her participants that she missed the salience of sexual orientation for several of her participants, who identified as queer or even as heterosexual. That type of interrogation of your own work as you write not only builds trustworthiness with your audience but also simultaneously gives your writing the freedom and permission to become more complex and interesting without becoming stilted in the process.

In addition, be sure to write about the way in which you sampled your participants. This is a good place to, again, invite complexity into your writing. Tell the audience what the sampling approach was and how it was used, in addition to its appropriateness for your phenomenon of interest. See Case Example 12.2 for a student example of a good beginning of the Participant section. In this example, the student is writing a proposal for whom she would sample for her study.

CASE EXAMPLE 12.2. The Participant Section of Your Report

Julie F. Byers, *Exploring Teacher Candidates' Reflections of Instructor Picture Book Usage in Teacher Education Programs.*

Stratified purposeful sampling was used to select participants. Participant selection was criterion based and thus came from a pool of students that had taken an education course in which a professor used a picture book in the college classroom. It was intended to gather participants with similar picture book experiences from various instructors. However, convenience sampling was the most logical choice due to the fact that the researcher utilizes picture books in her college classroom. From those chosen from the initial pool, an anticipated 6–10 participants would then be selected in a way that would be most representative of the demographics of the students currently in the education program at [university]. This was determined by analyzing the current statistics of enrollment of education courses. Selection will include sampling representativeness in terms of age, race, and sex of participant. Age was included due to the variety of age in current programs. Age differences between traditional and nontraditional students would add a richer range of lived experiences in regard to this study. (p. 12)

The Procedure Section of Your Report

When your audience reads the Procedure section of your report, it should be 100% clear to them what the procedural steps of your study "looked like." You should write about the setting and context of your study. The overall steps and approach to data collection should also be included, such as the type of instruments used (e.g., semi-structured interviews, focus groups, art). Sometimes the instruments of a section can be a subheading of your Procedure section if you need to define them further. This is especially important if you are using an innovative instrument of which a general audience might not be aware. Other times, the overall description of your instruments will be sufficient as you detail the steps of your study in the Procedure section. We include a good example of the beginning of a Procedure section in Case Example 12.3.

CASE EXAMPLE 12.3. The Procedure Section of Your Report

Bouck, E. C. (2008). Exploring the enactment of functional curriculum in self-contained cross-categorical programs: A case study. *Qualitative Report, 13*(3), 495–530.

"Data from the case study was collected through multiple means in an effort to triangulate (Stake, 1995). At each site data was collected through full school day classroom observations for two days a week for three months (Bogdan & Biklen, 2003). A total of 85 hours was spent at Harborville and 70 hours spent at River Bend. During classroom observations, the researcher took fieldnotes and observed the events within the classroom. Decisions about what to observe and when were based on purposeful sampling (Patton, 1980), such that observations were selected to present the greatest opportunity to understand and gain insight into the case (i.e., each program). In addition, document reviews were conducted. Students' CA-60 files were analyzed and data was gathered on students' IQ, achievement test scores, disability classification, years in special education, age, and other pertinent information. Prior to any data collection, the researcher collected student assent and parental consent for the collection of all data" (p. 500).

As you can see, Bouck (2008) included the basic information and the steps of how she secured the informed consent and assent of participants. This is a very important component of the Procedure section that we often see qualitative report writers omit. Don't make that same mistake!

Your Reflexive Statement as a Researcher

We have emphasized throughout this volume how critical it is to be able to clearly identify your researcher positionality. We discussed researcher reflexivity in Chapter 5 extensively and have referred to its importance repeatedly. When writing about your researcher positionality, we encourage you to use the concept of "getting real" with your audience. Throughout your data collection and analysis, you know how your researcher positionality has influenced your writing. Ideally, you have documented your positionality, interrogated it, and sought to identify how it influenced the findings and understanding of your topic. Don't leave all that work behind! Write about this process. There may have been times in the data collection and analysis where your positionality took an unexpected turn or remained steady. Write about that process as well.

In our experience in reading both student qualitative reports and the manuscripts of more established qualitative researchers, we see authors touch lightly on their positionality. To some extent, this is due to the limits of journal page space in journal publications. As much as you can, however, don't skimp on this section. Ideally, we would love to read thick description on researcher positionality in every qualitative report. However, we can be realistic as well. Take a look at Case Example 12.4 so you can see how much researcher positionality you can pack into a brief one or two paragraphs when you "get real" in writing reflexively for your audience.

CASE EXAMPLE 12.4. Reflexive Statement/Research Positionality

Joseph W. Davis, *Experiences of Gay, Bisexual, Queer, and Questioning Greek Students.*

In relation to qualitative research, the issue of bias must be addressed to promote the ideal of trustworthiness. For the proposed study, the primary researcher is a 25-year-old white man who is working toward a doctorate in counselor education. The researcher identifies as gay and is actively involved in a Greek letter organization at his academic institution. He is at a level of complete disclosure within his organization in regard to his sexual orientation. The researcher has been involved with the interest area of sexual-minority students in Greek letter organizations for 5 years and has brought a national speaker to his academic institution to present on the subject material. The researcher holds the belief that Greek letter organizations have the potential to be beacons of acceptance for GBQQ individuals. However, this belief exists in that the potential for acceptance has rarely been met. He has experienced homophobic insults and derogatory jokes from within his own fraternity as well as others at his academic institution. These experiences have led to the occasional belief that the Greek system does not represent itself in an acceptable manner to incoming sexual-minority students. Along with what he has witnessed, the researcher also recognizes the acceptance he has gained from the majority of the other people in his respective organizations. (This proposal can be found in Appendix B.)

The Data Collection and Analysis Section

We do believe that every section of your qualitative report is incredibly important. And there is something about your data collection and analysis section that we think demands critical attention to detail. For those of you who love structure, this section should be pretty straightforward to write, whereas for those of you who are more fluid writers, this section might drive you a bit nuts. Essentially, your data collection and analysis section should not only showcase your most concise writing but also requires you to metaphorically hold your reader's hand and walk him or her step by step through what you did with your data.

The key word here is *step*. We actually advise you to use linear words such as *step, phase, stage,* and so on. We are not encouraging you to eliminate any recursivity that occurred in your data collection and analysis—quite the opposite. We are asking you to write in detail, step by step, about each component of your data collection and analysis. We include an excerpt from the beginning of a data collection and analysis section by Frankel and Levitt (2009; "Clients' Experiences of Disengaged Moments in Psychotherapy: A Grounded Theory Analysis") as an example of how detailed your writing should be in your data collection and analysis section:

The transcribed data collected in the interviews was divided into meaning units (MUs). MUs are segments of texts that each contain one main idea (Giorgi, 1970). In the initial stages of the analysis, the MUs were labeled in a manner that remained very close to the language used by the participants. The MUs were compared with each other and organized according to their similarities, creating descriptive categories. MUs could be assigned to more than one category, as dictated by the meanings contained therein. Once the initial descriptive categories were placed into higher order categories based on their commonalities. This process was repeated and, in this way a hierarchy of categories was developed. At the top of the hierarchy one core category was formed that represented the central interpretation drawn from the analysis. (p. 175)

Frankel and Levitt (2009) have begun discussing their analytic steps. We like that they did not talk about the data analysis process using words such as *emerged*. Rather, they used action verbs, such as *developed*, to acknowledge the power they had as researchers to identify patterns in the data. Next, as grounded theory designs require, the authors discuss the recursivity of data collection and analysis:

The process of collected data continued until the categories became "saturated," that is new descriptive categories did not appear to be present in additional interviews. This analysis became saturated at the sixth interview—meaning that the last three interviews did not add any new categories and that the analysis appeared to be comprehensive. (p. 175)

Our only critique of their writing in this section is their use of the word *appeared*. Whereas in their previous paragraph they acknowledged their researcher power in the data analysis, here they slip into a passive voice with this word. A better word to strengthen their writing here would be *identified* or even the word *developed*, which they used in the previous paragraph. However, they move into a strong section of writing in discussing their role as researchers in the data collection and analysis as they wrap up this section:

A detailed record of the researchers' intuitions, suspicions, feelings and thoughts about the interviews and analysis was maintained throughout the study. By noting these assumptions via memoing, an attempt was made to minimize any biasing effect they might have on the interviewing and analytic process, in order to keep the conceptualization of the phenomenon closely tied to the data and to keep a careful record of the procedures and theoretical developments of the analysis. (p. 175)

Again, we think the authors' writing is concise, is detailed, and helps the reader understand their steps. Our only suggestion here would be to give even more detail about the specific steps of *how* they minimized the "biasing effect" they reference. Without that information, although the writing is concise, it lacks some clarity as to what steps regarding their biases they actually took.

There may be other components of your data collection and analysis that you want to include in your writing so that the audience can understand the scope of your study. Although you cannot share the entire set of data management tools you might have used with your audience in your qualitative report, we do encourage you to share your codebook with your audience (as either an appendix or a table). See Table 12.5 for a student example by Ann Wendle Barnes of her codebook from her qualitative report.

TABLE 12.5. A Sample Codebook by a Student, Ann Wendle Barnes, for a Study on "Lived Experiences of a Few Who Forged Women's Programming"

Term	Meaning
Alone	Cut off, disconnected, invisible, isolated, nothing, scattered, starved
Barriers	Traditions, prohibit, block, different, differences, difficulty, discouragement, shut down, threatening atmosphere, overcome by environment, old, not welcome, not allowed, feeling guilty
Beginning	Start of change, paving the way, infant stages, infancy, didn't happen overnight
Change	Community movement, student involvement, consciousness, funding
Climate	Negative, tolerated, understood, change in the room, across the board, institutionalized
Control	Funding, traditions, assistance refusal, acknowledgment refusal, work credit refusal, recognition refusal, domestic, elitist, unacceptable female course of study
Discrimination	Anti-equal rights, discriminated against, disparate treatment, disrespect, intentionally embarrassed, irrational treatment by others, shouted down, sneered at, thrown out, thrown away, automatic "F"
Harassment	Blatant, appalling, eyeing, innuendo, looking a female up and down, mockery, sexual comments, wouldn't look at completed female student work, wouldn't give female students explicit directions, resentment of female students, demeaning word *deary*, degrading
Minority	Not necessarily population number, could be race other than white, gender other than male, religion other than Christian, nationality other than American
Strength	Brave, confident, hard work, independent, rise above, sacrifice, struggle, stubborn, work twice as hard
Support	Community, accomplishments, achieve, assisted, connected, encouraged, encouragement, sameness, secure, security, sense of connection, support, supported, supportive, uplifting, strong, warm, welcome, opportunity

The Findings Section

When you write your Findings section, you should demonstrate the same coherence and congruence Kline (2008) discussed (see earlier section on Writing a Quality Proposal). In other words, if you are writing a grounded theory study, do not switch to a phenomenological portrayal of your findings, or vice versa. In addition, there are several ways you can portray your findings. You might decide to use a table to summarize your findings or some type of visual portrayal of your model. However, again, keep in mind the ideas of coherence and congruence. If you are doing a grounded theory, your reader will expect to see some type of visual model that portrays your findings in a way that might be transferable to other groups. Yet, you might also use a visual model to portray phenomenological findings. You just want to be careful to clearly state that this is not a model you expect readers to transfer to other groups, but that it is representative of the group of participants involved in your study. Although an extensive exploration of writing up your findings is beyond the scope of this chapter, we refer you to Table 12.6 on page 406 which reproduces Chenail's (1995) suggestions for presenting data both within the qualitative report and to professional audiences is in Table 12.7 on page 408.

The Discussion Section

Ah—you have made it to the Discussion section! It is quite a feat to have made it to this point. And by now, you are likely tired—maybe tired of your topic in general or tired in terms of the work you have already put into your study. Heppner and Heppner (2004) discussed three challenges they see students experience by the time they get to the actual writing of the Discussion section. First, they discuss that you might feel like you have run out of ideas and/or momentum at this point. We both have experienced this challenge quite a bit in our own qualitative manuscript writing. We have found it helpful to grab some time with one another or other colleagues who "get" our topic and are willing to lend a listening ear. Sometimes, when addressing this challenge, one of us will actually become a note taker for the other. So, the one who is having some trouble writing her Discussion section will do some brainstorming of ideas out loud, while the other one takes notes.

The second challenge Heppner and Heppner (2004) discuss is feeling some insecurity or doubt about the relevance of one's research. If you are a novice researcher, this feeling is to be expected. A good way to combat these feelings of doubt is to return to why you decided to study this topic in the first place. You can also reread some of your participant transcripts to remember the importance of their voices. Sometimes this approach can backfire, though. Your participants, remember, are *real* people. And so are you. You definitely want to seek to represent their voices in the most truthful, accurate way you can; however, don't let perfectionism in seeking to do so get you stuck. We have a feeling your participants would want you to do the *best job* you could, *not the perfect job.*

The third challenge Heppner and Heppner (2004) address is a researcher's hesitance or even fear of putting his or her work in front of an audience. If this happens to you, the authors suggest recognizing that making one's research public is actual a significant component of the research process. Once you have put all of that work into your study, it is now time to share it with others to receive feedback, stimulate the literature, and come out of the more solitary actions of being a researcher to interacting with the public about your findings.

Now that we have discussed some of the challenges you might experience, let's look at specific steps you want to take in your Discussion section. Below is a potential draft outline you could follow to get the "bones" of your Discussion section in place:

    I. Restate research problem.

    II. Interpret each of your findings in terms of your conceptual framework.

    III. Describe any intersections among your findings that were unexpected or expected.

    IV. Explore the implications of your findings both within and outside of your field.

    V. Write about the future research directions regarding your topic based on your findings.

    VI. Discuss the limitations of your study.

    VII. Write a brief conclusion summarizing your entire study.

PRESENTING YOUR FINDINGS
IN STUDENT AND PROFESSIONAL SETTINGS

Presenting your findings can definitely be a great precursor to writing your final qualitative report. However, numerous scholars have written about the complications that come when presenting your study to the public (e.g., Chenail, 1995; Constas, 1992). Writing up your study for a class or professional presentation is, in actuality, an entirely different beast to wrestle with than writing your entire report. We suggest that you present your findings early and often to your classmates, peers, instructors, and even people in your personal life. By presenting your findings often to diverse audiences, you will benefit from a variety of feedback and questions that you may have never otherwise considered when writing up your study. This means you may be presenting at different points during your study. In this section we discuss presenting your findings from the perspective of having completed your entire study. However, if you have not completed your study and are presenting on one aspect of your findings, just delve into each of the components we discuss more deeply.

By the time you are thinking about presenting your findings, you have already sorted through immense amounts of literature, theory, research paradigms, data collection and analytic tools, and management techniques—just to name a sampling! So, where do you even begin in thinking about presenting your data? The simplest answer and approach we have found may sound a bit, well, simple. *Start at the beginning.* Why did you decide to conduct your qualitative study in the first place? There is probably a personal and a professional rationale; we encourage you to share both. The personal reason invites your audience to care about your study, and the professional reasons begin to build your credibility with your audience. After you have established your rationale, begin to inform your audience of the important constructs in your study. Define these constructs and make certain that you are grounding these definitions in the previous literature. We often see writers omit this step. It might seem obvious what a construct such as self-esteem means. You might even have a great definition of your own of self-esteem. However, your audience may have their own ideas of what self-esteem is, and those ideas may be drastically different from yours. Plus, and we know this is not a fun thing to think about—your definition is probably not an original one. It is more likely that a construct such as self-esteem has been defined repeatedly in the literature, possibly for a long period of time. Cite these previous definitions, especially any incongruence and debates among scholars about how to define the constructs you aim to understand in your study.

Take the same approach for your literature review. Depending on the time you have to present your findings, you may not have the luxury of elegantly articulating all the gaps in knowledge in the literature. Give your audience members the most important basics, though, so that they can understand the major underpinnings of your study. Next, be sure to let them know about your research paradigm and the essential demographics of your participants, the procedure for your study, and the details of your data collection and analysis. You may not be able to share all of the findings in your study. Again, select participant quotes that are thick and rich in description of the phenomenon you have studied. Don't forget to present your Discussion section, including the link back to earlier literature and your interpretation of your findings. This should include exploring the implications and limitations of your study.

We provide an outline for organizing your presentation in Table 12.6, to which you can refer as an example. Also, take a look at the student exemplar (Ann Wendle Barnes) for a class presentation of findings in Appendix B. Finally, no matter how much time you have to present, try to balance your time so that you can do justice to each section you have planned to present. Common challenges we have observed in qualitative study presentations include the following:

- Skipping over construct definition
- Neglecting to state researcher positionality
- Neglecting data analytic techniques to account for researcher bias
- Overlooking details of the researcher paradigm and tradition(s)
- Passing too quickly over identified findings
- Making assumptions about participants that are not grounded in the data
- Running out of time to discuss the implications and limitations of the study

TABLE 12.6. Sample Outline for a PowerPoint Presentation of Your Findings

Slide and number of slides	Description
Title (1 slide)	Includes your study's title, your name and credentials related to your field, and the date and place of your presentation.
Rationale (1 or 2 slides)	Ground this in statistics and any other important information related to the *why* of your study's topic.
Literature Review (2 or 3 slides)	Showcase the gaps in the literature. Define the constructs in your study and any consistencies and inconsistencies important for your audience to be aware of in understanding your study.
Method (2–5 slides)	Include the most significant aspects of your conceptual framework in this section. Identify research paradigm and tradition(s). Discuss your participant demographics, study's procedure, and data collection and analysis techniques used according to your tradition.
Findings (5–9 slides)	This is the bulk of your presentation if you are presenting an entire study. Consider using some type of visual portrayal of your findings either before or after you present them in order to help the audience understand their importance. Make certain to include thick, rich description from participants in the form of direct quotes and key observations you have as a result of analyzing how your researcher biases influenced your interpretation of your data.
Discussion (3–5 slides)	Summarize your findings and refer back to your earlier literature review in terms of how your findings either aligned or did not align with your topic. Discuss the implications of your study for your field and possibly other disciplines. Detail your study's limitations and possible ways future research might address these.
References (1 or 2 slides)	You might not include your entire reference list for the audience. You can highlight the most salient references or refer your audience to your e-mail so that they may e-mail you for your reference list.

Note. In this table we provide a sample outline for presenting your study in an hour format. You can think of each section in the left column as the "title" that can be listed at the top of each of your PowerPoint slides.

The main point you want to keep in mind when you present your findings is that just as in writing up your qualitative report, you are taking the role of storyteller. So, remember to make sure you have a beginning, middle, and end to your presentation. Invite your audience to give you feedback. Be comfortable with saying "I don't know" if you are stumped by a question (and then say that you will find out and get back to them!). Do whatever stress management techniques you need to do ahead of time and during your presentation so that you do not distract your audience with too many "umms" or excessive movements of your hands. We have found that even taking a few deep belly breaths before presenting can calm the nerves, activate the parasympathetic relaxation system, and set us up for a successful presentation. And, finally, try to enjoy the moment. You have accomplished a good deal to get to the stage of presenting your findings. Congrats!

Preparing a Poster of Your Qualitative Study

Up until now, we have discussed a general approach for presenting your findings at various student settings and professional conferences. One format that you may consider using is a poster presentation of your qualitative study. This type of presentation is often called a "Poster Session," wherein many researchers present their work simultaneously within the same time slot, while attendees walk through the poster session. The word *poster* indicates that your work may be compiled in a PowerPoint slide or other format, which is then printed on a large poster-size sheet and displayed on a large stand-alone bulletin board or a trifold poster board. No matter what the specific setup may be, posters are often arranged in rows so that attendees can walk through a poster session and either glance at your study's findings from afar or approach you to hear more about your study. See Table 12.7.

The most helpful aspect of poster sessions is that you are informally presenting to a potential mix of your peers and other more senior researchers and practitioners in your field. Many people are initially confused about how a poster session "works," but it really is an informal presentation wherein you may select to tailor your "presentation" to those who visit your poster. Some attendees may only be interested in your topic and in your handouts that summarize your study. Other attendees will stop and want to discuss particular aspects of your study, perhaps your findings or the methodology you selected for your study. We believe that poster presentations are an ideal vehicle to gather feedback from others about your research study at various stages (e.g., literature review, method, findings) of the project or at its completion. These informal discussions and feedback can help you view your study from different perspectives and ultimately strengthen it.

 ACTIVITY 12.1. Presenting Qualitative Research

Select a topic of research. What are the journals and conferences (local, regional, national, international) that are most suited to presenting your research?

TABLE 12.7. Suggested Formats for Presenting Your Qualitative Report

Natural	The data are presented in a shape that resembles the phenomenon being studied. For instance, if the data are excerpts from a therapy session, present them in a sequential order or in an order that represents the flow of the session itself.
Most simple to most complex	For sake of understanding, start the presentation of data with the simplest example you have found. As the complexity of each example or exemplar presented increases, the reader will have a better chance of following the presentation.
First discovered/constructed to last discovered/constructed	The data are presented in a chronicle-like fashion, showing the course of the researcher's personal journey in the study. This style is reminiscent of an archeological style of presentation: What was the first "relic" excavated, then the second, and so forth.
Quantitative-informed	In this scheme data are presented according to strategies commonly found in quantitative or statistical studies. Data are arranged along lines of central tendencies and ranges, clusters, and frequencies.
Theory-guided	Data arrangement is governed by the researcher's theory or theories regarding the phenomenon being represented in the study. For instance, a Marxist-informed researcher might present data from a doctor–patient interview in terms of talk which shows who controls the means for producing information in the interaction, talk which illustrates who is being marginalized, and so forth. In clinical qualitative research, this approach is quite prevalent as clinicians organize the data in terms of their understandings of how doctor–patient, or nurse–patient, and therapist–client interact.
Narrative logic	Data are arranged with an eye for storytelling. Researchers plot out the data in a fashion which allows them to transition from one exemplar to another just as narrators arrange details in order to best relate the particulars of the story.
Most important to least important or from major to minor	Like the journalistic style of the inverted pyramid, the most important "findings" are presented first and the minor "discoveries" come last.
Dramatic presentation	This one is the opposite of the inverted pyramid style. With the dramatic arrangement scheme, researchers order their data presentation so as to save the surprises and unforeseen discoveries for last.
No particular order	As it sounds, data are arranged with no particular, conscious pattern in mind, or the researcher fails to explain how or why the data are displayed the way they are.

Source: Chenail (1995). Reprinted with permission from *The Qualitative Report*.

 ACTIVITY 12.2. Presenting Your Qualitative Proposal

Conduct a 20-minute presentation in small groups of your research proposal and any initial findings. Evaluate your group members using criteria developed in earlier chapters.

PUBLISHING YOUR FINDINGS

Now that you have put a good deal of time and energy into your entire manuscript, you might be considering finding a publication outlet for your work. Heppner and Heppner (2004) identified two approaches that are helpful in selecting a journal. First, find journals that are appropriate for your topic and type of research; then, identify the best quality journals available. Their first suggestion is a relatively easy one. A good way to begin identifying appropriate journals is to ask your professors and to pay attention to where qualitative articles you like have been published. We think it is a good idea to brainstorm with your peers as well.

You want to identify at least five journals you might consider within your field. You may never have read some of these journals before. So, take some time to examine the typical manuscripts they publish. Often, you will stumble upon a journal that has issued a call for manuscripts or proposal submissions for a special issue for which your study might be a good match. An example of this from my own (Singh) publications was the call for a special issue by the *International Journal of Traumatology* on LGBTQ issues and trauma. When I read the call, I knew little about the journal's quality and its typical submissions. First I took a look at some of its past issues. I saw that the journal published qualitative work—not often, but the ones it did publish were of good quality. The bonus was that I had just wrapped up a phenomenological study of the resilience strategies of transgender people of color who had survived traumatic life events.

There can be surprises as you identify the list of potential journals to which you might submit. Once you have identified a list within your field, then take your search even wider than your field to identify additional journals that fit the scope of your topic. For instance, there are journals that specifically focus on qualitative articles (e.g., *Qualitative Inquiry, The Qualitative Report*). A good listing of journals that accept qualitative manuscripts can be found at *www.slu.edu/organizations/qrc/QRjournals.html*. Some of these journals are published online and some are in paper, whereas others are simultaneously published in online and paper formats.

In thinking about the Heppners' (2004) second suggestion to identify the highest quality journals, there are several ways to proceed. Impact factor, which is measured in a few ways, might be a primary concern for you. Traditionally, *impact factor* refers to the Institute for Scientific Information (ISI) rating. This rating is calculated yearly for journals in the Thomson Reuters *Journal Citation Reports* and is linked to the number of times manuscripts published in journals are cited (Craig, 2009). This type of impact factor might be more important to you if you are thinking of building an academic career. Other times, you might be more concerned with reaching a large number of practitioners through your research. In this case, you want to be curious about the subscription rate (i.e., the number of people who receive a journal). For example, there are about 50,000 members of the American Counseling Association (ACA) who receive the ACA's flagship journal (*Journal of Counseling and Development*). That is a huge audience that will potentially read your work!

Once you select a journal to submit to, check online to see if there are any existing guidelines for writing a qualitative manuscript. If guidelines are not available online, contact the editor. You might also locate a stand-alone article on guidelines for submitting qualitative research to a journal. See Table 12.8 for an excerpt from an article on guidelines. It may seem obvious, but we suggest, if this type of document exists for a journal in which you really want to publish your study, following those guidelines to the "t." And if you do not follow some of the guidelines, you might consider acknowledging this point and your reasons so that the editor does not decide to toss your manuscript submission without sending it out for review.

There are some politics involved with publishing; however, the topic of politics is beyond the scope of this chapter (we refer you to Rowena Murray's [2005] book *Writing for Academic Journals* for a comprehensive discussion of academic writing). It can be easy to stress out about the process of submitting your written manuscript for publication. We like to think about your submission as the first step in building a relationship with a particular journal. That means writing a cover letter introducing your manuscript to the journal's editor. We list a few tips and key words and phrases you may want to include in your cover letter here:

TABLE 12.8. Guidelines for Writing a Qualitative Manuscript

I. Background

   A. Review the theory and research underpinning of a study, to clearly present a solid conceptual framework for the study.

   B. Provide a succinct and coherent articulation of the research approach used in conducting the study, focusing on uncovering an emic perspective rather than proving etic hypotheses.

II. Method

   A. Present sufficient information on the process of data collection, with explicit articulation of how participants and/ or sites were selected; the kinds of questions asked; and the documentation of observations, all of which allow the reader to judge the trustworthiness of the research.

   B. Establish some form of dependability through the articulation of triangulation, reflexive journaling, multiple viewpoints and sources, and length of engagement.

   C. Include a self-reflexive description of the investigator(s) role, location, and perspective because this may have relevance to the conduct of the research, the participant responses, or the relationship with the data.

III. Data Analysis

   A. Give a description of the inductive approach used in the study.

   B. Present evidence of careful, recursive analysis with enough detail about the steps involved for a reader to determine the validity of the findings. For instance, demonstrating the links from codes to categories, from subthemes to themes, is helpful in determining whether the themes emerged from the data or were imposed on the data.

IV. Findings

   A. Communicate interpretations and conclusions that are rooted in the data, through the use of examples that can allow the reader to determine the transferability and depth of the findings.

   B. Trace the meaning of emerging patterns across all the contexts in which they are embedded, with an articulation of the limitations.

Source: Choudhuri, Glauser, and Peregoy (2004). Reprinted with permission from the American Counseling Association.

1. This is a formal letter. Therefore, use formal language that upholds the respect of the academic review process.

2. Include the title of your manuscript in the first sentence of your cover letter.

3. Describe anything that is unique about your study—*briefly*. For instance, is it the first qualitative study on a topic? Try not to be too editorial in this letter. Avoid saying you are studying a "serious" issue, for example.

4. Identify the section within the journal that your qualitative manuscript would fall under—often a research section.

5. Refer to your research ethics. Was there an ethics code that guided your writing within your field (we hope so)? Briefly note that you followed this code in preparing the manuscript.

6. Identify up front any ways that you may not be in accordance with the journal's submission guidelines. Did you go over their suggested page limit (an easy thing to do with a qualitative manuscript). Say so. Own it, build a rationale for doing so, and explicitly give concrete details (e.g., number of words or pages over the page limit for manuscripts) to the editor.

7. Be brief.

8. Thank the editor for his or her time in the review process. It's a real, live person who is the journal's editor, and chances are that he or she has been working terribly hard to ensure that each submission is handled in a timely, ethical, and respectful manner. Be appreciative.

We provide a sample cover letter (see Figure 12.5) to bring these tips for writing a good submission cover letter to life. If you have done a strong job in preparing your manuscript for the review process, you will hopefully get a favorable decision from the editor. The range of editorial decisions includes the following: (1) reject, with no invitation to revise and resubmit (ouch!); (2) reject, with an invitation to revise and resubmit; (3) accept, with major revisions; (4) accept, with minor revisions; and (5) accept, with no revisions (very, very rare). *All* of the possible editorial decisions from 2 to 5 are good news. Even the unequivocal rejection can be a good thing and can be helpful for you in making revisions. We suggest that you strengthen your manuscript based on these revisions, and *as soon as possible, submit the manuscript to another publication outlet.* Of course, give yourself time to process the sting of rejection. And then get right back up on that metaphorical publishing horse and revise and submit again!

Editorial decisions 2–5 also require immediate attention. These editorial decisions come with deadlines the editor has set for receiving your revised manuscript, in addition to the specific reviews from the editor and review team. Sometimes reviewer feedback can be confusing, brief, and/or actually conflicting. It is fine to contact the editor with specific questions—just don't overdo this contact. You do not want the editor to feel like he or she should be made an additional author on your manuscript because of the amount of feedback and time he or she has poured into your manuscript. Plus, your manuscript (believe it or not) is *not* the only one he or she is managing. A critical last step (really, an ongoing one as you are revising your manuscript) is to detail how you responded to each of the reviewer comments and any feedback offered by the editor.

We like to include this information as a bulleted list at the end of the cover letter we send when we resubmit an article.

The last steps of the publication process (and we are still continually surprised by this) involve a dramatic process of ... *waiting.* You wait. And *wait some more.* And possibly even *wait* some more. The publication process in academic journals is rarely a quick-footed beast. Rather, it operates more at a turtle's pace—and don't think of the story of the turtle and the hare, where there is a fantastic ending replete with meaning. You usually just wait and wait. Eventually, you get proofs of your manuscript (exciting!) to review; in this final step you ensure that your citations are all in your reference list, and vice versa, and you double-check things like the spelling of your name and your organizational affiliation. At some point, usually many years later, you get a journal containing an article with your name beside a fantastic study and with much improved writing as a result of the review process. We suggest celebrating every step along the road to publication, *including* the waiting.

Throughout this chapter we have discussed various writing tips. We summarize some of these in Wild Card 12.1 as reminders for you as seek to make your writing "sing" off the page and draw the audience into your qualitative study.

Dear Dr. Auger,

  Attached please find the manuscript "School Counselors' Strategies for Social Justice Change: A Grounded Theory of What Works in the Real World" for publication review in the Research section of the *Professional School Counseling* (PSC) journal. This is the first grounded theory inquiry into the interventions of school counselors who identify as successful social justice advocates within their school to achieve success in improving their school settings. In preparing this manuscript for submission to PSC, we followed the standards for research set by the ethics codes of the American Counseling Association (ACA) and the American School Counselor Association (ASCA).
  We would like to thank you in advance for the time and energy involved in the review of this manuscript. We look forward to your review. Please do not hesitate to contact us at *asingh@uga.edu* if you have any questions or concerns.

                                    Sincerely,
                                    Anneliese Singh, PhD, LPC
                                    Danica G. Hays, PhD, LPC

FIGURE 12.5. Sample cover letter to a journal editor when submitting your manuscript.

REFLEXIVE ACTIVITY 12.1.
Exploring Presenting and Publishing Your Findings

In your journal, explore your answers to the following questions:

- What are the strengths and challenges you may face in presenting and publishing your findings?

- What resources will you need to bring your study to completion and to publish your findings?

⚠ WILD CARD 12.1. CAUTIONS FOR THE WRITING ROAD

1. Refuse to give into "writer's block"! If you are not writing, identify the reasons why and address them so that you do not suffer in silence.

2. Do not write in the passive voice (Wolcott, 2008).

3. Use simple language that is accessible, inviting, and clear for your readers.

4. Mix it up! Do a word search for any words or phrases that you use too many times or that are somewhat stale.

5. Take your writing one section at a time, especially if thinking about the entire manuscript overwhelms you. Sometimes just taking it one sentence at a time helps us when we feel stuck.

6. Watch out for editorializing your participants' thick descriptions (Wolcott, 2008). Don't let your writing imply that you know more about participants' experiences than they do.

7. Be clear in your writing about your researcher interpretation. It is perfectly fine to say, for example, "From the researcher's perspective ... " or "The researcher interprets this as. ... " That way, you are transparent about where your participants "end" and your researcher perspective begins.

8. Keep the exemplars of qualitative writing whom you admire close by while you are writing. That way, when you are confused about how to transition to a new section, or are unsure about how to write a section, you have an example of good writing nearby.

9. Be open and actively seek feedback on your writing. We know that you may not be keen on joining a writing group, but if not, do not avoid getting commentary on your writing because it will be to your detriment in the end. Writing can feel like a vulnerable act; we feel less vulnerable and more open to feedback about our writing when we practice receiving (and giving) feedback on writing.

10. Remember the "uncle" test at every stage of your writing.

CHAPTER SUMMARY

In this chapter we discussed the essential components of writing and publishing your research findings. Quality is a huge aspect of your writing to which you want to pay attention throughout your report. There are also specific words you may want to use in terms of academic writing, and there is language that you will want to avoid in order to build trustworthiness with your reader. Overall, we recommend that you pay attention to how you write best—in a group or alone—and take the necessary steps in advance to avoid distractions to your writing process and/or writer's block. The key to writing quality reports also involves engaging feedback from your professors, colleagues, and peers—and even that "uncle" we like to refer to—in order to strengthen your report. Move through any fear you might have and share your writing with others. We promise that you will then end up with a report of which you are proud!

RECOMMENDED READINGS

Golden-Biddle, K. G., & Locke, K. (2007). *Composing qualitative research* (2nd ed.). Thousand Oaks, CA: Sage.

Wolcott, H. F. (2008). *Writing up qualitative research* (3rd ed.). Thousand Oaks, CA: Sage.

Glossary of Key Terms

Abductive Analysis: The generation of new concepts through qualitative data analysis.

Action Research: Corresponds to the purpose of solving specific problems and engaging individuals in solving those problems. The researcher focuses on a specific site, collaborates with individuals with a relationship to the topic, and works to resolve key issues to improve the lives of those at the site.

Analysis: A second step of qualitative data analysis in ethnography whereby the description of the first step in ethnographic analysis is sorted, displayed, and collapsed into patterns. Analysis involves identifying themes and patterns for the culture-sharing group as well as the group relative to groups, norms, and standards outside the group. During analysis, the researcher examines situated meanings, or ways that a local culture experiences and makes meaning of the events within their group.

Analytic Induction: The process by which qualitative data analysis moves from exploratory to confirmatory or verification methods. Verification involves seeking out cases to disconfirm present codes and themes in order to strengthen emerging models.

Applied Research: A type of research whereby a researcher seeks specialized knowledge about a specific problem in order to intervene in the problem.

Archival Data: An unobtrusive, often secondary data source such as written materials (e.g., case records, data sets, applications, forms) or statistics maintained typically by government or educational institutions. Archival data can be a helpful supplement to primary data collection.

Attributional Coding: Analysis of public attributions individuals make during spoken or written discourse; their understanding of the causes of various events of interest.

Auditor: An individual without a conflict of interest who reviews the audit trail (a trustworthiness strategy; see *Audit Trail*) to determine the extent to which the researcher or research team(s) completed a comprehensive and rigorous study.

Audit Trail: Physical evidence of systematic data collection and analysis procedures. Audit trails provide evidence of the research process for an auditor or any other consumer to review.

Authenticity: Criteria of trustworthiness, similar to confirmability (see *Confirmability*) in that clinicians and educators strive to represent participant perspectives authentically, using theoretical versus methodological criteria.

Autobiographical Case Study: Identified as a research approach of the case study tradition. The autobiographical case study is one written by researchers about themselves.

Autoethnography: Type of research tradition that involves a first-person account of events, interactions, and relationships within a cultural context. Autoethnographers use their own thoughts, feelings, documentation of field notes, and other personal experiences they have in response to their ethnographic examination of a culture as data.

Axial Coding: Second phase of analysis in the grounded theory tradition, wherein a researcher refines and examines relationships among open codes. This process collapses open codes into broader categories or codes for theory building.

Axiology: A philosophy of science that refers to values in the research process; the role of researcher, participant, and setting values in the research design; and the degree to which the research relationship is prioritized.

Background Question: A type of interview question about the participant, setting, or phenomenon to which the interviewer seeks an answer during the interview itself. Background questions tend to be solicited in written form, such as a demographic questionnaire.

Basic Research: A type of research whereby a researcher serves to expand the scope and depth of knowledge of a case for the sake of contributing knowledge to a particular discipline.

Behavior Questions: Behavior or experience questions are the "*what* versus *why*" questions; as an interviewer you are concerned with gathering a thick description of *what* occurred by and for the participants rather than *why* things occurred.

Belmont Report: A national report attending to three key research ethics: respect for persons (i.e., informed consent, voluntariness of participation), beneficence (i.e., maximizing participant benefits with minimal risk), and justice (i.e., representative and equitable participation and representation in the research process and reports).

Biographical Case Study: Identified as a research approach of the case study tradition. The researcher documents the history of an individual by using primarily archival data and other information sources about the person.

Blurred Genres:	A historical moment of qualitative research between approximately 1970 and 1986. The phase represented greater attention to the act of writing qualitative reports, with researchers no longer viewing a report as free from their values; reports were now considered to be interpretations of interpretations.
Bracketing:	Typically viewed as the first step in phenomenological data analysis. The researcher examines and sets aside preconceived beliefs, values, and assumptions about the research topic and proposed research design.
Case:	An individual or individuals, setting, process, or event that is the focus of a study. Cases have boundaries around them in that they can be explored as a unique and independent entity. Although in some instances a case could be classified as all four of these types, it is likely that one form of case best exemplifies an area of inquiry.
Case Description:	An aspect of qualitative data analysis in the case study tradition. Examination of the details and facts of a case and identification of the major findings to assist an audience in understanding the phenomenon, its boundaries, and its context more fully.
Case Display:	Qualitative data management tool that involves a graphic depiction of reduced (and chunked) data. Case displays are initially created for each individual case (within-case display) and then are later consolidated to examine concepts and variables across cases (cross-case display) for increased understanding of themes and patterns and to enhance generalizability.
Case Study:	A research tradition known as the universal tradition. Case studies are distinguished from other qualitative traditions because cases are researched in depth and the data are delineated by time period, activity, and place, using multiple data sources and methods.
Categorical Aggregation:	First phase of data analysis in the case study tradition. The researcher examines several occurrences of critical incidents, concerns, and issues within the data collected.
Causal Conditions:	A component of analysis in the grounded theory tradition. Causal conditions are factors influencing the phenomenon being studied.
Causal Network:	A form of case display (see *Case Display*) that allows for explanation and prediction of data. A causal network is a display of the most important variables, showing directions and sequences rather than relationships. In cross-case displays, this allows for a comparative analysis of individual cases, using the most influential variables to account for a particular outcome as the organizing principle. This type of display rates antecedents found across cases and links variables and processes.

Code: A label, tag, or "chunk" of various sizes based on the defined case or unit of analysis (see *Case*; *Unit of Analysis*). It can be referred to by many other terms, including *domain*, *factor*, *theme*, *subtheme*, and *item*, to name a few. Codes can be descriptive or interpretive, and they can be labeled by participants themselves (emic codes) and/or by the researcher (etic codes).

Coherence: Criterion of trustworthiness that refers to the degree of consistency of an epistemological perspective throughout the research design. The researcher is responsible for infusing the chosen perspective throughout the research process and describing it thoroughly in the research report.

Collective Case Study: Term defined by Robert Stake wherein multiple cases are used to investigate more general or broader phenomena or population.

Colonial Ethnography: A historical moment of qualitative research within the 17th, 18th, and 19th centuries. During this period one camp of researchers had an interest in studying and colonizing "primitives" and another camp had an interest in liberating colonized peoples.

Comparative Pattern Analysis: A qualitative data analysis technique in which researchers move back and forth through chunked data to compare categories. Comparative pattern analysis creates meta-codes that are not likely visible from directly reviewing data. Researchers consider the processing and sequencing of data and attend to where, how, why, and by whom that data occurred. Researchers seek and examine sequences and changes across time while triangulating data sources.

Comprehensive Sampling: Purposeful sampling method used to represent a sample. The researcher selects an entire group of people by an established set of criteria.

Concept Map: An aspect of the conceptual framework (see *Conceptual Framework*) and a visual display of an evolving theory and/or researcher assumptions about an area of inquiry, developed before data collection and revised throughout the research process. Concept maps can be categorized as *variance* or *process* maps (display of causal links or relationships between particular constructs or variables, and descriptive display of specific events or situations rather than variables, respectively).

Conceptual Framework: A network of concepts, theories, personal and professional assumptions, exploratory studies, and alternative explanations that collectively inform a research topic. The four major components of a conceptual framework are experiential knowledge (researcher assumptions, expectations, and biases), prior theory and research, pilot and exploratory studies, and thought experiments (alternative models or frameworks).

Conceptually Ordered Case Display:	A case display that explores and describes a concept (see *Case Display*). Conceptually ordered case displays can be created for individual case displays (e.g., thematic conceptual matrix, cognitive map, and folk taxonomy) or for several case displays (e.g., content-analytic summary table and the decision tree model).
Confirmability:	A criterion of trustworthiness similar to authenticity (see *Authenticity*) that refers to the degree, from a methodological perspective, that findings are genuine reflections of the participants investigated. This concept is most similar to the constructs of *objectivity* and *neutrality* in quantitative research.
Confirming and Disconfirming Sampling:	Purposeful sampling method associated with theory development and verification. As patterns emerge, the researcher looks for confirming cases to add depth to the study and seeks cases to disconfirm the pattern.
Consensual Qualitative Research:	Research tradition that integrates phenomenological, grounded theory, and other approaches. Consensus is key to this approach, as qualitative researchers use rigorous methods to facilitate agreement in interpretations among themselves, participants, as well as the general audience.
Consensus Coding:	Use of multiple researchers wherein each independently codes a data source, and then reach agreement as a team, discussing and agreeing on an operational definition of a code.
Consequences:	A component of analysis in the grounded theory tradition. Consequences are the results of intervening conditions for participants (see *Intervening Conditions*).
Constant Comparison:	A qualitative data analysis technique useful in developing a codebook. It refers to the continuous process of using earlier coding systems to code future data sources and revise the coding system.
Contact Summary Sheet:	A qualitative data management tool that summarizes a single contact with a case and serves as an initial step to qualitative data analysis. Contact summary sheets help researchers capture their own reflections about the data, outline initial salient themes based on the interview process, and jot down additional questions to be asked of a participant or setting.
Content Analysis:	A process of examining content and themes, typically from written documents. When used in ethnography (see *Ethnography*), researchers seek to identify relationships and patterns among words, phrases, and ideas within the data.
Convenience Sampling:	Purposeful sampling method used to represent a sample. Convenience sampling is the least representative sampling strategy, whereby researchers sample those to whom they have relatively easy access.

GLOSSARY

Creative Synthesis: The final qualitative data analysis phase of the heuristic inquiry tradition. The researcher seeks the best way to portray the findings as a composite whole, integrating his or her role and experience with the phenomenon.

Creativity: A criterion of trustworthiness that refers to implementing novel methodological designs, including imaginative ways of organizing, presenting, and analyzing data, and demonstrating flexibility in the overall research process.

Credibility: A criterion of trustworthiness that refers to the "believability" of a study. Credibility is somewhat analogous to *internal validity* in quantitative research. It is one of the major criterion qualitative researchers use to determine if conclusions make sense for a qualitative study.

Crisis of Representation: A historical moment of qualitative research within the mid-1980s. In this period there was a rise in feminism, constructivism, and critical theory paradigms, and a subsequent realization that qualitative researchers may not be representing themselves and their participants in an accurate way. During this historical moment, researchers begin to examine more closely the role of gender, class, and race in participants', as well as in their own, lives.

Criterion Sampling: Purposeful sampling method used to describe a phenomenon. Researchers sample participants who meet an important, predetermined criterion. The purpose is to review all cases that meet a criterion.

Critical Case Sampling: Purposeful sampling method used to describe a phenomenon. The researcher looks for experiences that are particularly significant because of their intensity or irregularity in order to serve as a benchmark or "cutoff score" for other participants.

Critical Reflection: A major characteristic of participatory action research. It refers to Freire's work that provided a critical analysis of power holders as a way to generate social and systemic change.

Critical Theory: A research paradigm that extends social constructivism (see *Social Constructivism*). Critical theorists assume that participants' experiences and thus constructions of various phenomena may be influenced by social injustices and work to change participant experiences within and outside the research process.

Cross-Analysis: The third phase of analysis for the consensual qualitative research tradition. Research team members meet and attempt to reach consensus on core ideas. Categories are developed by team members through a consensus-building process, examining each category for evidence across all, some, and/or none of the participants. The cross-analysis should result in a separate document that includes a list of domains and within-domain categories common to all participants and any participant data that were not common across participants and/or were not included in another domain or subdomain.

Dependability:	A criterion of trustworthiness that refers to the consistency of study results over time and across researchers, similar to the concept of *reliability* in quantitative research.
Description:	A qualitative data analysis technique of the biography and ethnography traditions. In the biography tradition, description focuses on the chronology of the participant's experiences in life. In the ethnography tradition, the ethnographer uses a chronological, sequential, or some other type of order to describe a culture-sharing group.
Dialogical Analysis:	A qualitative data analysis technique of the narratology tradition, with attention to dialogue in a participant narrative.
Direct Interpretation:	A qualitative data analysis technique of the case study tradition. The researcher directly interprets the meaning of singular critical incidents, concerns, and issues within the data.
Domain Abstraction:	The second phase of analysis for the consensual qualitative research tradition. The research team members abstract core ideas by reimmersing themselves in the data and keeping an eye out for core ideas that illuminate aspects of domains they have previously selected to examine.
Domain Development and Coding:	The initial phase of analysis for the consensual qualitative research tradition. Each research team member immerses him- or herself in all of the data, reading each participant transcript and identifying independently, then collectively, a list of large domains, categories, or themes based on the data.
Diaries:	An unobtrusive data source that shows change over a period of time and may showcase the context of participants' lived experiences. Diaries can be solicited as a form of qualitative data collection or obtained as a personal document (see *Personal Documents*).
Duty to Warn and Protect:	Ethical and legal responsibility to warn identifiable victims and protect others from dangerous individuals, or in some instances, from danger from themselves.
Early Ethnography:	A historical moment of qualitative research within the 15th, 16th, and 17th centuries. This period involved a comparison of diversity throughout the globe against an established theory of human diversity. Descriptions were made of how non-Western societies diverged from the "civilized" European nations.
Effects Matrix:	A form of case display (see *Case Display*) that explains and predicts data. Effects matrices can be developed as individual case displays (e.g., explanatory effects matrix and case dynamics matrix) or for several case displays (e.g., case-ordered effects matrix, case-ordered predictor–outcome matrix, and variable-by-variable matrix).
Epiphany:	Story or critical incident within the biography tradition.

Epistemology:	A philosophy of science that involves the process of knowing or the acquisition of knowledge. In qualitative research, epistemology encompasses the degree to which knowledge is believed to be, or not to be, constructed by the research process in general and by the context of the researcher–participant relationship in particular.
Epoche:	Analogous to bracketing (see *Bracketing*), it involves setting aside prior explanations of phenomena found in literature and acknowledging researchers' values and assumptions regarding phenomena. *Epoche* is a Greek word for refraining from judgment.
Ethical Validation:	A criterion of trustworthiness that refers to treating all aspects of the qualitative research process as a moral and ethical issue. It is the practice of engaging in research that provides insights to practical and meaningful real-world problems.
Ethics:	A set of guidelines established within a professional discipline to guide thinking and behavior. There are several types of ethics: *principle ethics*—minimal acts or choices that focus heavily on morality and obligations based on stated ethics codes; *utilitarian ethics*—a universal set of rules of morality that determine what we ought to do; *virtue ethics*—nonobligatory ideals and personal characteristics of the researcher and participants; *social ethics*—moral judgments as inevitable decisions seated in relationships and neutral espoused principles not as easily applied; and *communitarian ethics*—an ethic of care that challenges the mission of research to build community among researchers and participants, involving them in ethical decisions and research design.
Ethnography:	A qualitative research tradition in which the researcher describes and provides interpretations about the culture of a group or system. Participant observation is utilized by the researcher and involves prolonged engagement over a significant period of time with the group studied, in order to describe the process and experience of its culture.
Ethnomethodology:	A qualitative research tradition that seeks to study social order and patterns. The focus of study is on the informants' perspectives of the "everydayness" of their lives. Ethnomethodology typically involves investigating normative social attitudes by disrupting environments to create non-normative situations.
Evaluative Research:	A type of research that assesses the effectiveness of a program or intervention throughout its course. Two common forms of evaluative research, formative evaluation and summative evaluation, involve examining practices throughout a program or intervention in an effort to improve and shape it, and assessing the outcomes at the end of the program or intervention, respectively.
Experimental Setting:	The setting of a controlled experimental design that utilizes a quantitative or mixed methods approach (not a naturalistic setting).

Explication:	A qualitative data analysis technique of the heuristic inquiry tradition. The researcher uses self-reflection to further analyze structural and textural descriptions (see *Structural Description*; *Textual Description*).
External Audit:	A key component of consensual qualitative research analysis. A secondary research team assesses the accuracy of the cross-analysis (see *Cross-Analysis*) and the creation of domains and subdomains common to all participants. Auditors communicate their audit to the primary research team, suggesting alterations, revisions, and/or data that were not addressed by the original abstraction of core ideas and cross-analysis.
Extreme Sampling:	Also called deviant case sampling, a purposeful sampling method that selects participants whose experiences are characterized at either or both of the extremes.
Feeling Question:	A type of qualitative interview question that assesses participant affect regarding a phenomenon.
Feminism:	A research paradigm that places emphasis on the roles of affect and researcher–participant relationship in the research process. Gender and other social locations of participants are organizing principles in understanding and reporting research findings.
Field Notes:	Written records of field activities developed within an observational period (as possible) and continually expanded and revised after the observation has occurred. There are two types: descriptive field notes (i.e., detailed behavioral descriptions of what occurred in a setting) and reflective field notes (i.e., subjective aspects of data collection, including assumptions, impressions, attitudes, and ideas).
Fieldwork:	Research activities in which individuals engage when in a particular setting to gather a thick description of the context and to provide a deeper understanding of a particular phenomenon. Fieldwork is often associated with participant observation, but it can be used with a variety of methods.
Focus Groups:	A data collection method that results in data from interactions among participants who share a common experience or are homogeneous in some manner. This method often serves as a catalyst for participant disclosure, connecting with others, and expanding on or challenging perspectives in a synergistic manner.
Foreshadowed Problems:	A qualitative version of hypotheses in quantitative research where the research enters a setting with topics to explore.
Frequency Analysis:	The final qualitative data analysis technique of the consensual qualitative research tradition whereby research team members categorize domains into one of three categories: general, typical, and variant. A *general domain* reflects all or almost all of the participants' experiences. A *typical domain* is one that was identified

for the majority (over half) of the participants. A *variant theme* is one that has significance for participants, but was common to less than half of the participants' data. A *rare theme* is one that occurs for two to three participants in studies involving approximately 15 individuals.

Frequency Counting: A tally of the number of times a code occurs for a data source.

Gatekeeper: An individual who grants you access to participants and/or to a site of study.

Grounded Theory: A qualitative research tradition that seeks to generate theory that is "grounded" in data from participants' perspectives of a particular phenomenon. Characteristics include inductive approach, constant comparison (see *Constant Comparison*), and theoretical sampling (see *Theoretical Sampling*).

Hermeneutics: A qualitative research tradition that involves interpreting "sacred" texts, such as religious documents, mythology, history, art, and politics. With hermeneutics, the assumption is that texts and other documents are recorded expressions of human experience.

Heuristic Inquiry: A qualitative research tradition that is a variation of phenomenology. The purpose of heuristic inquiry is to emphasize the essence of experience and the person in relation to that experience.

Homogeneous Sampling: A purposeful sampling method that represents a sample by selecting those who share similarities to one another. Homogeneous sampling is common when a researcher is interested in gaining a depth of information about one specific subgroup.

Horizontalization: A phenomenological data analysis technique whereby researchers identify nonrepetitive, nonoverlapping statements in participants' transcripts.

Illumination: A qualitative data analysis technique of the heuristic inquiry tradition. Researchers identify categories, themes, and patterns of the phenomenon within the data.

Illustrative Question: A type of interview question whereby researchers communicate to interviewees that "you have heard it all." Response extremes are presented to participants to illustrate a range of potential responses.

Importance of Context: A qualitative research characteristic that refers to how participants create and give meaning to social experience. Phenomena are created and maintained by those in an environment, and social settings are self-organized in the sense that activities are structured for themselves.

Inductive Analysis: Analysis of qualitative data with the assumption that data drive theory or a deeper understanding of an issue or phenomenon. The research process involves collecting data to refine research questions and build theory, not test hypotheses.

Informed Consent:	An ethical and legal concept that clearly identifies and outlines research activity and rights and responsibilities of all parties involved. The researcher describes the purpose of the research and provides information about him- or herself, the extent of participation, limits of confidentiality, and any foreseeable risks and benefits of participation and nonparticipation, and emphasizes the voluntariness of participation. Furthermore, qualitative researchers indicate how and what data will be accessed and presented. Process consent is an important component of informed consent wherein consent is viewed as an ongoing, mutually negotiated and developed activity.
Institutional Review Board:	A team of institutional and outside members that reviews research applications and monitors federal compliance to aspects of the Belmont Report (see *Belmont Report*) to ensure protection of human subjects.
Intensity Sampling:	A purposeful sampling method wherein intense (but not extreme) cases are identified to demonstrate a phenomenon.
Interactive Interviewing:	Conversational interaction and exchange of narratives between interviewer and interviewee. Involves the interpretation of interview content by the interviewee and the complex interactions between the interviewee and interviewer.
Interpretivism:	Philosophical perspective that assumes "everything is relative." Interpretivists believe that criteria for determining the trustworthiness of research are socially constructed. This approach for evaluating research is most closely assigned with constructivist, critical theory, feminist, and queer theory paradigms.
Interrater Reliability:	Method for determining consistency or agreement among research team members. Interrater reliability is a ratio of the number of research team members who approve, to those who do not approve, the appropriateness of each code or pattern in textual or visual data.
Intervening Conditions:	A component of analysis in the grounded theory tradition. Intervening conditions are ways in which participants address influencing factors.
Instrumental Case Study:	Term defined by Robert Stake wherein the researcher seeks cases to assist in understanding a particular issue exterior to a specific case.
Intrinsic Case Study:	Term defined by Robert Stake wherein the researcher has an internally guided or intrinsic interest in a particular case.
Key Informants:	Individuals who provide important information that may shape qualitative inquiry.
Knowledge Question:	A type of interview question that solicits responses from participants about the amount of information they possess regarding a phenomenon as well as where that knowledge originated.

Life History:	A qualitative research tradition that follows the life of an individual, including the cultural norms that shape the person studied, and uses interviews with them as data collection. The life history tradition represents an account of a person's life situated in a broader social context.
Literature Map:	A display that visually organizes themes of the research literature.
Maximum Variation:	A purposeful sampling method that seeks to maximize diversity of characteristics within a sample to help illustrate the central aspects of the research topic.
Member Checking:	Ongoing consultation with participants to test the "goodness of fit" of developing findings as well as final reports.
Memos:	A data collection, management, and analysis tool whereby extensive thoughts or reflections are jotted down. Memos can be integrated into field notes at a later point in the research process.
Mind Maps:	Visual diagrams that organize a researcher's ideas about important players in the field and that document potential challenges and opportunities related to access and fieldwork (see *Fieldwork*).
Mixed Methods:	The integration of qualitative and quantitative research approaches that may occur concurrently (i.e., quantitative and qualitative data collection occurs at the same time) or sequentially (i.e., either quantitative or qualitative data collected first, depending on the research purpose and question). When researchers employ qualitative strategies first, the method is referred to as an *exploratory design*. When they introduce a study with quantitative measures, the method is referred to as an *explanatory design*.
Modernist Phase:	A historical moment in qualitative research that occurred between the 1940s and 1970s. This phase primarily involved the emergence of several new approaches as well as an increased attention to rigor and quality. This period was known as the "golden age of qualitative analysis."
Multiple Case Study:	Investigation of several cases that are similar in nature.
Narrative Process Coding System:	A qualitative data analysis technique of the narratology tradition that involves three analytic techniques. The first, *external narrative sequences*, describes events. The second, *internal narrative sequences*, builds on a description of clients' subjective experiences and expands these descriptions. The third, *reflexive narrative sequences*, analyzes the meaning of client narratives.
Narratology:	A qualitative research tradition similar to the hermeneutic and life history approaches. Narratology seeks to understand what stories or narratives reveal about an individual. With origins in social sciences and literature, it extends the hermeneutic approach by examining data sources such as interview transcripts, life history and other historical narratives, and creative nonfiction.

426

Naturalistic Generalizability:	A form of case study data analysis whereby the researcher actively interprets the data with an eye toward the ways in which an audience would be able to transfer or apply the broad categories or findings from the case study to another case(s).
Naturalistic Observation:	Method of observation that seeks to render the researcher's impact as negligible as possible so as to not upset naturally occurring phenomena.
Naturalistic Setting:	Qualitative inquiry in a naturalistic setting is important because researchers are interested in the role of context. The naturalistic setting affords practitioners and researchers with opportunities to examine how individuals interact with their environment through symbols, social roles, and social structures, to name a few.
Negative Case Analysis:	A trustworthiness strategy that refines a developing theme as additional information becomes available. A researcher constantly searches for data that go against current findings, or searches for cases that may be represented by the same findings but differ from the population of interest.
Nuremberg Code:	The first legal attempt to deal with controversies of research, specifically to those of the Nazi medical experiments. Established in 1947, it was an initial effort to put forth guidelines for social, medical, and behavioral research, with particular emphasis on informed consent.
Observer Bias:	The subjective manner in which an individual selectively observes preselected individuals, events, and activities within an observation period.
Observer Effect:	The unintentional effect an observer has on the research and participants.
Observer as Participant Role:	A point on the observation continuum that involves having a primary role as an observer with some interaction with study participants.
Observer Role:	One extreme of the observation continuum that refers to having minimal or no interactions with participants. In these cases, participants are often not aware that they are being observed.
One-Shot Question:	A type of interview question popular in opportunistic sampling (see *Opportunistic Sampling*) that refers to preparing one question to ask a key informant, should an opportunity to do so arise.
Online Focus Groups:	Application of the focus group method via the Internet. Individuals can share a common experience of a phenomenon that might be rare and/or a difficult subject to discuss face-to-face in a group of people.
Ontology:	A philosophy of science that refers to the nature of reality or the degree to which a "universal truth" is sought about a particular construct or process.

Open Coding:	The initial data analysis technique of the grounded theory tradition. General domains such as keywords or phrases provided by the participants or the researchers are identified.
Opinion Question:	A type of interview question that seeks participants' personal beliefs about a phenomenon.
Opportunistic Sampling:	Sometimes called *emergent sampling*, a purposeful sampling method that capitalizes on the appearance of new potential samples as the research process evolves.
Oral History:	A form of case study whereby the a researcher documents events, including cultural themes, emerging from individual interviews.
Otherness:	The degree of relationship between those inside and outside the research. There are four types of otherness that interact with one another: epistemological, societal, practical, and local. Epistemological and practical otherness refer to the distance between the researcher and the participant within the research context, whereas societal and local otherness refer to the social context that privileges or diminishes people—researchers and participants alike—in terms of social power.
Partially Ordered Display:	A data management tool used for exploring and describing data during the initial stages of data analysis. Types of partially ordered displays include the context chart, the checklist matrix, and the partially ordered meta-matrix.
Participant Observation:	The researcher's active involvement in the setting. Participant observation is often used in interviewing and other activities to negotiate tensions in a setting.
Participant as Observer Role:	A point on the observation continuum that involves becoming more a participant than an observer of others.
Participant Role:	An extreme on the observation continuum that refers to a researcher functioning both as a member of a community under investigation and as an investigator. Although "going native" is rare, it is most likely to occur with this role.
Participatory Action Research:	A qualitative research tradition that seeks to facilitate change in the participants and researcher in the process of the examination. Goals include emancipation and transformation, and the researcher is required to critically reflect on the power of research as a change agent.
Pattern Identification:	A form of data analysis of the case study tradition wherein the researcher examines broad categories within a case for their relationships or interactions.
Peer Debriefing:	A strategy of trustworthiness that refers to consultation with peers as another check outside a designated research team. Peers can be interested colleagues, classmates, or individuals within the community where the phenomenon is being investigated.

Persistent Observation:	A strategy of trustworthiness that allows for in-depth and focused data collection. May be a result of prolonged engagement in some cases.
Personal Documents:	A data source typically solicited to help the researcher understand the culture and context of participants' experiences of a phenomenon. Examples of personal documents include letters, books, health care records, diaries or journals, financial records, report cards or grading sheets, homework assignments, legal documents, and any other artifacts that may help elucidate the phenomenon.
Phenomenology:	A qualitative research tradition whose purpose is to discover and describe the meaning or essence of participants' lived experiences, or knowledge, as it appears to consciousness.
Philosophies of Science:	Five interrelated constructs that conceptualize the nature of scientific inquiry: ontology, epistemology, axiology, rhetoric, and methodology.
Photovoice:	A data collection strategy using photography as a way to document visual information.
Politically Important Case Sampling:	A purposeful sampling method that selects a critical case that draws political attention to the phenomenon.
Positionality:	How social and cultural power is distributed in the researcher–participant relationship and recognized when there are power differentials.
Positivism:	A research paradigm common in quantitative research based on the assumption that researchers can arrive at an objective, universal truth through direct observation and experience of phenomena.
Post-Positivism:	A research paradigm common in quantitative research. It is similar to positivism but assumes that a theory is strengthened when it is verified and falsified. Post-positivists assert that universal reality can never be fully realized because one cannot say with complete certainty that a theory fully describes a phenomenon or construct.
Practice Ethnography:	A variation of ethnography that explores how practice and theory interface in a setting or culture.
Presupposition Question:	A type of interview question that a researcher uses when it is relevant to assume some experience with the topic of a question and as a way to encourage participant elaboration.
Probing Questions:	The *who, what, when, where,* and *how* interview questions that help to expand an interviewee's responses. Probing questions can be verbal, such as elaboration and clarification questions, or they can be nonverbal, such as head nods.
Procedural Rigor:	A criterion of trustworthiness referring to how researcher bias impacts all components of the research design.

Prolonged Engagement: A strategy of trustworthiness involving "staying in the field" to build and sustain relationships with participants and settings in a way that fosters an accurate description of a phenomenon of interest.

Public Documents: An unobtrusive data source that includes official records, newspapers, newsletters, magazines, meeting minutes, public artifacts, reports, tax records, legal reports, and the like.

Purposeful Sampling: Selection of participants for the amount of detail they can provide about a phenomenon (i.e., information-rich cases).

Queer Theory: A research paradigm that attends to how sexual orientation as a participant characteristic influences experiences of various phenomena.

Random Purposeful Sampling: A purposeful sampling method used to increase the variation of cases within your study by randomly selecting from a preselected sample.

Realism: A view of science involving the notion that one can only know reality from one's own perspective. This view is also known as *subtle realism* and *modernism*.

Reciprocity: The idea that there is a relationship between researcher and participant wherein knowledge is shared and constructed, and new ideas are formed.

Referential Adequacy: A strategy of trustworthiness that involves checking preliminary findings and interpretations against archived raw data.

Reflexive Journal: A strategy of trustworthiness wherein the researcher records thoughts of how the research process is impacting him or her. The researcher reflects in writing on how the participants, data collection, and data analysis are impacting him or her personally and professionally.

Research Agenda: The development of a researcher's line of inquiry in a topic(s) area over time. The connection of the individual research studies within this line of inquiry to one another.

Researcher–Practitioner: Also termed *scientist–practitioner*, the perspective of having research and practice inform one another.

Rhetoric: A philosophy of science that refers to the content and voice (first, second, third) of qualitative data presentation. Rhetoric also involves the degree to which narratives, thematic categories, and/or numbers are presented as findings.

Role-Ordered Case Display: A data management tool used to explore and describe data. Role-ordered case displays depict social interactions for a setting or variable of interest, providing a "role occupant" view for each key participants. A role × time matrix, contrast table, and a scatter-plot display are examples of role-ordered displays.

Role-Playing Question:	A type of interview question that allows the participant to discuss a topic from a particular role of authority.
Sampling Adequacy:	A criterion of trustworthiness that refers to using the appropriate sample composition and size based on the research question(s) and research tradition(s).
Saturation:	Typically associated with the grounded theory tradition, a point where there are no new ideas identified in the newly collected data.
Selective Coding:	A grounded theory analysis technique used to further refine axial codes (see *Axial Coding*). Selective coding is the most complex coding process in grounded theory, wherein patterns, processes, and sequences are identified among axial codes to generate a theory about a phenomenon.
Semiotics:	A research tradition closely tied to symbolic interaction (see *Symbolic Interaction*). Codes and symbols regarding a culture or context surround the qualitative researcher. Semiotics is the search, description, and interpretation of these codes.
Semistructured Interview:	A form of interview that uses a protocol as a guide and starting point for the interview experience.
Sensory Question:	A sensory-based interview question (i.e., sight, hear, taste, smell, touch) seeking information from participants about their bodily experiences.
Siedman's Phenomenological Interview:	A phenomenological approach involving three interviews that describe the essence of an experience. With this focus on the lived meanings of a phenomenon across individuals, this form of interview is conducted in three phases, with each phase revolving around a central question with probes.
Simulation Question:	An interview question that requests that the participant verbally observe a phenomenon for the interviewer. That is, the interviewer asks the participant to place him- or herself in a situation.
Single Case Study:	The examination of one phenomenon that should meet the criteria for testing a theory with one case.
Snowball Sampling:	A purposeful sampling method also called *chain* or *network sampling*. This sampling method has a "snowball" or "chain" effect wherein the researcher solicits participants based on referrals from previous participants or gatekeepers, stakeholders, or key informants.
Social Constructivism:	A belief system that assumes that "universal truth" cannot exist because there are multiple contextual perspectives and subjective voices that can label truth in scientific pursuit. It also has been referred to as *postmodernism*.
Stability Reliability:	Analogous to test–retest reliability in quantitative research, refers to the extent that the same researcher codes text the same way more than once.

Stakeholder:	An individual or group who has an investment or "stake" in the findings of a study.
Stratified Purposeful Sampling:	A purposeful sampling method that allows a researcher to demonstrate the distinguishing features of subgroups (or strata) of a phenomenon.
Structural Description:	An aspect of phenomenological data analysis whereby the researcher creates a list or visual model that represents a framework of participant experiences that are a result of refining the horizontalization of data into a textural description of the phenomenon's essence (see *Horizontalization*; *Textural Description*). Structural description may be considered analogous to axial codes in the grounded theory tradition.
Structured Interview:	A form of interview that relies on a preestablished sequence and pace of questions that a researcher follows rigidly. Questions are asked exactly as written, and probes, if included, are also standardized.
Subjectivity:	The internal understandings of the qualitative researcher of his or her phenomenon.
Substantive Validation:	A criterion of trustworthiness that relates to the question "Do the research report and other products have substance"? It is the degree to which research either adds new knowledge or supports existing information about a phenomenon.
Symbolic Interaction:	A research tradition that asserts that only through social experience can individuals become self-identified. That is, individuals interpret their experiences and identities based on social interactions.
Textural Description:	A phenomenological analysis to refine data into new categories. The purpose of textural description is to understand the meaning and depth of the essence of an experience.
Thematic Analysis:	A narrative data analysis technique whereby the researcher identifies central themes and their subthemes to note a larger storyline in which these themes and subthemes are subsumed.
Theoretical Sampling:	A purposeful sampling method that assumes that the evolving theory of data collection should guide the sampling strategy.
Theory Development:	A criterion of trustworthiness that refers to generating tenets from data to describe and explain how a phenomenon operates.
Thick Description:	A strategy of trustworthiness that refers to creating a detailed account of the research process, participants, context, and outcome, usually evidenced in the qualitative report, but may also be included in an audit trail (see *Audit Trail*).
Time-Ordered Display:	A data management tool that is used to explore and describe data when time is the organizing principle. This display depicts a sequence or flow of events or processes of a phenomenon of

interest. Examples of time-ordered displays include event listing, a critical incident chart, an activity record, a decision model, and a scatterplot over time.

Traditional Period: A historical moment of qualitative research that extends from the early 1900s to the mid-1940s. Classic ethnography is prevalent at the beginning of this period, slowly shifting to what is known as modern ethnography. A major contribution of this period included a greater emphasis on conducting fieldwork, taking field notes, and writing theory. The traditional period includes works from the British School and Chicago School.

Traditionalism: A perspective of science also known as *positivist realism* and *naive realism* that represents a lens by which researchers verify a single truth for a phenomenon using the five physical senses. Through experimental methods and empirical verification, traditionalists look for rational, objective, and logical explanations to research questions.

Transferability: A criterion of trustworthiness similar to external validity in quantitative research. To demonstrate transferability researchers must provide detailed description of the research process.

Triangulation: A strategy of trustworthiness that involves using multiple forms of evidence (e.g., data sources, data methods, investigators, unit of analysis, theories). Triangulation seeks to strengthen evidence that a particular theme exists by looking for inconsistencies among these forms.

Triple Crisis: A historical moment in qualitative research during the mid-1980s to mid-1990s, during which qualitative researchers struggled to best represent their participants and phenomena, to be flexible in how they evaluated the rigor of qualitative design, and to consider alternative methods beyond writing to disseminate their findings.

Typical Case Sampling: A purposeful sampling method wherein researchers attempt to represent an average or typical example of the focus of their study.

Typological Analysis: A narrative data analysis technique that involve investigations into the typology of clients' narratives.

Unit of Analysis: The "angle" or perspective toward a case (see *Case*). Qualitative researchers can use various units of analysis to study a case.

Unstructured Interview: Occurs as part of participant observation and often associated with ethnography and perhaps other "in-the-field" research traditions. The label *unstructured* is misleading, since no interview can truly be unstructured and is more likely a "guided conversation." Unstructured interviews focus on the surrounding context at the time of the interview.

Use of Commentary: An interview strategy that elicits information from a participant by using a statement rather than an interview question. Unlike an interview question, a comment does not preestablish how an interviewee might respond or pressure him or her to respond.

Value Question: A type of interview question a researcher asks about social norms in relation to individual beliefs.

Visual Ethnography: Use of images (e.g., photographs, paintings) to understand a culture-sharing group. The external narrative serves as the context for the image, whereas the internal narrative is the interpretation of the image by those who view it.

Whole Client Narrative Analysis: A narrative data analysis technique whereby the whole client narrative is evaluated to illuminate the entire "case" of the narrative rather than its diverse parts.

Sample Qualitative Proposals

Experiences of Gay, Bisexual, Queer, and Questioning Greek Students

JOSEPH W. DAVIS
Old Dominion University

ABSTRACT

Gay, bisexual, queer, and questioning students who elect to become members of Greek organizations at academic institutions often face unique situations in terms of the Greek process (Windmeyer, 2005). The Greek system, particularly for students who identify as male, are enculturated to adhere to the masculine stereotype and may involve instances of hazing, alcohol consumption, and hypersexualization. This qualitative proposal includes findings from a pilot study that examined any barriers and benefits in regard to being a gay, bisexual, queer, or questioning member of a Greek organization. Interviews were conducted with two gay, bisexual, queer, or questioning members of a Greek affiliation and a text detailing the experiences of gay men in college fraternities was examined to assist in identifying the barriers and benefits of being a gay, bisexual, queer, or questioning member of a Greek organization. This research proposal also details plans for a larger-scale study on a similar topic.

Gay, bisexual, queer, and questioning (GBQQ) students have a unique perspective of campus life. These students are contending with adapting to a college environment, in addition to negotiating their sexual orientation within the new campus environment (Windmeyer, 2005). To assist with the adaptation to a college setting, one option students often consider is becoming a member of a Greek letter organization. Greek letter organizations provide opportunities for the formation of personal bonds, leadership activities, and community service (*Greek life*, n.d.). GBQQ students often must decide if and how they wish to disclose their sexual identity. In Gortmaker and Brown's (2006) survey analysis, a majority of participants who had not disclosed their sexual orientation (74%) often perceived the need to hide their sexual identity in an effort to avoid unfair treatment from the university community.

In a grounded theory study of fraternities (Stevens, 2004), the researcher's findings included that these organizations were characterized as being hypermasculine. Within this type of environment, this study found that participants who were GBQQ felt the need to hide their sexual orientation from their organizations due to fear of rejection if they disclosed their sexual orientation. Stevens (2004) argued that this conflict and fear might produce a significant amount of stress for an individual. If the concept of brotherhood or sisterhood is taken literally, then the process of disclosure could be likened to that of disclosing to a biological family member. The researcher's findings suggested that a cornerstone to participants' sexual orientation identity development involved finding empowerment. Participants identified finding empowerment as being a personal process that relied on inner strengths. Even though this empowerment was a personal process, other factors such as environmental influences and disclosure to others influenced their experience of empowerment.

CHALLENGES FACED BY GBQQ FRATERNITY MEMBERS

A significant barrier for GBQQ individuals is the homophobia that may exist within fraternities. Homophobia is defined as the perceived threat to one's self-concept via homosexually oriented ideas (Moradi, van den Berg, & Epting, 2006). Moradi and colleagues (2006) concluded that increased levels of perceived threat from lesbian and gay individuals were related to increased levels of negative attitudes about the lesbian and gay population. The researchers argued that in order to retain a firm since of self, some individuals take action against what they deem to be a threatening group. These actions can include acts of violence (Moradi et al., 2006). If fraternities are often seen as hypermasculine (Stevens, 2004), then the fear to disclose or affiliate with a Greek organization might be due to a concern for physical safety.

In addition to homophobia as a barrier, GBQQ fraternity members may also experience internalized homophobia. Kimmel and Mahalik's (2005) survey analysis research suggested that gay individuals' mental well-being could be impacted by negative perceptions of their sexual orientation. An individual could develop a negative sense of self and act out in a potentially destructive manner. Windmeyer and Freeman (1997) suggested that homophobia could be destructive for both straight and GBQQ members of a Greek letter organization, as homophobia may manifest in hypermasculine activities. An individual may feel pressured to consume alcohol and engage in other potentially dangerous activities in order to appear masculine. They argue that this negatively impacts the ideal of fraternal bonds that the organization had worked to create.

Being a GBQQ member in a Greek letter organization does not imply constant barriers to acceptance. Ashworth (2001) related his comfort and trust in disclosing his sexual orientation to his Greek letter organization. He noted a sense of peace as well as stronger fraternal bonds following the disclosure (Ashworth, 2001). The act of his disclosure served to validate his position in his organization and also assisted in the idea that the bonds of a fraternity are beyond that of a typical friendship.

Adding more to the idea that sexual orientation can serve as both an obstacle as well as a positive influence is the qualitative work of Dilley (2005). Dilley's phenomenological interviews were conducted with nonheterosexual college men and found that college served as both an opportunity and obstacle in terms of personal development. His research resulted in categories of homosexual identification (Dilley, 2005). A person classified as *gay* would have an open support network of similar individuals. A persona classified *parallel* would, in essence, be leading two separate lives that did not intersect. While some of the participants in Dilley's research were able to integrate their identity and form positive male bonds in fraternities, others remained undisclosed and disaffiliated from their organization.

To further assess the campus climate for gay and lesbian students, Jurgens, Schwitzer, and Middleton's (2004) mixed methods approach to examining heterosexual students' attitudes toward gays and lesbians found that gays and lesbians were generally positively viewed in society, but were also seen with uncertainty in regard to more personal factors such as identity development. Although this finding suggests support for a warmer campus climate, the researchers note that the participants were less supportive in a public discussion group than in private survey submissions. If applied to the concept of Greek letter organizations, then, support is lent to Stevens's (2004) idea that gay individuals may be afraid to disclose due to fear of rejection. Even if GBQQ individuals are seen as generally positive, there might not be adequate visible support to assist with the disclosure decision.

Cass's (1979) model suggests that homosexual identity development occurs through six stages: identity confusion, identity comparison, identity tolerance, acceptance, pride, and synthesis. While there is no concrete time frame for the progression of these stages, college may be the first time that some individuals are able to examine their own lives. This compares with Stevens (2004, who noted individuals' fear of disclosure in fraternities; an individual may not be ready or willing to disclose at earlier stages of the model.

Liang and Alimo's (2005) survey analysis research examined the change in attitudes toward lesbian, bisexual, and gay populations after significant exposure to the population and found a positive correlation. While not a causal relationship, the results do lend support to a notion that increased exposure to the lesbian, bisexual, and gay population can foster a sense of acceptance (Liang & Alimo, 2005). In terms of Greek letter organizations, this could support the idea of familial bonds and acceptance from within the organization if a member was contemplating disclosing his or her sexual orientation.

In Troiden, Kahn, and Rhoads's research (as cited in Evans, Forney, & Guido-DiBrito, 1998) there is an emphasis on the role of personal support in the development and well-being of a homosexual identity. This support can be found through the bonds with family and friends. These bonds and their assistance with personal development resemble the mission of several Greek letter organizations as they strive to provide true and lasting bonds for each of their members (*Greek life*, n.d.). Individuals seeking acceptance and such bonds through a Greek letter organization have the potential to experience the positive support to assist in their personal development.

PURPOSE AND CONCEPTUAL FRAMEWORK OF CURRENT STUDY

In regard to the proposed study, the ontology of this social constructivist approach involved each participant's subjective reality consisting of varied experiences and personal relationships. Individuals' perspectives regarding sexual orientation and Greek letter organizations were varied. Salience is individualistically based, and each narrative will fluctuate with unique life experience. Epistemologically, knowledge about perspectives of being a GBQQ member of a Greek letter organization will be constructed jointly with the participants and the researcher. While there will be no set end to the amount of knowledge to be gained from individual perspectives, a general working knowledge about the topic can be acquired. In regard to axiology, the voices and experiences of the participants will be of high importance. The study will be designed to examine these perspectives and will respect individual differences. The data gained from this study will be presented via thematic groupings involving the use of participant narrative where appropriate.

The purpose of this grounded theory will be to examine and build theory about the perspectives of GBQQ undergraduate students in Greek letter organizations. The primary research question to be answered involves the depiction of any obstacles and benefits to being a GBQQ member of a Greek letter organization. Additionally, the research team will examine what role, if any, disclosure of sexual orientation plays in the Greek letter system. The participants in this study identified as GBQQ. Undergraduate students will consist of students enrolled in a 4-year baccalaureate institution. The term *Greek letter organization* refers to single-sexed and socially based student organizations at baccalaureate institutions. *Disclosure* refers to the process of informing others about one's sexual orientation.

METHOD

Participants

Participants to be involved in this study will be recruited via snowball and criterion sampling and with the requested assistance from the Lambda 10 Project, a national clearinghouse for gay, lesbian, bisexual, and transgendered issues relating to Greek letter organizations. Utilizing the Lambda 10 Project's resources assists the researcher in leading toward a sense of maximum variation in regard to gender and geographical location. Additionally, the researcher will use recruitment methods seeking a broad range of experience levels and time spent inside of Greek letter organizations. These actions will develop trustworthiness as the sample will come from multiple academic institutions in several geographical areas. A total of 25 participants will be recruited in hopes of reaching saturation. Additional participants will be recruited to establish saturation. Eligible participants are undergraduate students in a 4-year baccalaureate institution, identify as GBQQ, and are members of a Greek letter organization at their respective academic institution. There are no age or ethnicity requirements for eligibility. To assist with negative case analysis, five heterosexual members of Greek letter organizations will be recruited via snowball sampling from the 25 participants.

Research Team

In relation to qualitative research, the issue of researcher bias must be addressed to promote the ideal of trustworthiness. For the proposed study, the primary researcher is a 25-year-old white individual who identifies as male and who is working toward a doctorate in counselor education. The researcher identifies as gay and is actively involved in a Greek letter organization at his academic institution. He is at a level of complete disclosure within his organization in regard to his sexual orientation. The researcher has been involved with the interest area of GBQQ students in Greek letter organizations for 5 years and has brought a national speaker to his academic institution to present on the subject material. The researcher holds the belief that Greek letter organizations have the potential to be beacons of acceptance for GBQQ individuals. However, this belief exists in that the potential for acceptance has rarely been met. He has experienced homophobic insults and derogatory jokes from within his own fraternity as well as others at his academic institution. These experiences have led to the occasional belief that the Greek system does not represent itself in an acceptable manner to incoming GBQQ students. Along with what he has witnessed, the researcher also recognized the acceptance he has gained from the majority of the other people in his organization.

The primary researcher will use a team of at least three other individuals to assist in developing the interview protocol, coding processes, and triangulation for this pilot study. A diverse research team will be recruited to allow for variation in gender, ethnicity, sexual orientation, and Greek letter organization experience. This action will help the researcher further document researcher bias by providing multiple perceptions on the data.

Data Sources

The primary source of data will be individual interviews. The individuals will each be interviewed once and the interviews will be semistructured to allow for participant elaboration and exploration. The questions focus on the experiences of perceived obstacles and benefits to being a GBQQ member of a Greek letter organization and the process of sexual identity disclosure from within the same organization. The interviews will be approximately 40 minutes and consisted of approximately 10 questions. Due to the wide geographical area range, the interviews will be conducted and recorded via telephone. The primary researcher will transcribe each participant interview verbatim.

Additionally, texts depicting the firsthand experiences of GBQQ students in Greek letter organizations will be utilized as a source of data. Windmeyer's (2005) text examined the narratives of gay and bisexual men inside of fraternities. In a separate text, Windmeyer (2001) displayed narratives from lesbian and bisexual women in sororities. Four narratives will be randomly selected from each text and utilized in the proposed study.

Data Analysis

The research team members will recursively immerse themselves in the produced transcripts. Open coding will be conducted after each interview. The initial codebooks will serve as a framework for coding future transcripts. The unit of analysis for the initial set of coding will be at the sentence level. Once open coding has been completed for each interview, the researchers will use axial coding to relate thematic concepts and categories across the data sets. During this process, the researchers will revisit the original transcripts to ensure accuracy in coding. As the cyclical process of constant comparison continues, the researchers will use selective coding to identify core categories and several interacting subcategories. The research team will continue to revisit the original data to search for variation from the core category. The researchers, in regard to the projected sample size, will continue adding data sets until saturation of findings has been reached.

Alongside the interviews, the researchers will use document analysis on the two texts. This process will occur after interview data collection and coding. A similar process of open coding, axial coding, and selective coding will occur with the narrative texts, as the researchers create a separate codebook for the text analysis. Cross-coding will occur to search for thematic groupings between the multiple forms of data. Additionally, researchers will code five interviews from non-GBQQ members of Greek letter organizations to provide negative case analysis.

Strategies for Trustworthiness

Several strategies will be utilized to increase trustworthiness for this proposed study. Negative case analysis will be used to confirm data presented by the participants. In the case of this study, the primary researcher will interview heterosexual Greek letter organization members. In order to further establish confirmability, the research team will engage in member checking and solicit feedback from participants on their transcripts.

The researchers will use reflexive journaling to identify and address researcher bias and to document thought processes as the research progresses. The research team also will use memoing after each data collection in an effort to increase the dependability of the research. As the data are collected, analysis will occur. This will allow for the process of constant comparison between the data sets. The researcher has prolonged engagement with the subject matter. The primary researcher has identified as a gay for over 12 years and has been a member of a Greek letter organization for the past 5 years.

The research team will additionally use triangulation in an effort to increase trustworthiness. Triangulation between research team members will be used to ensure coding validation. Weekly team coding meetings will help structure this process. Additionally, a similar process will be used across multiple data sources and allow for a wide range of variance and cross-checking. For this proposed study, an auditor from an unaffiliated academic institution will work with the research team. The enlisted auditor has an interest in the target research populations and is selected on the basis of ensuring that the participants have an accurate voice in the research.

As is the purpose of grounded theory, the focus on this research will be on the development of theory. This will be done via the process of open, axial, and selective coding and will search for a core category (Strauss & Corbin, 2008). Close attention must be paid to the accurate perceptions of the participants and replicated until saturation.

PILOT STUDY

To further support the proposed study, a pilot study was conducted that observed the perceptions of any obstacles and benefits to being a GBQQ member of a Greek organization.

Participants

For the pilot study, individual interviews were conducted with two individuals. The participants were recruited via convenience sampling. Each interview lasted between 20 and 25 minutes. The interviews were semistructured and consisted of 10 predetermined questions (Figure A-1). The researcher was allowed to ask follow-up or probing questions to further engage the participant and to get a more complete understanding of the participant's experience. Each participant provided informed consent and completed a participant demographic form (Figure A-2). After the interviews, both participants were sent their respective transcripts for review. The participants were each given the opportunity to provide feedback and both chose to provide many comments on their transcripts.

The first participant was 18 years old and a white male. He was a freshman communications major at his academic institution and was in the process of becoming a member of his fraternity. He identifies as bisexual. The second participant was 21 years old and a white male. He was an engineering major at his academic institution and held a leadership position in his fraternity. This participant identifies as homosexual. Both participants came from the same large mid-Atlantic institution.

The second form of data came from Windmeyer's (2005) edited book, *Brotherhood: Gay Life in College Fraternities*. Two narratives were randomly selected from the text and were used in data analysis.

Research Team

The primary researcher for this pilot study was a 25-year-old white male. He was a doctoral student in a counselor education program at a large, mid-Atlantic academic institution. He identified as gay and was a member of a Greek letter organization. His biases are based on his prolonged exposure to both populations. The researcher has had experiences with discrimination via derogatory insults from individuals in multiple Greek letter organizations. Even with these negative experiences, he still holds to a positive ideal of what these specific organizations could aspire to become in the future. Additionally, he has had several positive experiences that have facilitated bonding and development within his own organization.

The research team consisted of three female doctoral-level students enrolled in a qualitative methods course at the same institution as the primary researcher. Their involvement with the pilot study consisted of several meetings throughout the course of the study about the logistics and design of the study. Only the primary researcher was involved in the interviews, coding of the participant interviews, and document analysis.

Data Analysis

For the pilot study, the researcher created memos after each data collection. Due to the nature of the study and instructional design, coding could not be accomplished immediately after transcription. An initial codebook was created via open coding for the first interview of the data collection. The unit of analysis was based on the multiple-sentence level. This codebook served as the guide for future codebooks. Upon completion of the initial codebook for the second interview, the first data set was reviewed again to begin the process of constant comparison. With both interviews complete, axial coding began while attempting to observe any emerging core concept or category.

In Windmeyer's (2005) narrative compilation, each of the two stories served as a separate source of data. The unit of analysis for these data sets was on the paragraph level. An initial codebook was created for each narrative, using open coding. The codebook from the participant interviews serves as a guide for narrative coding. Upon completion of open coding using constant comparison with the two narratives, axial coding was used to begin the search for thematic categories. Comparison occurred at the between-story level as well as between the written narratives and the participant interviews. Three final codebooks were developed over the course of this pilot study. The participant interviews and text-based narratives were maintained in their own codebooks as they are separate forms of data. A final codebook (Figure A-3) that attempted to combine the emerging core categories and potential theory was also produced. A case display (Table A-1) was produced to summarize key concepts in relation to each participant. Finally, a concept map was constructed to assist with the organization of project ideas (Figure A-4).

Strategies for Trustworthiness

Trustworthiness was assisted by the use of several methods. Member checking was attempted via soliciting feedback from the interview participants on their transcripts. However, none of the participants returned any comments on their transcripts.

Reflexive journaling was performed by the primary researcher prior to and after several of the data collections to assist in reducing bias and in organizing researcher thoughts and opinions. Memos were created for each set of the data to assist in the organization process and to support the process of coding. Constant comparison was available on a limited extent, due to the number of data sources and the delay for coding opportunities present within the design.

The role of the research team was not to interact with the collected data. The research team was used to assist in development of the interview protocol and to reduce personal bias in designing the pilot study.

Just as in the proposed study, the researcher established prolonged engagement with the subject material and the population. The researcher identified as a homosexual for over 12 years. Additionally, the researcher has been a member of a Greek letter organization for over 5 years. Furthermore, the interviewer has known one of the participants for over 3 years.

While emerging theory could not be fully developed by the conclusion of the pilot study, emerging core categories could be observed as well as several smaller intervening categories.

FINDINGS

At the conclusion of the pilot study, several thematic groups had emerged as a result of the constant comparison of the data. The idea of acceptance had emerged as a core category. This central category involved two subsets. The acceptance of oneself as a GBQQ male was found across all data sets. Included in this are thoughts about self and admittance to self of GBQQ status. Additionally, these groupings consisted of thoughts related to self-knowledge and adequacy.

For an example, Participant PA010 noted:

> I guess they do say, you know, college is a big time, you know, when you discover ... you finally know who you are. And I guess, this is, your views change all the time. You learn new things about yourself and this is just one of those things. Uh, it's been a real growing experience for me, I guess you could say. Um, I guess I feel more. It's not a fact that I try to hide. Kind of. Um, I'm happy with it. I guess, I realize it's nothing to be ashamed of, it's just who I am.

Additionally, the core category of acceptance involves a sense of being accepted within the organization. In the text-based narratives (Windmeyer, 2005), the stories often revolved around a fear of disclosure to their respective fraternities. There was often the concern about how a GBQQ member would be viewed in the fraternity. For one of the text examples, the individual commented that even though he had disclosed his sexual orientation to the entire Greek system, he was still concerned about finding acceptance within the organization.

In both sets of text narratives (Joseph, 2005; Shumake, 2005), acceptance was found only after personal disclosure of sexual orientation had occurred. Disclosure is an intervening category of acceptance. Also of note here is that emphasis was placed on being accepted by the fraternity and the importance of self-acceptance had been marginalized. The text narratives begin with what can be described as internalized homophobia. In Joseph's (2005) story, he commented, "Deep down, I thought, I could never let my fraternity brothers down. I could never let them see who I really am" (p. 12). This lends support to the idea that there is not a strong sense of self-acceptance prior to finding acceptance with a fraternity due to disclosure.

Along with the category of acceptance, there also seems to be a community of GBQQ students within the Greek letter organizations. Both interviewed participants as well as the written texts referenced the other GBQQ students involved in the Greek system. The text narratives appeared to reference this community as something to be kept as a secret. While the GBQQ community was referenced as a positive source of support and acceptance in the participant interviews, there was no mention of keeping such connections hidden.

Intervening with the core category of acceptance is the idea of being masculine via a macho stereotype. Appearing across the data sets was the idea that fraternities were to fill the masculine stereotype. One participant (PA010), who identified himself as bisexual, claimed that he felt like just another "skirt-chasing guy" when he was with his fraternity. Another participant quickly recognized the hypermasculine stereotype and debunked it within his own organization. However, he did mention that the masculine stereotype was active in other organizations on this campus.

The role of diversity also serves as an intervening category in the participant interviews. Both participants noted diversity as the joining together and the learning that happens between different cultures. Diversity was cited as a dominant motivation for both participants throughout their lives. Inside of this category rests the idea that the participants' home institution values diversity. While both participants lack knowledge of university policies on matters of sexual orientation, they both attribute the positive climate to the academic institution.

DISCUSSION

The findings of this proposed grounded theory would ultimately lead to a core category that would assist in the development of theory regarding the benefits and obstacles, if any, of being a GBQQ member of a Greek letter organization. In the proposed study, idea of acceptance could be a recurring theme as a major benefit to being a GBQQ member of a Greek letter organization. Because the pilot data showed strong connections to both ideas of acceptance of self and acceptance from the organization, it is expected that the proposed study would expand upon this category. Because this proposed study would involve multiple aspects of diversity, such as gender and geographical region, there is the possibility for more negative experiences to be expressed as students search for acceptance of themselves and from their respective Greek letter organizations. An additional area of interest became disclosure strategies, if any, of these students to their respective organizations. The results would likely lend support to the idea of disclosing as a means to seek acceptance. Disclosure, on the other hand, may serve as an obstacle that inhibits the feeling of acceptance.

Additionally, expanding the research to other diverse areas could continue to highlight the inner community of Greek members who are also GBQQ. With this more diverse study, different groups of organizations and individuals could be examined as sororities, lesbians, and bisexual women would all be afforded the opportunity to participate. All four data sources in the pilot study were able to express some recognition regarding others in their respective organizations that were of similar sexual orientations.

POTENTIAL IMPLICATIONS OF FUTURE DATA COLLECTION AND ANALYSIS

The issues facing GBQQ populations in Greek letter organizations are often seen as a side result in larger studies regarding college student development and sexual orientation (Dilley, 2005; Gortmaker & Brown, 2006; Jurgens et al., 2004; Stevens, 2004). However, little research has

444

been conducted to examine this exact population. The conducted pilot study lends support to the larger proposed study and can assist in filling the gap in research that had previously only been touched upon. As Windmeyer and Freeman (1997) noted, there are potential negative consequences for both heterosexuals and GBQQ members in Greek letter organizations if homophobia is present.

The central idea of acceptance needs to be expanded upon to fully gain an adequate understanding of its dimensions. The dimensions might possibly include different geographic areas, different Greek letter organizations, gender, and different variations of sexual orientation. This study could assist in further describing how GBQQ individuals make sense of their sense of self as well as well as how Greek letter organizations can work to promote or hinder the developing sense of self through support and understanding.

In terms of supporting and advocating for GBQQ individuals in Greek letter organizations, this research has the potential to provide rationale and open discussion within organizations and school settings about acceptance and the traditional stereotypes about Greek letter organizations. Freeman (2005) suggests that bringing these stories out into the open can assist in giving voice to an otherwise invisible issue in society. Perhaps the shame that Joseph (2005) felt in his personal narrative would no longer be a relevant issue. Much like Joseph's case, suicide can become an option for some individuals who are unable to come to terms with their sexual identity. As consistent with Cass's (1979) model of sexual identity development, these students may need support as they transition toward a state of identity acceptance.

There are several potential limitations with the proposed study. The first potential threat to trustworthiness would come from sampling adequacy. While the initial 25 interviews may be enough to reach saturation on a given topic, it may not be enough to reach saturation across multiple levels such as both fraternities and sororities. Adequate sampling must also be given to the varying forms of sexual identity.

Another possible limitation would be the transferability of the resulting theory. The acceptance described in this study would only be applicable to the Greek system on college campuses. Acute awareness must be paid to ensure that any findings are made specific to the target populations. Along with this notion is the idea of substantive validation. The proposed study may not be considered worthwhile due to the narrow target population. However, the individual voices and chance for life improvement assist this study in becoming worthwhile.

There are ethical limitations to this study. Participants must be willing to disclose their sexual orientation. If they are not at a point of disclosure to others, then the interview has the potential for harming their sense of security. While including informed consent and making concerted efforts to protect confidentiality can ease this, the individual choice to disclose must be unique. Individuals may not want there to be any possible method of their responses being traced back to their respective Greek organizations or any other individuals. To assist in this process, the names of the individual Greek letter organizations will not be solicited. As seen in the pilot data, participants may not want to represent their experiences within a Greek organization in a negative fashion.

One additional consideration comes in terms of the other forms of sexual identities. The proposed study only covers gay men, lesbian women, and bisexual men and women. No attempts will be made to seek out transgender or asexual individuals. The rationale for this is due to the rarity of these individuals inside of Greek letter organizations.

Cultural considerations also provide another potential limitation. There are several types of fraternities and sororities. There are traditionally African American and multicultural fraternities and sororities and are governed by their own standards. The focus of this proposed study is open to all forms of social Greek letter organizations; however, special attention must be paid to ensure adequate representation is allotted to different forms of fraternities and sororities. Additionally, religious differences must be considered as a cultural difference in analyzing the results. Attention must be given to ensure that religion is given the opportunity to exist as a cultural entity.

By the use of grounded theory, a general understanding is to be developed that depicts any possible obstacles or benefits to being a GBQQ member of a Greek letter organization. Special attention to the idea of acceptance and the disclosure process furthers the understanding of individual perspectives regarding the subject matter. While generating theory on a target population is not destined to cause massive changes in world paradigms, it does have the potential to change lives on an individual level.

REFERENCES

Ashworth, J. (2001). At home in Sigma Nu–Gay relations in college: Brief article. *The Advocate, 847*. Retrieved from *www.thefreelibrary.com/At+home+in+Sigma+Nu*. *(gay+relations+in+college)(Brief+Article)-a078682381*.

Cass, V. (1979). Homosexual identity formation: A theoretical model. *Journal of Homosexuality, 4*(3), 219–235. Retrieved from *www.informaworld.com/smpp/title~content=t792306897~db=all*.

Dilley, P. (2005). Which way out?: A typology of non-heterosexual male collegiate identities. *Journal of Higher Education, 76*(1), 56–88. Retrieved from *www.ohiostatepress.org/Journals/JHE/jhemain.htm*.

Evans, N. J., Forney, D. D., & Guido-DiBrito, F. (1998). *Student development in college: Theory, research, and practice.* San Francisco: Jossey-Bass.

Freeman, P. (2005). How to use stories as educational tools. In S. Windmeyer (Ed.), *Brotherhood: Gay life in college fraternities* (pp. 261–271). New York: Alyson Books.

Gortmaker, V. J., & Brown, R. D. (2006). Out of the college closet: Differences in perceptions and experiences of out and closeted lesbian and gay students. *College Student Journal, 40*(3), 606–619. Retrieved from *www.projectinnovation.biz/csj.html*.

Greek life. (n.d.). Retrieved from *studentaffairs.odu.edu/osal/greeklife/index.shtml*.

Joseph, E. (2005). Cry freedom. In S. Windmeyer (Ed.), *Brotherhood: Gay life in college fraternities* (pp. 10–17). New York: Alyson Books.

Jurgens, J. C., Schwitzer, A. M., & Middleton, T. (2004). Examining attitudes towards college students with minority sexual orientations: Findings and suggestions. *Journal of College Student Psychotherapy, 19*(1), 57–75.

Kimmel, S. B., & Mahalik, J. R. (2005). Body image concerns of gay men: The roles of minority stress and conformity to masculine norms. *Journal of Consulting and Clinical Psychology, 73*(6), 1185–1990.

Liang, C. T. H., & Alimo, C. (2005). The impact of white heterosexual students' interactions on attitudes toward lesbian, gay, and bisexual people: A longitudinal study. *Journal of College Student Development, 46*(3), 237–250. Retrieved from *www.jcsdonline.org*.

Moradi, B., van den Berg, J. J., & Epting, F. R. (2006). Intrapersonal and interpersonal manifestations of antilesbian and gay prejudice: An application of personal construct theory. *Journal of Counseling Psychology, 53*(1), 57–66.

Shumake, T. C. (2005). Change takes time. In S. Windmeyer (Ed.), *Brotherhood: Gay life in college fraternities* (pp. 63–71). New York: Alyson Books.

Stevens, R. A. (2004). Understanding gay identity development within the college environment. *Journal of College Student Development, 45*(2), 185–206. Retrieved from *www.jcsdonline.org*.

Strauss, A., & Corbin, J. (2008). *Basics of qualitative research: Techniques for developing grounded theory* (3rd ed.). Thousand Oaks, CA: Sage.

Windmeyer, S. L. (Ed.). (2001). *Secret sisters: Stories of being lesbian and bisexual in college sororities.* New York: Alyson Books.

Windmeyer, S. L. (Ed.). (2005). *Brotherhood: Gay life in college fraternities.* New York: Alyson Books.

Windmeyer, S. L., & Freeman, P. W. (1997). *How homophobia hurts the college fraternity.* Retrieved from *www.lambda10.org/outgreek/ L10HowHomophobiaHurts.pdf*.

FIGURE A-1. INTERVIEW PROTOCOL

1. How do you define diversity?

2. What role, if any, has diversity played in your life?

3. Can you describe your personal experiences with being a member of a Greek letter organization?

4. If all of your attributes, sexual orientation included, were made into characters for a play about your life, what would the sexual orientation character's role be like?

5. How, if at all, has your sexual orientation interacted with being a member of a Greek organization?

6. What perceptions do you have about the climate for GLBT individuals inside of your Greek organization?

7a. If a new and "out" GLBT student were to express interest in joining a Greek letter organization, what possible obstacles or challenges would he or she face?

7b. What possible benefits would this same person experience?

8. How would you describe your personal growth while going through the Greek system?

9. What university or fraternity policies are in place about GLBT individuals?

10. Is there anything that you would like to comment on that we did not cover?

FIGURE A-2. PARTICIPANT DEMOGRAPHIC FORM

ID Number (to be completed by researcher): _____

PARTICIPANT DEMOGRAPHIC SHEET

Age: _____ Race/Ethnicity: _____

Marital/Relationship Status: _____ Job: _____

Sexual Orientation: _____ Gender: _____

Number of Years in College: _____

Years in Greek Organization: _____

Annual Household Income: _____

Religious/Spiritual Orientation: _____

Please circle the groups of people, if any, with whom you have disclosed your sexual orientation:

                Friends   Family   Greek Brothers/Sisters   Coworkers

Other (Please Specify): _____

May we contact you for follow up? Circle one: Yes   No

How do you want to be contacted?:   Phone   E-mail   Other (Please specify)

Phone number: _____

E-mail: _____

Please provide any additional information you would like for us to know about you.

_____

_____

Thank You!

FIGURE A-3. FINAL CODEBOOK

Codebook: Final Codebook
Text One and Text Two
PA005 and PA010

Code	Meaning	Example
Disclosure	Talking about disclosing identity	63: Being gay might not mix with the traditional ideas of fraternal brotherhood. 70: None of the brothers had any idea what was going on. 14: Solidly slammed my closet door shut. 16: It felt so good to be coming out of the closet. 81: This kind of snuck up on me. 91–92: I hadn't really discovered myself until I moved to college.
Acceptance—Others	Accepted by organization	63: The brothers all seemed eager to meet me. 71: Knew where I belonged. 16: Someone who could just listen to me. 13: Let's not forget the gay 10% rule. 215: Brothers are able to look past that. 126–127: Candidates are openly gay and it's typically not an issue. 146–147: Oh, you're my brother. And no matter what, I'll be here for you. 150: I don't think they would care about my orientation.
Macho	Masculine stereotyping	64: A punch on the arm from one, a strong handshake from another. 69: Fraternity life was no place for an openly gay guy. 12: I do not need friends this badly. 12: I could never let my fraternity brothers down. I could never let them know who I am. 12: Fear of being labeled gay by association. 122: There is a very macho stereotype of Greeks. 109: Just another skirt-chasing guy.
Gay community within organization	Depicts gay community within organization	69: I never suspected that it was Cole. 12: Rob was openly bisexual. 90: Meeting fellow gays of the family. 119–120: Around some of the other brothers who, uh, we of uh, the same orientation as myself.
Diversity	Working together with people from different backgrounds	8–9: The collaboration, coordination of different types, groups of people. 21: Raised to be a more understanding and appreciative person. 13–14: Mixing or intermingling like, a social uh, a social background. 265–266: Diversity is alive, it is growing. It is just a genuinely good thing.
Self-Acceptance	Learning about and appreciating self	39: Taught me a lot about myself and others. 162–163: You learn so much more about yourself. 255: A great growing experience for me. 283–284: Acceptance in my orientation is a huge difference.

Created: 12/1/2009

PROPOSAL 1

448

TABLE A-1. CASE DISPLAY

Data	Acceptance of self	Acceptance: Organization	Diversity	Disclosure	Macho stereotype	Gay community
PA005	Accepted, but not integral to identity.	Acknowledges that some are not keen, but also lacking understanding. Has acceptance.	Collaboration of many groups of people. Learning environment. Always a part of life.	Ambivalent brothers. Mostly neutral reactions.	Sees some organizations and members subscribing to the fraternity stereotype.	Numerous individuals mentioned within organization and Greek system.
PA010	Conflicted; accepts self but can see as a negative attribute.	Brothers as accepting. Goes with the flow. Unsure about candidate class.	Learning of other groups, particularly religious. Growing sense of awareness.	Feels no need to hide, but sees how it can be stressful. Keeping a secret challenging.	Occasionally identifies with the stereotype as "just one of the guys."	Numerous individuals mentioned within own organization.
Text 1	Accepted, but initially low form. Accepts more as organization accepts.	Fear of rejection. Witness of negative remarks. Feeling of belonging.	N/A	Avoidant of disclosure initially. Would rather die than disclose. Disclosure met with acceptance.	Doesn't need friends this badly (hazing). Initial thoughts.	Hidden members mentioned in organization. Outside community referenced.
Text 2	Accepted, but cautious of reactions of others.	Rejected by two organizations before accepted by the first. Earned acceptance.	N/A	Never hidden within Greek system, but never on the front lines of knowledge.	Stereotypical roles. Punch on the arm. Firm handshakes.	Hidden member mentioned within organization.

FIGURE A-4. CONCEPT MAP

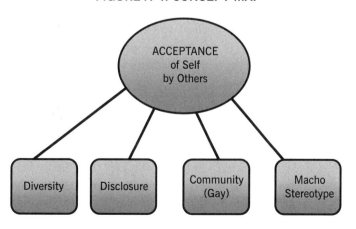

The Experience of Success for Adolescents Diagnosed with Attention-Deficit/Hyperactivity Disorder

ANNE M. P. MICHALEK
Old Dominion University

ABSTRACT

This qualitative study describes the experience of success for adolescents with ADHD. For the pilot study, the author used a phenomenological paradigm, tradition, and method of analysis. The primary researcher conducted two semistructured interviews in order to gather data. Results of this pilot study suggest that adolescents with ADHD had negative self-efficacy with regard to success and that their effort is linked to internal level of worth. Implications and future research directions are provided.

Attention-deficit/hyperactivity disorder (ADHD) is one of the most frequently cited medical/behavioral conditions and the most common childhood disorder (Barkley, 1997). Barkley (1997) describes ADHD as a developmental disorder affecting a child's ability to regulate behavior, control behavior, or keep future goals and consequences in mind. These deficits are manifested and demonstrated through a variety of behaviors, including an inability to sustain attention, effectively regulate levels of activity according to the situation, and effectively plan and complete tasks.

The specific criteria for diagnosing ADHD in children is outlined in the *Diagnostic and Statistical Manual of Mental Disorders*–IV—Text Revised (DSM-IV-TR; American Psychiatric Association, 2000) and divides ADHD into three specific subtypes: the inattentive type, the hyperactive type, and the combined type. The purpose of these criteria is to ensure that a diagnosis is made based on observable behaviors that are manifested before the age of 7 in two or more settings, thereby impacting the child's ability to function, and are not due to another disorder (American Psychiatric Association, 2000). These descriptions are meant to ensure the accurate and consistent diagnosis of ADHD in children. Today, between 3 and 5% of children have been diagnosed with a form of ADHD (Schmitz, Filippone, & Edelman, 2003). Although the prevalence of ADHD in the pediatric population is growing, there remains a significant debate regarding the existence and relevance of the ADHD diagnosis (Kendall, Hatton, Beckett, & Leo, 2003).

Over the past 10 years, ADHD has been the topic of numerous research articles and news stories. The media has taken the stance that ADHD is grossly overdiagnosed, resulting in the irresponsible prescription of the stimulant methylphenidate in young children (Brazelton & Sparrow, 2003; LeFever, Dawson, & Morrow, 1999; Vatz & Weinberg, 2001). The evidence for this argument is essentially rooted in prevalence studies, anecdotal stories of misdiagnosis, and passed-down misperceptions developed from personal bias and belief systems (Brazelton & Sparrow 2003; LeFever et al., 1999; Scuitto & Eisenberg, 2007; Vatz & Weinberg, 2001). Scholars and researchers contend that ADHD is not overdiagnosed, basing their argument on the same prevalence studies, current diagnostic criteria, and semantic nuances of the word *overdiagnosis* (Scuitto & Eisenberg, 2007; Singh, DelBello, Kowatch, & Strakowski, 2006). Regardless of position, researchers and news commentators agree that clinical science continues to recognize ADHD as a serious problem with serious consequences (Barkley, 1997).

Consequences of ADHD are experienced by parents, educators, and child. Often, quantitative and qualitative studies summarize the effects of ADHD from the perspective of parent, caregiver, and/or educator. Rarely do quantitative or qualitative studies explain or give voice to the child or adolescent diagnosed with ADHD. In 2003, Kendall and colleagues discussed the consequences of ADHD from the children's perspectives. Through this qualitative study, the researchers identified six common themes regarding how ADHD had impacted the lives of the children interviewed. These themes included (1) cognitive, affective, and behavioral problems; (2) meaning and identity of ADHD; (3) taking pills; (4) significance of maternal support; (5) causes of ADHD; and (6) lack of racial/ethnic differences. In general, children with ADHD consistently experienced problems with learning, thinking, feeling, and behaving (Kendall et al., 2003). The children also described ADHD in terms of emotion words (i.e., feeling *ashamed*, *sad*, *frustrated*, and *mad*). In general, the authors noted that the children interviewed had developed an ADHD identity that was characterized by the following descriptors: *hyper*, *bad*, *trouble*, and *weird*. Although the children reported learning problems, the research team did not seek information regarding how the children experienced, recognized, and predicted failure or success.

Success is a subjective concept that can be defined and described differently depending on the person's profession and point of reference. According to Schindler and Jones (2009), there are three main variables of success: having an internal locus of control, self-acceptance, and orientation toward goal setting (Schindler & Jones, 2009). *Internal locus of control* refers to an individual's belief that he or she is able to influence results so that he or she has control over outcomes. According to Schindler and Jones (2009), self-acceptance is judged according to how well a person likes themselves. The third variable of success, orientation toward goal setting, refers to an individual as either avoiding failure or seeking success (Schindler & Jones, 2009). These variables, combined, set the internal stage for a person's ability to successfully attain goals.

The purpose of the current pilot study is to develop an understanding of how ADHD impacts an adolescent's ability to recognize and plan for academic success in order to improve service delivery. In addition, the study will identify the overt and covert variables that influence the success of an adolescent with ADHD in the academic setting. The overarching research question guiding this study is: How do adolescents with ADHD experience academic success? For the purposes of this study, adolescents are defined as between the ages of 13 and 17 years old. ADHD is operationalized as the DSM-IV criteria: a persistent pattern of inattention or hyperactivity/impulsivity that is frequent and severe, as determined by a physician or psychologist. Academic failure is defined as one or more of the following: a *D* or below in one or more academic subjects, recommended accommodations/modifications/strategies found to be ineffective, few interpersonal relationships, and several parental concerns. Academic success is defined as one or more of the following: a *C* or above in more than two academic subjects, recommended accommodations/modifications/strategies found to be effective, several interpersonal relationships, and/or few parental concerns.

METHOD

This study will use an emergent design within a theoretical framework synthesized from the five philosophies of science. For the purposes of this study, the first philosophy, the research team's ontological perspective is that there are multiple truths regarding how success and failure are experienced. Epistemologically, the research team will recognize that an individual's knowl-

451

edge of success is unlimited and context specific. With regard to axiology, the research team will recognize that participants' and researchers' beliefs and values will impact and influence the research process. Rhetorically, the researchers agree that once multiple individuals share their experiences, an essence of the experience can be categorized and organized (Patton, 2002). With regard to methodology, the researchers will embrace the social constructivism paradigm that contends that multiple realities are constructed through social interactions, thereby generating knowledge of a phenomenon. Based on this paradigm that multiple realities of the phenomenon *success* are recognized, phenomenology will be the tradition used to capture and describe how a distinct group of people experience (i.e., adolescents) the phenomenon success (Patton, 2002).

Research Team and Researcher Bias

The research team for this study will be comprised of five scholars: three doctoral-level students and two professors. The doctoral-level students will have varying educational backgrounds and professional experiences. One student will have a master's degree in counseling and be working toward her doctorate. A second student will have a master's degree in special education and be working toward her PhD. The third student will have a master's degree in speech–language pathology and be working toward her PhD. All three students will be white and will be familiar with ADHD. The research team members are female. There will be one primary researcher responsible for data collection, transcription, and initial analysis. Both professors will oversee the research project and provide support and guidance as necessary. Like the students, the professors have varied areas of expertise. One professor specializes in counseling, while the other is an aphasia expert.

A very important step of a qualitative study is to acknowledge and explain researcher bias. Since this is a phenomenological study, these biases will also be bracketed throughout data collection and analysis. Specifically, the primary researcher recognizes that she has had work experiences that have influenced her core beliefs regarding how ADHD impacts an individual's ability to recognize and experience success. In addition, she has witnessed the importance of effective remediation and treatment for children with ADHD. A former patient sustained multiple traumatic brain injuries due to inconsistent and ineffective management of ADHD behaviors, resulting in additional, long-term cognitive deficits and eventual incarceration.

Participants

Participants for the study will be selected using criterion sampling of typical cases in order to facilitate a diverse sample. A total of 30–40 adolescents diagnosed with ADHD will be selected for the study if they are also experiencing academic failure. These adolescents may have the following co-diagnoses: learning disability, oppositional defiant disorder, and/or conduct disorder.

Data Collection

This study will be expected to take between a year and a year and a half to complete. Participants will be recruited through word of mouth and flier distributions to schools, other speech–language pathologists, and psychologists. The international review board will examine and approve all research methods and materials before the primary researcher will initiate participant recruitment. In addition, before interviewing participants, they will provide their assent as evidenced by signing the assent document. Furthermore, the adolescent's parent and/or caregiver will be required to provide parental consent by signing the parental consent document. Once the team has received proper consent and assent, the primary researcher will be responsible for conducting individual interviews with each adolescent participant. The interviews will be semistructured and designed using a variety of question types. These types include, but are not limited to, experience/behavior, opinion, knowledge, feeling, and probing questions. The interview protocol will be reviewed and agreed upon by research team members before administered to participants.

In addition to adolescent interviews, the primary researcher will conduct participant observations in the home and school environments. The primary researcher will thoroughly document her observations using field notes. It should be noted that these observations will only be completed if permission from all parties (i.e., school, parents, adolescents) is granted.

Data Analysis

The primary researcher will be responsible for transcribing each participant interview individually. Once transcribed, the interviews will be coded. The following coding procedure will be implemented. First, the primary researcher will bracket her assumptions, noting her biases and their influence on the coding process. Second, the primary researcher will use horizontalization. This essentially refers to the process of identifying direct quotes from the individual transcripts that may answer or provide more information regarding the research questions. Third, the primary researcher will use textual themes. This means that the researcher will thickly describe the identified quotes using key words in order to generate codes. Finally, the primary researcher will use structural themes. This means that the researcher will collapse textual themes into patterns. These patterns will be axial coded as either general, typical, or variant.

Throughout this procedure, the primary researcher will be reading and reviewing the transcripts and simultaneously reviewing, comparing, and collapsing themes. This will continue while the research team reviews the generated codes. Coding will be considered conclusive once the team has reached a point of saturation where no other codes or themes emerge and there is 95% agreement on the resulting codebook.

Strategies for Trustworthiness

For the purposes of this study, trustworthiness will be defined according to four categories: credibility, transferability, dependability, and confirmability. Credibility will be demonstrated through the use of memos, member checking, a thorough audit trail, and prolonged observation. Transferability will be demonstrated through the use of a diverse sample that meets the predetermined criteria and the use of thick description. Dependability will be demonstrated by the use of multiple coders and/or readers, triangulating the data sources, and using member checking. Finally, confirmability will be demonstrated by bracketing the researcher's assumptions.

PILOT STUDY

In order to generate preliminary information and assess the viability of the research project, a pilot study was completed. Two participants were selected for the pilot study and one unobtrusive method of data collection was facilitated. From this, several textual and structural themes were identified. These results indicate several potential contributions and suggest that the research project has value.

The pilot study was conducted through a larger research project. Initially, IRB approval had been obtained and several fliers were distributed announcing the recruitment of adolescents diagnosed with ADHD. To date, two participants have provided their assent in addition to parental consent. These participants are siblings. The first participant is described as a White male whose chronological age is 15 years, 6 months. He has a confirmed, medical diagnosis of ADHD and was referred to the research project by his guidance counselor due to academic failure. Finally, this participant takes prescription medication (Adderall) to help alleviate ADHD symptomology.

Participant two is described as a white female whose chronological age is 14 years, 7 months. She has a confirmed, medical diagnosis of ADHD and was also referred to the research project by her mother due to academic failure. This participant also takes Adderall to help alleviate ADHD symptomology.

The primary research collected data over the course of 2 days. Each research participant was interviewed individually using the interview protocol attached as Table A-2. These interviews were semistructured with varied questions and were approximately 35–40 minutes in length. The interviews took place at a child study center in a university setting. Once completed, the primary researcher transcribed each interview individually. Once transcribed, the primary researcher bracketed her assumptions, noting her biases and their influence on the coding process. Second, the primary researcher used horizontalization. Third, the primary researcher used textual themes. Finally, the primary researcher generated structural themes. Throughout this procedure, the primary researcher was reading, reviewing, comparing, and collapsing codes and themes. For the purposes of the pilot study, coding concluded once the primary researcher subjectively determined that she had reached saturation. The research team did not reach consensus during this process. The resulting codebook is included as Figure A-3.

In order to maintain trustworthiness, the primary researcher aligned selected data collection and analysis procedures with the following four categories: credibility, transferability, dependability, confirmability. The primary researcher used memos, member checking, and an audit trail to demonstrate credibility, and thick description when coding to demonstrate transferablility. To demonstrate dependability, the primary researcher used member checking. Finally, the primary researcher bracketed her assumptions in order to demonstrate confirmability.

Pilot Findings

The primary researcher identified several textual and structural themes in the pilot study test data. An attached codebook outlines these results in detail and is labeled Figure A-3. In summary, 34 textual themes were generated and defined according to the communicative purpose they served and the research question they answered. Once identified, these themes were studied for similarities that would allow them to be collapsed into structural themes. From this, six structural themes were identified and defined according to previous literature and/or the meaning gleaned from the interview. These six structural themes serve as the basis of the discussion and of the potential implications. The structural themes were motivation, self-esteem, language, family connection, hot executive functions, and cold executive functions (Barry & Welsh, 2007). It should be noted that data generated through individual interviews were confirmed when reviewing Internet blogs posted by parents and guardians of adolescents with ADHD.

Discussion

Several interesting, independent, and relevant conclusions were made based on the identified structural themes. With regard to executive functions, the female participant demonstrated deficits with hot executive functions (i.e., tasks with affective components involving reward and punishment) such as impulsivity and response inhibition, whereas the male participant demonstrated deficits with cold executive functions (i.e., cognitive aspects such as memory and attention). Although the researcher is unable to say that this information is generalizable, it is valuable for the participants' educators, counselors, and parents. Recognizing and responding to differences in executive function ability have significant consequences with regard to academic performance and interpersonal relationships. Both participants would benefit from direct and intense instruction to develop insight regarding the impact that hot and cold executive functions have on their activities of daily living.

In addition to profiling specific aspects of executive functions, the results support the existing literature that suggests that hot and cold executive functions impact an individual's ability to use verbal and nonverbal feedback to successfully self-evaluate (Barry & Welsh, 2007). The participants consistently demonstrated a lack of insight regarding how to use environmental cues to change their behavior. In the face of old problems, they continue to make choices that have negative consequences. This continued cycle makes it difficult for individuals to use lessons learned from previous experiences to effectively make choices when confronted with new problems. These deficits are closely related with the ability to plan effectively. That is, not only do individuals use feedback to respond differently but to make accurate, realistic, and concise plans. The results of this pilot study indicate that not only do cold executive functions impact planning skills but so do motivation and self-esteem. Unfortunately for our participants, all three of these areas were judged to be weaknesses making it very difficult for them to plan effectively.

In addition to planning, self-esteem appears to impact the participants' level of motivation. Both participants communicated a decreased level of value for their individual characteristics as evidenced by self-deprecating comments. This, combined with their decreased level of motivation or desire to achieve, gave the general impression of hopelessness. At a young age, these participants already seemed to have waved the white flag and surrendered to their inherent challenges. They have yet to internalize success, making it very difficult for them to embrace challenging or difficult academic tasks. Most importantly, it appears that these participants can recognize consequences, but their self-esteem influences their ability to recognize their worthiness for success. That is, they know what will happen if they are successful, but they do not believe they are good enough to succeed. It appears that these participants believe that they are only good enough for failure and, therefore, their worth has become inextricably linked to their effort.

In the area of language, both participants demonstrated unique and different language profiles. The female participant had average to above average expressive and receptive language skills, whereas the male participant demonstrated average receptive language with significant expressive language deficits. Specifically, the male participant has difficulty elaborating, creating syntactically and semantically complex sentences, and producing narratives. It should be noted that although the male participant had significant language deficits, he demonstrated a decreased level of apathy. His sister, however, demonstrated an increased level of apathy.

Finally, both participants consistently communicated a poor family connection. This is a structural theme identified and defined by the primary researcher. It refers to the influence immediate family members (i.e., mother, father, siblings) have had on the participants. Both participants communicated a strong desire to avoid their home environment, indicating that their caregivers may not provide adequate support.

IMPLICATIONS

This study has the potential to contribute to the field of education. Specifically, this research will give a voice to an otherwise voiceless population. It is very rare for researchers to ask adolescents themselves about their experience with success. This research project provides a great starting point for future discussions with adolescents who are diagnosed with ADHD in order to understand their deficits, and more importantly, what academic strategies are functional and beneficial. Finally, this study contributes preliminary information regarding the relationship between executive functions and ADHD.

FUTURE RESEARCH DIRECTIONS AND LIMITATIONS

Specifically, the pilot study completed provided the following as future research topics: the language profile of adolescents with ADHD, the impact of parental interactions on adolescents with ADHD, the characterization of hot and cold executive functions in this population, and the impact of interpersonal relationships on adolescents with ADHD.

This study has several limitations. The language profile of the participants may interfere with effective communication; therefore, provided verbal responses may not be a true representation of individual experiences. The study did not represent various cultures or races/ethnicities.

The primary researcher had a working relationship with the participants, and this may have influenced their responses. In addition, the primary researcher used her knowledge about participants when coding interviews and drawing conclusions. The primary researcher did not account for the impact of comorbidity, specifically, depression, on the experience of participants. It is unknown if these participants had another mental health diagnosis. This variable needs to be accounted for, since the literature suggests that there is a high rate of comorbidity for this population. Also, this study did not address medication or the impact medication may have on the participants' level of functioning.

The primary researcher did not interview teachers, which makes it difficult to triangulate results. Some neuropsychological literature argues that there is poor construct validity for executive functions. This information was not discussed during the literature review, making the review limited in its scope. Finally, with regard to cultural limitations, this study is not culturally representative. In addition, the researcher is a speech language pathologist who completed this research from that perspective.

REFERENCES

American Psychiatric Association. (2000). *Diagnostic and statistical manual of mental disorders* (4th ed., text rev.). Washington, DC: Author.

Barkley, R. A. (1997). *ADHD and the nature of self-control.* New York: Guilford Press.

Barry, P. G., & Welsh, M. (2007). The BrainWise Curriculum: Neurocognitive development intervention program. In D. Romer & E. Walker (Eds.), *Adolescent psychopathology and the developing brain* (pp. 42–440). New York: Oxford University Press.

Brazelton, T. B., & Sparrow, J. (2003, April 24). Overdiagnosis is a major problem with ADHD. *Deseret News.* Retrieved October 3, 2008, from *www.findarticles.com/p/articles/mi_qn4188/is_20030424/ai_nl1386912.*

Kendall, J., Hatton, D., Beckett, A., & Leo, M. (2003). Children's accounts of attention-deficit/hyperactivity disorder. *Advances in Nursing Science, 26*(2), 114–130.

LeFever, G. B., Dawson, K. V., & Morrow, A. L. (1999). The extent of drug therapy for attention deficit-hyperactivity disorder among children in public schools. *American Journal of Public Health, 89*(9), 1359–1364.

Patton, M. Q. (2002). *Qualitative research and evaluation methods* (3rd ed.). Thousand Oaks, CA: Sage.

Schindler, J., & Jones, A. (2009). A three-factor operational definition of success psychology. Retrieved August 2, 2009, from *www.calstatela.edu/faculty/jshindl/cm/success%20Psych%201pg.htm.*

Schmitz, M. F., Filippone, P., & Edelman, E. M. (2003). Social representations of attention deficit/hyperactivity disorder, 1988–1997. *Culture and Psychology, 9,* 383–406.

Scuitto, M. J., & Eisenberg, M. (2007). Evaluating the evidence for and against the overdiagnosis of ADHD. *Journal of Attention Disorders, 11*(2), 106–113.

Singh, M. K., DelBello, M. P., Kowatch, R. A., & Strakowski, S. M. (2006). Co-occurrence of bipolar and attention-deficit hyperactivity disorders in children. *Bipolar Disorders, 8,* 710–720.

Vatz, R. E., & Weinberg, L. S. (2001, March 1). Problems in diagnosing and treating ADD/ADHD (attention deficit disorder, attention deficit hyperactivity disorder). *USA Today Magazine.* Retrieved October 4, 2008, from *www.findarticles.com/p/articles/mi_m1272/is-2670-129/ai-72272577.*

TABLE A-2. THE INTERVIEW PROTOCOL

Research questions	Categories	Interview questions
How do students with ADHD and EF deficits experience academic success and/or failure?	Social experiences	Describe a time of success. Describe a time of failure. Describe your school day.
	Identification of failure/success	How do you know you are/are not doing good? Tell the me about what causes you to do good/not do good? What would help you do better, if anything?
	Reaction to failure/success	When I am not doing well in school , I ... What happens when you are doing good/not doing good? What advice would you give other kids who might not be doing good?
	Perception of school	Thinking about school makes me. ... What would a great school day be like?
	Consequences	If you are doing well, what kinds of things happen? If you are not doing well, what kinds of things happen? How do you think other students like you feel? Why is it important to do well?
What is the relationship between theory of mind and executive functions?	*Note:* Not used for this interview	

TABLE A-3. CODEBOOK

Textual Themes

Code	Description
Consequence _ success	Participant indicated understanding of what would happen if successful
Recognition _ success	Participant recognizes when success happens
Example _ success	Participant provided an example of success
Consequence _ failure	Participant indicated understanding of what would happen if he or she failed
Recognition _ failure	Participant recognizes failure
Example _ failure	Participant provided an example of failure
Incongruent exp _ success	Participant identified an example of success, which was not indicative of something positive
Self-perception _ neg	Participant made a statement that was a "put-down" or reflected poor self-acceptance
Incongruent nonverbals	Participant demonstrated nonverbal communication that was not aligned with the verbal message
Congruent nonverbal	Participant demonstrated nonverbal communication that matched the verbal message
Demeanor nonverbals	Participant demonstrated nonverbal communication that gave the impression of being bored, irritated, indifferent, and uninterested
Canned phrase	Participant made a comment that appeared to be repetitive of something heard by another person or adult
Elaboration _ el	Participant had difficulty elaborating
Self-perception nonverbal	Participant demonstrated nonverbal communication that indicated poor self-acceptance

457

Code	Description
Mlu _ el	Participant produced a sentence that was not the appropriate mean length of utterance for his chronological age
Problem solving	Participant response indicated difficulty with problem solving
Planning	Participant response indicated poor planning
Incongruent response	Participant response did not match something previously said or the question presented
Learning _ prob	Participant response evidenced a problem learning or using academic strategies
Appropriate response	Participant answered the question appropriately
Interpersonal _ prob	Participant response revealed a problem getting along with peers, siblings, or parents
Clarification	Participant response was an effort to get or provide clarification
Apathy _ other	Participant response communicated a lack of interest or concern regarding something
Apathy _ interp	Participant response communicated a lack of interest or concern regarding peers, parents, siblings
Apathy _ school	Participant response communicated a lack of interest or concern regarding school
Avoidance _ home	Participant indicated he or she tries to get away from home
Avoidance _ school	Participant response indicated he or she tries to get away from school and school-related activities
Avoidance _ answer	Participant response indicated he or she tried to avoid answering the question
Insight _ own	Participant response indicated difficulty with understanding own motives or thought processes
Insight _ others	Participant response indicated difficulty understanding someone else's motives or thought processes
Personal account	Participant response described a personal story or situation

Structural Themes—Identified as Collapsed Themes

Collapsed theme	Description
Motivation	Desire to achieve; moving them into action
Self-esteem	Valuing individual characteristics; feeling good about those characteristics
Language	Expressive language; syntax, semantics, and pragmatics
Family connection	Mother, father, siblings, and their influence on participants; use of them for support
Hot executive functions	Self-monitoring and self-regulation of emotion
Cold executive functions	Planning, problem solving, predicting, consequences

References

Adler, P. A., & Adler, P. (1987). *Membership roles in field research.* Newbury Park, CA: Sage.

Adler, P. A., & Adler, P. (2008). Of rhetoric and representation: The four faces of ethnography. *Sociological Quarterly, 49*(1), 1–30.

Agar, M. (2006, September). An ethnography by any other name ... *Forum: Qualitative Social Research, 7*(4), Art. 36. Retrieved February 2, 2011, from *www.qualitative-research.net/index/php/fas/article/view/177/396.*

Ahern, K. J. (1999). Ten tips for reflexive bracketing. *Qualitative Health Research, 9*(3), 407–411.

Alaggia, R., & Millington, G. (2008). Male child sexual abuse: A phenomenology of betrayal. *Clinical Social Work Journal, 36,* 265–275.

Alerby, E. (2003). "During the break we have fun": A study concerning pupils' experience of school. *Educational Research, 45,* 17–28.

Allport, G. W., Bruner, J., & Jandorf, E. (1941). Personality under social catastrophe: An analysis of 90 German refugees' life histories. *Character and Personality, 10,* 1–22.

Altheide, D. L. (1987). Ethnographic content analysis. *Qualitative Sociology, 10*(1), 65–77.

Amatea, E. S., & Clark, M. A. (2005). Changing schools, changing counselors: A qualitative study of administrators' conceptions of the school counselor role. *Professional School Counseling, 9,* 16–27.

American Association for Marriage and Family Therapy. (2001). AAMFT code of ethics. Retrieved January 25, 2011, from *www.aamft.org/resources/lrm.../ethics/ethicscode2001.asp.*

American Counseling Association. (2005). *ACA code of ethics.* Alexandria, VA: Author.

American Education Research Association. (2006). Ethical standards of AERA. Retrieved September 5, 2009, from *www.aera.net.*

American Psychiatric Association. (2000). *Diagnostic and statistical manual of mental disorders* (4th ed., text rev.). Washington, DC: Author.

American Psychological Association. (2002). Ethical principles of psychologists and code of conduct. Retrieved February 4, 2010, from *www.apa.org/ethics/code/index.aspx.*

American Psychological Association. (2010). *Publication manual of the American Psychological Association* (6th ed.). Washington, DC: Author.

Ames, G. M., & Grube, J. W. (1999). Alcohol availability and workplace drinking: Mixed method analyses. *Journal of Studies on Alcohol, 60*(3), 383–393.

Anderson, L. (2006). Analytic autoethnography. *Journal of Contemporary Ethnography, 35*(4), 373–395.

Angen, M. J. (2000). Evaluating interpretive inquiry: Reviewing the validity debate and opening the dialogue. *Qualitative Health Research, 10*(3), 378–395.

Angus, L. E., Levitt, H., & Hardtke, K. (1999). The narrative processes coding system: Research applications and implications for psychotherapy. *Journal of Clinical Psychology, 55*(10), 1255–1271.

Anzaldua, G. (1987). *Borderlands/La frontera: The new mestiza.* San Francisco: Aunt Lute Press.

Arber, A. (2006). Reflexivitiy: A challenge for the researcher as practitioner? *Journal of Research in Nursing, 11*(2), 147–157.

Armstrong, N. (2005). Resistance through risk: Women and cervical cancer screening. *Health, Risk and Society, 7*(2), 161–176.

Atkinson, J. M., & Heritage, J. (1984). *Garfinkel and ethnomethodology.* Cambridge, UK: Polity Press.

Atkinson, P. (2006). Rescuing autoethnography.

Journal of Contemporary Ethnography, 35, 400–404.

Au, W. (2004, Fall). No child left untested. *Rethinking Schools.* Available at *www.rethinkingschools.org/archive/19_01/nclb191.shtml.*

Auxier, C. R., Hughes, F. R., & Kline, W. B. (2003). Identity development in counselors-in-training. *Counselor Education and Supervision, 43,* 23–38.

Avdi, E., & Georgaca, E. (2007). Narrative research in psychotherapy: A critical review. *Psychology and Psychotherapy: Theory, Research, and Practice, 80,* 407–419.

Bakhtin, M. M. (1984). *Problems of Dostoevsky's poetics* (C. Emerson, Ed. & Trans.). Minneapolis: University of Minnesota Press.

Banks, J., & Cochran-Smith, M. (2005). Teaching diverse learners. In L. Darling-Hammond & J. Bransford (Eds.), *Preparing teachers for a changing world: What teachers should learn and be able to do* (pp. 232–275). Mahwah, NJ: Erlbaum.

Banks, M. (2001). *Visual methods in social research.* London: Sage.

Barkley, R. A. (1997). *ADHD and the nature of self-control.* New York: Guilford Press.

Bays, D. A., & Crockett, J. B. (2007). Investigating instructional leadership for special education. *Exceptionality, 15,* 143–161.

Becker, H. S. (1970). Field work evidence. In H. Becker, *Sociological work: Method and substance* (pp. 39–62). New Brunswick, NJ: Transaction Books.

Becker, H. S., Geer, B., Hughes, E. C., & Strauss, A. L. (1961). *Boys in white: Student culture in medical school.* Chicago: University of Chicago Press.

Bell, J. (2005). *Doing your research project: A guide for first-time researchers in education, health and social science.* Berkshire, UK: Open University Press.

Benner, P. (1994). *Interpretative phenomenology: Embodiment, caring and ethics in health and illness.* London: Sage.

Berg, B. L. (2004). *Qualitative research methods for the social sciences* (5th ed.). Boston: Allyn & Bacon.

Berger, P. L., & Luckmann, T. (1966). *The social construction of reality: A treatise in the sociology of knowledge.* Garden City, NY: Doubleday.

Beshai, J. A. (2008). Are cross-cultural comparisons of norms on death anxiety valid? *Omega: Journal of Death and Dying, 57*(3), 299–313.

Blalock, H. (1967). *Toward a theory of minority-group relations.* New York: Wiley.

Blank, J. (2009). Life in the village: Teacher community and autonomy in an early childhood education center. *Early Childhood Education Journal, 36,* 373–380.

Bloland, P. A., & Edwards, P. B. (1981). Work and leisure: A counseling synthesis. *Vocational Guidance Quarterly, 30,* 101–108.

Bogar, C. B., & Hulse-Killacky, D. (2006). Resiliency determinants and resiliency processes among female adult survivors of childhood sexual abuse. *Journal of Counseling and Development, 84,* 318–327.

Bogdan, R. C., & Biklen, S. K. (2003). *Qualitative research for education: An introduction to theories and methods* (4th ed.). Boston: Allyn & Bacon.

Bonomi, C. (2005). Was Freud afraid of flying? *International Forum of Psychoanalysis, 14,* 49–53.

Borland, K. W., Jr. (2001). Qualitative and quantitative research: A complementary balance. *New Directions for Institutional Research, 112,* 5–13.

Bouck, E. C. (2008). Exploring the enactment of functional curriculum in self-contained cross-categorical programs: A case study. *Qualitative Report, 13*(3), 495–530.

Brinkmann, S., & Kvale, S. (2005). Confronting the ethics of qualitative research. *Journal of Constructivist Psychology, 18,* 157–181.

Brotherson, M. J. (1994). Interactive focus group interviewing: A qualitative research method in early intervention. *Topics in Early Childhood Special Education, 14,* 101–118.

Brown, P. U., Rogers, K. M., Feuerhelm, C., & Chimblo, S. (2007). The nature of primary teaching: Body, time, space, and relationships. *Journal of Early Childhood, 28,* 3–16.

Brownlow, C., & O'Dell, L. (2002). Ethical issues for qualitative research in on-line communities. *Disability and Society, 17*(6), 685–694.

Brydon-Miller, M. (1997). Participatory action research: Psychology and social change. *Journal of Social Issues, 53,* 657–666.

Bubany, S. T. (2008). College students' perspectives on their career decision-making. *Journal of Career Assessment, 16,* 177–197.

Burgess, R. G. (1991). *In the field: An introduction to field research.* London: Routledge.

Burnes, T. R. (2006). Opening the door of a bigger closet: An analysis of sexual orientation identify development for lesbian, bisexual, and queer college women of color. *Dissertation Abstracts International*, B, 67/07.

Burstow, B. (2003). Toward a radical understanding of trauma and trauma work. *Violence Against Women, 9,* 1293–1317.

Buzan, T., & Buzan, B. (1996). *The mind map book: How to use radiant thinking to maximize your brain's untapped potential.* New York: Penguin Books.

Caldwell, K., & Atwal, A. (2005). Non-participant observation: Using video tapes to collect data in nursing research. *Nurse Researcher, 13*(2), 42–54.

Campbell, R., Adams, A. E., Wasco, S. M., Ahrens, C. E., & Sefl, T. (2010). "What has it been like for you to talk with me today?": The impact of participating in interview research on rape survivors. *Violence against Women, 16,* 60–83.

Casterline, G. L. (2009). Heuristic inquiry: Artistic science for nursing. *Southern Online Journal of Nursing Research, 9*(4), 1–8.

Chandler, D. (2002). *Semiotics: The basics.* New York: Routledge.

Charmaz, K. (2005). *Grounded theory: Methods for the 21st century.* London: Sage.

Charmaz, K., & Mitchell, R. G. (2001). Grounded theory in ethnography. In P. Atkinson, A. Coffey, S. Delamount, & J. Lofland (Eds.), *Handbook of ethnography* (pp. 160–174). London: Sage.

Chenail, R. J. (1995). Presenting qualitative data. *Qualitative Report, 2*(3). Retrieved from *www.nova.edu/ssss/QR/QR2-3/presenting.html.*

Chiu, L. F. (2006). Critical reflection: More than nuts and bolts. *Action Research, 4,* 183–203.

Choudhuri, D. D. (2003). Qualitative research and multicultural counseling competency: An argument for inclusion. In D. B. Pope-Davis, H. L. K. Coleman, W. M. Liu, & R. L. Toporek (Eds.), *Handbook of multicultural competencies in counseling and psychology* (pp. 267–281). Thousand Oaks, CA: Sage.

Choudhuri, D. D., Glauser, A., & Peregoy, J. (2004). Guidelines for writing a qualitative manuscript for the *Journal of Counseling and Development. Journal of Counseling and Development, 82,* 443–446.

Christians, C. G. (2003). Ethics and politics in qualitative research. In N. K. Denzin & Y. S. Lincoln (Eds.), *The landscape of qualitative research: Theories and issues* (2nd ed., pp. 208–243). Thousand Oaks, CA: Sage.

Chwalisz, K., Shah, S. R., & Hand, K. M. (2008). Facilitating rigorous qualitative research in rehabilitation psychology. *Rehabilitation Psychology, 53*(3), 387–399.

Clarke, A. E. (2005). *Situational analysis: Grounded theory after the postmodern turn.* Thousand Oaks, CA: Sage.

Cochran-Smith, M., & Zeichner, K. (2005). Executive summary: The report of the AERA panel on research and teacher education. In M. Cochran-Smith & K. Zeichner (Eds.), *Studying teacher education* (pp. 1–36). Mahwah, NJ: Erlbaum.

Code of Federal Regulations (CFR). (1991). Title 21 Code of Federal Regulations Part 56. Retrieved January 26, 2011, from *www.irb-irc.com/section6/21_CFR_56_(01)_Peds.pdf.*

Code of Federal Regulations (CFR). (2001). *Title 45 public welfare Department of Health and Human Services Part 46—Protection of human subjects (45 CFR 46).* Washington, DC: U.S. Government Printing Office.

Cole, A. L., & Knowles, J. G. (2008). Arts-informed research. In J. G. Knowles & A. L. Cole (Eds.), *Handbook of the arts in qualitative research* (pp. 55–70). Thousand Oaks, CA: Sage.

Constas, M. A. (1992). Qualitative analysis as a public event: The documentation of category development procedures. *American Educational Research Journal, 29,* 253–266.

Corbin J., & Strauss, A. (2008). *Basics of qualitative research* (3rd ed.). Thousand Oaks, CA: Sage.

Corbin, J., & Strauss, A. (2008). *Basics of qualitative research: Techniques and procedures for developing grounded theory* (3rd ed.). Thousand Oaks, CA: Sage.

Corey, G., Corey, M. S., & Callanan, P. (2003). *Issues and ethics in the helping professions* (6th ed.). Pacific Grove, CA: Brooks/Cole.

Cornett-DeVito, M. M., & Worley, D. W. (2005). A front row seat: A phenomenological investigation of learning disabilities. *Communication Education, 54*(4), 312–333.

Craig, I. D. (2009). Impact factor redux: New indicators, new challenges. *Journal of Sexual Medicine, 6*(11), 2976–2978.

Creswell, J. W. (2003). *Research design: Qualitative, quantitative, and mixed methods approaches* (2nd ed.). Thousand Oaks, CA: Sage.

Creswell, J. W. (2006). *Qualitative inquiry and re-*

search design: Choosing among five traditions (2nd ed.). Thousand Oaks, CA: Sage.

Creswell, J. W. (2008). Research design: Qualitative, quantitative, and mixed methods approaches (3rd ed.). Thousand Oaks, CA: Sage.

Creswell, J. W., & Plano Clark, V. L. (2011). Designing and conducting mixed methods research. Thousand Oaks, CA: Sage.

Creswell, J. W., Plano Clark, V. L., Gutmann, M. L., & Hanson, W. E. (2003). Advanced mixed methods research designs. In A. Tashakkori & C. Teddlie (Eds.), Handbook of mixed methods in social and behavioral research (pp. 209–240). Thousand Oaks, CA: Sage.

Creswell, J. W., Shope, R., Plano-Clark, V., & Green, D. O. (2006). How interpretive qualitative research extends mixed methods research. Research in the Schools, 13, 1–11.

Cullen, J. E. (2009). "Some friends and I started talking … ": A participatory action research project to deconstruct white privilege among student affairs practitioners. Dissertation Abstracts International Section A: Humanities and Social Sciences, 69(8-A), 3057.

Cutliffe, J. R., & McKenna, H. P. (1999). Establishing the credibility of qualitative research findings: The plot thickens. Journal of Advanced Nursing, 30(2), 374–380.

Daly, J., Willis, K., Small, R., Green, J., Welch, N., Kealy, M., et al. (2007). A hierarchy of evidence for assessing qualitative health research. Journal of Clinical Epidemiology, 60, 43–49.

Danes, S. M. (1998). Multiple roles, balance between work and leisure, and satisfaction with level of living. Family and Consumer Sciences Research Journal, 26, 401–424.

Daniels, J. A., Bradley, M. C., Cramer, D. P., Winkler, A., Kinebrew, K., & Crockett, D. (2007). In the aftermath of a school hostage event: A case study of one school counselor's response. Professional School Counseling, 10, 482–489.

Darbyshire, P., MacDougall, C. J., & Shiller, W. (2005). Multiple methods in qualitative research with children: More insight or just more? Qualitative Research, 5(4), 417–436.

Daud, R., & Caruthers, C. (2008). Outcome study of an after-school program for youth in a high-risk environment. Journal of Parks and Recreation Administration, 26, 95–114.

Davison, J. (2004). Dilemmas in research: Issues of vulnerability and disempowerment for the social worker/researcher. Journal of Social Work Practice, 18, 379–383.

Deegan, M. N. (2001). Handbook of ethnography. Thousand Oaks, CA: Sage.

de Kok, B. C. (2008). The role of context in conversation analysis: Reviving an interest in ethnomethods. Journal of Pragmatics, 40(5), 886–903.

de Laine, M. (2000). Fieldwork, participation and practice: Ethics and dilemmas in qualitative research. London: Sage.

Denzin, N. K. (1989). Interpretive biography. Newbury Park, CA: Sage.

Denzin, N. K. (1997). Interpretive ethnography: Ethnographic practices for the 21st century. Thousand Oaks, CA: Sage.

Denzin, N. K. (2003). Performance ethnography: Critical pedagogy and the politics of culture. Thousand Oaks, CA: Sage.

Denzin, N. K. (2006). Analytic autoethnography, or déjà vu all over again. Journal of Contemporary Ethnography, 35, 419–428.

Denzin, N. K., & Lincoln, Y. S. (1998). Collecting and interpreting qualitative materials. Thousand Oaks, CA: Sage.

Denzin, N. K., & Lincoln, Y. (Eds.). (2000). Handbook of qualitative research (2nd ed.). Thousand Oaks, CA: Sage.

Denzin, N. K., & Lincoln, Y. S. (2005). Introduction: The discipline and practice of qualitative research. In N. K. Denzin & Y. S. Lincoln (Eds.), The Sage handbook of qualitative research (pp. 1–42). Thousand Oaks, CA: Sage.

Department of Health and Human Services. (1996). Health information privacy. Retrieved January 26, 2011, from www.hhs.gov/ocr/privacy/.

de Rivera, J. (2006). Conceptual encounter: The experience of anger. In C. T. Fischer (Ed.), Qualitative research methods for psychologists: Introduction through empirical studies (pp. 213–245). Burlington, MA: Academic Press.

Devers, K. J., & Frankel, R. M. (2000). Study design in qualitative research—2: Sampling and data collection strategies. Education for Health, 13(2), 263–271.

DiCicco-Bloom, B., & Crabtree, B. F. (2006). The qualitative research interview. Medical Education, 40, 314–321.

Dickey, L. M., Burnes, T. R., & Singh, A. A. (2011). Sexual identity development of female-to-male transsexuals: A grounded theory inquiry. Manuscript submitted for publication.

Diekelmann, N., & Ironside, D. M. (2005). Hermeneutics. In J. J. Fitzpatrick & M. Wallace (Eds.), *Encyclopedia of nursing research* (pp. 260–262). New York: Springer.

Dimaggio, G., & Semerari, A. (2001). Psychopathological narrative forms. *Journal of Constructivist Psychology, 14*, 1–23.

DiSalvo, P. L. (2009). Leadership "in the moment": How effective education leaders play their respective roles by employing theatrical acting and improvisation as an education leadership tool: A study of a strategic communication model. *Dissertation Abstracts International Section A: Humanities and Social Sciences, 69*(8-A), 2959.

Dollard, J. (1946). *Criteria for the life history.* New Haven, CT: Yale University Press.

Donovan, F. (1920). *The woman who waits.* Boston: Gorham Press.

Donovan, F. (1929). *The saleslady.* Chicago: University of Chicago Press.

Doyle, B. W. (1937). *The etiquette of race relations in the South: A study in social control.* Chicago: University of Chicago Press.

Drapeau, M. (2002, September). Subjectivity in research: Why not? But … *Qualitative Report, 7*(3). Retrieved November 15, 2008, from *www.nova.edu/ssss/QR/QR7-3/drapeau.html.*

Drisko, J. W. (1997). Strengthening qualitative studies and reports: Standards to promote academic integrity. *Journal of Social Work Education, 33*(1), 185–197.

Duncan, M. (2004). Autoethnography: Critical appreciation of an emerging art. *International Journal of Qualitative Methods, 3*(4), 1–4. Retrieved May 14, 2009, from *www.ualberta.ca/~iiqm/backissues3_4/html.*

Duncombe, J., & Jessop, J. (2002). "Doing rapport" and the ethics of "faking friendship." In M. Mauthner, M. Birch, J. Jessop, & T. Miller (Eds.), *Ethics in qualitative research* (pp. 107–121). Thousand Oaks, CA: Sage.

Dwyer, S. C., & Buckle, J. L. (2009). The space between: On being an insider–outsider in qualitative research. *International Journal of Qualitative Methods, 8*(1), 54–63.

Eagan, J., Chenoweth, L., & McAuliffe, D. (2006). Email-facilitated qualitative interviews with traumatic brain injury survivors: A new and accessible method. *Brain Injury, 20*(12), 1283–1294.

Ebbs, C. A. (1996). Qualitative research inquiry: Issues of power and ethics. *Education, 117*(2), 217–222.

Edwards, D., & Potter, J. (1992). *Discursive psychology.* London: Sage.

Eger, K. S. (2008). Powerless to affect positive change for the gifted students in an urban school district as revealed through one teacher's heuristic inquiry. *Dissertation Abstracts International Section A: Humanities and Social Sciences, 69*(3-A), 827.

Eisner, E. (1991). *The enlightened eye: Qualitative inquiry and the enhancement of educational practices.* New York: Macmillan.

Elder, N. C., & Miller, W. L. (1995). Reading and evaluating qualitative research studies. *Journal of Family Practice, 41*(3), 279–285.

Elliott, E. (2003). Moving in the space between researcher and practitioner. *Child and Youth Care Forum, 32*(5), 299–303.

Ellis, C. (1991). Sociological introspection and emotional experience. *Symbolic Interaction, 14*, 23–50.

Ellison, N. B., & Wu, Y. (2008). Blogging in the classroom: A preliminary exploration of student attitudes and impact on comprehension. *Journal of Educational Multimedia and Hypermedia, 17*(1), 99–122.

Emden, C., & Sandelowski, M. (1998). The good, the bad and the relative, part one: Conceptions of goodness in qualitative research. *International Journal of Nursing Practice, 4*, 206–212.

Emerson, R. M., Fretz, R. I., & Shaw, L. L. (1995). *Writing ethnographic fieldnotes.* Chicago: University of Chicago Press.

Ercikan, K., & Roth, W. (2006). What good is polarizing research into qualitative and quantitative? *Educational Researcher, 35*(5), 14–23.

Erikson, E. (1963). *Childhood and society* (2nd ed.). New York: Norton.

Espino, M. E. (2008). *Seeking the "truth" in the stories we tell: An approach to constructing counter-storytelling in higher education research.* Unpublished manuscript.

Esterberg, K. G. (2002). *Qualitative methods in social research.* Boston: McGraw-Hill.

Estrella, K., & Forinash, M. (2007). Narrative inquiry and arts-based inquiry: Multinarrative perspectives. *Journal of Humanistic Psychology, 47*(3), 376–383.

Etherington, K. (2004). Heuristic research as a vehicle for personal and professional development. *Counseling and Psychotherapy Research, 4*(2), 48–63.

Etziono, A. (2009, Winter). The common good and rights: A neo-communitarian approach. *Georgetown Journal of International Affairs,* 113–119.

Farberman, H. A. (1985). The foundations of symbolic interaction: James, Cooley, and Mead. *Foundations of Interpretive Sociology: Original Essays in Symbolic Interaction, Studies in Symbolic Interaction, Supplement 1,* 13–27.

Fassinger, R. E. (2005). Paradigms, praxis, problems, and promise: Grounded theory in counseling psychology research. *Journal of Counseling Psychology, 52,* 156–166.

Fawcett, B., & Hearn, J. (2004). Researching others: Experience, participation and material reflexivity. *International Journal of Social Science Methodology, 7*(3), 201–218.

Fielding, N. (1994). Varieties of research interviews. *Nurse Researcher, 1*(3), 4–13.

Fielding, N., & Lee, R. (1991). *Using computers in qualitative research.* London: Sage.

Finley, S. (2008). Arts-based research. In J. G. Knowles & A. L. Cole (Eds.), *Handbook of the arts in qualitative research* (pp. 71–82). London: Sage.

Fisher, C. B. (2000). Relational ethics in psychological research: One feminist's journey. In M. M. Brabeck (Ed.), *Practicing feminist ethics in psychology* (pp. 125–142). Washington, DC: American Psychological Association.

Flint's Youth Violence Prevention Center. (2009). Photovoice. Retrieved April 15, 2009, from *www.sph/umich.edu/yvpc/projects/photvoice/index/shtml.*

Floersch, J. (2004). Practice ethnography: A case study of invented clinical knowledge. In D. K. Padgett (Ed.), *The qualitative research experience* (pp. 79–99). Belmont, CA: Wadsworth.

Flyvbjerg, B. (2004). Five misunderstandings about case-study research. In C. Seale, G. Giampietro, J. F. Gubrium, & D. Silverman (Eds.), *Qualitative research practice* (pp. 420–434). Thousand Oaks, CA: Sage.

Ford, G. G. (2006). *Ethical reasoning for mental health professionals.* Thousand Oaks, CA: Sage.

Forman, J. (2009). *The perceptions of agency: Sexual assault counselors on self-care, vicarious trauma, and counselor burnout.* Manuscript submitted for publication.

Fossey, E., Harvey, C., McDermott, F., & Davidson, L. (2002). Understanding and evaluating qualitative research. *Australian and New Zealand Journal of Psychiatry, 36,* 717–732.

Frankel, R. M., & Devers, K. J. (2000). Study design in qualitative research—1: Developing questions and assessing resource needs. *Education for Health, 13,* 251–261.

Frankel, Z., & Levitt, H. M. (2009). Clients' experiences of disengaged moments in psychotherapy: A grounded theory analysis. *Journal of Contemporary Psychotherapy, 39,* 171–186.

Freebody, P. (2001). Re-discovering practical reading activities in homes and schools. *Journal of Research in Reading, 24*(3), 222–234.

Friere, P. (1972). *Pedagogy of the oppressed.* Harmondsworth, UK: Penguin.

Fryer, E. M. (2004). Researcher–practitioner: An unholy marriage? *Educational Studies, 30*(2), 175–185.

Galuzzo, G. R., Hilldrup, J., Hays, D. G., & Erford, B. T. (2008). The nature of research and inquiry. In B. T. Erford (Ed.), *Research and evaluation in counseling* (pp. 2–24). Boston: Lahaska Press.

Garfinkel, H. (1967). *Studies in ethnomethodology.* Englewood Cliffs, NJ: Prentice Hall.

Gay, G., & Howard, T. (2000). Multicultural teacher education for the 21st century. *Teacher Educator, 36*(1), 1–16.

Gee, J. P. (1991). A linguistic approach to narrative. *Journal of Narrative and Life History, 1,* 15–39.

Geertz, C. (1973). *The interpretation of cultures.* New York: Basic Books.

Geertz, C. (1983). *Local knowledge: Further essays in interpretive anthropology. New York: Basic Books.*

Giddens, A. (1990). *The consequences of modernity.* Stanford, CA: Stanford University Press.

Gilgun, J. F. (1994). Hand into glove: The grounded theory approach and social work practice research. In E. Sherman & W. J. Reid (Eds.), *Qualitative research in social work* (pp. 115–125). New York: Columbia University Press.

Gill, G. (2006). Asynchonous discussion groups: A use-based taxonomy with examples. *Journal of Information Systems Education, 17*(4), 373.

Gillies, J. L. (2007). Staying grounded while being uprooted: A visual and poetic representation of the transition from university to community for graduates with disabilities. *Leisure Sciences, 29*(2), 175–179.

Gillies, V., & Alldred, P. (2002). The ethics of intention: Research as a political tool. In M. Mauthner, M. Birch, J. Jessop, & T. Miller

(Eds.), *Ethics in qualitative research* (pp. 32–52). Thousand Oaks, CA: Sage.

Giorgi, A. (1970). *Psychology as a human science: A phenomenological approach.* New York: Harper & Row.

Gladding, S. T. (2008). *Group work: A counseling specialty* (5th ed.). New York: Merrill.

Gladstone, B. M., & Volpe, T. (2008, April 23). *Qualitative secondary analysis: Asking "new" questions of "old" data.* Paper presented at the Qualitive Research Interest Group, Athens, GA.

Gladstone, B. M., Volpe, T., & Boydell, K. (2007). Issues encountered in a qualitative secondary analysis of help-seeking in the prodrome to psychosis. *Journal of Behavioral Health Services and Research, 34*(4), 431–442.

Glaser, B. (1992). *Basics of grounded theory analysis: Emergence versus forcing.* Mill Valley, CA: Sociology Press.

Glaser, B. J. (1978). *Theoretical sensitivity: Advances in the methodology of grounded theory.* Mill Valley, CA: Sociology Press.

Glaser, B. J., & Strauss, A. (1967). *The discovery of grounded theory: Strategies for qualitative research.* Chicago: Aldine.

Glesne, C. (2006). *Becoming qualitative researchers: An introduction.* Boston: Pearson.

Gnisci, A., Bakeman, R., & Quera, V. (2008). Blending qualitative and quantitative analyses in observing interaction: Misunderstandings, applications and proposals. *International Journal of Multiple Research Approaches, 2*(1), 15–30.

Goffman, E. (1972). *Encounters: Two studies in the sociology of interaction.* London: Allen Lane.

Golden-Biddle, K. G., & Locke, K. (2007). *Composing qualitative research* (2nd ed.). Thousand Oaks, CA: Sage.

Gorin, S., Hooper, C., Dyson, C., & Cabral, C. (2008). Ethical challenges in conducting research with hard to reach families. *Child Abuse Review, 17,* 275–287.

Gosnell, H. F. (1935). *Negro politicians.* Chicago: University of Chicago Press.

Graff, J. M. (2007). *The literary lives of marginalized readers: Preadolescent girls' rationale for book choice and experiences with self-selected books.* Gainesville: University of Florida.

Graham, D. S. (1998). Consultation effectiveness and treatment acceptability: An examination of consultee requests and consultant responses. *School Psychology Quarterly, 13,* 155–168.

Graneheim, U. H., & Lundman, B. (2004). Qual-itative content analysis in nursing research: Concepts, procedures and measures to achieve trustworthiness. *Nurse Education Today, 24*(2), 105–112.

Grant, P. S., & Boersma, H. (2005). Making sense of being fat: A hermeneutic analysis of adults' explanations for obesity. *Counselling and Psychotherapy Research, 5*(3), 212–220.

Grbich, C. (2007). *Qualitative data analysis: An introduction.* Thousand Oaks, CA: Sage.

Greenwood, D. J., & Levin, M. (2005). Reform of the social sciences and of universities through action research. In N. K. Denzin & Y. S. Lincoln (Eds.), *The Sage handbook of qualitative research* (pp. 43–64). Thousand Oaks, CA: Sage.

Groenewald, T. (2004). A phenomenological research design illustrated. *International Journal of Qualitative Methods, 3,* 1–26.

Guajardo, M., Guajardo, F., & Del Carmen Casaperalta, E. (2008). Transformative education: Chronicling a pedagogy for social change. *Anthropology and Education Quarterly, 39*(1), 3–22.

Guba, E. G., & Lincoln, Y. S. (1989). *Fourth-generation evaluation.* Newbury Park, CA: Sage.

Guba, E. G., & Lincoln, Y. S. (2005). Paradigmatic controversies, contradictions, and emerging confluences. In N. K. Denzin & Y. S. Lincoln (Eds.), *The Sage handbook of qualitative research* (3rd ed., pp. 191–215). Thousand Oaks, CA: Sage.

Guelzow, M. G., & Bird, G. W. (1991). An exploratory path analysis of the stress process for dual-career men and women. *Journal of Marriage and the Family, 53,* 151–164.

Guest, G., Bunce, A., & Johnson, L. (2006). How many interviews are enough?: An experiment with data saturation and variability. *Field Methods, 181,* 59–82.

Hadjistavropoulos, T., & Smythe, W. E. (2001). Elements of risk in qualitative research. *Ethics and Behavior, 11,* 163–174.

Halbrook, B., & Ginsberg, R. (1997). Ethnographic countertransference in qualitative research: Implications for mental health counseling research. *Journal of Mental Health Counseling, 19*(1), 87–93.

Hamilton, R. J., & Bowers, B. J. (2006). Internet recruitment and e-mail interviews in qualitative studies. *Qualitative Health Research, 16*(6), 821–835.

Hammersley, M. (1992). *What's wrong with ethnography?* London: Routledge.

Hammersley, M. (1995). Theory and evidence in qualitative research. *Quality and Quantity, 29,* 55–66.

Hammersley, M. (2004). Toward a usable past for qualitative research. *International Journal of Social Research Methodology, 7*(1), 19–27.

Hammersley, M. (2008). *Questioning qualitative inquiry: Critical essays.* Thousand Oaks, CA: Sage.

Hammersley, M., & Atkinson, P. (2007). *Ethnography: Principles in practice* (3rd ed.). New York: Taylor & Francis.

Hansen, J. T. (2004). Thoughts on knowing: Epistemic implications of counseling practice. *Journal of Counseling and Development, 82,* 131–138.

Haverkamp, B. E. (2005). Ethical perspectives on qualitative research in applied psychology. *Journal of Counseling Psychology, 52*(2), 146–155.

Haverkamp, B. E., & Young, R. A. (2007). Paradigms, purpose, and the role of the literature: Formulating a rationale for qualitative investigations. *The Counseling Psychologist, 35,* 265–294.

Hayes, J. A., McCracken, J. E., McClanahan, M. K., Hill, C. E., Harp, J. S., & Carozonni, P. (1998). Therapist perspectives on countertransference: Qualitative data in search of a theory. *Journal of Counseling Psychology, 45,* 468–482.

Hays, D., Forman, J., & Sikes, A. (2009). Use of visual data to explore adolescent females' perceptions of dating relationships. *Journal of Creativity in Mental Health, 4*(4), 295–307.

Hays, D. G. (2010). Introduction. *Counseling Outcome Research and Evaluation, 1*(1), 1–7.

Hays, D. G., Chang, C. Y., & Chaney, M. P. (2011). *Becoming social advocates: Counselor trainees' social justice knowledge, attitudes and behaviors.* Manuscript submitted for publication.

Hays, D. G., Chang, C. Y., & Dean, J. K. (2004). White counselors' conceptualization of privilege and oppression: Implications for counselor training. *Counselor Education and Supervision, 43,* 242–257.

Hays, D. G., Cole, R. F., Emelianchik-Key, K., Forman, J., Lorelle, S., McBride, R., et al. (2011). *A qualitative investigation of adolescent females' reflections on dating violence.* Manuscript in review.

Hays, D. G., & Emelianchik, K. M. (2009). A content analysis of intimate partner violence assessments. *Measurement and Evaluation in Counseling and Development, 42,* 139–153.

Hays, D. G., McLeod, A. L., & Prosek, E. A. (2009). Diagnostic variance among counselors and counselor trainees. *Measurement and Evaluation in Counseling and Development, 42,* 3–14.

Hays, D. G., & Newsome, D. (2008). Qualitative research designs. In B. T. Erford (Ed.), *Research and evaluation in counseling* (pp. 107–128). Boston: Lahaska Press.

Hecht, L. M. (2001). Role conflict and role overload: Different concepts, different consequences. *Sociological Inquiry, 71,* 111–121.

Hellawell, D. (2006). Inside-out: Analysis of the insider–outsider concept as a heuristic device to develop reflexivity in students doing qualitative research. *Teaching in Higher Education, 11*(4), 483–494.

Henwood, K., & Pidgeon, N. (2006). Grounded theory in psychological research. In P. M. Camic, J. E. Rhodes, & L. Yardley (Eds.), *Qualitative research in psychology: Expanding perspectives in methodology and design* (pp. 131–155). Washington, DC: American Psychological Association.

Heppner, P. P., & Heppner, M. J. (2004). *Writing and publishing your thesis, dissertation, and research: A guide for students in the helping professions.* New York: Thomson/Brooks Cole.

Heritage, J. (1984). *Garfinkel and ethnomethodology.* Cambridge, UK: Polity Press.

Herr, E. L., Cramer, S. H., & Niles, S. G. (2004). *Career guidance and counseling through the life span: Systematic approaches* (6th ed.). New York: HarperCollins.

Hesse-Biber, S. N., & Leavy, P. (2006). *The practice of qualitative research.* Thousand Oaks, CA: Sage.

Hill, C. E., Knox, S., Thompson, B. J., Williams, E. N., Hess, S. A., & Ladany, N. (2005). Consensual qualitative research: An update. *Journal of Counseling Psychology, 52,* 196–205.

Hill, C. E., Thompson, B. J., & Williams, E. N. (1997). A guide to conducting consensual qualitative research. *The Counseling Psychologist, 25,* 517–572.

Ho, B. S. (2002). Application of participatory action research to family–school intervention. *School Psychology Review, 31*(1), 106–121.

Hollander, J. A. (2004). The social contexts of focus groups. *Journal of Contemporary Ethnography, 33*(5), 602–637.

Hollins, E., & Torres Guzman, M. (2005). Research on preparing teachers for diverse populations. In M. Cochran-Smith & K. Zeichner (Eds.), *Studying teacher education* (pp. 477–548). Mahwah, NJ: Erlbaum.

Hood, J. C. (2006). Teaching against the text: The case of qualitative methods. *Teaching Sociology, 34*, 207–223.

hooks, b. (2000). *Feminist theory: From margin to center.* London: Pluto Press.

Hookway, N. (2008). "Entering the blogosphere": Some strategies for using blogs in social research. *Qualitative Research, 8*(1), 91–113.

Horsburgh, D. (2003). Evaluation of qualitative research. *Journal of Clinical Nursing, 12*, 307–312.

Huisman, K. (2008). "Does this mean you're not going to come visit me anymore?": An inquiry into an ethics of reciprocity and positionality in feminist ethnographic research. *Sociological Inquiry, 78*(3), 372–296.

Hummelvoll, J. K., & Severinsson, E. (2001). Coping with everyday reality: Mental health professionals' reflections on the care provided in an acute psychiatric ward. *Australian and New Zealand Journal of Mental Health Nursing, 10*, 156–166.

Hutchby, I., & Wooffitt, R. (1998). *Conversation analysis.* Cambridge, UK: Polity Press.

INCITE! Women of Color Against Violence. (2008). Participatory action research. Retrieved April 10, 2010, from *www.incite-national.org/index.php?s=129.*

Insch, G. S., Moore, J. E., & Murphy, L. D. (1997). Content analysis in leadership research: Examples, procedures, and suggestions for future use. *Leadership Quarterly, 8*(1), 1–25.

Internet World Stats. (2010). Internet usage statistics. Retrieved January 27, 2011, from *www.internetworldstats.com/stats.htm.*

Ireland, L., & Holloway, I. (1996). Qualitative health research with children. *Children and Society, 10*, 155–164.

James, A. (2001). Ethnography in the study of children and childhood. In P. Atkinson, A. Coffey, S. Delamont, J. Lofland, & L. Lofland (Eds.), *Handbook of ethnography* (pp. 246–257). Thousand Oaks, CA: Sage.

James, N. (2003). *Teacher professionalism, teacher identity: How do I see myself?* Unpublished doctoral thesis, University of Leicester, Leicester, UK.

James, N. (2007). The use of email interviewing as a qualitative method of inquiry in educational research. *British Educational Research Journal, 33*(6), 963–976.

James, N., & Busher, H. (2007). Ethical issues in online educational research: Protecting privacy, establishing authenticity in email interviewing. *International Journal of Research and Method in Education, 30*(1), 101–113.

Janesick, V. J. (1994). The dance of qualitative research design: Metaphor, methodolatry, and meaning. In N. K. Denzin & Y. S. Lincoln (Eds.), *Handbook of qualitative research* (pp. 209–219). Thousand Oaks, CA: Sage.

Jennings, J. L. (1986). Husserl revisited: The forgotten distinction between psychology and phenomenology. *American Psychologist, 41*(11), 1231–1240.

Johnson, A. S. (2007). An ethics of access: Using life history to trace preservice teachers' initial viewpoints on teaching for equity. *Journal of Teacher Education, 58*, 299–314.

Johnson, C. W. (2008). "Don't call him a cowboy": Masculinity, cowboy drag, and a costume change. *Journal of Leisure Research, 40*(3), 385–403.

Johnson, M. (2006). Preparing reading specialists to become competent travelers in urban settings. *Urban Education, 41*(4), 402–426.

Johnson, P. (1998). Analytic induction. In G. Symon & C. Cassell (Eds.), *Qualitative methods and analysis in organizational research: A practical guide* (pp. 28–50). London: Sage.

Johnson, R. B. (1997). Examining the validity structure of qualitative research. *Education, 118*(2), 282–292.

Jones, R. E. J., & Cooke, L. (2006). A window into learning: Case studies of online group communication and collaboration. *Research in Learning Technology, 14*, 261–274.

Jones, S. (2006). *Girls, social class, and literacy: What teachers can do to make a difference.* Portsmouth, NH: Heinemann.

Jones, S. R. (2002). (Re)Writing the word: Methodological strategies and issues in qualitative research. *Journal of College Student Development, 43*(4), 461–473.

Jorgensen, D. L. (1989). *Participant observation: A methodology for human studies.* Newbury Park, CA: Sage.

Kando, T. M., & Summers, W. C. (1971). The impact of work on leisure: Toward a paradigm and research strategy. *Pacific Sociological Review, 14*, 310–327.

Kanter, R. M. (1977). Some effects of proportions on group life: Skewed sex ratios and responses to token women. *American Journal of Sociology, 82*, 965–990.

Karp, S. (2003, November 7). *The No Child Left Behind hoax.* Speech presented at Portland Area Rethinking Schools, Portland, OR.

Karp, S. (2006, Spring). Bulldozers or band aids. *Rethinking Schools.* Available at *www.rethinking-schools.org/special_reports/bushplan/band203.shtml.*

Kasturirangan, A., & Williams, E. (2003). Counseling Latina battered women: A qualitative study in the Latina perspective. *Journal of Multicultural Counseling and Development, 31*, 162–178.

Kaufman, J. E. (1988). Leisure and anxiety: A study of retirees. *Activities, Adaptation and Aging, 11*, 1–10.

Kelly, T., & Howie, L. (2007). Working with stories in nursing research: Procedures used in narrative analysis. *International Journal of Mental Health Nursing, 16*, 136–144.

Kezar, A. (2003). Transformational elite interviews: Principles and problems. *Qualitative Inquiry, 9*(3), 395–415.

Kidd, S. A., & Kral, M. J. (2005). Practicing participatory action research. *Journal of Counseling Psychology, 52*(2), 187–195.

Kimchi, J., Polivka, B., & Stevenson, J. S. (1991). Triangulation: Operational definitions. *Nursing Research, 40*(6), 364–366.

King, N. (1998). Template analysis. In G. Symon & C. Cassell (Eds.), *Qualitative methods and analysis in organizational research: A practical guide* (pp. 118–134). London: Sage.

Kitchener, K. S. (1984). Intuition, critical evaluation, and ethical principles: The foundation for ethical decisions in counseling psychology. *The Counseling Psychologist, 12*(3), 43–55.

Kline, W. B. (2008). Developing and submitting credible qualitative manuscripts. *Counselor Education and Supervision, 47*(4), 210–217.

Klopfenstein, K. (2005). Beyond test scores: The impact of black teacher role models on rigorous math taking. *Contemporary Economic Policy, 23*(3), 416–428.

Koch, T., Mann, S., Kralik, D., & van Loon, A. M. (2005). Reflection: Look, think and act cycles in participatory action research. *Journal of Research in Nursing, 10*(3), 261–278.

Koliba, C. J., Campbell, E. K., & Shapiro, C. (2006). The practice of service learning in local school–community contexts. *Educational Policy, 20*, 683–717.

Kress, V. E., & Shoffner, M. F. (2007). Focus groups: A practical and applied research approach for counselors. *Journal of Counseling and Development, 85*, 189–195.

Ku, H., Lahman, M. K. E., Yeh, H., & Cheng, Y. (2008). Into the academy: Preparing and mentoring international doctoral students. *Education Technology Research Development, 56*, 365–377.

Kvale, S., & Brinkmann, S. (2009). *InterViews: Learning the craft of qualitative research interviewing* (2nd ed.). Thousand Oaks, CA: Sage.

Lalor, J. G., Begley, C. M., & Devane, D. (2006). Exploring painful experiences: Impact of emotional narratives on members of a qualitative research team. *Journal of Advanced Nursing, 56*(6), 607–616.

Lambert, P. (2007). Client perspectives on counseling: Before, during and after. *Counseling and Psychotherapy Research, 7*(2), 106–113.

Lambert, S. D., & Loiselle, C. G. (2008). Combining individual interviews and focus groups to enhance data richness. *Journal of Advanced Nursing, 62*, 228–237.

Lapadat, J., & Lindsay, A. C. (1999). Transcription in research and practice: From standardization of technique to interpretive positionings. *Qualitative Inquiry, 5*(1), 64–86.

Lather, P. (1991). *Getting smart: Feminist research and pedagogy within the postmodern.* New York: Routledge.

Lather, P. (2007). *Getting lost: Feminist efforts toward a double(d) science.* Albany: State University of New York Press.

Lease, S. H. (1999). Occupational role stressors, coping, support, and hardiness as predictors of strain in academic faculty: An emphasis on new and female faculty. *Research in Higher Education, 40*, 285–307.

LeBosco, K. (2004). Managing visibility, intimacy, and focus in online critical ethnography. In M. D. Johns, S. L. S. Chen, & G. J. Hall (Eds.), *Online social research* (pp. 63–80). New York: Peter Lang.

LeCompte, M. D., & Preissle, J. (1993). *Ethnography and qualitative design in educational research* (2nd ed.). Orlando, FL: Academic Press.

LeCompte, M. D., & Schensul, J. J. (1999). *The ethnographer's toolkit.* Lanham, MD: Altamira.

Levinson, D. (1978). *The season of a man's life.* New York: Knopf.

Lewis, J., Arnold, M. S., House, R., & Toporek, R. (2003). *Advocacy competencies.* [Electronic version]. Retrieved April 15, 2010, from *www.counseling.org/Publications.*

Lewis, R. B., & Maas, S. M. (2007). QDA Miner 2.0: Mixed-model qualitative data analysis software. *Field Methods, 19,* 87–108.

Lincoln, Y. S., & Guba, E. G. (1985). *Naturalistic inquiry.* Beverly Hills, CA: Sage.

Lincoln, Y. S., & Guba, E. G. (1995). *Naturalistic inquiry* (2nd ed.). Thousand Oaks, CA: Sage.

Liu, W. M., Stinson, R., Hernandez, J., Shepard, S., & Haang, S. (2009). A qualitative examination of masculinity, homelessness, and social class among men in a transitional shelter. *Psychology of Men and Masculinity, 10*(2), 131–148.

Lofland, J., & Lofland, L. H. (1984). *Analyzing social settings: A guide to qualitative observation and analysis* (2nd ed.). Belmont, CA: Wadsworth.

Lofland, J. L., & Lofland, L. H. (1995). *Analyzing social settings: A guide to qualitative observation and analysis* (3rd ed.). Belmont, CA: Wadsworth.

Loutzenheiser, L. W. (2007). Working alterity: The impossibility of ethical research with youth. *Educational Studies, 41*(2), 109–127.

Lynd, R. S., & Lynd, H. M. (1929). *Middletown: A study in American culture.* New York: Harcourt Brace.

Lynd, R. S., & Lynd, H. M. (1937). *Middletown in transition: A study of cultural conflicts.* New York: Harcourt Brace.

Lysaker, P. H., Lancaster, R. S., & Lysaker, J. T. (2003). Narrative transformation as an outcome in the psychotherapy of schizophrenia. *Psychology and Psychotherapy: Theory, Research and Practice, 76,* 285–299.

MacDonald, S. (2001). British social anthropology. In P. Atkinson, A. Coffey, S. Delamont, J. Lofland, & L. Lofland (Eds.), *Handbook of ethnography* (pp. 60–79). Thousand Oaks, CA: Sage.

MacIntyre, A. (1984). *After virtue: A study in moral theory* (2nd ed.). Notre Dame, IN: University of Notre Dame Press.

Mackrill, T. (2008). Solicited diary studies of psychotherapy in qualitative research: Pros and cons. *European Journal of Psychotherapy and Counselling, 10*(1), 5–18.

Magee, C., & Huriaux, E. (2008). Ladies' night: Evaluating a drop-in programme for homeless and marginally housed women in San Fran-

cisco's mission district. *International Journal of Drug Policy, 10*(2), 113–121.

Malinowski, B. (1922). *Argonauts of the western Pacific: An account of native enterprise and adventure in the archipelagoes of Melanesian New Guinea.* London: Routledge & Kegan Paul.

Malone, R. E., Yerger, V. B., McGruder, C., & Froelicher, E. (2006). "It's like Tuskegee in reverse": A case study of ethical tensions in institutional review board review of community-based participatory research. *American Journal of Public Health, 96*(11), 1914–1919.

Manning, K. (1992). A rationale for using qualitative research in student affairs. *Journal of College Student Development, 33,* 132–136.

Mantzoukas, S. (2008). Facilitating research students in formulating research questions. *Nurse Education Today, 28,* 371–377.

Marshall, C. (1990). Goodness criteria: Are they objective or judgment calls? In E. G. Guba (Ed.), *The paradigm dialog* (pp. 188–197). Newbury Park, CA: Sage.

Marshall, C., & Rossman, G. B. (1999). *Designing qualitative research* (3rd ed.). Thousand Oaks, CA: Sage.

Maso, I. (2001). Phenomenology and ethnography. In P. A. Atkinson, S. Delamont, A. J. Coffey, J. Lofland, & L. H. Lofland (Eds.), *Handbook of ethnography* (pp. 136–144). Thousand Oaks, CA: Sage.

Mason, J. (2002). *Qualitative researching.* London: Sage.

Maxwell, J. A. (1992). Understanding and validity in qualitative research. *Harvard Educational Review, 62,* 279–300.

Maxwell, J. A. (2005). *Qualitative research design: An interactive approach* (2nd ed.). Thousand Oaks, CA: Sage.

Maxwell, J. A. (2010). Using numbers in qualitative research. *Qualitative Inquiry, 20,* 1–8.

Maxwell, J. A., & Miller, B. A. (2008). Categorizing and connecting strategies in qualitative data analysis. In P. Leavy & S. N. Hesse-Biber (Eds.), *Handbook of emergent methods* (pp. 461–477). New York: Guilford Press.

Mays, N., & Pope, C. (2000). Qualitative research in health care: Assessing quality in qualitative research. *British Medical Journal, 320,* 50–52.

Mazzei, L. A. (2009). An impossibly full voice. In A. Y. Jackson & L. A. Mazzei (Eds.), *Voice in qualitative inquiry: Challenging conventional, interpretative, and critical conceptions in qualitative research* (pp. 45–62). New York: Routledge.

Mazzei, L. A., & Jackson, A. Y. (2009). Introduction: The limit of voice. In A. Y. Jackson & L. A. Mazzei (Eds.), *Voice in qualitative inquiry: Challenging conventional, interpretative, and critical conceptions in qualitative research* (pp. 1–14). New York: Routledge.

McBride, A. B. (1990). Mental health effects of women's multiple roles. *American Psychologist, 45,* 381–384.

McBride, R. (2008). *Survival on the streets: The experience and perceived unmet needs of the homeless population.* Unpublished manuscript.

McDaniels, C. (1984). The work/leisure connection. *Vocational Guidance Quarterly, 33,* 35–43.

McDaniels, C., & Gysbers, N. C. (1992). *Counseling for career development: Theories, resources, and practice.* San Francisco: Jossey-Bass.

McIntyre, A., Chatzipoulos, N., Politi, A., & Roz, J. (2007). Participatory action research: Collective reflections on gender, culture, and language. *Teaching and Teacher Education, 23,* 748–756.

McKenzie, K. B., & Scheurich, J. J. (2004). Equity traps: A useful construct for preparing principals to lead schools that are successful with racially diverse students. *Educational Administration Quarterly, 40,* 601–632.

McLeod, A. L., Chang, C. Y., Hays, D. G., Orr, J. J., & Uwah, C. (2011). *Attention to cultural issues in multicultural supervision: Supervisors' and supervisees' perspectives.* Manuscript under review.

McLeod, J. (2001). *Qualitative research in counseling and psychotherapy.* London: Sage.

McLeod, J., & Lynch, G. (2000). This is our life: Strong evaluation in psychotherapy narrative. *European Journal of Psychotherapy, Counselling and Health, 3*(3), 389–406.

McMahan, E., M., & Rogers, K. L. (1994). *Interactive oral history interviewing.* Hillsdale, NJ: Erlbaum.

McMillan, J. H., & Schumacher, S. (2006). *Research in education: Evidence-based inquiry* (6th ed.). Boston: Pearson.

McNeil, K. (2005). *Through our eyes: The shared experiences of growing up attention deficit hyperactivity disordered.* Doctoral dissertation, Seattle University, Seattle, WA.

McTaggart, R. (1997). Guiding principles for participatory action research. In R. McTaggart (Ed.), *Participatory action research: International contexts and consequences* (pp. 1–24). Albany: State University of New York Press.

Meara, N. M., Schmidt, L. D., & Day, J. D. (1996). Principles and virtues: A foundation for ethical decisions, policies, and character. *The Counseling Psychologist, 24*(1), 4–77.

Melton, J. L., Nofzinger-Collins, D., Wynne, M. E., & Susman, M. (2005). Exploring the affective inner experiences of therapists in training: The qualitative interaction between session experience and session content. *Counselor Education and Supervision, 45,* 82–96.

Merriam, S. B. (2002). Introduction to qualitative research. In S. B. Merriam (Ed.), *Qualitative research in practice: Examples for discussion and analysis* (pp. 3–16). San Francisco: Jossey-Bass.

Merton, R. (1972). Insiders and outsiders: A chapter in the sociology of knowledge. *American Journal of Sociology, 78*(1), 9–47.

Miles, M. B., & Huberman, A. M. (1994). *Qualitative data analysis: An expanded sourcebook* (2nd ed.). Thousand Oaks, CA: Sage.

Miller, T., & Bell, L. (2002). Consenting to what?: Issues of access, gate-keeping, and "informed" consent. In M. Mauthner, M. Birch, J. Jessop, & T. Miller. (Eds.), *Ethics in qualitative research* (pp. 53–69). Thousand Oaks, CA: Sage.

Mishler, E. G. (1986). *Research interviewing: Context and narrative.* Cambridge, MA: Harvard University Press.

Mishler, E. G. (1997). Narrative accounts in clinical and research interviews. In B. L. Gunnarsson, P. Linell, & B. Norberg (Eds.), *The construction of professional discourse* (pp. 223–244). London: Longman.

Mitchell, C., & Allnutt, S. (2008). Photographs and/as social documentary. In J. G. Knowles & A. L. Cole (Eds.), *Handbook of the arts in qualitative research* (pp. 251–264). Thousand Oaks, CA: Sage.

Molee, K. (2009). *School reform from a legislator's point of view.* Unpublished manuscript.

Moloney, M. F., Dietrich, A. S., Strickland, O., & Myerburg, S. (2003). Using Internet discussion boards as virtual focus groups. *Advances in Nursing Science, 26*(4), 274–286.

Moon, S. J. (2009). *The subsistence and impact of tokenism on the doctoral experiences of African American females.* Unpublished manuscript.

Moore, S., & Murphy, M. (2005). *How to be a student: 100 great ideas and practical habits for students everywhere.* Maidenhead, UK: Open University Press.

Morgan, D. L. (1988). *Focus groups as qualitative research.* Thousand Oaks, CA: Sage.

Morgan, D. L. (1997). *Focus groups as qualitative research* (2nd ed.). Newbury Park, CA: Sage.

Morris, C. W. (Ed.). (1934). *Mind, self, and society.* Chicago: University of Chicago Press.

Morrison, J. (2002). Developing research questions in medical education: The science and the art. *Medical Education, 36,* 596–597.

Morrow, S. L. (2005). Quality and trustworthiness in qualitative research in counseling psychology. *Journal of Counseling Psychology, 52*(2), 250–260.

Morrow, S. L. (2007). Qualitative research in counseling psychology: Conceptual foundations. *The Counseling Psychologist, 35*(2), 209–235.

Morse, J. M. (1995). The significance of saturation. *Qualitative Health Research, 5,* 147–149.

Morse, J. M. (1999). Silent debates in qualitative inquiry. *Qualitative Health Research, 9,* 163–165.

Morse, J. M., Barrett, M., Mayan, M., Olson, K., & Spiers, J. (2002). Verification strategies for establishing reliability and validity in qualitative research. *International Journal of Qualitative Methods, 1*(2), 1–19.

Moustakas, C. E. (1990). *Heuristic research: Design, methodology, and applications.* Newbury Park, CA: Sage.

Moustakas, C. E. (1994). *Phenomenological research methods.* Thousand Oaks, CA: Sage.

Murphy, E., & Dingwall, R. (2001). The ethics of ethnography. In P. Atkinson, A. Coffey, S. Delamont, J. Lofland, & L. Lofland (Eds.), *Handbook of ethnography* (pp. 339–351). Thousand Oaks, CA: Sage.

Murphy-Berman, V., Berman, J. J., & Melton, G. B. (2008). Transformative change: An analysis of the evolution of special events within three communities. *Family and Community Health, 31,* 136–149.

Murray, M. (2003). Narrative psychology and narrative analysis. In P. M. Camic, J. E. Rhodes, & L. Yardley (Eds.), *Qualitative research in psychology: Expanding perspectives in methodology and design* (pp. 95–112). Washington, DC: American Psychological Association.

Murray, R. (2005). *Writing for academic journals.* Berkshire, UK: Open University Press.

Namaste, V. K. (2000). *Invisible lives: The erasure of transsexual and transgendered people.* Chicago: University of Chicago Press.

Narayan, K. (1993). How native is a "native" anthropologist? *American Anthropologist, 85,* 671–686.

Nastasi, B. K. (1998). A model for mental health programming in schools and communities. *School Psychology Review, 27,* 165–174.

Nastasi, B. K., Moore, R. B., & Varjas, K. M. (2004). *School-based mental health services: Creating comprehensive and culturally specific programs.* Washington, DC: American Psychological Association.

Nastasi, B. K., Varjas, K., Schensul, J. J., Schensul, S. L., Silva, K. T., & Ratnayake, P. (2000). The participatory intervention model: A framework for conceptualizing and promoting intervention acceptability. *School Psychology Quarterly, 15,* 207–232.

Nastasi, B. K., Varjas, K. M., Sarkar, S., & Jayasena, A. (1998). Participatory model of mental health programming: Lessons learned from work in a developing country. *School Psychology Review, 27,* 260–276.

National Association of Social Workers. (1996/2008). Code of ethics of the National Association of Social Workers. Retrieved January 31, 2010, from *www.socialworkers.org/pubs/code/code.asp.*

National Commission for the Protection of Human Subjects of Biomedical and Behavioral Research. (1979). The Belmont report: Ethical principles and guidelines for the protection of human subjects in research. Retrieved February 4, 2010, from *ohsr.od.nih.gov/guidelines/belmont.html.*

Nelson, M. L., & Quintana, S. M. (2005). Qualitative clinical research with children and adolescents. *Journal of Clinical Child and Adolescent Psychology, 34*(2), 344–356.

Noblet, A., Rodwell, J., & McWilliams, J. (2001). The job strain model is enough for managers: No augmentation needed. *Journal of Managerial Psychology, 16,* 635–649.

Nunkoosing, K. (2005). The problems with interviews. *Qualitative Health Research, 15,* 698–706.

Oates, G. L. St. C. (2003). Teacher–student racial congruence, teacher perceptions, and test performance. *Social Science Quarterly, 84*(3), 508–525.

O'Byrne, K. R., & Goodyear, R. K. (1997). Client assessment by novice and expert psychologists: A comparison of strategies. *Educational Psychology Review, 9*(3), 267–278.

O'Connor, D. B., O'Connor, R. C., White, B. L., & Bundred, P. E. (2000). The effect of job strain on British general practitioners' mental health. *Journal of Mental Health, 9,* 637–654.

Okech, J. E. A., & Kline, W. B. (2004). A qualitative exploration of group co-leader relationships. *Journal for Specialists in Group Work, 30*(2), 173–190.

Okubo, Y., Yeh, C. J., Lin, P. Y., Fujita, K., & Shea, J. M. Y. (2007). The career decision-making process of Chinese American youth. *Journal of Counseling and Development, 85,* 440–448.

Onwuegbuzie, A. J., & Leech, N. L. (2007). Validity and qualitative research: An oxymoron? *Quality and Quantity, 41*(1), 233–249.

Paden, S. L., & Buehler, C. (1995). Coping with the dual-income lifestyle. *Journal of Marriage and the Family, 57,* 101–110.

Padgett, D. K. (2004). Finding a middle ground in qualitative research. In D. K. Padgett (Ed.), *The qualitative research experience* (pp. 1–18). Belmont, CA: Wadsworth.

Palmer, K., & Shepard, B. (2008). An art inquiry into the experiences of a family of a child living within a chronic pain condition. *Canadian Journal of Counseling, 42,* 7–23.

Park, R. E. (1950). *Race and culture.* Glencoe, IL: The Free Press.

Park, R. E. (1955). *Society.* Glencoe, IL: The Free Press.

Park, R. E. Burgess, E. W., & McKenzie, R. D. (1925). *The city.* Chicago: University of Chicago Press.

Parker, L., & Stovall, D. (2004). Actions following words: Critical race theory connects to critical pedagogy. *Educational Philosophy and Theory, 36,* 167–182.

Patton, M. Q. (1980). *Qualitative evaluation methods.* Newbury Park, CA: Sage.

Patton, M. Q. (1991). Qualitative research on college students: Philosophical and methodological comparisons with the quantitative approach. *Journal of College Student Development, 32,* 389–396.

Patton, M. Q. (2002). *Qualitative research and evaluation methods* (3rd ed.). Thousand Oaks, CA: Sage.

Paulus, T. M., Horvitz, B., & Shi, M. (2006). "Isn't it just like our situation?": Engagement and learning in an online story-based environment. *Educational Technology Research and Development, 54*(4), 355–385.

Pawson, R., Boaz, A., Grayson, L., Long, A., & Barnes, C. (2003). *Types and quality of knowledge in social care.* London: Social Care Institute for Excellence.

Pearson, Q. M. (1998). Job satisfaction, leisure satisfaction, and psychological health. *Career Development Quarterly, 46,* 416–426.

Pearson, Q. M. (2008). Role overload, job dissatisfaction, leisure satisfaction, and psychological health among employed women. *Journal of Counseling and Development, 86,* 57–63.

Pedro, J. Y. (2005). Reflection in teacher education: Exploring re-service teachers' meanings of reflective practice. *Reflective Practice, 6,* 49–66.

Pennington, J. L. (2007). Silence in the classroom/whispers in the halls: Autoethnography as pedagogy in White pre-service teacher education. *Race, Ethnicity, and Education, 10*(1), 93–113.

Peronne, K. M. (1999/2000). Balancing life roles to achieve career happiness and life satisfaction. *Career Planning and Adult Development Journal, 15,* 49–58.

Peshkin, A. (1988). Virtuous subjectivity: In the participant observer's I's. In D. Berg & K. Smith (Eds.), *The self in social inquiry: Researching methods* (pp. 267–281). Newbury Park, CA: Sage.

Pettinger, D. J. (2003). Internet research: An opportunity to revisit classic ethical problems in behavioral research. *Ethics and Behavior, 13*(1), 45–60.

Pitts, M. J. (2007). Upward turning points and positive rapport-development across time in researcher–participant relationships. *Qualitative Research, 7*(2), 177–201.

Plummer, K. (2001). The call of life stories in ethnographic research. In P. A. Atkinson, S. Delamont, A. J. Coffey, J. Lofland, & L. H. Lofland (Eds.), *Handbook of ethnography* (pp. 395–406). Thousand Oaks, CA: Sage.

Poland, B. D. (1995). Transcription quality as an aspect of rigor in qualitative research. *Qualitative Inquiry, 1*(3), 290–310.

Polit, D. F., & Beck, C. T. (2003). *Nursing research: Principles and methods* (7th ed.). Philadelphia: Lippincott Williams & Wilkins.

Polkinghorne, D. E. (1988). *Narrative knowing and the human sciences.* Albany: State University of New York Press.

Polkinghorne, D. E. (1989). Changing conversations about human science. In S. Kvale (Ed.), *Issues of validity in qualitative research* (pp. 13–46). Lund, Sweden: Studentlitteratur.

Polkinghorne, D. E. (2005). Language and

meaning: Data collection in qualitative research. *Journal of Counseling Psychology, 52*(2), 137–145.

Pollner, M., & Emerson, R. M. (2001). Ethnomethodology and ethnography. In P. A. Atkinson, A. J. Coffey, S. Delamont, J. Lofland, & L. H. Lofland (Eds.), *Handbook of ethnography* (pp. 118–135). Thousand Oaks, CA: Sage.

Pomerantz, A., & Fehr, B. J. (1997). Conversation analysis: An approach to the study of social action as sense making practices. In T. A. van Dijk (Ed.), *Discourse as social interaction* (pp. 64–91). London: Sage.

Ponterotto, J. G. (2005). Qualitative research in counseling psychology: A primer on research paradigms and philosophies of science. *Journal of Counseling Psychology, 52*, 126–136.

Porter, S. (2007). Validity, trustworthiness and rigor: Reasserting realism in qualitative research. *Journal of Advanced Nursing, 60*(1), 79–86.

Potter, J., & Wetherell, M. (1987). *Discourse and social psychology: Beyond attitudes and behaviour.* London: Sage.

Powell, P. J. (2006). *The effects of grade retention: Life histories of adults who were retained as children.* Doctoral dissertation, Northern Arizona University, Flagstaff, AZ.

Pratt, M. G. (2009). From the editors—for the lack of a boilerplate: Tips on writing up (and reviewing) qualitative research. *Academy of Management Journal, 52*(5), 856–862.

Project South. (1996). *The Olympic Games and our struggles for justice: A people's story.* Atlanta, GA: Author.

Quimby, E. (2006). Ethnography's role in assisting mental health research and clinical practice. *Journal of Clinical Psychology, 62*(7), 859–879.

Quinlan, N. (2009). *A phenomenological case study of the multicultural counseling experience of students and faculty in relation to their perceptions of their multicultural competency and CACREP standards.* Doctoral dissertation, Old Dominion University, Norfolk, VA.

Radford, L. (2003). Gestures, speech, and the sprouting of signs: A semiotic–cultural approach to students' types of generalizations. *Mathematical Thinking and Learning, 5,* 37–70.

Rager, K. B. (2005). Compassion stress and the qualitative researcher. *Qualitative Health Research, 15*(3), 423–430.

Rapley, T. (2007). *Doing conversation, discourse analysis and document analysis: Qualitative research kit.* London: Sage.

Rashid, S. F. (2007). Accessing married adolescent women: The realities of ethnographic research in an urban slum environment in Dhaka, Bangladesh. *Field Methods, 19*(4), 369–383.

Ratts, M., D'Andrea, M., & Arredondo, P. (2004). Social justice counseling: "Fifth" force in field. *Counseling Today, 47,* 28–30.

Reason, P. (1994). Three approaches to participative inquiry. In N. K. Denzin & Y. S. Linocoln (Eds.), *The Sage handbook of qualitative research* (pp. 324–339). Thousand Oaks, CA: Sage.

Reed-Danahay, D. (2001). Autobiography, intimacy, and ethnography. In P. Atkinson, A. RefWorks. About us. Retrieved October 20, 2008, from *www.refworks.com.*

Reinharz, S. (1992). *Feminist methods in social research.* New York: Oxford University Press.

Reis, S. M., & Diaz, E. (1999). Economically disadvantaged urban female students who achieve in schools. *Urban Review, 31*(1), 31–54.

Rennie, D. (2000). Grounded theory methodology as methodical hermeneutics: Reconciling realism and relativism. *Theory Psychology, 10*(4), 481–502.

Rennie, D. L. (1994). Clients' deference in psychotherapy. *Journal of Counseling Psychology, 41,* 427–437.

Rennie, D. L. (1998). Grounded theory methodology: The pressing need for a coherent logic of justification. *Theory and Psychology, 8,* 101–119.

Resnik, D. B., & Zeldin, D. C. (2008). Environmental health research on hazards in the home and the duty to warn. *Bioethics, 22*(4), 209–217.

Rhodes, T., & Fitzgerald, J. (2006). Visual data in addictions research: Seeing comes before words? *Addiction Research and Theory, 14*(4), 349–363.

Richardson, L. (1994). Writing: A method of inquiry. In N. K. Denzin & Y. S. Lincoln (Eds.), *The Sage handbook of qualitative research* (pp. 923–948). Thousand Oaks, CA: Sage.

Richardson, L. (2003). Writing: A method of inquiry. In Y. S. Lincoln & N. K. Denzin (Eds.), *Turning points in qualitative research: Tying knots in a handkerchief* (pp. 379–396). Lanham, MD: Rowman & Littlefield.

Ricouer, P. (1984). *Time and narrative, Vol. I* (K. McLaughlin & D. Pellauer, Trans.). Chicago: University of Chicago Press.

Ricouer, P. (1985). *Time and narrative, Vol. II* (K. McLaughlin & D. Pellauer, Trans.). Chicago: University of Chicago Press.

Riel, M. (2007). Understanding action research: Center for Collaborative Action Research. Retrieved on May 10, 2009, from *www.cadres.pepperdine.edu/ccar/define.html*.

Riemenschnieder, A., & Harper, K. V. (1990). Women in academia: Guilty or not guilty? Conflict between caregiving and employment. *Initiatives, 53,* 27–35.

Roberts, D. A. (1996). What counts as quality in quantitative research? *Science Education, 80*(3), 243–248.

Rogers, C. (1961). *On becoming a person: A therapist's view of psychotherapy.* London: Constable & Robinson.

Rolfe, G. (2006). Validity, trustworthiness and rigor: Quality and the idea of qualitative research. *Journal of Advanced Nursing, 53*(3), 304–310.

Ronai, C. R. (1996). My mother is mentally retarded. In C. Ellis & A. P. Bocner (Eds.), *Composing ethnography: Alternative forms of qualitative writing* (pp. 109–131). Walnut Creek, CA: AltaMira Press.

Rowan, J. (2000). Research ethics. *International Journal of Psychotherapy, 5*(2), 103–111.

Runte, R. (2008). Blogs. In J. G. Knowles & A. L. Cole (Eds.), *Handbook of the arts in qualitative research* (pp. 313–322). Thousand Oaks, CA: Sage.

Ruth, J. E., & Öberg, P. (1996). Ways of life: Old age in a life history perspective. In J. E. Birren, G. Kenyon, J. Ruth, J. Schroots, & T. Svensson (Eds.), *Aging and biography: Explorations in adult development* (pp. 167–186). New York: Springer.

Sacks, H. (1992). *Lectures on conversation.* Oxford, UK: Blackwell.

Sanchez, B., Reyes, O., & Singh, J. (2006). Makin' it in college: The value of significant individuals in the lives of Mexican American adolescents. *Journal of Higher Education, 5,* 48–67.

Sandage, S. J., Cook, K. V., Hill, P. C., Strawn, B. D., & Reimer, K. S. (2008). Hermeneutics and psychology: A review and dialectical method. *Journal of General Psychology, 12*(4), 344–364.

Sandelowski, M. (1993). Rigor or rigor mortis: The problem of rigor in qualitative research revisited. *Advances in Nursing Science, 16*(2), 1–8.

Sandelowski, M. (1995). Sample size in qualitative research. *Nursing and Health, 18,* 179–183.

Sandelowski, M. (1996). Using qualitative methods in intervention studies. *Research in Nursing and Health, 19,* 359–364.

Sandelowski, M. (1998). Writing a good read: Strategies for re-presenting qualitative data. *Research in Nursing and Health, 21,* 375–382.

Sandelowski, M. (2002). Reembodying qualitative inquiry. *Qualitative Health Research, 12,* 104–115.

Saris-Gallhofer, I. N., Saris, W. E., & Morton, E. L. (1978). A validation study of Holsti's content analysis procedure. *Quality and Quantity, 12,* 131–145.

Schegloff, E. A. (1968). Sequencing in conversational openings. *American Anthropologist, 70,* 1075–1995.

Schensul, J. J. (1998). Community-based risk prevention with urban youth. *School Psychology Review, 27,* 233–245.

Schneider, K. J. (1999). Multiple-case depth research. *Journal of Clinical Psychology, 55*(12), 1531–1540.

Schwandt, T. A. (2001). *Dictionary of qualitative inquiry* (2nd ed.). Thousand Oaks, CA: Sage.

Sells, S. P., Smith, T. E., Coe, M. J., Yoshioka, M., & Robbins, J. (1994). An ethnography of couple and therapist experiences in reflecting team practice. *Journal of Marital and Family Therapy, 20,* 247–266.

Selwyn, D. (2007). Highly qualified teachers: NCLB and teacher education. *Journal of Teacher Education, 58*(2), 124–137.

Seo, S., & Koro-Ljungberg, M. (2005). A hermeneutical study of older Korean graduate students' experiences in American higher education: From Confucianism to Western educational values. *Journal of Studies in International Education, 9,* 164–187.

Sharf, B. (1999). Beyond netiquette: The ethics of doing naturalistic discourse research on the Internet. In S. Jones (Ed.), *Doing Internet research: Critical issues and methods for examining the net* (pp. 243–257). Thousand Oaks, CA; Sage.

Shaw, C. (1930). *The jack-roller: A delinquent boy's own story.* Chicago: University of Chicago Press.

Shaw, C. (1931). *The natural history of a delinquent career.* Chicago: University of Chicago Press.

Shaw, C. (1938). *Brothers in crime.* Chicago: University of Chicago Press.

Shiflett, C. (2008). *Mainstreaming students with autism in the art classroom: An exploration of participant experiences.* Unpublished manuscript.

Shoffner, M. F., Newsome, D. W., & Barrio, C. A. (2005). *Young adolescents' outcome expectations: A qualitative study.* Unpublished manuscript.

Siedman, I. (2006). *Interviewing as qualitative research: A guide for researchers in education and the social sciences* (3rd ed.). New York: Teachers College Press.

Silverman, D. (1993). *Interpreting qualitative data: Methods for analyzing talk, text, and interaction.* Newbury Park, CA: Sage.

Silvester, J. (1998). Attributional coding. In G. Symon & C. Cassell (Eds.), *Qualitative methods and analysis in organizational research: A practical guide* (pp. 73–93). London: Sage.

Singh, A. (2010). "Just getting out of bed is a revolutionary act": The resilience of transgender people of color who have survived traumatic life events. *Traumatology, 16*(4).

Singh, A., Hays, D. G., & Watson, L. (2011). Strength in the face of adversity: Resilience strategies of transgender individuals. *Journal of Counseling and Development, 89*, 20–27.

Singh, A., Hofhess, C. D., Boyer, E. M., Kwong, A., Lau, A. S. M., McLain, M., et al. (2010). Social justice and counseling psychology: Listening to the voices of doctoral trainees. *Counseling Psychologist, 38*(6), 766–795.

Singh, A. A., Hays, D. G., Chung, Y. B., & Watson. L. (2010). South Asian immigrant women who have survived child sexual abuse: Resilience and healing. *Violence Against Women, 16*(4), 444–458.

Singh, A. A., Urbano, A., Haston, M., & McMahon, E. (2010). School counselors' strategies for social justice change: A grounded theory of what works in the real world. *Professional School Counseling, 13*, 135–145.

Smythe, W. E., & Murray, M. J. (2000). Owning the story: Ethical considerations in narrative research. *Ethics and Behavior, 10*, 311–336.

Snow, D. A., Zurcher, L. A., & Sjoberg, G. (1982). Interviewing by comment: An adjunct to the direct question. *Qualitative Sociology, 5*(4), 462–476.

Snow, M. S., Hudspeth, E. F., Blake, G., & Seale, H. A. (2007). A comparison of behaviors and play themes over a six-week period: Two case studies in play therapy. *International Journal of Play Therapy, 16*(2), 147–159.

Solis, C. M., Meyers, J., & Varjas, K. (2004). A qualitative case study of the process and impact of filial therapy with an African American parent. *International Journal of Play Therapy, 13,* 99–118.

Solórzano, D. (1998). Critical race theory, racial and gender microaggressions, and the experiences of Chicana and Chicano scholars. *International Journal of Qualitative Studies in Education, 11,* 121–136.

Solórzano, D., Ceja, M., & Yosso, T. (2000). Critical race theory, racial microaggressions and campus racial climate: The experiences of African American college students. *Journal of Negro Education, 69,* 60–73.

Solórzano, D., & Yosso, T. (2000). Critical race and LatCrit theory and method: Counterstorytelling Chicana and Chicano graduate school experiences. *International Journal of Qualitative Studies in Education, 14,* 471–495.

Solorzano, D. G., & Delgado Bernal, D. (2001). Examining transformational resistance through a critical race and LatCrit theory framework: Chicana and Chicano students in an urban context. *Urban Education, 36*(3), 308–342.

Sommers, I., & Baskin, D. (2006). Methamphetamine use and violence. *Journal of Drug Issues, 36,* 77–96.

Soobrayan, V. (2003). Ethics, truth and politics in constructivist qualitative research. *Westminster Studies in Education, 26*(2), 107–123.

Sortino, D. P. (1999). *The experience of attempting to understand behavior-disordered students: A heuristic inquiry.* Doctoral dissertation, Saybrook Institute, San Francisco.

Spall, S. (1998). Peer debriefing in qualitative research: Emerging operational models. *Qualitative Inquiry, 4*(2), 280–292.

Sperandio, J. (2008). Alternative mentoring of street girls in Bangladesh: New identities and non-traditional opportunities. *Mentoring and Tutoring: Partnership in Learning, 16*(2), 207–221.

Spillett, M. A. (2003, Fall). Peer debriefing: Who, what, when, why, how. *Academic Exchange Quarterly.* Retrieved on November 20, 2008, from *findarticles.com/p/articles/mi_hb3325/is_3_7/ai_n29051739/pg_4?tag=artBody;col1.*

Spradley, J. (1979). *The ethnographic interview.*

Florence, KY: Wadsworth Group/Thomas Learning.

Stake, R. (1990). Situational context as influence on evaluation design and use. *Studies in Educational Evaluation, 16,* 231–246.

Stake, R. (1995). *The art of case study research.* Thousand Oaks, CA: Sage.

Stake, R. (2005). Qualitative case studies. In N. K. Denzin & Y. S. Lincoln (Eds.), *The Sage handbook of qualitative research* (3rd ed., pp. 443–466). Thousand Oaks, CA: Sage.

Stake, R. E. (2006). *Multiple case study analysis.* New York: Guilford Press.

Stanford, S. L. (2009). Twenty-nine mixtures: Adult postsecondary learners' writing self-efficacy perceptions in a first-term composition course. *Dissertations Abstracts International Section A: Humanities and Social Sciences, 69*(7-A), 2564.

Stanley, L. (2001). Mass-observation's fieldwork methods. In P. A. Atkinson, S. Delamont, A. J. Coffey, J. Lofland, & L. H. Lofland (Eds.), *Handbook of ethnography* (pp. 92–108). Thousand Oaks, CA: Sage.

Stewart, K., & Williams, M. (2005). Researching online populations: The use of online focus groups for social research. *Qualitative Research, 5*(4), 395–416.

Stoecker, R. (2005). *Research methods for community change: A project-based approach.* Thousand Oaks, CA: Sage.

Strauss, A. (1987). *Qualitative research for social scientists.* Cambridge, UK: Cambridge University Press.

Strauss, A., & Corbin, J. (1998). *Basics of qualitative research: Techniques and procedures for developing grounded theory* (2nd ed.). Thousand Oaks, CA: Sage.

Stricker, G. (2002). What is a scientist–practitioner anyway? *Journal of Clinical Psychology, 58,* 1277–1283.

Sue, D. W., Lin, A. I., Tornio, G. C., Capodilupo, C. M., & Rivera, D. P. (2009). Racial microaggressions and difficult dialogues on race in the classroom. *Cultural Diversity and Ethnic Minority Psychology, 15*(2), 183–190.

Super, D. E. (1980). A life-span, life-space approach to career development. *Journal of Vocational Behavior, 16,* 282–298.

Super, D. E. (1984). Leisure: What it is and might be. *Journal of Career Development, 11,* 71–80.

Super, D. E. (1990). A life-span, life-space approach to career development. In D. Brown, L. Brooks, & Associates (Eds.), *Career choice and development: Applying contemporary theories and practice* (2nd ed., pp. 197–261). San Francisco: Jossey-Bass.

Sutherland, E. H. (1937). *The professional thief.* Chicago: University of Chicago Press.

Suzuki, L. A., Ahluwalia, M. K., Mattis, J. S., & Quizon, C. A. (2005). Ethnography in counseling psychology research: Possibilities for application. *Journal of Counseling Psychology, 52*(2), 206–214.

Sword, W. (1999). Accounting for presence of self: Reflections on doing qualitative research. *Qualitative Health Research, 9*(2), 270–278.

Thomas, W. I., & Znaniecki, F. (1927). *The Polish peasant in Europe and America* (2nd ed.). Oxford, UK: Knopf.

Thomson Reuters. (n.d.). About us. Retrieved October 20, 2008, from *www.endnote.com.*

Tiedje, L. B., & Wortman, C. B. (1990). Women with multiple roles: Role-compatibility perceptions, satisfaction, and mental health. *Journal of Marriage and the Family, 52,* 63–72.

Tinker, C., & Armstrong, N. (2008). From the outside looking in: How an awareness of difference can benefit the qualitative research process. *Qualitative Report, 13*(1), 53–60.

Tobin, G. A., & Begley, C. M. (2004). Methodological rigor within a qualitative framework. *Journal of Advanced Nursing, 48*(4), 388–396.

Trenberth, L., & Dewe, P. (2002). The importance of leisure as a means of coping with work related stress: An exploratory study. *Counselling Psychology Quarterly, 15,* 59–72.

van den Hoonaard, W. (2001). Is research-ethics review a moral panic? *Canadian Review of Sociology and Anthropology, 38*(1), 19–36.

VanDorn, N., Van Zoonen, L., & Wyatt, S. (2007). Writing from experience: Presentations of gender identity on weblogs. *European Journal of Women's Studies, 14*(2), 143–159.

van Eeden-Moorefield, B., Proulx, C., & Pasley, K. (2008). A comparison of Internet and face-to-face qualitative methods in studying gay couples. *Journal of GLBT Family Studies, 2,* 181–204.

van Kaam, A. (1959). Phenomenological analysis: Exemplified by a study of the experience of "really feeling understood." *Journal of Individual Psychology, 15,* 66–72.

van Kaam, A. (1966). *Existential foundations of psychology.* Pittsburgh, PA: Duquesne University Press.

VanWynsberghe, R., & Khan, S. (2007). Redefining case study. *International Journal of Qualitative Methods, 6*(2), 80–94. Retrieved January 27, 2011, from *www.ualberta.ca/~iiqm/back-issues/6_2/vanwynsberghe.pdf.*

Varjas, K., Graybill, E., Mahan, W., Meyers, J., Dew, B. J., Marshall, M., et al. (2006). Urban service providers' perspectives on school responses to gay, lesbian, and questioning students: An exploratory study. *Professional School Counseling, 11*(2), 113–119.

Vidich, A. J., & Lyman, S. M. (2001). Qualitative methods: Their history in sociology and anthropology. In N. K. Denzin & Y. S. Lincoln (Eds.), *The landscape of qualitative research* (2nd ed., pp. 55–129). Thousand Oaks, CA: Sage.

Vryan, K. D. (2006). Expanding analytic autoethnography and enhancing its potential. *Journal of Contemporary Ethnography, 35*, 405–409.

Waldrop, D. P. (2004). Ethical issues in qualitative research with high-risk populations: Handle with care. In D. K. Padgett (Ed.), *The qualitative research experience* (pp. 236–249). Toronto: Thomson.

Waldrop, D. P. (2007). Caregiver grief in terminal illness and bereavement: A mixed methods study. *Health and Social Work, 32*(3), 197–206.

Wall, S. (2008). Easier said than done: Writing an autoethnography. *International Journal of Qualitative Methods, 7*(1), 38–53.

Wanat, C. L. (2008). Getting past the gatekeepers: Differences between access and cooperation in public school research. *Field Methods, 20*, 191–208.

Wang, C., & Burris, M. A. (1997). Photovoice: Concept, methodology, and use for participatory needs assessment. *Health Education and Behavior, 24*(3), 369–387.

Watson, D., & Slack, A. K. (1993). General factors of affective temperament and their relation to job satisfaction over time. *Organizational Behavior and Human Decision Processes, 54*, 181–202.

Watt, D. (2007). On becoming a qualitative researcher: The value of reflexivity. *Qualitative Report, 12*(1), 82–101.

Weber, R. P. (1990). *Basic content analysis.* Newbury Park, CA: Sage.

Wentling, R. M. (1998). Work and family issues: Their impact on women's career development. *New Directions for Adult and Continuing Education, 80*, 15–24.

Werle, G. D. (2004). The lived experience of violence: Using storytelling as a teaching tool with middle school students. *Journal of School Nursing, 20*(2), 81–87.

Wertz, F. J. (2005). Phenomenological research methods in counseling psychology. *Journal of Counseling Psychology, 52*, 167–177.

Wester, K. L. (2009). Key ethical issues in research and evaluation. In American Counseling Association (Ed.), *The ACA encyclopedia of counseling* (pp. 451–453). Alexandria, VA: American Counseling Association.

Westerlund, J. F., & Barufaldi, J. P. (1997). *Reform and reality: A two year study. Observations of Texas teachers on the biology I end of course examination* (ERIC Document Reproduction Service No. ED406159)

White, M., & Epston, D. (1990). *Narrative means to therapeutic ends.* New York: Norton.

Whittemore, R., Chase, S. K., & Mandle, C. L. (2001). Validity in qualitative research. *Qualitative Health Research, 11*(4), 522–537.

Wiersma, W., & Jurs, S. G. (2009). *Research methods in education* (9th ed.). Boston: Pearson.

Wilkinson, S. (2003). Focus groups. In J. A. Smith (Ed.), *Qualitative psychology: A practical guide to research methods* (pp. 184–204). Thousand Oaks, CA: Sage.

Williams, G. T., & Ellison, L. (2009). Duty to warn and protect. In American Counseling Association (Ed.), *The ACA encyclopedia of counseling* (pp. 163–165). Alexandia, VA: American Counseling Association.

Williams, J. H., Horvath, V. E., Wei, H., Dorn, V., & Jonson-Reid, M. (2007). Teachers' perspectives of children's mental health service needs in urban elementary schools. *Children and Schools, 29*(2), 95–107.

Williams, S. M. (2007). The dynamics of adolescent friendships: An investigation of school, classrooms, and peer groups—implications for educational policy. *Dissertation Abstracts International*, A, 68/04.

Williams, S. W., Dilworth-Anderson, P., & Goodwin, P. Y. (2003). Caregiver role strain: The contribution of multiple roles and available resources in African-American women. *Aging and Mental Health, 7*, 103–112.

Wilson, S., & Youngs, P. (2005). Research on accountability processes in teacher education. In M. Cochran-Smith & K. Zeichner (Eds.), *Studying teacher education* (pp. 549–590). Mahwah, NJ: Erlbaum.

Winefield, A. H., Tiggemann, M., & Winefield,

H. R. (1992). Spare time use and psychological well-being in employed and unemployed young people. *Journal of Occupational and Organizational Psychology, 65*, 307–313.

Wolcott, H. F. (1994). *Transforming qualitative data: Description, analysis, and interpretation.* Thousand Oaks, CA: Sage.

Wolcott, H. F. (2008). *Writing up qualitative research* (3rd ed.). Thousand Oaks, CA: Sage.

Wolkomir, M., & Powers, J. (2007). Helping women and protecting the self: The challenge of emotional labor in an abortion clinic. *Qualitative Sociology, 30*, 153–169.

Wright, T. A., & Bonett, D. G. (1992). The effect of turnover on work satisfaction and mental health: Support for a situational perspective. *Journal of Organizational Behavior, 13*, 603–615.

Yeh, C. J., Inman, A. G., Kim, A. B., & Okubo, Y. (2006). Asian American families' collectivistic coping strategies in response to 9/11. *Cultural Diversity and Ethnic Minority Psychology, 12*(1), 134–148.

Yin, R. K. (1984). *Case study research: Design and methods* (Applied Social Research Methods Series, Vol. 5). Beverly Hills, CA: Sage.

Yin, R. K. (2003). *Case study research: Design and methods* (3rd ed.). Thousand Oaks, CA: Sage.

Yin, R. K. (2008). *Case study research: Design and methods* (4th ed.). Thousand Oaks, CA: Sage.

Zumwalt, K., & Craig, E. (2005). Teachers' characteristics: Research on the demographic profile. In M. Cochran Smith & K. Zeichner (Eds.), *Studying teacher education* (pp. 111–156). Mahwah, NJ: Erlbaum.

Zunker, V. G. (2002). *Career planning: Applied concepts of life planning* (6th ed.). Pacific Grove, CA: Brooks/Cole.

Author Index

Subject Index

Page numbers followed by *f* indicate figure, *t* indicate table

486

Objectivity, 90
Observation rubrics, 227
Observational records, 228. *See also* Field notes
Observational research, steps in, 237
Observations, 223–237
    benefits of, 224
    continuum of, 226–227, 226*f*
    developing protocol for, 224
    field notes and, 228–236
    naturalistic, 224
    participant, 6, 227
    persistent, as trustworthiness strategy, 207
    suitable use of, 226
    through fieldwork, 225–226
Observer, as participant, 226
Observer bias, defined, 232
Observer effect, defined, 232
Observer role, variations on, 226–227, 226*f*
One-shot questions, 248
Online mask, 268
Online research
    ethical issues in, 93–94
    See also Internet data collection; Internet research
Ontology, 34–35
    purpose statement and, 127–128
    and research on career aspirations of Latino
        students, 38*f*
Open coding, in grounded theory study, 345–346
Opinion questions, 241
Opportunistic sampling, 169
    one-shot questions and, 248
Oral history, 46
Otherness, types of, 141–142
"Other/outsider"
    early qualitative research on, 15
    Eurocentric perspectives on, 16*t*, 17–18
    lone ethnographer and, 18
    researcher as, 94
Outrageous comments, 243
Outsider research, versus insider research, 140–141
    proposal development for, 144

Paradigms. *See* Research paradigms
Partially ordered case displays, 320*t*
Partially ordered displays, 318–319, 320*t*
    examples of, 319, 320*f*, 321*f*, 322*f*
Partially ordered meta-matrix, 318, 322*f*
Participant
    artwork of, 282, 282*f*
    characteristics of, informed consent and, 82
    deception of, 83
    holistic understanding of, 7
    intentionality of, 50
    journals and diaries of, 284–285
    leaving research products with, 186
    as observer role, 226
    prolonged engagement with, 206–207
    protection of, 72–73
    reactions to recorders, 256–257
    researcher bias and, 198
    researcher positionality and, 142
    respect for, 71–72

    and risk of harm, 79
    voice of, 37
        in research, 70
        understanding, 148–150
Participant demographic form, in sample qualitative
        proposal, 447
Participant effect, 198
Participant observation, 6, 227
    Chicago School and, 19
    ethnography and, 60
    modern ethnography and, 18
    See also Participant–researcher relationship
Participant recruitment
    for focus groups, 255–256
    online, 266–270
Participant role
    observer as, 226–227
    planning, 227–228
Participant section
    of research report, 398–399
        case example, 399
    in sample qualitative proposal, 452
Participant voice, in research report, 397–398
Participant–researcher relationship, 6–7
    characteristics of, 8
    ethical issues in, 91–92
    in focus groups, 255
    negative effects of, 197–198
    Pitts's stage model of, 181*t*
    positionality in, 186
    post-study evaluation of, 184, 186
    reciprocity in, 186
Participatory action research (PAR), 23, 63–65
    basic principles of, 25*t*
    data analysis in
        case study, 370–371
        cultural/contextual variables and, 370
        recursive nature of, 369–370
        reflection in, 369
        researcher–participant involvement in, 370
        tips for, 371*t*
        visual portrayal of, 369, 369*f*
    general and unique characteristics, 46*t*
    online recruitment for, 269
    research design for, action components in, 372
    research questions and, 132
    selection criteria for, 64
    in study of dual-career families, 59*t*
Pattern analysis, 300, 302–303, 339
    comparative, 303
Pattern codes, 300, 302
Pattern identification, 341
    in ethnography, 363
Peer debriefers, 146*t*
    use of, 151–152
Peer debriefing
    defined, 151
    prompts for, 152
    techniques for, 143
    as trustworthiness strategy, 208*t*, 211
Persistent observation, as trustworthiness strategy,
        207, 208*t*

About the Authors

Danica G. Hays, PhD, LPC, NCC, is Associate Professor of Counseling and Chair of the Department of Counseling and Human Services at Old Dominion University. She is a recipient of the Outstanding Research Award, Outstanding Counselor Educator Advocacy Award, and Glen E. Hubele National Graduate Student Award from the American Counseling Association as well as the Patricia B. Elmore Excellence in Measurement and Evaluation Award and President's Special Merit Award from the Association for Assessment in Counseling and Education (AACE). Dr. Hays is the Founding Editor of the journal *Counseling Outcome Research and Evaluation*, a national peer-refereed publication of the AACE. Her research interests include qualitative methodology, assessment and diagnosis, trauma and gender issues, and multicultural and social justice concerns in counselor preparation and community mental health. She has published numerous articles and book chapters in this area and has coauthored or coedited three books to date: *Developing Multicultural Counseling Competence: A Systems Approach, Mastering the National Counselor Exam and the Counselor Preparation Comprehensive Exam*, and *The ACA Encyclopedia of Counseling*. Her primary teaching responsibilities are master's- and doctoral-level research courses, assessment, and supervision.

Anneliese A. Singh, PhD, LPC, is Assistant Professor in the Department of Counseling and Human Development Services at the University of Georgia. She is a past president of the Association for Lesbian, Gay, Bisexual and Transgender Issues in Counseling (ALGBTIC), where her Presidential Initiatives included the development of counseling competencies. She has received numerous awards for the integration of her research and community organizing work with historically marginalized groups, including the Ramesh and Vijaya Bakshi Community Change Award, Counselors for Social Justice O'Hana Award, American Counseling Association Kitty Cole Human Rights Award, and Asian American Psychological Association Division on Women Award. Dr. Singh's clinical, research, and advocacy interests include LGBT youth, Asian American/Pacific Islander counseling and psychology, multicultural counseling and social justice training, qualitative methodology with historically marginalized groups (e.g., people of color, LGBT individuals, immigrants), and feminist empowerment interventions with survivors of trauma.